MEDICINE:
A Competency-Based Companion

Jessica L. Israel MD

Chief, Division of Geriatrics and Palliative Medicine
Medical Director, Inpatient Hospice Unit
Monmouth Medical Center
Long Branch, New Jersey
Clinical Associate Professor of Medicine
Drexel University College of Medicine
Philadelphia, Pennsylvania

Allan R. Tunkel MD, PhD, MACP

Chair, Department of Internal Medicine
Monmouth Medical Center
Long Branch, New Jersey
Professor of Medicine
Drexel University College of Medicine
Philadelphia, Pennsylvania

Series Editor:
Barry D. Mann MD

Chief Academic Officer
Main Line Health System
Wynnewood, Pennsylvania

ELSEVIER
SAUNDERS

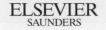

1600 John F. Kennedy Blvd.
Ste 1800
Philadelphia, PA 19103-2899

Notices

Knowledge and best practice in this field are constantly changing. As new research and experience broaden our understanding, changes in research methods, professional practices, or medical treatment may become necessary.

Practitioners and researchers must always rely on their own experience and knowledge in evaluating and using any information, methods, compounds, or experiments described herein. In using such information or methods they should be mindful of their own safety and the safety of others, including parties for whom they have a professional responsibility.

With respect to any drug or pharmaceutical products identified, readers are advised to check the most current information provided (i) on procedures featured or (ii) by the manufacturer of each product to be administered, to verify the recommended dose or formula, the method and duration of administration, and contraindications. It is the responsibility of practitioners, relying on their own experience and knowledge of their patients, to make diagnoses, to determine dosages and the best treatment for each individual patient, and to take all appropriate safety precautions.

To the fullest extent of the law, neither the Publisher nor the authors, contributors, or editors, assume any liability for any injury and/or damage to persons or property as a matter of products liability, negligence or otherwise, or from any use or operation of any methods, products, instructions, or ideas contained in the material herein.

Library of Congress Cataloging-in-Publication Data
Medicine : a competency-based companion / [edited by] Jessica L. Israel,
Allan R. Tunkel.—1st ed.
     p. ; cm.—(Competency based companion)
  Includes bibliographical references and index.
  ISBN 978-1-4160-5351-4 (pbk. : alk. paper)
  I. Israel, Jessica L.   II. Tunkel, Allan R.   III. Series: Competency-based companion.
  [DNLM: 1. Internal Medicine—methods—Case Reports.   2. Clinical Competence—Case
Reports.   3. Patient Care—Case Reports. WB 115]
  LC classification not assigned
  616—dc23
                                                                    2012001434

Senior Content Strategist: James Merritt
Content Developmental Specialist: Christine Abshire
Publishing Services Manager: Pat Joiner-Myers
Project Manager: Marlene Weeks
Designer: Lou Forgione

Working together to grow
libraries in developing countries
www.elsevier.com | www.bookaid.org | www.sabre.org

ELSEVIER   BOOK AID International   Sabre Foundation

Printed in China

Last digit is the print number: 9   8   7   6   5   4   3   2   1

For Benjamin and Matthew
And for Adam
JLI

For Randy,
Lindsay, and Emily
ART

Foreword

What constitutes an effective clinician?

Medical schools recognize the importance of defining the qualities, knowledge, and skills their graduates must achieve by graduation. Educators realize that to become effective clinicians, students must achieve a variety of competencies; all the organizations that regulate medical education have adopted competency language. The Accreditation Council for Graduate Medical Education (ACGME) has articulated six general competencies that residency programs must teach and assess, and many medical schools have been influenced by this framework. These competencies are:

1. **Patient Care.** Residents must be able to provide patient care that is compassionate, appropriate, and effective for the treatment of health problems and the promotion of health.
2. **Medical Knowledge.** Residents must demonstrate knowledge of established and evolving biomedical, clinical, epidemiological and social behavioral sciences, as well as the application of this knowledge to patient care.
3. **Practice-Based Learning and Improvement.** Residents must demonstrate the ability to investigate and evaluate their care of patients, to appraise and assimilate scientific evidence, and to continuously improve patient care based on constant self-evaluation and life-long learning.
4. **Interpersonal and Communication Skills.** Residents must demonstrate interpersonal and communication skills that result in the effective exchange of information and collaboration with patients, their families, and health professionals.
5. **Professionalism.** Residents must demonstrate a commitment to carrying out professional responsibilities and an adherence to ethical principles.
6. **Systems-Based Practice.** Residents must demonstrate an awareness of and responsiveness to the larger context and system of health care, as well as the ability to call effectively on other resources in the system to provide optimal health care.*

*From ACGME Competency definitions: Used with permission of Accreditation Counsel for Graduate Medical Education © ACGME 2011. Please see the ACGME website: www.acgme.org for the most current version.

There is a problem, though. Over the years, medical education has proved most successful in teaching knowledge and technical skills and less successful in teaching and assessing competencies, such as skills in medical interviewing, behavioral change counseling, advanced communication (such as giving bad news), and clinical reasoning. Medical curricula often put too little emphasis on practice-based learning and improvement and on systems-based practice. Critical aspects of professionalism, such as maintaining altruism, integrity, and respect for patients, may be undermined by the "hidden curriculum" imparted by negative role models and the lack of adequate mentorship. The stresses of ward routines and sick and dying patients challenge values and emotions. Often there is little time or no appropriate venue for fruitful reflection and discussion. Because you use yourself as an instrument of diagnosis and therapy, you must know how your own attitudes, values, and biases may influence your clinical decisions. You must have balance and equanimity in your life so that you can be emotionally available and truly present for your patients. To do all this, you must develop into a reflective practitioner, always assessing your actions and thoughts in the light of the ideals of care you want to achieve. If you are to become a physician who can cure disease while healing illness, you must pay attention to multiple dimensions of learning.

The editors and authors of this book have done us all a great service in directing us to think about clinical problem solving in the context of the six competencies, which is necessary to provide the best patient care. When you care for a patient, you work to take an excellent history that helps you understand the factors in the patient's personal history and social context that have contributed to the illness; you perform a skillful physical examination; you create a robust differential diagnosis and work it through in your mind with the help of appropriate testing; you communicate with the patient and family members; you talk with consultants; you work within a multidisciplinary team to ensure coordination and continuity of care; you treat your patient with compassion and respect; you think about your decisions and make mid-course corrections; and you advocate for your patient with insurance companies and others involved in care.

In this gem of a book, the authors guide you in thinking in multiple dimensions of learning that are available in caring for every one of your patients. If you can learn to think in this multidimensional way, and intentionally work on enhancing multiple competencies, you will grow as an individual and as a professional. You will become an effective clinician who will be an asset to your patients and a credit to our profession.

Dennis H. Novack MD
Professor of Medicine
Associate Dean of Medical Education
Drexel University College of Medicine

Series Preface

When the Accreditation Council for Graduate Medical Education (ACGME) initiated the six competency categories a decade ago, it was left to the discretion of individual program directors to define and develop competency content and then to evaluate the ability of each trainee to achieve the competency. Elsevier's *Competency-Based Companion Series* represents the publisher's goal of demonstrating that the ACGME competencies are indeed important components of what makes the art and science of doctoring a multidimensional profession. I congratulate Elsevier for fostering the concept of exploring the value of a competency-based textbook in four different fields.

In *Surgery: A Competency-Based Companion,* the first volume of the series, physician educators defined the specifics of what is meant by each competency. When editing the surgery volume, I personally called upon more than 100 surgical educators, asking them to offer specific examples of how they defined behaviors in the six ACGME competency categories. Early in the process, it became clear that authors had different understandings of what might be meant by each of the competencies. We recognized that defining this six-pronged curriculum with concrete examples would prove to be an interesting educational journey.

Even as *Surgery: A Competency-Based Companion* was being compiled, the editors of the subsequent volumes struggled with another fundamental educational question: "Why crowd a book addressed to students and residents, who are hungry for *clinical* science, with the issues of Interpersonal and Communication Skills, Professionalism, or how to make one's practice Systems-Based?" In compilation of the chapters for *Obstetrics and Gynecology: A Competency-Based Companion,* the second book of the series, Dr. Michael Belden and his colleagues demonstrated that these hard-to-measure competencies are actually quite *integral* to the clinical science of a women's health curriculum.

In *Pediatrics: A Competency-Based Companion,* Drs. Maureen McMahon and Glenn Stryjewski studied the integration of the six competencies into pediatric cases. In doing so, they recognized that communication in pediatrics is a **triangulation**: physician, child, and family. Surely specific skills are required for communication with a child, but one always needs to communicate with parents and with families; special skills may even be required to bring the child and family "in sync" with each other. McMahon and Stryjewski also demonstrated that making the **system** work in pediatrics has an additional moral mandate: the system must work for the less fortunate, for the indigent, for children hampered by congenital problems and disabilities, and for those whose chronic illnesses require significant system support.

In *Medicine: A Competency-Based Companion*, the fourth and final volume of the *Competency-Based Companion Series*, Drs. Jessica L. Israel and Allan R. Tunkel demonstrate how the ACGME competencies are applicable to common clinical problems in Internal Medicine. In so doing, they remind students that optimal clinical practice requires the integration of knowledge with interpersonal skills, ethical values, and continued self-assessment, demonstrating that the ACGME competency categories represent an intelligent and rationally chosen set of the pillars of practice.

I am indebted to Drs. Israel and Tunkel for editing this volume, as I am indebted to the nearly 600 authors who have, during the past decade, helped define concrete examples of the ACGME competencies and applied them to clinical scenarios. We all hope that the *Competency-Based Companion Series* has set forth a model that will encourage students to integrate their medical knowledge with the skills, attitudes, behaviors, values, and continual self-assessment that will make them competent and caring physicians who serve the best interests of their patients and society.

Barry D. Mann MD

Preface

The approach to graduate medical education (i.e., residency training) changed dramatically in 1999 when the Accreditation Council for Graduate Medical Education (ACGME) introduced the requirement for competency-based education. These new ACGME requirements mandated that residency training programs define the specific knowledge, skills, and attitudes that their residents needed to demonstrate to be deemed competent in their specialty area. The six ACGME competencies are Patient Care, Medical Knowledge, Practice-Based Learning and Improvement, Interpersonal and Communication Skills, Professionalism, and Systems-Based Practice (see Appendix 1 of Section I for detailed definitions for each competency as defined by the ACGME). These competencies now provide the basis for how all Internal Medicine residents are evaluated. This ACGME requirement was later followed by a mandate from The Joint Commission, the body that accredits hospitals throughout the United States, that hospitals are now required to develop a process for Ongoing Physician Performance Evaluation (OPPE) built around the ACGME competencies and to demonstrate that they have a process of ongoing competency-based evaluation of the physicians who practice at their hospitals.

With the mandate for competency-based education at the residency level and beyond, there is also a need for competency-based education to begin in an organized way in medical school so that students will understand that it is just as important to foster interpersonal skills and professionalism as it is to acquire medical knowledge and that practice-based learning and systems-based practice are critically important to preparing the student for self-directed learning. This book is the fourth in a series (that also includes Surgery, Obstetrics and Gynecology, and Pediatrics) that attempts to provide medical students with the clinical framework to understand and utilize the competencies as they encounter patients during the junior clerkships.

The Medicine Clerkship is somewhat unique in the breadth and depth of information that the student must master. Although the acquisition of medical knowledge and the approach to differential diagnosis has been considered the mainstay of learning on the clerkship for decades, a competency-based approach has the benefit of better preparing the student for a lifetime of medical practice. The book begins with a few chapters that introduce the student to the competencies and provides some tips for success on the clerkship; these are followed by 58 chapters in 11 sections in which the competency-based approach to adult patients is oriented around clinical presentation of specific laboratory abnormalities. The section on practice-based learning will help the student understand the value of acquisition of skills and knowledge based on the best evidence. The "vertical read" format of these sections on interpersonal and communication skills, professionalism, and systems-based practice will assist the student in mastering these concepts across a wide range of clinical diagnoses.

Medicine: A Competency-Based Companion has been written by experts in their fields and will be a useful and practical compendium in educating and training students during the Junior Medicine Clerkship.

Jessica L. Israel MD
Allan R. Tunkel MD, PhD, MACP

Acknowledgments

Medicine: A Competency-Based Companion is being published as the fourth book in the Competency-Based Companion series, which was originally conceived by Barry Mann. We wish to acknowledge Barry's extraordinary vision at the outset of this project and also express our gratitude for his assistance with both ideas and editing throughout the entire process. As medical education evolves for today's student, inspiring and visionary clinician educators will carry their knowledge and experience to the next level. Barry has been that kind of mentor and teacher for us. We thank Barry for entrusting this final part of his series to the two of us.

We also wish to acknowledge the valuable insight and help from Christine Abshire and James Merritt at Elsevier. Their support for this book has made this process exciting from start to finish. We feel lucky to have had the opportunity to work with both of them.

In addition, we wish to thank Peggy Gordon for her assistance with organizing the production phase of our book, James Alexander for his help in supplying data on Medicare reimbursement for diagnostic tests and studies, and Samantha Nagengast for her assistance with referencing the medical information in our text. Sam did this work in record-breaking time while learning the ropes during her brand new fellowship in a new city, and we are very grateful.

Finally, we are grateful to our section editors and chapter authors for what we truly recognize as hard work and an above and beyond commitment to medical education. It has been a privilege to work with such a talented and bright group of contributors.

Jessica L. Israel, MD
Allan R. Tunkel, MD, PhD, MACP

Contributors

Eva Aagaard MD
Associate Professor of Medicine, Vice Chair for Education, Department of Medicine, University of Colorado School of Medicine; Department of Medicine, University of Colorado Hospital, Aurora, Colorado

John Abramson MD
Clinical Associate Professor of Medicine, Thomas Jefferson University Hospital, Philadelphia; Chief, Section of Nutrition; Attending Physician, Lankenau Hospital, Wynnewood, Pennsylvania

Kavita Ahuja DO
Physician, Nephrology–Private Practice, Robert Wood Johnson University Hospital; St. Peters University Hospital, New Brunswick, New Jersey

Zonera Ali MD
Attending Physician, Department of Hematology/Oncology, Lankenau Medical Center, Wynnewood, Pennsylvania

Akhtar Ashfaq MD
Clinical Research Medical Director, Amgen, Inc., Thousand Oaks, California

Shadi Barakat MD
Endocrinologist, Director, The Diabetes Center, Department of Medicine, Baltimore, Maryland

Sameer Bashey MD
Postdoctoral Medical Fellow, Department of Cutaneous Oncology, Stanford University, Stanford, California

Cindy Baskin MD
Assistant Professor of Medicine, Department of Internal Medicine, Weill Cornell Medical Center, New York Hospital, New York, New York

Alessandro Bellucci MD
Associate Professor of Medicine, Division of Kidney Diseases, Hofstra; Executive Vice Chair of Department of Medicine, North Shore–Long Island Jewish Health System, North Shore University Hospital, Manhasset; Long Island Jewish Medical Center, New Hyde Park, New York

Tami Berry MD
Resident, Department of General Surgery, Lankenau Medical Center, Wynnewood, Pennsylvania

James G. Bittner IV MD
Instructor in Surgery, Department of Surgery, Section of Minimally Invasive Surgery, School of Medicine, Washington University in St. Louis, St. Louis, Missouri

Isai Gopalakrishnan Bowline MD
Instructor, Wake Forest University School of Medicine, Winston-Salem, North Carolina

Elizabeth Briggs MD
Endocrinologist, Maryland Endocrine, PA, Columbia, Maryland

Ari D. Brooks MD
Vice Chair for Research, Associate Professor, Surgery, Drexel University College of Medicine; Chief, Surgical Oncology, Department of Surgery, Hahnemann University Hospital, Philadelphia, Pennsylvania

Patricia D. Brown MD
Associate Professor of Medicine, Division of Infectious Diseases, Wayne State University School of Medicine; Chief of Medicine, Detroit Receiving Hospital, Detroit, Michigan

M. Susan Burke MD
Clinical Assistant Professor of Medicine, Thomas Jefferson University Medical School, Philadelphia; Senior Advisor, Internal Medicine Clinical Care Center, Lankenau Medical Center, Wynnewood, Pennsylvania

Esaïe Carisma DO
Attending Physician, Department of Critical Care Medicine, Memorial Regional Hospital, Hollywood, Florida

Elie R. Chemaly MD, MSc
Research and Clinical Fellow, Cardiovascular Research Center, Mount Sinai School of Medicine; Cardiovascular Institute, Mount Sinai Medical Center, New York, New York

Bridgette Collins-Burow PhD, MD
Assistant Professor, Department of Medicine, Section of Hematology and Medical Oncology, Tulane Medical School, New Orleans, Louisiana

Byron E. Crawford MD
Assistant Dean of Academic Affairs, Vice Chair and Professor of Pathology, Department of Pathology and Laboratory Medicine, Tulane School of Medicine; Medical Director, Tulane Medical Center Pathology Laboratories, Tulane Medical Center, New Orleans, Louisiana

Amy L. Curran MD
Physician, Penn Care-Hematology/Oncology, Cancer Center at Phoenixville Hospital, Phoenixville, Pennsylvania

Mary Denshaw-Burke MD
Clinical Assistant Professor of Medicine, Department of Medicine, Thomas Jefferson University, Philadelphia; Program Director, Hematology/Oncology Fellowship, Department of Medicine, Lankenau Medical Center; Clinical Assistant Professor, Affiliated Clinical Faculty, Lankenau Institute for Medical Research, Wynnewood, Pennsylvania

Minal Dhamankar MD
Fellow, Department of Hematology/Oncology, Lankenau Medical Center, Wynnewood, Pennsylvania

Shamina Dhillon MD
Staff Attending, Department of Gastroenterology, Monmouth Medical Center, Long Branch; Chief of Gastroenterology, Department of Gastroenterology, Jersey Shore Medical Center, Neptune, New Jersey

Robin Dibner MD
Clinical Associate Professor of Medicine, Department of Medicine, New York University School of Medicine; Associate Chairman, Education, Residency Program Director, Department of Medicine, Lenox Hill Hospital, New York, New York

Tamara Donatelli DO
Resident, Department of General Surgery, Lankenau Hospital, Wynnewood, Pennsylvania

Jennifer Elbaum MD
Bronx, New York

Bob Etemad MD
Medical Director of Endoscopy, Main Line Health System, Departments of Gastroenterology and Hepatology, Lankenau Medical Center, Main Line Health System, Wynnewood, Pennsylvania

Michelle Fabian MD
Assistant Professor, Department of Neurology, Mount Sinai School of Medicine; Attending Physician, Corinne Goldsmith Center for Multiple Sclerosis, Mount Sinai Medical Center, New York, New York

Arzhang Fallahi MD
Resident, Department of Medicine, Mount Sinai School of Medicine, New York, New York

Christopher P. Farrell DO
Gastroenterology Fellow, Department of Gastroenterology, Lankenau Medical Center, Wynnewood, Pennsylvania

Rabeena Fazal MD
Physician, Internal Medicine and Nephrology, Brooklyn, New York

Dennis Finkielstein MD
Assistant Professor of Medicine, Department of Medicine, Albert Einstein School of Medicine, Bronx; Director, Cardiovascular Diseases Fellowship; Director, Ambulatory Cardiology, Division of Cardiology, Beth Israel Medical Center, New York, New York

Erica S. Friedman MD
Professor of Medicine and Medical Education; Associate Dean for Education Assessment and Scholarship, Medical Education and Medicine, Mount Sinai School of Medicine; Department of Medicine, Mount Sinai Medical Center, New York, New York

Paul Gilman MD
Clinical Assistant Professor, Department of Hematology/Oncology, Thomas Jefferson University, Philadelphia; Chief, Division of Hematology/Oncology, Department of Hematology/Oncology, Lankenau Medical Center; Adjunct Professor, Department of Oncology, Lankenau Institute for Medical Research, Wynnewood, Pennsylvania

Michael Gitman MD
Assistant Professor of Medicine, Department of Medicine, Hofstra North Shore–LIJ School of Medicine, New York; Associate Chairman of Medicine, Department of Medicine, North Shore University Hospital, Great Neck, Long Island Jewish Hospital, New Hyde Park, New York

Christopher Greenleaf MD
Resident, Department of Surgery, Lankenau Medical Center, Wynnewood, Pennsylvania

Azzour Hazzan MD
Director of Clinical Trials/Division of Nephrology, Department of Medicine, Hofstra North Shore–LIJ Health System, Great Neck; Attending, Department of Medicine, Division of Nephrology, North Shore University Hospital, Manhasset; Long Island Jewish Medical Center, New Hyde Park, New York

Austin Hwang MD
Gastroenterology Fellow, Department of Gastroenterology, Lankenau Hospital, Wynnewood, Pennsylvania

Jessica L. Israel MD
Chief, Division of Geriatric and Palliative Medicine, Medical Director, Inpatient Hospice Unit, Monmouth Medical Center, Long Branch, New Jersey; Clinical Associate Professor of Medicine, Drexel University College of Medicine, Philadelphia, Pennsylvania

Kavita Iyengar MD
Fellow, Department of Endocrinology, Union Memorial Hospital, Baltimore, Maryland

Joan R. Johnson MD, MMS
Resident, Department of Surgery, Georgia Health Sciences University, Augusta, Georgia

Marc J. Kahn MD, MBA
Professor and Senior Associate Dean, Department of Medicine, Hematology/Medical Oncology, Tulane University School of Medicine, New Orleans, Louisiana

Maya Katz MD
Movement Disorders Fellowship, University of California San Francisco, San Francisco, California

Michael Kim MD
Assistant Professor of Medicine, Mount Sinai Heart, Department of Medicine/Cardiology, Mount Sinai School of Medicine; Director, Coronary Care Unit, Department of Cardiology, Mount Sinai Medical Center, New York, New York

Stephen Krieger MD
Assistant Professor, Department of Neurology, Mount Sinai School of Medicine; Attending Neurologist, Department of Neurology, Mount Sinai Medical Center, New York, New York

Rebecca Kruse-Jarres MD, MPH
Assistant Professor, Department of Medicine, Tulane University, New Orleans, Louisiana

Jennifer LaRosa MD
Assistant Professor of Medicine, Internal Medicine, Division of Pulmonary and Critical Care Medicine; Associate Director, Division of Pulmonary and Critical Care Medicine; Director, Pulmonary and Critical Care Medicine Fellowship Program; Director, Intensive Care Unit, Internal Medicine, Division of Pulmonary and Critical Care Medicine, Newark Beth Israel Medical Center, Newark, New Jersey

Bradley W. Lash MD
Hematology/Medical Oncology Fellow, Department of Medicine, Division of Hematology/Oncology, Lankenau Medical Center, Wynnewood, Pennsylvania

D. Scott Lind MD
Professor and Chair, Department of Surgery, Drexel University College of Medicine; Service Chief, Hahnemann University Hospital, Philadelphia, Pennsylvania

Ellena Linden MD
Assistant Professor, Department of Medicine, Mount Sinai Medical Center, New York; Attending Nephrologist, Department of Medicine, Elmhurst Hospital Center, Elmhurst, New York

Joel Mathew MD
Resident, Department of Medicine, Lenox Hill Hospital, New York, New York

Frank C. McGeehin III MD
Chief, Clinical Cardiology, Main Line Health Hospitals; Lankenau Medical Center, Wynnewood, Pennsylvania

Giancarlo Mercogliano MD, MBA, AGA
Associate Clinical Professor of Medicine, Department of Medicine, Jefferson University School of Medicine, Philadelphia; Chief of Gastroenterology, Department of Medicine, Main Line Health System, Lankenau Medical Center, Wynnewood, Pennsylvania

Christina Migliore MD
Associate Director, Lung Transplant and Pulmonary Hypertension, Department of Pulmonary and Critical Care Medicine, Newark Beth Israel Medical Center, Newark; Attending Physician, Department of Pulmonary and Critical Care Medicine, St. Barnabas Medical Center, Livingston, New Jersey

Ilene Miller MD
Medical Director, North Shore–Long Island Jewish Health System, North Shore University Hospital, Manhasset, New York

Richard H. Miranda MD
Assistant Professor of Medicine, Department of Medicine, University of Colorado School of Medicine, Aurora; Department of Graduate Medical Education, Presbyterian/St. Luke's Hospital; Assistant Professor of Medicine, Department of Graduate Medical Education, The Colorado Health Foundation, Denver, Colorado

Melissa Morgan DO
Gastroenterology Fellow, Department of Gastroenterology, Lankenau Medical Center, Wynnewood, Pennsylvania

Joseph J. Muscato MD
Clinical Associate Professor of Medicine, Department of Hematology and Medical Oncology, University of Missouri School of Medicine, Columbia, Missouri

Ranjit Nair MD
Attending Physician, Pulmonary/Critical Care, Newark Beth Israel Medical Center, Newark, New Jersey

Smitha Gopinath Nair DO
Physician, Department of Pulmonary/Critical Care Medicine, Robert Wood Johnson University Hospital; Saint Peter's University Hospital, New Brunswick; Raritan Bay Medical Center, Perth Amboy and Old Bridge, New Jersey

Sudheer Nambiar MD
Physician, Pulmonary Critical Care, T. J. Samson Community Hospital, Glasgow, Kentucky

Gary Newman MD
Attending Physician, Department of Gastroenterology, Lankenau Medical Center, Wynnewood, Pennsylvania

Benjamin Ngo MD
Gastroenterology Fellow, Department of Gastroenterology, Lankenau Medical Center, Wynnewood, Pennsylvania

Dennis H. Novack MD
Professor of Medicine, Associate Dean of Medical Education, Office of Educational Affairs, Drexel University College of Medicine, Philadelphia; Physician, Department of Internal Medicine, Abington Memorial Hospital, Abington; Hahnemann University Hospital, Philadelphia, Pennsylvania; American Academy on Communication in Healthcare, Chesterfield, Missouri

Pratik Patel MD
Associate Director, Pulmonary and Critical Care Fellowship; Director, Interventional Pulmonology, Department of Pulmonary and Critical Care Medicine, Newark Beth Israel Medical Center, Newark; Attending Physician, Pulmonary and Critical Care Medicine, St. Barnabas Medical Center, Livingston, New Jersey

Clifford H. Pemberton MD
Main Line Oncology/Hematology, Lankenau Medical Center, Wynnewood, Pennsylvania

Nils Petersen MD
Clinical Fellow in Vascular Neurology, Department of Neurology, Columbia University, New York, New York

Julie Robinson-Boyar MD
Assistant Professor, Department of Neurology, Albert Einstein College of Medicine, Montefiore Hospital, Bronx, New York

Deena K. Roemer
Volunteer, The Walter and Leonore Annenberg Conference Center for Medical Education, Lankenau Medical Center, Main Line Health System, Wynnewood, Pennsylvania

Amy Rogstad MD
Department of Endocrinology, Rockville Internal Medicine Group, Rockville, Maryland

David Rudolph DO
Gastroenterology Fellow, Department of Gastroenterology, Lankenau Medical Center, Wynnewood, Pennsylvania

Joseph Rudolph MD
Fellow, Department of Neurology, Mount Sinai Medical Center, New York, New York

Kathleen F. Ryan MD
Associate Professor of Medicine; Director, Medical Simulation Center, Drexel University College of Medicine, Philadelphia, Pennsylvania

Lana Zhovtis Ryerson MD
Resident, Department of Neurology, Mount Sinai School of Medicine, New York, New York

Jennifer Sabol MD
Assistant Professor of Surgery, Department of Surgery, Jefferson Medical College, Thomas Jefferson University, Philadelphia; Director of the Breast Care Program, Lankenau Hospital, Wynnewood, Pennsylvania

Paul Sack MD
Clinical Assistant Professor of Medicine, Department of Endocrinology, Diabetes, and Nutrition, University of Maryland; Attending Physician, Department of Endocrinology, Union Memorial Hospital, Baltimore, Maryland

Madelaine R. Saldivar MD, MPH
Associate Program Director, Ambulatory Medicine, Department of Internal Medicine, Lankenau Medical Center, Wynnewood, Pennsylvania

Henry Schoonyoung MD
Resident, Department of General Surgery, Lankenau Medical Center, Wynnewood, Pennsylvania

Pamela R. Schroeder MD, PhD
Assistant Professor, Department of Medicine, Division of Endocrinology, Johns Hopkins University School of Medicine; Co-Director of Thyroid Clinic, Department of Medicine, Diabetes and Endocrine Center, Union Memorial Hospital, Baltimore, Maryland

Michael Share MD
Jefferson Medical College, Thomas Jefferson University, Philadelphia, Pennsylvania

Irtza Sharif MD
*Pulmonary and Critical Care Medicine Fellow, Department of Medicine,
Newark Beth Israel Medical Center, Newark, New Jersey*

Aarti Shevade MD
*Resident, Department of Internal Medicine, Lankenau Hospital,
Wynnewood, Pennsylvania*

Jennifer Sherwood MD
Executive Health Resources, Newtown Square, Pennsylvania

Mansur Shomali MD
*Clinical Assistant Professor, Department of Medicine, University of Maryland
School of Medicine; Associate Director, Diabetes and Endocrine Center;
Fellowship Program Director, Endocrinology Program, Med Star Union
Memorial Hospital, Baltimore, Maryland*

Cynthia D. Smith MD
*Senior Medical Associate for Content Development, Department of Medical
Education, American College of Physicians, Philadelphia, Pennsylvania*

Sean M. Studer MD, MSc
*Clinical Associate Professor of Medicine, Department of Medicine, Drexel
University College of Medicine, Philadelphia, Pennsylvania; Director,
Division of Pulmonary and Critical Care, Department of Medicine, Newark
Beth Israel Medical Center, Newark, New Jersey*

Nishanth Sukumaran MD
*Fellow, Department of Hematology/Oncology, Lankenau Medical Center,
Wynnewood, Pennsylvania*

William D. Surkis MD
*Clinical Assistant Professor of Medicine, Department of Internal Medicine,
Jefferson Medical College, Philadelphia; Interim Program Director, Internal
Medicine Residency Program, Lankenau Medical Center, Wynnewood,
Pennsylvania*

Michele Tagliati MD
*Professor, Department of Neurology, Cedars-Sinai Professorial Series;
Vice Chairman and Director of the Movement Disorders Program,
Department of Neurology, Cedars-Sinai Medical Center, Los Angeles,
California*

James Thornton MD
*Clinical Associate Professor of Medicine, Department of Medicine, Thomas
Jefferson University, Philadelphia; Associate in Medicine; Emeritus Chief of
Gastroenterology, Department of Medicine, Lankenau Medical Center,
Wynnewood, Pennsylvania*

Owen Tully MD
Department of Gastroenterology, Lankenau Medical Center, Wynnewood, Pennsylvania

Allan R. Tunkel MD, PhD, MACP
Chair, Department of Internal Medicine, Monmouth Medical Center, Long Branch, New Jersey; Professor of Medicine, Drexel University College of Medicine, Philadelphia, Pennsylvania

Spirithoula Vasilopoulos MD
Physician, Nephrology and Internal Medicine, North Syracuse, New York

Roxane Weighall DO
Clinical Assistant Professor, Department of Surgery, Wright State University Boonshoft School of Medicine, Dayton, Ohio

Kelly J. White MD
Associate Professor, Department of Internal Medicine, University of Colorado, Denver, Colorado

Brian Wojciechowski MD
Hematology/Oncology Fellow, Department of Medicine, Lankenau Medical Center, Wynnewood, Pennsylvania

Sidharth Yadav DO
Associate Director, Division of Cardiology, The New York Methodist Hospital, Brooklyn, New York

Edward H. Yu MD
Department of Neurology, Staten Island University Hospital, Staten Island, New York

Erik L. Zeger MD
Attending Physician, Department of Hematology/Oncology, Lankenau Medical Center, Wynnewood, Pennsylvania

Marc Zitin MD
Attending Physician, Department of Gastroenterology, Lankenau Medical Center, Wynnewood, Pennsylvania

Contents

Section I INTRODUCTION   1
Section Editor: *Allan R. Tunkel MD, PhD, MACP*

Chapter 1 How to Study This Book   3
Allan R. Tunkel MD, PhD, MACP and Jessica L. Israel MD

Chapter 2 The Competencies   5
Erica S. Friedman MD

Chapter 3 Tips for the Medicine Clerkship   8
Kathleen F. Ryan MD

Appendix 1 ACGME General Competencies   12

Appendix 2 Competency Self-Assessment Form: Medicine   15

Section II AMBULATORY INTERNAL MEDICINE   17
Section Editor: *Cynthia D. Smith MD*

Chapter 4 Tips for Learning on the Ambulatory Clerkship   19
Kelly J. White MD, Richard H. Miranda MD, and Eva Aagaard MD

Chapter 5 Preventive Medicine (Case 1)   24
Cynthia D. Smith MD and Brian Wojciechowski MD

**Chapter 6 Common Problems in Ambulatory Internal Medicine
(Case 2: A Problem Set of Five Common Cases)   35**
Madelaine R. Şaldivar MD, MPH and M. Susan Burke MD

Chapter 7 The Patient with Complex Problems (Case 3)   56
William D. Surkis MD

Section III CARDIOVASCULAR DISEASES   63
Section Editor: *Michael Kim MD*

Chapter 8 Chest Pain (Case 4)   65
Arzhang Fallahi MD and Michael Kim MD

Chapter 9 Teaching Visual: Coronary Angiography   81
Sidharth Yadav DO and Frank C. McGeehin III MD

Chapter 10 Congestive Heart Failure (Case 5)   90
Sameer Bashey MD and Michael Kim MD

Chapter 11 Palpitations and Arrhythmias (Case 6)   103
Arzhang Fallahi MD and Michael Kim MD

Chapter 12 Teaching Visual: How to Interpret an Electrocardiogram   117
Jessica L. Israel MD

Chapter 13 Hypertension (Case 7)   123
Elie R. Chemaly MD, MSc and Michael Kim MD

Section IV PULMONARY DISEASES   143
Section Editor: *Sean M. Studer MD, MSc*

Chapter 14 Dyspnea (Case 8)   145
Esaïe Carisma DO and Christina Migliore MD

Chapter 15 Cough (Case 9)   155
Ranjit Nair MD and Sean M. Studer MD, MSc

Chapter 16 Hemoptysis (Case 10)   166
Sudheer Nambiar MD and Pratik Patel MD

Chapter 17 Pulmonary Nodule (Case 11)   177
Smitha Gopinath Nair DO and Jennifer LaRosa MD

Chapter 18 Teaching Visual: How to Interpret a Chest Radiograph   188
Irtza Sharif MD and Sean M. Studer MD, MSc

Section V RENAL DISEASES AND ELECTROLYTE DISORDERS   197
Section Editor: *Michael Gitman MD*

Chapter 19 Acute Kidney Injury (Case 12)   199
Isai Gopalakrishnan Bowline MD and Akhtar Ashfaq MD

Chapter 20 Edema (Case 13)   211
Ellena Linden MD and Dennis Finkielstein MD

Chapter 21 Acid-Base Disorders (Case 14)   219
Kavita Ahuja DO and Ilene Miller MD

Chapter 22 Abnormal Electrolytes (Case 15)   232
Rabeena Fazal MD and Alessandro Bellucci MD

Chapter 23 Hematuria (Case 16)   244
Spirithoula Vasilopoulos MD and Michael Gitman MD

Chapter 24 Dysuria (Case 17)   256
Cindy Baskin MD and Michael Gitman MD

Chapter 25 Renal Mass (Case 18)   269
Azzour Hazzan MD

Section VI GASTROINTESTINAL AND LIVER DISEASES   279
Section Editors: *Giancarlo Mercogliano MD, MBA, AGA and Barry D. Mann MD*

Chapter 26 Abdominal Pain (Case 19)   281
Shamina Dhillon MD, Henry Schoonyoung MD, and Jessica L. Israel MD

Chapter 27 Nausea and Vomiting (Case 20)   293
Owen Tully MD and Bob Etemad MD

Chapter 28 Esophageal Dysphagia (Case 21) 305
Benjamin Ngo MD and John Abramson MD

Chapter 29 Gastrointestinal Bleeding (Case 22) 312
Melissa Morgan DO, Michael Share MD, and Marc Zitin MD

Chapter 30 Constipation (Case 23) 324
Christopher P. Farrell DO and Gary Newman MD

Chapter 31 Diarrhea (Case 24) 334
David Rudolph DO and James Thornton MD

Chapter 32 Jaundice (Case 25) 346
Austin Hwang MD and Giancarlo Mercogliano MD, MBA, AGA

Section VII HEMATOLOGIC DISEASES 359
Section Editor: *Marc J. Kahn MD, MBA*

Chapter 33 Elevated Blood Counts (Case 26) 361
Marc J. Kahn MD, MBA

Chapter 34 Teaching Visual: The Importance of the Peripheral Blood Smear 368
Aarti Shevade MD and Paul Gilman MD

Chapter 35 Pancytopenia (Case 27) 375
Byron E. Crawford MD

Chapter 36 Excessive Bleeding or Clotting (Case 28) 387
Rebecca Kruse-Jarres MD, MPH

Chapter 37 Lymphadenopathy and Splenomegaly (Case 29) 396
Bridgette Collins-Burow PhD, MD

Section VIII ONCOLOGIC DISEASES 407
Section Editor: *Mary Denshaw-Burke MD*

Chapter 38 Breast Mass (Case 30) 409
*Tamara Donatelli DO, Jennifer Sabol MD, Roxane Weighall DO,
Ari D. Brooks MD, and Mary Denshaw-Burke MD*

Chapter 39 Prostate Mass (Case 31) 421
Amy L. Curran MD and Clifford H. Pemberton MD

Chapter 40 Testicular Mass (Case 32) 431
*Christopher Greenleaf MD, Tamara Donatelli DO, Jennifer Sherwood MD,
and Mary Denshaw-Burke MD*

Chapter 41 Neck Mass (Case 33) 439
Bradley W. Lash MD and Erik L. Zeger MD

Chapter 42 Pigmented Skin Lesions (Case 34) 449
James G. Bittner IV MD, Joan R. Johnson MD, MMS, and D. Scott Lind MD

Chapter 43 Incidentally Discovered Mass Lesions (Case 35) 459
Tami Berry MD and Joseph J. Muscato MD

Chapter 44 Oncologic Emergencies (Case 36: A Problem Set of Three Common Cases)   470
Minal Dhamankar MD and Zonera Ali MD

Chapter 45 Paraneoplastic Syndromes (Case 37: A Problem Set of Three Common Cases)   483
Nishanth Sukumaran MD and Mary Denshaw-Burke MD

Section IX ENDOCRINE DISEASES   495
Section Editor: *Mansur Shomali MD*

Chapter 46 Polyuria and Polydipsia (Case 38)   497
Kavita Iyengar MD

Chapter 47 Hypoglycemia (Case 39)   507
Shadi Barakat MD

Chapter 48 Weight Gain and Obesity (Case 40)   519
Elizabeth Briggs MD

Chapter 49 Weight Loss (Case 41)   529
Pamela R. Schroeder MD, PhD

Chapter 50 Amenorrhea (Case 42)   538
Amy Rogstad MD

Chapter 51 Fragility Fracture (Case 43)   553
Paul Sack MD

Section X RHEUMATOLOGIC DISEASES   567
Section Editor: *Allan R. Tunkel MD, PhD, MACP*

Chapter 52 Acute Joint Pain (Case 44)   569
Robin Dibner MD, Joel Mathew MD, and Jessica L. Israel MD

Chapter 53 Chronic Joint Pain (Case 45)   578
Robin Dibner MD, Joel Mathew MD, and Jessica L. Israel MD

Section XI INFECTIOUS DISEASES   593
Section Editor: *Patricia D. Brown MD*

Chapter 54 Infections Presenting with Rash (Case 46)   595
Patricia D. Brown MD

Chapter 55 Skin and Soft-Tissue Infections (Case 47)   604
Patricia D. Brown MD

Chapter 56 Upper Respiratory Tract Infections (Case 48)   616
Patricia D. Brown MD

Chapter 57 Genital Ulcers (Case 49)   625
Patricia D. Brown MD

Chapter 58 Vaginitis and Urethritis (Case 50)   635
Patricia D. Brown MD

Chapter 59 Fever in the Hospitalized Patient (Case 51)   647
Patricia D. Brown MD

Section XII NEUROLOGIC DISEASES   661
Section Editors: *Michele Tagliati MD and Stephen Krieger MD*

Chapter 60 Altered Mental Status (Case 52)   663
Nils Petersen MD

Chapter 61 Dementia (Case 53)   675
Jessica L. Israel MD

Chapter 62 Seizures (Case 54)   687
Julie Robinson-Boyer MD

Chapter 63 Abnormal Movements (Case 55)   698
Joseph Rudolph MD and Michele Tagliati MD

Chapter 64 Headache (Case 56)   710
Michelle Fabian MD and Jennifer Elbaum MD

Chapter 65 Dizziness and Vertigo (Case 57)   726
Lana Zhovtis Ryerson MD and Stephen Krieger MD

Chapter 66 Weakness (Case 58)   737
Edward H. Yu MD and Maya Katz MD

Index   751

Section I
INTRODUCTION

Section Editor
Allan R. Tunkel MD, PhD, MACP

Section Contents

1 **How to Study This Book**
Allan R. Tunkel MD, PhD, MACP and Jessica L. Israel MD

2 **The Competencies**
Erica S. Friedman MD

3 **Tips for the Medicine Clerkship**
Kathleen F. Ryan MD

Appendix 1 **ACGME General Competencies**

Appendix 2 **Competency Self-Assessment Form: Medicine**

Chapter 1
How to Study This Book

Allan R. Tunkel MD, PhD, MACP and Jessica L. Israel MD

Patients on the inpatient medicine services run the gamut of complaints that may require not only care by primary care physicians but also involvement of a number of specialty services—some within internal medicine such as cardiology, nephrology, or infectious diseases, and others from a variety of non–internal medicine specialties (e.g., surgery). Furthermore, the majority of the medical care of adult patients now occurs primarily in the outpatient setting, and coordination of ambulatory care and preventive medicine fall within the purview of the general internist. Based on the shift of care to the outpatient setting, most Internal Medicine Clerkships and Internal Medicine Residencies include significant time in the ambulatory setting.

This book is not meant to be an exhaustive approach to all aspects of Internal Medicine. Rather, the book serves as a framework to introduce students and residents to patient care utilizing a competency-based approach. Information surrounding each patient's diagnosis, or consideration of additional aspects of clinical presentation, diagnosis, and management, should be supplemented by the reading of standard internal medicine textbooks (such as *Andreoli and Carpenter's Cecil Essentials of Medicine*, 8e). It is also critically important that students and residents utilize the principles of self-directed learning to ensure that they develop the attitudes and skills to learn medicine for the rest of their careers.

STRUCTURE OF THE BOOK

The book begins with several introductory chapters that provide an overview into the organizational structure, consideration of the principles surrounding the Accreditation Council for Graduate Medical Education (ACGME) competencies, and "Tips for the Medicine Clerkship." These are followed by 58 case-based chapters that are divided into the following 11 sections:

Ambulatory Internal Medicine
Cardiovascular Diseases
Pulmonary Diseases
Renal Diseases and Electrolyte Disorders
Gastrointestinal and Liver Diseases
Hematologic Diseases
Oncologic Diseases
Endocrine Diseases

Rheumatologic Diseases
Infectious Diseases
Neurologic Diseases

Within each section are individual chapters in which disease states are considered based on symptoms or syndromes, or abnormal laboratory findings, to assist the reader in considering a broad range of possibilities based on a patient's clinical presentation. In some sections there are also teaching visuals on specific topics: interpretation of electrocardiograms, chest radiographs, and peripheral blood smears; and coronary angiography and colonoscopy.

CHAPTER ELEMENTS AND VERTICAL READS

Each chapter begins with a representative **Case** that includes the pertinent aspects of the patient's subjective complaints and physical examination findings; some data are also provided if pertinent to consideration of a **Differential Diagnosis** (generally four to eight likely conditions to consider, but only the more common entities and not an exhaustive list). The next paragraph, termed **Speaking Intelligently**, sums up the clinical overview in language that is representative of a physician speaking to a colleague. This is followed by **Patient Care**, consisting of bulleted sections on **History**, **Physical Examination**, and **Tests for Consideration**; each section includes pertinent information that may assist the student and resident in consideration of a specific diagnosis. A section on **Imaging Considerations** (if applicable) follows. In these latter sections, the reimbursements for specific diagnostic tests and imaging modalities are provided. These are taken from the Medicare payments listed in the Clinical Diagnostic Laboratory Fee Schedule and the Ambulatory Payment Classification for 2012, and are provided only to give guidance to the reader in considering cost and reimbursement when ordering specific diagnostic tests; exact amounts are subject to multiple variables and will likely change in the future. The listed reimbursements do not include payments to physicians. For readers who have acquainted themselves with the other volumes in the series, you will note that the listed costs are different than those in this volume; in the other books, the authors and editors provided best estimates gleaned from difficult-to-obtain hospital charges. This discrepancy highlights the great variability in charges, as well as differences in reimbursements for tests and procedures from Medicare and commercial payers.

The **Clinical Entities** section then takes each of the more common, but not all, disease states listed as part of the **Differential Diagnosis** and reviews pertinent information on pathogenesis and pathophysiology, clinical features, diagnosis, and management. Unusual diagnoses are considered in the **Zebra Zone**.

Each chapter has a section on **Practice-Based Learning and Improvement**, which presents and critiques an important publication from the literature. For the student and resident, this illustrates how clinical trials have been designed to evaluate clinical questions and how evidence-based medicine has been utilized to change medical practice.

Finally, there are sections on **Interpersonal and Communication Skills**, **Professionalism**, and **Systems-Based Practice**. These three sections begin with an important principle in each competency that relates to the patient's clinical situation or diagnosis. Across chapters these competencies can be organized into a "vertical read" to allow the reader to develop a complete understanding of these competencies as they pertain to the Medicine Clerkship and during the Internal Medicine Residency; these vertical reads are available online at http://www. studentconsult.com. In addition, suggested websites for most chapters are available online on Student Consult.

We are optimistic that this competency-based approach to learning internal medicine will be productive for you on the clerkship or during your residency, and will prepare you for a successful career in the discipline of your choice.

Chapter 2
The Competencies

Erica S. Friedman MD

Medicine: A Competency-Based Companion is part of a series for medical students and residents designed to guide you through an expert clinician's thought process when encountering a particular patient or clinical problem; it uses a competency-based framework to approach the problem.

Competencies are an educational paradigm helpful in clarifying for the teacher and the learner the outcomes-based performance expectations. Competencies identify behaviors as opposed to knowledge or skills, and they require synthesis and integration of information to achieve the outcome. They define what physicians must be able to achieve for effective practice and to meet the needs of their patients. Defining competencies also helps guide curriculum development, teaching, learning, and assessment.

Medical education has experienced a major paradigm shift from structure- and process-based to competency-based education and measurement of outcomes. Structure- and process-based education focuses on knowledge acquisition in a fixed time frame, has the teacher responsible for the content and dissemination of knowledge, and, in general, evaluates success by defining the norm and failing anyone whose performance falls more than two standard deviations below the mean. In contrast, competency-based education focuses on knowledge application, and the learner is the driving force for the process, equally responsible with the teacher for the content. It utilizes multiple evaluations in real time and, in general, applies a standard for developing the criteria for competence. It allows and expects variability in time for mastery of these competencies.

In the latter part of the 20th century, the public expectation for accountability and responsibility around physician competency became a driving force for the Accreditation Council for Graduate Medical Education (ACGME) to establish the competencies. The ACGME shifted its focus from a structure and process system of graduate medical education to one that is outcomes-based and since 1999 has required all residents in training to achieve competence in six broad domains.

The ACGME's six core competencies are as follows:

1. **Patient Care.** Residents must be able to provide patient care that is compassionate, appropriate, and effective for the treatment of health problems and the promotion of health.
2. **Medical Knowledge.** Residents must demonstrate knowledge of established and evolving biomedical, clinical, epidemiological and social behavioral sciences, as well as the application of this knowledge to patient care.
3. **Practice-Based Learning and Improvement.** Residents must demonstrate the ability to investigate and evaluate their care of patients, to appraise and assimilate scientific evidence, and to continuously improve patient care based on constant self-evaluation and life-long learning.
4. **Interpersonal and Communication Skills.** Residents must demonstrate interpersonal and communication skills that result in the effective exchange of information and collaboration with patients, their families, and health professionals.
5. **Professionalism.** Residents must demonstrate a commitment to carrying out professional responsibilities and an adherence to ethical principles.
6. **Systems-Based Practice.** Residents must demonstrate an awareness of and responsiveness to the larger context and system of health care, as well as the ability to call effectively on other resources in the system to provide optimal health care.*

These six competencies are intentionally general, because it is expected that each residency will define the specific knowledge, skills, and attitudes required to meet these competencies in that specific specialty.

---

*From ACGME Competency definitions: Used with permission of Accreditation Counsel for Graduate Medical Education © ACGME 2011. Please see the ACGME website: www.acgme.org for the most current version.

Medical students in the 21st century are also now expected to graduate with a set of competencies or skills and qualities that prepare them for residency training. The challenge is in coordinating and aligning medical student and residency curricula and competencies so there is a seamless developmental transition.

Being an exemplary physician requires more than knowing how to diagnose and manage patients. It requires a constellation of skills, attitudes, and abilities that include the ability to communicate effectively, understand and embody the expectations of the profession, and use the literature in an evidence-based fashion to improve patient care and outcomes, as well as to evaluate one's own practice.

Organizing this book around the competencies is novel and assists the learner in developing clinical reasoning and in understanding the required competencies for each patient care scenario. The chapters are structured around a case presentation leading to an explanation of the preliminary differential diagnoses, why specific information is relevant (history, physical exam, and diagnostic testing) and should be collected, and how to interpret this information so as to decide upon a patient diagnosis. Each chapter provides a discussion of the presentation and key diagnostic features of each possible diagnosis, the underlying pathophysiology, and general concepts around management. This part of each chapter addresses the ACGME Medical Knowledge and Patient Care competencies. Each chapter then addresses the requisite Interpersonal and Communication Skills to care for the patient, and identifies a Professionalism issue from the Advancing Medical Professionalism to Improve Health Care (ABIM) professionalism principles charter that is relevant to the case. It also provides best evidence around a patient care issue (Practice-Based Learning and Improvement), and identifies and discusses a Systems-Based Practice issue that impacts on the care of the patient.

Most medical student educational materials provide information on medical knowledge and patient care. This resource goes further in identifying what issues relate to systems-based practice and practice-based learning. It also concisely provides an explanation for the reasoning behind potential diagnoses and helps prioritize them based upon the key features of each one. In short, it is the equivalent of a functional magnetic resonance imaging scan, providing a road map of the path of an expert's diagnostic reasoning.

It is exceedingly helpful for medical students and residents to approach taking care of patients using a competency-based framework in preparation for directing their learning both during medical school and residency training and beyond, and this resource supports development of the skills required for development of an exemplary physician.

Competency definitions according to the ACGME are provided in Appendix 1 to this section.

Chapter 3
Tips for the Medicine Clerkship

Kathleen F. Ryan MD

The Internal Medicine Clerkship is the educational experience during which students are expected to gain the basic knowledge, skills, and attitudes needed to care for adult patients with medical disorders. Traditionally, the clerkship has been hospital-based and geared to the diagnosis and management of acutely ill inpatients. With changes in the delivery of health care in the United States, clerkships at many medical schools have also included some training time in the ambulatory environment. The clerkship can be an anxiety-provoking time for some students as they move from the objective evaluation system (i.e., tests and quizzes) of the preclinical years to the subjective evaluation system of the clinical years, which is based on day-to-day knowledge and care of patients. That is not to say that students will never encounter a written examination, as many schools administer the National Board of Medical Examiners (NBME) Shelf Examination in Medicine at the end of the clerkship, which may account for a significant portion of the student's final grade. This chapter provides a few pointers to hopefully ensure success in this very exciting, but sometimes intimidating, clinical journey.

KNOW THE GOALS

There are levels of proficiency throughout medical school and during the clerkship that are usually linked to the goals and objectives. Schools either distribute the goals and objectives or have a website devoted to the clerkship where they can be found. In addition, many schools have adopted the national *Clerkship Directors in Internal Medicine—Society of General Internal Medicine Core Medicine Clerkship Curriculum;* the national goals, objectives, and syllabus can be accessed at the Alliance for Academic Internal Medicine's website (http://www.im.org). These elucidate what the learner will need to master, as the goals and objectives are usually tied in some way into the final evaluation for the Internal Medicine Clerkship.

GREAT EXPECTATIONS: THE DUTIES OF A JUNIOR CLERK

Many students struggle with what is expected of them as junior clerks. It is optimal for students to discuss the expectations of their resident and attending physician early during the first week of the rotation. The following are examples of basic duties and responsibilities that are commonly suggested across a wide variety of medical schools and other clerkships.

Timeliness

Always be on time; in fact, try to be a bit early. This includes lectures, teaching rounds, and other required activities. Timeliness is a part of being a professional and working within a profession. If you need to be late or absent, you should immediately notify the attending physician, resident, and the person responsible for the clerkship at that site (director or administrator). It is also important to realize that if illness is the reason you are absent, you may need a doctor's note to return. This is not because your supervisors don't believe you but instead because if your absence is related to an infection, you may need to be deemed noninfectious before returning, as many of your patients may have depressed or absent immune systems such that close contact can expose them to serious illness.

Be Aware of How You Look to Others

Professional dress is a must. What may be the latest fashion trend may not be appropriate for patient care. Attire can matter from a safety standpoint: open-toed shoes may allow access of resistant organisms to your skin or even allow for an unexpected needle stick injury. Improper dress can also cause a communication barrier. Many patients encountered on the Internal Medicine Clerkship are older and may not feel comfortable opening up about their medical conditions to someone with tricolor hair. As it is critical to get the information from the patient so as to provide appropriate care, a medical clerk may have to conform to more conservative dress while involved in patient care activities. Also be aware of the rules concerning scrubs! Unlike what one sees on TV, most hospitals prefer that scrubs are worn only in the operating room and while you are on night call.

There Is No "I" in Team: Working as Part of the Medical Team

You will now be working with others for the good of the patient. The medical team consists of doctors, nurses, pharmacists, respiratory therapists, physical therapists, case managers, social workers, students, and even environmental staff. Each has duties and responsibilities in the care of the patient. Each member of the team should be treated with respect. When writing sign-out instructions or documenting information in the medical record, handwriting should be legible and the contact information of the author should clearly be visible. For the student to be kept abreast of changes in the patient's condition, prompt answering via any communication device is a must. Many institutions have moved to the use of cell phones instead of beepers, so it is imperative that the preferred method of communication is identified on the first day of the rotation. When answering calls or pages, make sure people know who you are and what role you have on the team. Many students feel more comfortable using terms such as "medical student" or "student doctor." It is important to realize, however, that in the eyes of the patient you are a doctor on the care team. Therefore, if a question is posed that you feel uncomfortable answering, explain that you will get an answer from a more senior member of the team. A patient's condition can sometimes change very rapidly in the hospital, and the team will not be able to spend time looking for you. Be available to help the members of the team any way you can, even if it is not concerning one of your patients. Students sometimes underestimate how helpful they can be to the team.

Speak No Evil: What Happens in the Hospital Stays in the Hospital

Since the 5th century BCE Hippocratic Oath, patient confidentiality has been an integral part of medicine. Students experience many privileged conversations and hear test results of their patients. It is imperative that patient information not be shared in public venues such as the cafeteria, hallways, or elevators. In addition, one must be aware that pictures and stories regarding patients should never be shared on public forums such as Facebook. Even if the patient's name or other identifying information is excluded, any posted information or photos will be in violation of the Health Insurance Portability and Accountability Act of 1996 (HIPAA; http://www.hhs.gov/ocr/privacy).

LEARNING EFFECTIVELY ON THE CLERKSHIP

One of the most exciting aspects of the Internal Medicine Clerkship is that now the world is your classroom! Learning will mostly be "on the fly," and your patients and your team will be your teachers, although there may be some foundation lectures that will be part of your clerkship experience. Also a larger portion of learning will be moved to the student and become self-directed. Carving out time each night to read about your patients and their medical conditions is very important. When approaching topics, always cover the basics, as follows:

1. Who gets the condition?
2. What do they complain of?
3. What do they look like on examination?
4. What other conditions are commonly confused with this one?
5. How does one diagnose and treat it?

When you are on teaching rounds, keep track of the types of questions that arise, as it is likely they will come up again. Make sure you look them up. Use an evidence-based approach applying practice guidelines that have the support of the literature. One should strive to practice medicine founded upon sound scientific evidence. You should know the most about your patients. You will generally be following from two to four patients at any given time, and your other team members will have considerably more than that. You will be an integral member of the patient care team and have important contributions to make in the care of your patients. This will allow you to actively participate on teaching rounds, which will foster evaluation of your performance.

FEEDBACK: ASK AND ASK OFTEN

Since the evaluation process on the clerkship is very subjective, it is very important that you obtain useful feedback to improve your performance. This concept is sometimes tricky for attending staff and residents to convey to medical students. Be wary of simple phrases such as "You are doing great!" or "There is no need to improve." One always can improve on something, and this is especially true when a student is first starting on clinical rotations. One of the ways students can ask for feedback, without seeming to nag, is by approaching a supervisor more directly, as follows:

"Hi, Dr Smith! I was wondering if you had time to give me some feedback? Could you tell me in what areas I might improve on the clerkship?"

This phrasing makes it more difficult to give one-word or simple-phrase answers and may allow Dr. Smith to give meaningful feedback to the student. If you are provided feedback but are not sure what the person is speaking about, ask for an example. Always be courteous and thank the person offering feedback—even if it is difficult for you to accept what he or she is saying. Feedback is an opinion, and it is important for you as the learner to know the opinions of others. You may not believe it, but if you start to see patterns of similar feedback from different people, you need to consider what you are doing to make multiple persons observe the same behavior. Remember that the goal of feedback is to assist you in improving your performance to the best that it can be. It is also not inappropriate to get weekly feedback from both the resident and the attending physician. At the very least, you should inquire about feedback by the halfway mark of working together to ensure that you have time to make any necessary changes in your performance.

The Internal Medicine Clerkship is one of the most important you will experience, because what you learn will be applicable to patients regardless of your eventual area of focus. Patients with diseases such as hypertension and diabetes mellitus will be encountered in many different disciplines. Therefore, you should take advantage of all of the learning opportunities and use this time to hone your clinical and deductive reasoning skills. Enjoy yourself and cherish your patients, as they truly are your greatest teachers.

Appendix 1
ACGME General Competencies

ACGME GENERAL COMPETENCIES

The program must integrate the following ACGME competencies into the curriculum.

1. Patient Care

Residents must be able to provide patient care that is compassionate, appropriate, and effective for the treatment of health problems and the promotion of health. Residents:

- [As further specified by the Review Committee]

2. Medical Knowledge

Residents must demonstrate knowledge of established and evolving biomedical, clinical, epidemiological and social behavioral sciences, as well as the application of this knowledge to patient care. Residents:

- [As further specified by the Review Committee]

3. Practice-Based Learning and Improvement

Residents must demonstrate the ability to investigate and evaluate their care of patients, to appraise and assimilate scientific evidence, and to continuously improve patient care based on constant self-evaluation and life-long learning. Residents are expected to develop skills and habits to be able to meet the following goals:

- identify strengths, deficiencies, and limits in one's knowledge and expertise;
- set learning and improvement goals;
- identify and perform appropriate learning activities;
- systematically analyze practice using quality improvement methods, and implement changes with the goal of practice improvement;
- incorporate formative evaluation feedback into daily practice;
- locate, appraise, and assimilate evidence from scientific studies related to their patients' health problems;
- use information technology to optimize learning; and,
- participate in the education of patients, families, students, residents and other health professionals.
- [As further specified by the Review Committee]

4. Interpersonal and Communication Skills

Residents must demonstrate interpersonal and communication skills that result in the effective exchange of information and collaboration with patients, their families, and health professionals. Residents are expected to:

- communicate effectively with patients, families, and the public, as appropriate, across a broad range of socioeconomic and cultural backgrounds;
- communicate effectively with physicians, other health professionals, and health related agencies;
- work effectively as a member or leader of a health care team or other professional group;
- act in a consultative role to other physicians and health professionals; and,
- maintain comprehensive, timely, and legible medical records, if applicable.
- [As further specified by the Review Committee]

5. Professionalism

Residents must demonstrate a commitment to carrying out professional responsibilities and an adherence to ethical principles. Residents are expected to demonstrate:

- compassion, integrity, and respect for others;
- responsiveness to patient needs that supersedes self-interest;
- respect for patient privacy and autonomy;
- accountability to patients, society and the profession; and,
- sensitivity and responsiveness to a diverse patient population, including but not limited to diversity in gender, age, culture, race, religion, disabilities, and sexual orientation.
- [As further specified by the Review Committee]

6. Systems-Based Practice

Residents must demonstrate an awareness of and responsiveness to the larger context and system of health care, as well as the ability to call effectively on other resources in the system to provide optimal health care. Residents are expected to:

- work effectively in various health care delivery settings and systems relevant to their clinical specialty;
- coordinate patient care within the health care system relevant to their clinical specialty;
- incorporate considerations of cost awareness and risk-benefit analysis in patient and/or population-based care as appropriate;
- advocate for quality patient care and optimal patient care systems;
- work in interprofessional teams to enhance patient safety and improve patient care quality; and,
- participate in identifying system errors and implementing potential systems solutions.
- [As further specified by the Review Committee]

Appendix 2
Competency Self-Assessment Form: Medicine

Competency Self-Assessment Form: Medicine

Patient Summary:

Dx:

Patient Care

Was I complete in my history and physical exam? Was my clinical reasoning appropriate and sound?

Medical Knowledge

Do I understand the basics of the patient's most likely disease processes?

Practice-Based Learning and Improvement

Did I utilize evidence-based medicine? Did I increase my fund of knowledge regarding internal medicine?

Interpersonal and Communication Skills

Did I work well with the team providing care? Was I respectful and compassionate in my interactions with the patient?

Professionalism

Did I function at the highest possible level? What can I do to improve my medical professionalism?

Systems-Based Practice

Did the medical system work at its best for the welfare of the patient? How can I facilitate improvements?

Section II
AMBULATORY INTERNAL MEDICINE

Section Editor
Cynthia D. Smith MD

Section Contents

4　Tips for Learning on the Ambulatory Clerkship
Kelly J. White MD, *Richard H. Miranda* MD, *and Eva Aagaard* MD

5　Preventive Medicine (Case 1)
Cynthia D. Smith MD *and Brian Wojciechowski* MD

6　Common Problems in Ambulatory Internal Medicine
(Case 2: A Problem Set of Five Common Cases)
Madelaine R. Saldivar MD, MPH *and M. Susan Burke* MD

7　The Patient with Complex Problems (Case 3)
William D. Surkis MD

Section II
AMBULATORY
INTERNAL MEDICINE

Section Editor
Cynthia D. Smith, MD

SECTION CONTENTS

4 Tips for Learning on the Ambulatory Clerkship
   Kelly J. White, L.J. Kleppel, R. Michael Gendron, and Eva Aagaard

5 Preventive Medicine (Case 1)
   Cynthia D. Smith, MD and Brian Hyett-Brown, MD

6 Common Problems in Ambulatory Internal Medicine
   (Case 6: A Problem Set of Five Common Cases)
   Madeline R. Solomon, MD and M. Susan Burke, MD

7 The Patient with Complex Problems (Case 5)
   William B. Burnside

Chapter 4
Tips for Learning on the Ambulatory Clerkship

Kelly J. White MD, Richard H. Miranda MD, and Eva Aagaard MD

As clinical medicine has progressively shifted to the outpatient setting, the Ambulatory Clerkship has become an increasingly important component of the clinical curriculum. Most medical schools in the United States have at least one required outpatient primary care experience in the core clinical year. This may be associated with the inpatient Internal Medicine Clerkship, a Family Medicine Clerkship, or a Pediatric Clerkship. Alternatively, it may be an integrated or longitudinal outpatient experience with multiple specialties or may function independently. The goal of the Ambulatory Clerkship is to expose students to the health care setting in which the majority of health care is provided—the outpatient clinic. In the Ambulatory Clerkship, students will have the opportunity to practice patient-centered care, focus on health promotion and disease prevention, and understand the pathophysiology, presentation, and management of common illnesses. While most students will have been exposed to primary care as a component of their preparatory doctoring curriculum, the expectations for students on the Ambulatory Clerkship are generally significantly different from that prior experience and often pose new challenges to learning. This chapter aims to provide the student with the proper tools to have a successful learning experience on the Ambulatory Clerkship.

When you meet your preceptor during your clerkship orientation, you should make sure to learn the basic expectations of the clerkship. Be aware of the learning goals, specific project work, examination dates, and all recommended reading. Learn what time you should be in the clinic, what you are expected to wear, if you can see patients independently, how much access you have to the patient chart or electronic health record, with whom else you might be working, what presentation style is preferred, whether you are responsible for documentation, and any other expectations the administrator(s) might have. If the expectations of your preceptor are vastly different from those of your clerkship director, speak to the clerkship director early in the rotation.

PATIENT CARE

The ambulatory care setting offers students an abundance of opportunities to interact with patients with a wide variety of disease processes and diverse backgrounds and to learn about unique approaches to health care provision. Patients present to their primary care provider with a variety of acute, chronic, and preventive care needs. These needs are addressed in brief appointment slots (often 20 minutes or less). This can often be a daunting task for even the most seasoned provider. As a result, students in this environment will often feel hurried, and patient care may seem incomplete. Students may not have the opportunity to provide continuity of care for their patients in these settings and often feel the need to address every complaint or problem on a patient's problem list. This is not possible and can cause frustration for your preceptor, the patients, and the clinic staff. Thus, developing skills to identify and target the most important concerns is the best approach.

One highly effective technique is to review the patient's medical record before the visit and identify one or two issues (often chronic or preventive care issues) that you hope to address. After entering the room, discuss with the patient his or her major concerns for that day. Together you can negotiate the two to four most important issues to be addressed at that visit. Begin with open-ended questions, but quickly direct your questioning to formulate an appropriate differential diagnosis. Perform a focused physical examination relevant to the patient's primary complaint to narrow your differential diagnosis. After discussing the relevant information with your supervising preceptor either outside or inside the room, you will then discuss your findings and negotiate an appropriate plan with your patient. Patient encounters will be effective and efficient when they provide resources for further information as well as ensure timely and appropriate follow-up. Finally, early recognition of findings of concern must be addressed immediately with the preceptor to prevent delays in initiation of diagnostic or therapeutic interventions. If the patient looks ill or shows worrisome symptoms or signs of a potentially acute life-threatening event, stop the interview and notify your preceptor immediately.

MEDICAL KNOWLEDGE

The outpatient setting provides a remarkable opportunity to increase your medical knowledge. You will repeatedly see patients with common chronic and acute illnesses, such as diabetes or back pain. You may also have the opportunity to see patients with rare diseases or acute presentations of severe illnesses. You cannot possibly anticipate everything, but familiarizing yourself with common symptoms and diseases will certainly help. Another large part of primary care practice is disease prevention. This includes screening tests, immunizations, and patient education. Take time to learn the evidence-based recommendations for commonly used vaccinations and screening tests. Organizations such as the United States Preventive Service Task Force (USPSTF), American Cancer Society (ACS), and Centers for Disease

Control and Prevention (CDC) have easily accessible published guidelines that are utilized in everyday practice. There are also evidence-based treatment guidelines for common diseases such as hypertension and diabetes. You can use the following website to easily identify different evidence-based guidelines: http://www.guidelines.gov/. Many of these guidelines are also available on handhelds for easy reference (see list at http://www.studentconsult.com). Utilize both your patients and your clerkship learning objectives to guide your reading. Use every opportunity available to you to increase your knowledge; ask questions, observe your teachers, read, and listen to your patients.

PRACTICE-BASED LEARNING AND IMPROVEMENT

The clinical rotations bring many opportunities for self-directed learning. Reading about your patients at the end of each day will allow you to focus on the subjects about which you need to learn more. Keep a notebook, a working document, or another tracking system with you in the clinic. Write down questions or issues that came up during your clinic day. These questions may come from your preceptor, patients, colleagues, or yourself. One important goal is to try to read about at least one patient-related complaint, condition, or preventive strategy each night. Resources such as online cases (SIMPLE, DXR, CLIPP) can also be valuable resources for learning. Use your clerkship manual to help guide your reading and set goals for the depth of knowledge required. You may have the opportunity to share your learning with your patients, your preceptor, or even the clinic team, providing you with more opportunities to further your learning. If you are having trouble identifying areas to work on, ask your preceptor for feedback and use this information as a guide.

In addition to increasing your medical knowledge, use the Ambulatory Clerkship to help you improve your clinical skills. Ask for feedback from your supervising preceptor, nurses, or other members of the interdisciplinary team. When asking for feedback, make sure the timing is appropriate. Ask specific questions about things you can work on to improve (e.g., How was my oral presentation? Would you have done anything differently on that physical examination? Are there parts of the history I left out that you thought were important?), helping your preceptor to provide specific and constructive feedback. Listen and incorporate the feedback into your practice.

INTERPERSONAL AND COMMUNICATION SKILLS

Oral presentation skills are important in any setting, and they become essential for success in the clinic. Because of the time constraints of the preceptor's schedule, you must present your findings succinctly and maintain focus on the issues that have to be dealt with during that visit. Many patients present with both acute and chronic concerns, which need to be prioritized and addressed appropriately. The *SNAPPS* approach to oral presentation has been successfully utilized in the outpatient setting. This acronym stands for (1) *S*ummarize the history and physical exam findings, (2) *N*arrow the differential diagnosis, (3) *A*nalyze the differential diagnosis, (4) *P*robe the preceptor with questions about the diagnosis, (5) *P*lan management of the patient's problems, and (6) *S*elect a relevant issue for self-directed learning.*

Your communication skills are important not only when presenting to your preceptor but also when talking with patients and to the health care team. In patient communication, be sure to speak clearly, make eye contact, and use terms that are easily understood by nonmedical professionals. If your management plans are complicated, make sure to write them down. Ensure that your patient understands the problems and treatment plans by asking questions and having the patient explain the information you have provided.

Written communication is a vital component of outpatient medicine. It is how we document our findings, clinical decision making, and plans for treatment. It is the way we communicate this information to ourselves (so we can remember at the next visit) and often the way we communicate to our partners, interdisciplinary team members, and consultants. *SOAP* notes (i.e., subjective, objective, assessment, and plan) are the most common form of written communication, although consultant letters are also quite common. Review the guidelines in your clerkship syllabus—and ask your preceptor his or her expectations of you—for note writing, including format, length, and whether or not these notes will become an official part of the medical record.

PROFESSIONALISM

In your role as a third-year medical student, patients are seeing you as a treating provider, a professional. This requires you to exhibit professional behavior at all times, both in and out of the clinic. Dress professionally, and show compassion and respect for others. Be on time, or even early, as you might be able to help someone. Arrive eager to work and learn, putting the patient's needs above your own. Respect patient privacy by following the guidelines from the Health Insurance Portability and Accountability Act (HIPAA). Appreciate diversity and leave judgment behind. Communicate with your preceptor and the clinic staff about any potential absences or tardiness. Demonstrate respect for your clinic and patients by operating efficiently. Learn names and roles of team members, treating all with the same respect you give your patients and preceptor. Know your limitations as a student, and do not be afraid to ask for help.

SYSTEMS-BASED PRACTICE

Ambulatory practices vary dramatically in the services and approach afforded to patients during their visit. Many practices are converting to an electronic health record for documentation, while others still rely on paper charts. Understanding the system in which you will be working is vital to ensure efficiency and accuracy. Take the time to familiarize yourself with the systems and people who make the clinic work before embarking on your own patient encounter. Be sure to recognize and identify all the members of the health care team, learning their roles and how they can help you provide care for your patients. Be aware of how much time you have for your encounter, as it may be only 10 minutes. Finally, have an understanding of some of the patient-related resources. There are many easily accessible, reputable web-based resources to provide to patients when time is of the essence and extended discussions are not feasible. Providing such educational resources will help reinforce important concepts.

KEY POINTS

- Time is of essence in the outpatient setting.
- Look at your preceptor's schedule in advance to identify patients with problems about which you want to learn more.
- Discuss expectations with your preceptor at the beginning of the rotation. Find out how he or she likes to work and when feedback will be provided. Uncover any other expectations the preceptor might have.
- Familiarize yourself with the goals and expectations of the clerkship, and make sure you are meeting them.
- Ask to see patients independently so you can have the first attempt at formulating the differential diagnosis and plan.
- Briefly review the patient's chart before the visit, and choose one or two issues on which to focus.
- Impress your preceptor with your knowledge of common diseases and screening guidelines.
- Try to fit into the practice as best you can. Take the time to get to know the names and roles of office staff.
- Be on time and eager to work.
- Keep your appearance professional, and get to know the medical team caring for the patients.
- Enjoy the opportunity to work with patients who have a trusting relationship with their doctors.
- Learn, have fun, and work hard.

*From Wolpaw TM, Wolpaw DR, Papp KK: SNAPPS: A Learner-centered Model for Outpatient Education, Academic Medicine, September 2003, vol. 78, no. 9, 893–898; by permission of Wolters Kluwer Health.

Suggested Readings

Dent JA. AMEE Guide No 26: clinical teaching in ambulatory care settings: making the most of learning opportunities with outpatients. Med Teacher 2005;27:302–315.

Kernan WN, Hershman W, Alper EJ, et al. Disagreement between students and preceptors regarding the value of teaching behaviors for ambulatory care settings. Teach Learn Med 2008;20:143–150.

Chapter 5
Preventive Medicine (Case 1)

Cynthia D. Smith MD and Brian Wojciechowski MD

Case: A 60-year-old female kindergarten teacher presents for a checkup. She has no complaints and has not seen a physician for over 10 years. She has no significant past medical history, takes no medications, and has no allergies. She lives with her husband and has two grown children who are married and six grandchildren who live nearby. She occasionally drinks alcohol (one to two drinks per week) and has smoked one pack of cigarettes per day for 30 years. She has a younger sister who was recently diagnosed with breast cancer at the age of 53 years. She comes today because she is worried that she might have breast cancer.

Screening and Prevention Options

Breast cancer screening	Aspirin for prevention of ischemic strokes	Immunizations
Colon cancer screening	Blood tests: total cholesterol/ high-density lipoprotein (HDL) cholesterol or fasting lipid profile, HIV Fasting glucose, hemoglobin A_{1c} (HgA$_{1c}$), thyroid-stimulating hormone (TSH)	Tobacco use and alcohol misuse counseling
Cervical cancer screening		Healthy diet and exercise
	Hypertension/obesity	Depression screening

Speaking Intelligently

When asked to perform a routine physical exam on a middle-aged female smoker, it is best to first try to choose the highest impact areas to focus on in the time allotted. It helps to find out right away the patient's greatest concern and if there is a particular area of prevention on which he or she would most like to focus. This can help in maximizing impact and outcomes during the visit. In this patient, high-impact areas would be breast cancer screening, colon cancer screening, and tobacco cessation.

PATIENT CARE

Clinical Thinking

- Your first task is to figure out why the patient chose to come in to see you for preventative care after 10 years without a physician encounter.
- Your second task is to identify a select number of high-impact screening tests and counseling strategies that have the best evidence to keep this woman healthy.
- As you proceed with the history, review of systems (ROS), and physical exam, try to identify additional items that may motivate the woman to quit smoking (e.g., family history of lung cancer or chronic obstructive pulmonary disease, smoker's cough, financial strain) or motivate her to get colon/breast cancer screening or vaccinations.
- Use the time to make a personal connection with her and to communicate your desire to work together as a team to keep her healthy.
- Finally, create a prioritized list of recommendations to negotiate with her at the end of the encounter. This list cannot be too long or overwhelming, or it will discourage her from following through with the testing and/or coming back for follow-up.

History

- Take a complete past medical history and past surgical history, and include a history of vaccinations, travel, and possible exposures.
- Inquire about over-the-counter medications and herbal supplements.
- Take a thorough obstetrics-gynecologic history, as this will help you calculate her breast cancer risk score and provide counseling with regard to HIV testing and safe sex. That she is 60 years old doesn't mean she's not sexually active!
- Use the time you have to flesh out her social history in detail. The more you know about her as a person, the better prepared you will be to help her make decisions to improve her health. This will also help you decide how to best spend the time counseling her at the end of the visit.

- Family history has a large impact on timing and strength of recommendation of screening tests. Focus particularly on family history of cancer, including age at diagnosis, and family history of heart disease in the 40s or 50s. Focus only on first-degree relatives (parents, siblings).
- Don't forget to do a complete ROS.

Physical Examination
- Check blood pressure, weight, and height, then calculate a body mass index (BMI).
- Carefully examine lymph nodes and lungs, given the smoking history.
- Examine breast and axillary lymph nodes.
- Do a pelvic exam and Papanicolaou (Pap) smear.
- Although there is little evidence that doing a complete physical examination on an asymptomatic person is a valuable screening tool, people who go to the doctor expect to be examined, and this is a good opportunity to do a simultaneous ROS.

Tests for Consideration
- Colonoscopy $655
- Fecal occult blood testing $5
- Pap smear $15
- Fasting lipid profile or nonfasting total cholesterol/HDL $19
- Fasting glucose/HgA$_{1C}$ $14
- TSH $24
- HIV $13

IMAGING CONSIDERATIONS

→ Mammogram $130
→ Dual-energy x-ray absorptiometry (DXA) scan $104

Screening and Prevention Strategies   Medical Knowledge

Breast Cancer Screening	
Estimating risk	Large, well-conducted trials have shown reduction in mortality from breast cancer from screening mammography with the greatest benefit in women aged 50–74 years.

Estimating risk	Determine a patient's risk of developing breast cancer using a detailed history and a risk prediction tool such as the Gail model (www.cancer.gov/bcrisktool/). An average-risk woman has a less than 15% lifetime risk for developing invasive breast cancer.
Mammography	For an **average-risk woman**, screening should be discussed beginning at age 40 years. The risks and benefits should be reviewed, and a decision should be made based on the patient's values and her level of risk. Women aged 50–74 years should undergo screening mammography every 1 to 2 years. For women over age 74 years (this age group not included in randomized trials so no data are available), screening should be based on individual discussions regarding risk vs. benefit with the patient and life expectancy.
Clinical breast exam	Clinical breast exam may be used as an adjunct to mammographic screening (insufficient evidence of additional benefit above mammography).
Breast self-exam	The benefit of breast self-exam (BSE) has not been proven, and the United States Preventive Services Task Force (USPSTF) recommends against teaching BSE, citing the lack of proven benefit. Women who express interest may be instructed in how to differentiate normal from abnormal tissue. BSE should not substitute for mammography. **High-risk women**, with Gail model risk scores above 20%, should be referred for genetic counseling. They may choose an intensified surveillance strategy with annual magnetic resonance imaging and mammogram, clinical breast exams every 3–6 months, and breast self-exams every month starting at age 25 years.

Colorectal Cancer Screening	
Colonoscopy	Screening with colonoscopy has been shown to decrease mortality from colorectal cancer; screening should be performed in average-risk patients starting at age 50 years and continuing at least until age 75 years.

FOBT (fecal occult blood testing)	Biannual home FOBT screening, followed by colonoscopy for positive results, has also been shown to decrease mortality from colorectal cancer. This should be done with three cards mailed in and rehydrated. No mortality benefit has been found for a single test in the office.
Computed tomography (CT) colonography Double-contrast barium enema Sigmoidoscopy	Screening options that directly visualize the entire colon are preferred (colonoscopy). If a patient opts for flexible sigmoidoscopy, CT colonography, or double-contrast barium enema, the interval is every 5 years. Please note that women are more likely to have right-sided lesions that may be missed on these studies.
High-risk patients	Patients with a first-degree relative with colorectal cancer should be screened 10 years before the age at which the relative was diagnosed.

Cervical Cancer Screening

| Pap smear | Risk factors for cervical cancer include history of abnormal Pap smears, cervical cancer, in utero exposure to DES (diethylstilbestrol), immunocompromise, early onset of sexual activity, and multiple sexual partners.

Cervical cytologic examination via the Pap smear has been shown to decrease mortality from cervical cancer.

Immunocompetent, average-risk women should begin screening at age 21 years, whether or not they are sexually active.

Screening should occur every 2 years, and women over 30 years with three consecutive normal Pap smears may undergo screening every 3 years.

For patients after total hysterectomy for benign disease, there is no evidence for benefits of obtaining vaginal smears. |

Aspirin for Prevention of Ischemic Strokes in Women and Coronary Artery Disease (CAD) in Men

Calculate 10-year stroke risk for patient and if above net benefit threshold, start ASA 81 mg daily	Use a calculator to input the patient's data and calculate the 10-year risk of ischemic stroke; compare this with threshold value and decide if the net benefit is positive for your patient. http://www.westernstroke.org
	Our patient's 10-year stroke risk is 10%. Because this is above the net benefit threshold of 8% for her age group, she may benefit from empiric aspirin (ASA) therapy (81 mg daily).

Screening Tests to Consider

DXA	A DXA scan is recommended for women age 65 years and older every 2 years and for women aged 60–64 years who are at high risk (weight under 70 kg or 154 pounds, tobacco use, prior fracture) for osteoporosis and pathologic fractures.
Lipids	A lipid panel should be obtained in all males 35 years or older and all women 20 years or older who are at increased risk for cardiovascular disease.
	Nonfasting total cholesterol/HDL levels can be obtained as an initial screening test. If total cholesterol is >200 mg/dL and HDL is <40 mg/dL, patient will need a fasting lipid profile.
	Fasting lipid profile is obtained after a 12-hour fast, if nonfasting screen is elevated, or as first screening test. Repeat every 5 years if normal.
HIV	Voluntary **HIV testing** for all persons aged 13–64 years
Diabetes	Should consider **fasting glucose** or **HgA$_{1c}$** in patients with blood pressure (BP) > 135/80 mm Hg or patients with hyperlipidemia.
Thyroid	Insufficient evidence to recommend for or against routine screening for thyroid disease

Hypertension and Obesity Screening

BP Check BP every 2 years if <120/80 mm Hg, yearly if 120–139/80–89 mm Hg. This recommendation is based on the reduction in all-cause mortality for patients who are diagnosed and treated for hypertension (decreased death due to stroke and heart failure).

BMI Measure height and weight, and calculate the BMI.

BMI = body weight (in kg)/height (in meters) squared.

Underweight: BMI < 18.5 kg/m^2; normal weight: BMI ≥ 18.5–24.9 kg/m^2; overweight: BMI ≥ 25.0–29.9 kg/m^2; obesity: BMI ≥ 30 kg/m^2. For patients who are overweight or obese, discuss their eating habits and activity level, and find out if they are open to meeting with a nutritionist. Identify high-calorie foods they can cut out easily (juices, sugar sodas, sweets), and ask them to start walking. Starting a food diary is also helpful for them before seeing the nutritionist.

Immunization

Influenza vaccine	Recommended for all adults. This vaccine is given every year in the autumn. (Avoid if egg allergy or a history of Guillain-Barré syndrome within 6 weeks of having received an influenza vaccine.)
Pneumococcal vaccine	For adults 65 years and older give pneumococcal polysaccharide vaccine once to prevent 60% of bacteremic disease from pneumococcal infection. Administer to adults < 65 years of age with chronic conditions. One-time revaccination at 5 years. The 13-valent pneumococcal conjugate vaccine has recently been approved by the FDA for use in adults 50 years of age and older.
Meningococcal vaccine	Meningococcal conjugate vaccine is preferred for adults ≤ 55 years of age and in those with risk factors; meningococcal polysaccharide vaccine is preferred for adults > 55 years of age. Revaccinate with conjugate vaccine after 5 years for those at increased risk of infection.
Tetanus-diphtheria-pertussis (Tdap) vaccine	Td vaccine should be administered every 10 years; substitute a one-time dose of Tdap for the Td booster for adults 19–64 years of age.

Zoster vaccine	Live attenuated vaccine. Use in patients ≥60 years to prevent shingles and postherpetic neuralgia whether or not they report a prior episode of herpes zoster.

Tobacco Use and Alcohol Misuse

Tobacco	All patients must be screened for tobacco use. Two simple questions: "Do you smoke?" "Do you want to quit?" Patients who want to quit smoking should be offered pharmacologic therapy in addition to counseling, as this increases cessation rates from 50% to 70%.
Alcohol	Routine screening in all patients is recommended by USPSTF. One single question: "How many times in the past have you had four (women)/five (men) or more drinks in a day?"

Diet and Exercise

Healthy diet	Adults with hyperlipidemia and other risk factors for CAD should be counseled about a healthy diet.
Physical inactivity	Insufficient evidence for routinely discussing this with every patient. Need to know that asymptomatic adults who are interested in being physically active do not need to be cleared before starting. Recommendations should include 30 minutes of moderate aerobic exercise 5 days per week. Keep it simple!

Depression

Depression	All adults over the age of 18 years should be screened for depression provided staff-assisted depression care supports are in place. Use the quick two-question screen: "Over the past 2 weeks have you felt down, depressed, or hopeless?" and "Over the past 2 weeks, have you felt little interest or pleasure in doing things?"

ZEBRA ZONE

Zone of Controversy

a. Prostate cancer screening: Controversy exists regarding the role of prostate-specific antigen (PSA) screening, chiefly because prostate cancer can be a very indolent, not clinically relevant problem, and most men who are diagnosed with prostate cancer will live to die of another disease. Men may suffer the burden of additional testing, unnecessary treatment, and anxiety for a problem that may never have become clinically relevant. Unnecessary testing and treatments are expensive, may have severe side effects, and may also be ultimately unnecessary. On the other hand, a very large European trial showed a 20% decrease in prostate cancer mortality from screening; however, to save one life, you would need to screen 1410 men and treat 48 of them.[1] Men in high-risk groups (African American or positive family history) may have the most to gain from PSA screening.

Practice-Based Learning and Improvement: Evidence-Based Medicine

Title
An analysis of the effectiveness of interventions intended to help people stop smoking

Authors
Law M, Tang JL

Institution
Department of Environmental and Preventive Medicine, Wolfson Institute of Preventive Medicine, London, UK

Reference
Arch Intern Med 1995;155:1933–1941

Problem
It takes time to counsel a patient about stopping smoking. What is the cost of this per life saved?

Intervention
Personal advice and encouragement to stop smoking should require less than or equal to 5 minutes given by physicians during a single routine consultation.

Quality of evidence
Systematic review of 20 studies in primary-care settings

Outcome/effect
An estimated 2% (95% confidence limits, 1%, 3%; $P < 0.001$) of all smokers stopped smoking and did not relapse for up to 1 year as a direct consequence of the advice. The effect is modest but cost-effective: the cost of saving a life is about $1500.

Historical significance/comments
This systematic review showed that a one time, 5-minute intervention could save lives.

Interpersonal and Communication Skills

Educate Patients about HIV Testing
The Centers for Disease Control and Prevention now recommends routinely screening for HIV at least once for everyone between the ages of 13 and 64 years. There is no need to identify risk factors for HIV before screening, but you must counsel and obtain consent from patients before obtaining the test. Laws vary by state regarding the amount of pre- and post-test counseling required. The key message is that HIV is a treatable disease, and the sooner it is diagnosed and treated, the better the outcomes. Additionally, early identification diminishes the likelihood that the virus will be spread to others. If patients have multiple risk factors or new high-risk exposures, they may require repeated HIV testing. Be sure to schedule a follow-up appointment to give patients their results in person. You do not want to inform patients that they are HIV positive over the telephone.

Professionalism

Professionalism Challenges in the Electronic Age
The modern era of communication has changed the way doctors communicate with each other and the way doctors can communicate with their patients, and has given patients potential access to their doctors as never before. In so doing, numerous issues of professionalism are raised.

Although many physicians still use beepers, especially in the hospital, cell phones make it possible for doctors to be reached around the clock. E-mail and social media (such as Facebook, Twitter, and Linked-in) add additional ways for physicians to be accessed at all hours. Whereas telephone access outside of the hospital has traditionally been left to physician preference, many physicians now share their private cell phone numbers with patients for after-hours emergencies, particularly for very sick patients; other physicians, however, still feel strongly that the patient should contact the answering service to reach them or the doctor on call. Regardless of the choice, it is important for doctors to set professional boundaries and to practice self-care with respect to time off and maintenance of a personal life outside of their practice. Such guidelines are preferably established at the onset of the doctor-patient relationship.

The **Internet** not only gives patients access to incredible amounts of current medical information (of varying reliability!), it also gives the physician and patient a new way to communicate: many physicians now use **e-mail** as an easy way to communicate with patients and their families when questions arise, or to follow up issues discussed during an office visit. Most doctors who prefer this approach use a professional or office-based e-mail address for these communications. It is important to note that all such written communications need to respect **Health Insurance Portability and Accountability Act (HIPAA)** regulations and should be encrypted and password protected.

Using **social media** to directly contact and interact with patients and their families is generally not recommended. Privacy issues are a problem, as well as the crossover and exposure that occur between the doctor's professional life and personal life. The posting of private information about your day at work, even to a friend list that does not include patients or families, is a clear HIPAA violation. Note, however, that from an advertising perspective, many practices and hospitals can be "followed" on Facebook or Twitter by the general public. These interactions are generally informational (e.g., listing of new programs and office services) and do not contain specific patient data or one-to-one doctor-patient interactions.

Systems-Based Practice

Limit Unnecessary Care
A difficult decision is when to stop screening patients for preventable diseases; guidelines often do not address an upper limit. A good standard is that if the patient's life expectancy is not greater than 10 years, there is probably little or no benefit to screening. A recent study published in *The Journal of the American Medical Association* used Medicare databases in conjunction with a tumor registry to compare cancer screening rates and found that up to 15% of patients with advanced cancer who did not have a meaningful likelihood of benefit continued to undergo screening tests.[2]

References

1. Schröder FH, Hugosson J, Roobol MJ, et al. Screening and prostate-cancer mortality in a randomized European study. N Engl J Med 2009;360:1320–1328.
2. Sima CS, Panageas KS, Schrag D. Cancer screening among patients with advanced cancer. JAMA 2010;304:1584–1591.

Suggested Readings

Boulware LE, Marinopoulos S, Phillips KA, et al. Systematic review: the value of the periodic health evaluation. Ann Intern Med 2007;146:289–300.

Elwood JM, Cox B, Richardson AK. The effectiveness of breast cancer screening by mammography in younger women. Online J Curr Clin Trials 1993;Feb 25; Doc No. 32.

Fenton JJ, Cai Y, Weiss NS, et al. Delivery of cancer screening: How important is the preventive health examination? Arch Intern Med 2007;167:580–585.

Chapter 6
Common Problems in Ambulatory Internal Medicine (Case 2: A Problem Set of Five Common Cases)

Madelaine R. Saldivar MD, MPH and M. Susan Burke MD

CASE 1

A 35-Year-Old Woman with Headache

The patient is a 35-year-old healthy woman who comes to the office with daily headache and dizziness for 6 weeks. Her only medication is an oral contraceptive. Her exam is unremarkable except for a blood pressure of 130/90 mm Hg and body mass index of 30.

Differential Diagnosis

Primary Headache	Secondary Headache
Migraine	Medication side effect
Tension	Inflammatory: systemic lupus erythematosus (SLE), temporal arteritis
	Infectious: meningitis, sinusitis
	Intracranial mass or hemorrhage

Speaking Intelligently

When we see this patient in the office, our first task is to determine whether she is well enough to continue her evaluation in the office. Signs and symptoms that warrant consideration for immediate transfer to the emergency department (ED) for emergent evaluation include sudden-onset severe headache, focal neurologic complaints, projectile vomiting, and severe hypertension. Headaches are common, and 90% of the time there will be a benign cause. A gradual onset of symptoms and a precipitating event, such as increased stress or a recent viral illness, make us consider benign causes.

PATIENT CARE

Clinical Thinking
- A careful history is the best tool to narrow the differential diagnosis.
- Migraine and tension-type headaches are the most common causes of cephalgia, but don't forget to look for warning signs that point to a more ominous cause.
- If there are no warning signs to serious disease, initial empirical treatment for one of these disorders is recommended.
- Radiologic studies are reserved for persistent or changed symptoms.
- Counseling on modifying environmental and lifestyle triggers is important.

History
Making sure there are no concerning symptoms is important. These are:
- Age over 50 years
- Accompanying systemic symptoms
- Headache brought on by exertion
- Visual changes or focal neurologic deficits
- Sudden onset of the worst headache of one's life
- Severe hypertension
- Change in the pattern of chronic headache
- Projectile vomiting

Physical Examination
- Concentrate on vital signs (fever, hypertension, or hypotension) and the neurologic exam, including a funduscopic exam, looking for papilledema and/or hemorrhages. Any abnormality should prompt immediate transfer to the ED for acute management and workup.

Tests for Consideration
• Computed tomography (CT) head	$334
• Magnetic resonance imaging (MRI) brain	$534

- Complete blood count (CBC) $11
- Basic metabolic profile (BMP) $12
- Serum human chorionic gonadotropin (hCG) $21
- Lumbar puncture $272
- Urinalysis $4
- Antinuclear antibody (ANA) $16
- Erythrocyte sedimentation rate (ESR) $4

Clinical Entities	Medical Knowledge

Migraine Headache

Pφ The pathophysiology of headaches is not well understood. However, experts agree that there are multiple factors that contribute to development of a headache:
1. Increased neuroexcitation with cortical spreading depression
2. Vascular dilation

TP Migraine can be distinguished from other types of primary headaches by its characteristics.

	Migraine Headache	Tension Headache	Cluster Headache
Location	Unilateral, though can be global	Bilateral	Always unilateral
Onset and duration	Gradual, reaching peak within hours; can last for a few days	Pressure-like; can be gradual over minutes to hours	Quick; reaches maximum intensity within minutes, but usually lasts only a few hours; intermittent for days in blocks of time usually less than 2 weeks
Associated symptoms	Nausea, vomiting, photophobia, preceded by aura, has trigger	None	Lacrimation and conjunctival erythema, rhinorrhea, sweating

Dx Making the diagnosis is based on history and physical. Secondary causes and warning signs of more serious causes should not be present.

Tx All of the headaches described above respond to acute management with analgesics. Acetaminophen and ibuprofen have been shown to be effective as first-line medications for tension and migraine headaches. Remove headache triggers—alcohol, chocolate, sweeteners, caffeine, nitrites, hormonal medications, stress, and schedule changes or sleep deprivation. If migraine headaches persist, consideration should be given to headache prophylaxis with daily suppressive therapy (e.g., amitriptyline, β-blocker, or topiramate). **See Cecil Essentials 119.**

Secondary headaches are discussed in Chapter 64, Headache.

ZEBRA ZONE

a. **Temporal arteritis:** It is a large-vessel vasculitis that affects the temporal artery, usually bilaterally. Associated symptoms include temporal headache, jaw claudication, and vision changes. It should be considered in any patient presenting with typical complaints, especially in patients over the age of 50 years. It is a medical emergency that requires treatment with immediate steroids. Diagnosis is made by temporal artery biopsy.

b. **Subarachnoid hemorrhage:** This is usually due to trauma or rupture of a cerebral artery aneurysm. Typical symptoms include sudden onset of an excruciating headache with no history of headache in the past. The diagnosis should not be delayed. Emergent CT scan is warranted. Treatment is usually expectant management and blood pressure control in an intensive-care setting.

Practice-Based Learning and Improvement: Evidence-Based Medicine

Title
Practice parameter: evidence-based guidelines for migraine headache; report of the Quality Standards Subcommittee of the American Academy of Neurology

Authors
Silberstein SD

Problem
What are evidence-based approaches to treating migraine headache?

Intervention
Analgesic medications and prophylactic medications

Quality of evidence
Systematic review of class I studies for treatment, class I, II, and III studies for diagnosis and neuroimaging utility

Outcome/effect
Migraine is a chronic condition with episodic attacks that affects 18% of women and 6% of men. Treat acute attacks rapidly. Consider prophylactic medications to reduce disability, frequency, and severity associated with attacks.

Historical significance
Migraine headaches are common and are disabling at a significant cost to society due to lost work productivity.

CASE 2

A 43-Year-Old Man with Back Pain

The patient is a 43-year-old truck driver who presents with right lower back pain (LBP) that started about a week ago when he lifted a heavy load at work. He stopped working and has been resting ever since. He tried acetaminophen, which did not help; however, his brother's oxycodone with acetaminophen does provide him with relief.

Differential Diagnosis

Mechanical/nonspecific	Disk herniation	Compression fracture
Degenerative spine disorders	Spinal stenosis	

Speaking Intelligently

Back pain is the second most common symptom-related reason for which patients present to the doctor. The vast majority of low back pain is due to mechanical or nonspecific causes and does not require imaging. The goal of evaluation is to identify those patients needing urgent attention by looking for signs and symptoms (red flags) suggesting an underlying condition that may be more serious and by determining who may need urgent surgical evaluation. We also evaluate for psychosocial factors (yellow flags), because they are stronger predictors of LBP outcomes than either physical examination findings or severity and duration of pain.

PATIENT CARE

Clinical Thinking
- After a focused history and physical exam, place patients in one of three broad categories: nonspecific LBP, radicular back pain or spinal stenosis, and back pain from secondary causes.

History
- Concentrate on onset, location, radiation, exacerbating or alleviating factors, and failed treatments.
- Look for secondary gain, such as work disability and litigation.
- Evaluate for red flag symptoms that suggest more ominous causes requiring immediate evaluation.
- **Red flags include:**
  - Recent significant trauma, mild trauma with age over 50 years
  - Unexplained weight loss
  - Unexplained fever or recent urinary tract infection
  - Immunosuppression
  - Injection drug use
  - Osteoporosis
  - Prolonged use of glucocorticoids
  - Age over 70 years
  - Progressive motor or sensory deficit
  - Duration longer than 6 weeks
  - History of cancer
  - Saddle anesthesia, bilateral sciatica/weakness, urinary or fecal difficulties

Physical Examination
- Observe patient walking and changing position.
- Inspect and palpate the back and spine, noting any asymmetry, bruising, scars, deviation from the normal lordosis, or step-off between vertebrae.
- Check reflexes and sensation.
- Test for manual strength in both legs. Can the person walk on his or her heels (L5) and toes (S1)?
- Know how to do a proper straight-leg raising (SLR) test. With the patient supine, lift the leg up. For a positive SLR, the patient should note pain down the posterior or lateral leg below the knee (not just in the back) at less than 70 degrees of hip flexion. A herniated disk correlates with a positive SLR at a lower degree of elevation, is aggravated by ankle dorsiflexion, and is relieved with knee flexion. A crossover SLR produces pain in the affected leg when the unaffected side is raised and is more specific for nerve irritation.

Clinical Entities   **Medical Knowledge**

Mechanical Low Back Pain/Nonspecific

Pφ Complex and multifactorial; can involve any lumbar spine
elements including bones, ligaments, tendons, disks, muscle,
and nerve. Onset may be from an acute event or cumulative
trauma. Most common presentation of back pain. May be divided
into acute (<4 weeks), subacute (4–12 weeks), or chronic
(>12 weeks).

TP Pain can be hard for patient to localize because of the small
cortical region dedicated to the back.

Dx Clinical diagnosis; imaging is indicated only if red flags are
present or symptoms persist. More than 90% of symptomatic
lumbar disk herniations occur at the L4/L5 and L5/S1 levels.

Tx Most mechanical LBP resolves within 6 weeks. If it persists or
worsens (or both), consider imaging. For acute pain use heat,
nonsteroidal anti-inflammatory drugs (NSAIDs), muscle relaxants,
and/or spinal manipulation. For chronic pain, use exercise, heat,
NSAIDs, tricyclic antidepressants, and/or spinal manipulation.
May also consider acupuncture or cognitive behavioral therapy.
See Cecil Essentials 119.

Disk Herniation

Pφ Herniation is thought to result from a defect in the annulus
fibrosus, most likely due to excessive stress applied to the disk,
with extrusion of material from the nucleus pulposus. Herniation
most often occurs on the posterior or posterolateral aspect of the
disk.

TP Dermatomal distribution of sensory deficit, motor weakness, or
hyporeflexia.

Dx Clinical exam including SLR test. MRI is indicated only if
weakness or incontinence is present.

Tx Initial treatment is with analgesics and/or steroids. Surgery is
reserved for patients with refractory pain or with evidence of
motor deficits. Outcomes are similar at 5 years for patients
treated either way.

ZEBRA ZONE

a. **Inflammatory spondyloarthropathies:** This condition usually presents before age 40 years, has an insidious onset, and is associated with morning stiffness. It may also have systemic features (e.g., eye, skin).

b. **Spinal stenosis:** This is a degenerative disorder resulting from hypertrophy of facet joints and ligamentum flavum; it can be congenital. Pain is worsened with walking, improved by rest—"neurogenic claudication." Surgery is only for severe symptoms.

c. **Epidural abscess:** Usually there is sudden onset of severe pain that can progress rapidly to radicular symptoms, spinal cord dysfunction, and paralysis.

d. **Compression fracture:** This is associated with decreased bone density due to osteoporosis, bone tumors, or metastatic cancer. Low-level trauma can produce symptoms.

e. **Referred pain:** This may come from organs such as lung (pleuritis, pulmonary embolism), kidney (pyelonephritis, stone), aorta (aneurysm), or uterus (fibroids).

Practice-Based Learning and Improvement: Evidence-Based Medicine

Title
Diagnosis and treatment of low back pain: a joint clinical practice guideline from the American College of Physicians and the American Pain Society

Authors
Chou R, Qaseem A, Snow V, et al., for the Clinical Efficacy Assessment Subcommittee of the American College of Physicians/ American Pain Society Low Back Pain Guidelines Panel

Institution
American College of Physicians

Reference
Ann Intern Med 2007;147:478–491

Problem
Back pain is common, but there is little consensus among the different specialties as to the appropriate clinical evaluation and management.

Intervention
To present the available evidence for evaluation and management of acute and chronic back pain

Quality of evidence
The literature search for this guideline included studies from Medline (1966 through November 2006), Cochrane Database of Systematic Reviews, the Cochrane Central Register of Controlled Trials, and EMBASE.

Outcome/effect
Seven recommendations guide the clinician through the optimal approach to low back pain.

Historical significance/comments
The article provides joint recommendations from the ACP and APS.

Interpersonal and Communication Skills

Explore Underlying Reasons for Somatic Complaints
When a patient presents with multiple complaints, there are usually underlying social and psychological factors that should be explored. It is important to determine the patient's insight regarding how these factors might be contributing to his or her problems. Express empathy and validate the decision to seek medical care. Reassure the patient that he or she does not have any life-threatening cause for the symptoms. Offering a patient a good balance of appropriate pharmacologic treatment and lifestyle modification is the best approach. Be clear that you will be following up with him or her in the near future.

Professionalism

The Impaired Physician
Working in a busy outpatient clinic, physicians share the care of patients with many colleagues. There are times when the care that another physician provides raises concerns that the physician might be impaired. The American Medical Association defines an impaired physician as being unable to fulfill professional and personal responsibilities because of an alcohol or drug dependency, or a psychiatric illness. It is estimated that up to 15% of working

PATIENT CARE

Clinical Thinking

- Iron deficiency is the most common cause of microcytic anemia.
- It can be due to poor iron intake or chronic blood loss.
- The most sensitive test for iron deficiency is the serum ferritin, a measure of stored iron.
- In the United States, blood loss causes most cases of iron deficiency anemia; looking for a source of blood loss is imperative.

History

- With iron deficiency anemia, sources of blood loss can be identified with a good history.
- Menstrual history is imperative, including pad count, presence of clotted blood, and any menstrual irregularities.
- Gastrointestinal blood loss is the next consideration. Symptoms related to upper and lower gastrointestinal bleeding should be explored, including melena or hematochezia, hematemesis, epigastric pain, and changes in bowel habits. A history of weight loss should make one think of gastrointestinal malignancy.
- A careful family history is essential in making the diagnosis of thalassemia, an inherited disorder common in patients of Mediterranean, Asian, or African descent.

Physical Examination

- More acute blood loss can also be associated with hemodynamic instability, including orthostatic hypotension and tachycardia.
- Mild anemia (Hgb < 10 g/dL) usually is not associated with any physical findings.
- More severe anemia (Hgb < 7 g/dL) is usually associated with signs, including pale conjunctivae, slow capillary refill, and new cardiac systolic murmur ("flow murmur").
- "Koilonychia," or spooning of the nails, may also be present.
- Chronic blood loss is usually compensated even if the Hgb level is severely low.

Tests for Consideration

• Iron studies (serum iron, total iron-binding capacity [TIBC], and ferritin)	$40
• Reticulocyte count	$6
• Hgb electrophoresis, if family history present	$19
• Fecal occult blood testing	$5

Clinical Entities	Medical Knowledge

Iron Deficiency Anemia

Pφ Iron deficiency anemia is caused by either decreased intake or absorption of iron, or loss of iron-containing red blood cells through hemolysis or bleeding. Gastrointestinal hemorrhage is a frequent pathologic cause of iron deficiency anemia; other causes are malabsorption syndromes and gastric bypass.

TP In mild anemia, patients usually complain of fatigue, decreased exercise tolerance, and headaches. In more severe anemia, patients may have pica (a persistent desire to eat nonfood substances).

Dx Low serum ferritin is the most sensitive marker for iron deficiency anemia. Since ferritin can be falsely elevated or normal due to acute inflammation, also measure the transferrin ratio, serum iron, or TIBC. In iron deficiency states, this ratio is low. Serum iron alone is a poor measure of iron stores.

Tx Iron sulfate 325 mg three times a day is the treatment of choice. In patients with malabsorption problems, parenteral iron can be used. Hemoglobin levels should respond within several weeks. **See Cecil Essentials 49.**

Anemia of Chronic Disease

Pφ Patients with chronic inflammatory diseases have decreased secretion of erythropoietin and decreased responsiveness of erythroid precursors to erythropoietin.

TP This is usually a laboratory finding seen in patients with chronic diseases, such as SLE, malignancy, congestive heart failure, and diabetes mellitus.

Dx The typical iron study profile shows normal serum ferritin, low or normal serum iron, and low TIBC, resulting in normal transferrin saturation.

Tx Treat the underlying inflammatory disorder. Since iron stores are normal, iron supplementation is not necessary. Erythropoietin may be used if erythropoietin levels are low for the degree of anemia found. **See Cecil Essentials 49.**

Clinical Entities	Medical Knowledge

Atopic Dermatitis

Pφ Usually starts in childhood but can persist into adulthood; a result of genetic predisposition and environmental factors.

TP Pruritic, eczematous, poorly demarcated papulovesicular lesions located on wrists and on antecubital and popliteal fossae (flexor surfaces). Skin can become lichenified from chronic scratching. Excoriations are generally present. There is a general association with personal or family history of allergies, asthma, and allergic rhinitis. The history often includes sensitivity to certain products.

Dx Clinical presentation is usually typical. IgE levels and peripheral eosinophilia are usually present.

Tx Avoid exposure to irritating materials. Use emollients, such as hypoallergenic soap and lotion, daily. Mild- to moderate-potency steroids are effective. Antihistamines can help with pruritus.

Seborrheic Dermatitis

Pφ The cause is unclear, but the yeast *Malassezia* is implicated. Overgrowth causes a skin inflammatory response, resulting in seborrhea.

TP Erythematous scaly plaques in areas with sebaceous glands such as the scalp, nasolabial folds, eyebrows, and upper trunk. These plaques are not intensely pruritic. Commonly associated with HIV.

Dx Physical exam revealing the above distribution of plaques is enough to establish the diagnosis.

Tx For scalp lesions, shampoos containing tar, selenium sulfide, and zinc pyrithione are usually effective. Since *Malassezia* fungal infection is implicated in the inflammatory response, use of antifungal shampoo may also be useful. For face and skin lesions, topical low-potency steroids and antifungal creams have been used with success. **See Cecil Essentials 108.**

ZEBRA ZONE

a. **Allergic contact dermatitis:** This is a delayed, type IV cell-mediated hypersensitivity reaction requiring previous exposure. Common types are poison ivy, nickel jewelry, leather, and latex allergies. Treatment is with topical steroids and calamine lotion. Diffuse cases might require oral steroids.

b. **Nummular dermatitis:** This is characterized by round lesions that can occur on any part of the body. There may be a single lesion or there may be as many as 50 lesions. The cause is unknown. Patients complain of intense pruritus, oozing, and scaling. This condition is often confused with tinea corporis. Treatment is a moderate- to high-strength topical steroid and daily skin moisturizer.

c. **Psoriasis:** Psoriasis is an immune-mediated inflammatory disease that results in hyperproliferation of the epidermis. It can be distinguished from other causes of dermatitis, because it is not generally pruritic and often has associated systemic findings, such as nail pitting, distal interphalangeal joint deformity, symmetrical large-joint arthritis, and seronegative spondyloarthropathy. Treatment depends on the extent and severity of illness, and includes topical steroids, tar, ultraviolet radiation, oral steroids, retinoids, methotrexate, and other immunomodulatory drugs.

Practice-Based Learning and Improvement: Evidence-Based Medicine

Title
Atopic and non-atopic eczema

Authors
Brown S, Reynolds NJ

Historical significance: clinical review
Discussion of the pathophysiology and genetic factors important in the development of eczema. Also discusses common treatments for eczema.

Reference
BMJ 2006;332:584–588

CASE 5

A 57-Year-Old Man with a Cough
A 57-year-old man with hypertension, coronary artery disease, and obesity presents with dry cough for 4 weeks. He notes the cough is worse at night but also occurs during the day. He still smokes cigarettes (¼ pack per day). He denies chest pain. He is compliant with his medications, including lisinopril, simvastatin, loratadine, and aspirin. On exam he has a few scattered wheezes but no rales or rhonchi. He is obese. His cardiac exam is normal.

Differential Diagnosis

Bronchopulmonary infection	Congestive heart failure	Allergic rhinitis/postnasal drip
Asthma exacerbation	Gastroesophageal reflux disease (GERD)	Head and neck cancer
		Lung cancer

Speaking Intelligently

Take a detailed history, paying extra attention to the time frame of the cough. Acute infectious causes tend to resolve within 2 to 6 weeks, while more chronic causes will persist for months. Associated symptoms are very important, especially in the case of cardiac causes. Since this patient has a history of heart disease and ongoing risk factors, make sure to include an angina and heart failure history in questioning.

PATIENT CARE

Clinical Thinking
- The chronicity of the cough and the associated symptoms will help in narrowing the differential to just a few diseases.
- Keep in mind the patient's risk factors and age.
- Consider the most morbid conditions first, and try to eliminate them as possibilities based on history. If you cannot, initiate a workup on this initial visit.
- If the pretest probability of lung cancer or congestive heart failure is low based on the history, further testing can be delayed until the more common and benign diagnoses have been empirically treated.

History
Important red flags that should prompt early testing include:
- Cardiac: dyspnea on exertion, history of heart disease, chest pain, worsening orthopnea, paroxysmal nocturnal dyspnea
- Cancer: weight loss, hemoptysis, voice changes, worsening dyspnea, dysphagia
- Once these have been addressed, the history should include asking about other symptoms associated with each of your most likely causes: GERD, postnasal drip, and asthma.

Physical Examination
- Concentrate on the lung and head and neck exams.
- Are there any signs of allergic rhinitis (dark circles under the eyes, nasal crease, turbinate congestion)?
- Do you hear wheezing, stridor?
- Is there cervical lymphadenopathy?

Tests for Consideration
- Chest radiography if infection is a concern or red flags are present	$45
- Pulmonary function tests (PFTs)	$52
- CT of the chest and/or neck	$334
- Esophagogastroduodenoscopy (EGD)	$600

Clinical Entities	Medical Knowledge

Asthma

Pφ Immediate IgE-mediated bronchospasm followed by cell-mediated inflammatory response in prolonged symptoms and in chronic asthma.

TP Presents with acute onset of shortness of breath and dyspnea; may be audibly wheezing. Tachypnea and difficulty completing sentences may precede respiratory failure. Clinical exam will reveal wheezing.

Dx Chest radiograph is usually normal; peak expiratory flow rate and FEV_1 are decreased.

Tx Bronchodilators (albuterol, salmeterol); corticosteroids (inhaled and/or oral); immunomodulators (montelukast); other (theophylline). **See Cecil Essentials 17.**

Gastroesophageal Reflux Disease

Pφ Hyperacidity in the distal esophagus due to abnormal relaxation of the lower esophageal sphincter.

TP Heartburn symptoms; cough; association with certain foods, especially mint, spicy foods, fatty foods, alcohol.

Dx Response to empirical treatment with antacid therapy; esophagogastroduodenoscopy can show typical inflammatory changes; probe of the lower esophageal area shows acidic pH.

Tx Proton-pump inhibitor therapy; avoidance of foods that cause symptoms; weight loss; in severe cases, fundoplication surgery may be needed. **See Cecil Essentials 36.**

Allergic Rhinitis

Pφ IgE-mediated histamine release in response to environmental exposure.

TP Postnasal drip with nasal congestion, rhinorrhea, and cough.

Dx Typical symptoms respond to antihistamine treatment; in severe cases allergy skin and radioallergosorbent testing (RAST) may be necessary.

Tx Antihistamines; steroid nasal inhaler. **See Cecil Essentials 98.**

ZEBRA ZONE

a. **Head and neck cancer:** Cough can be a presenting symptom of vocal cord polyps and cancer. A smoking history and complaint of voice change should raise suspicion of this diagnosis. Diagnostic test of choice is direct laryngoscopy by an otolaryngologist.

b. **Pulmonary embolus:** Cough is usually associated with hemoptysis. Be suspicious with anyone with multiple risk factors and no other diagnosis that is more likely. Test of choice is a CT angiogram of the chest.

c. **Pertussis:** Pertussis is characterized by paroxysms of severe cough that sounds like a whoop. The cough is often associated with post-tussive vomiting. The cough usually lasts 6 weeks. This is highly contagious and requires treatment with antibiotics. Pertussis vaccination can help to prevent disease and is now included in the tetanus and diphtheria booster (Tdap); give as a one-time dose to adults from 19 through 64 years of age.

Practice-Based Learning and Improvement: Evidence-Based Medicine

Title
The diagnosis and treatment of cough

Authors
Irwin RS, Madison JM

Problem
What is the best approach to diagnosing cough?

Intervention
This is a discussion of common causes of cough and a stepwise approach to diagnosis and management, including suggested guidelines for treatment.

Outcome/effect
Using a systematic approach can lead to appropriate diagnosis and management of cough in 88% to 100% of cases while avoiding nonspecific therapy and costly diagnostic tests.

Reference
N Engl J Med 2000;343:1715–1721

Interpersonal and Communications Skills

Prepare Patients for the Possibility of Further Testing
Before you begin the evaluation of a patient, it is important to communicate the potential need for more invasive testing depending on the results of initial studies. Prepare the patient to consider the possible need for further testing, as it is important to be sure that he or she will be willing to undergo future tests, such as colonoscopy or CT scanning, if an abnormality is identified. If patients are unsure about their willingness to comply with additional testing, empathize with their concerns, but assist them in understanding the rationale for your management plan.

Systems-Based Practice

Use Practice Guidelines in Medical Decision Making
Practice guidelines are a useful tool in helping to treat chronic diseases such as asthma and anemia. The best practice guidelines are based on evidence and are endorsed by expert panels consisting of representatives from stakeholder organizations. Guidelines can be found easily by performing a web-based search: http://www.guideline.gov. This is an excellent link to the National Guideline Warehouse assembled by the Agency for Healthcare Research and

PATIENT CARE

Clinical Thinking

- This is a worrisome patient. She has a complex medical history and recent new issues.
- When confronted with such a situation, my general thought process is to isolate my highest priorities of concern:
  - She has had a recent hospitalization for a serious issue (stroke or TIA) without accurate knowledge of her medications.
  - For financial reasons, she has not been taking the antiplatelet agent (clopidogrel), which was apparently prescribed. *After the first TIA, 10% to 20% of patients will have a stroke within 90 days, and in 50% of patients, this stroke will take place 24–48 hours after the TIA.*
  - Obtaining paperwork from the hospital and pharmacy is always a priority.
  - I now put myself in the mindset to decipher the details of her hospitalization. (See details in history taking below.)

History

- Sort out acute matters first:
  - What changes may have brought her to her appointment today?
  - Try to determine if her symptoms resolved before she reached the hospital.
  - Does she still have any of the symptoms that brought her in?
  - Given her previous alleged diagnosis of TIA or stroke, ensure that she is having no neurologic symptoms at this time.
- Review the problems that you know about:
  - Ensure that she has been going to hemodialysis.
  - You know she has a history of cardiomyopathy, so you can ask about shortness of breath, swelling, orthopnea, and paroxysmal nocturnal dyspnea.
  - You know she had atrial fibrillation in the past, so you can ask about palpitations.
  - You know she has an implanted defibrillator, so you can ask about shocks.
  - She has a history of diverticulosis, so you can ask about melena or hematochezia, or symptoms of anemia such as fatigue or dyspnea.
- Work backwards using any clues provided:
  - If this patient indeed had a TIA or stroke, she probably received a head CT scan. If asked about imaging, she may state that she had an MRI, but this would be unlikely given the suspected diagnosis and in light of her pacemaker. To help clarify which test was performed, CT can be differentiated from MRI by asking about lying in a noisy tube (MRI) vs. lying on a table and moving back and forth through the middle of a quiet machine shaped like a doughnut (CT).
  - Inquire why she was taking clopidogrel (Plavix) and ask about the nature of her allergy to aspirin.

- This patient has been on warfarin in the past; ask her if she is back on warfarin or Coumadin (remember that many patients know medications by only one name; there are no guarantees if this is the brand or generic name!), or a "blood thinner."
- Ask about related problems for which she may be high risk.
- Ask about any symptoms of acute coronary syndrome while in the hospital—chest pain, dyspnea? Ask about delivery of cardiac-specific medications such as nitroglycerin or procedures like cardiac catheterization.

Physical Examination
- Start with vital signs and weight.
- Compare the patient's weight to her previous weights checked in the office.
- Cardiac exam should include assessment for jugular venous distension, arrhythmia (is she in atrial fibrillation?), murmurs, gallops.
- Listen for rales and evidence of pleural effusion.
- Look for lower extremity edema.
- Dialysis access must be examined at every visit. Fistulas should be palpated and auscultated, examining for thrills or bruits, and line access sites should be visualized at their interface with the skin to ensure no erythema, pus, or other sign of infection. Line sites should always be addressed.
- For this patient in particular, a *thorough neurologic examination must be performed* including cranial nerves, looking for pronator drift, strength and sensation exam, cerebellar examination, reflexes, and evaluation of gait.

Tests for Consideration
My major caveat here is to recommend avoidance of ordering new lab tests or doing new radiologic studies at this time. It is likely that this patient has recently had numerous blood tests and multiple imaging studies during her recent hospitalization. As these results should be obtainable within 24 hours, in principle it is wise to refrain from ordering new (and potentially unnecessary) lab tests at this time unless another acute problem has appeared.

Follow-up
- Not only are this patient's problems complex, but also she has potentially evolving issues. I will see her soon, and as frequently as is required, to be sure her medical conditions are under good control. Her future visits can be spaced out further.
- In patients with complex baseline problems, common preventive care can be neglected. It is important to remember that these patients may still require basic screening measures such as mammograms, Pap smears, and colonoscopies as well as basic preventative measures such as immunizations. In such patients it would be ideal to plan for a future visit dedicated to discussing health maintenance and prevention.

Hajjar ER, Cafiero AC, Hanlon JT. Polypharmacy in elderly patients. Am J Geriatr Pharmacother 2007;5:345–351.

Hilliard AA, Weinberger SE, Tierney LM Jr, et al. Clinical problem-solving: Occam's razor versus Saint's Triad. N Engl J Med 2004;350:599–603.

Hohl CM, Dankoff J, Colacone A, Afilalo M. Polypharmacy, adverse drug-related events, and potential adverse drug interactions in elderly patients presenting to an emergency department. Ann Emerg Med 2001;38:666–671.

Johnston SC, Gress DR, Browner WS, Sidney S. Short-term prognosis after emergency department diagnosis of TIA. JAMA 2000;284:2901–2906.

Kuo Y, Sharma G, Freeman JL, Goodwin J. Growth in the care of older patients by hospitalists in the United States. N Engl J Med 2009;360:1102–1112.

Lindenauer PK, Rothberg MB, Pekow PS, et al. Outcomes of care by hospitalists, general internists, and family physicians. N Engl J Med 2007;357:2589–2600.

Makaryus AN, Friedman EA. Patients' understanding of their treatment plans and diagnosis at discharge. Mayo Clin Proc 2005;80:991–994.

Meisel S: Falling through the cracks: medication reconciliation at admission and discharge. Pharm World Sci 2008;30:92–98.

Section III
CARDIOVASCULAR DISEASES

Section Editor
Michael Kim MD

Section Contents

8 **Chest Pain (Case 4)**
   Arzhang Fallahi MD and *Michael Kim* MD

9 **Teaching Visual: Coronary Angiography**
   Sidharth Yadav DO and *Frank C. McGeehin III* MD

10 **Congestive Heart Failure (Case 5)**
   Sameer Bashey MD and *Michael Kim* MD

11 **Palpitations and Arrhythmias (Case 6)**
   Arzhang Fallahi MD and *Michael Kim* MD

12 **Teaching Visual: How to Interpret an Electrocardiogram**
   Jessica L. Israel MD

13 **Hypertension (Case 7)**
   Elie R. Chemaly MD, MSc and *Michael Kim* MD

Chapter 8
Chest Pain (Case 4)

Arzhang Fallahi MD and Michael Kim MD

Case: A 54-year-old man with a history of smoking, hypertension, and hyperlipidemia comes to the emergency department complaining of chest pain. He has had hypertension for 20 years but is poorly compliant with his antihypertensive regimen. He complains of chest pain while exercising and can make it up only two flights of stairs before having to rest. The day of presentation, he was walking up the stairs when he noticed a sudden onset of chest pressure radiating down the left arm associated with diaphoresis, shortness of breath, and nausea. The patient forgot to bring in his medications but says he is not taking what he was given, which was hydrochlorothiazide 25 mg daily, atorvastatin 20 mg daily, and aspirin 81 mg daily. He has a family history of hypertension, and his father died at the age of 45 from a myocardial infarction (MI). On examination he is a diaphoretic man weighing 150 kg, his pulse is 110 beats per minute (bpm), and his blood pressure (BP) is 170/95 mm Hg. His exam is notable for elevated neck veins, coarse breath sounds bilaterally, an S_3 gallop, and 1+ edema in his lower extremities.

Differential Diagnosis*

Cardiac Causes	Pulmonary Causes	GI Causes	Chest Wall Causes
Coronary heart disease • ST-elevation myocardial infarction • Non-ST-elevation myocardial infarction • Stable angina pectoris • Unstable angina Aortic dissection Pericarditis	Pulmonary embolism Pneumothorax	Gastroesophageal reflux Mediastinitis	Chest wall pain

*The differential diagnosis of chest pain is quite broad; this box is limited to the causes elucidated in the Clinical Entities section.

Speaking Intelligently

The assessment when approaching a patient with chest pain is as follows:

1. Assess airway, breathing, and circulation with intravenous access, oxygen administration, and cardiac monitoring, with initial blood work (including serum troponin).

2. Although acute coronary syndromes represent the leading cause of death in adults in developed countries, one should quickly assess and consider other immediately life-threatening conditions such as aortic dissection, pulmonary embolism, tension pneumothorax, pericardial tamponade, and mediastinitis (e.g., secondary to esophageal rupture).

3. Characterize the chest pain: onset (abrupt, gradual), position (localized to small area, diffuse), quality (tight/pressure, burning, fullness, knot, Levine sign [where the patient places his or her fist in center of chest]), radiation (to neck, throat, lower jaw, teeth, upper extremity, or shoulder), aggravating factors (association with eating, exertion or stress induced, positional, worse with cough or deep breathing), alleviating factors (relieved by antacids, nitroglycerin, or rest), associated symptoms (belching, vomiting, diaphoresis, dyspnea, cough, syncope, palpitations, underlying psychiatric disorders such as anxiety, depression, somatization).

4. Risk-stratify patients for coronary heart disease (Framingham: age, gender, high-density lipoprotein cholesterol [HDL], low-density lipoprotein cholesterol [LDL], systolic blood pressure, diabetes, smoking), as well as assessing thrombolysis in MI (TIMI) risk score, which categorizes a patient's risk of death and ischemic events, providing a basis for therapeutic decision making.

5. Depending on the patient's presentation, comorbidities, risk factors, and initial assessment, therapy can be conservative or invasive.

6. Quick and thorough assessment of the patient is of utmost importance. Often with acute coronary syndromes, the more time that passes the more myocardium is jeopardized. Remember that "time is myocardium."

PATIENT CARE

Clinical Thinking

- First and foremost, the patient must be quickly assessed systematically for airway, breathing, and circulation. Prompt intravenous access, administration of oxygen, and cardiac monitoring should be instituted. Always consider the immediate life-threatening causes of chest pain: MI, aortic dissection, pulmonary embolism, tension pneumothorax, pericardial tamponade, and mediastinitis (e.g., secondary to esophageal rupture).

- Given the clinical presentation, this patient's chest pain is most likely cardiac in nature. Angina can be broken down into two main subtypes: stable and unstable. Stable angina is defined as chest discomfort that occurs with exertion or stress and that is relieved by rest or nitroglycerin. Unstable angina is a type of acute coronary syndrome that encompasses myriad conditions including new-onset chest pain, rest angina, accelerating pattern of previously stable angina, post–myocardial infarction angina, and angina after a revascularization procedure.

- This patient's presentation is classic for an acute coronary syndrome (ACS), which can be divided into three main subtypes: ST-elevation MI (STEMI), non–ST-elevation MI (NSTEMI), and unstable angina (UA). Three primary presentations that suggest ACS are (1) rest angina usually lasting more than 20 minutes, (2) new-onset angina that significantly limits physical activity, and (3) increasing angina that is more frequent, is longer in duration, and occurs with less exertion that previous angina. UA can present as new angina, rest angina, early post-MI angina (chest pain occurring within 48 hours after an acute MI), and post-revascularization angina. UA and NSTEMI are often indistinguishable on initial evaluation, as elevation of serum troponins and/or creatine kinase–isoenzyme B (CK-MB) is needed to distinguish the two and takes as long as 4 to 6 hours post MI to show elevations. UA and NSTEMI differ in whether ischemia is severe enough to cause enough myocardial damage to release markers of myocardial injury. NSTEMI often shows ST-segment depression (defined for acute MI as new horizontal or down-sloping ST depression greater than or equal to 0.05 mV in two contiguous leads and/or T inversion greater than or equal to 0.1 mV in two contiguous leads with prominent R-wave or R/S ratio greater than 1). STEMI is defined as ST-segment elevation with serum cardiac biomarker elevation. On electrocardiogram (ECG), acute ST-elevation MI is defined as elevation at the J-point in two contiguous leads with cutoff points: greater than or equal to 0.2 mV in men or greater than or equal to 0.15 mV in women in leads V_2 to V_3 and/or greater than or equal to 0.1 mV in other leads.

Creatinine level assessment is helpful to assess renal function and whether the kidneys are being perfused. **$12**

- **Complete blood count:** It is important to determine if the patient has an underlying infection (suggested by an elevated white blood cell count), which may be contributing to ACS. Hemoglobin and hematocrit are important to determine if the patient is anemic, which could lead to cardiac ischemia as well as indicate a potential hemorrhage. **$11**
- **Liver function tests** may be helpful to ascertain if there is a gastrointestinal cause of the chest pain. **$12**
- **Coagulation tests** are helpful to determine if the patient is prone to thrombosis or if the patient is at high risk of bleeding. They are also helpful if the patient is to undergo an invasive procedure. **$15**

IMAGING CONSIDERATIONS

→ **Chest radiography** is helpful to assess if any pulmonary disease or process such as a pneumonia, effusion, or pneumothorax is present. Cardiomegaly can be assessed but poorly so with a portable chest radiograph often obtained in an emergency situation. This can also help determine whether there is a widened mediastinum, which may be suggestive of an aortic dissection. **$45**

→ **Echocardiography** is typically not used to evaluate chest pain but is used when a noncardiac cause such as aortic dissection, pulmonary embolus, pericarditis, or pericardial effusion is suspected. It also can be used to visualize wall motion abnormalities within seconds of coronary artery occlusion. **$393**

→ **Nuclear imaging** with thallium-201 and technetium-99m sestamibi is helpful in certain clinical situations, as these agents accumulate proportional to myocardial perfusion. The 2003 joint task force of the American College of Cardiology (ACC), American Heart Association (AHA), and American Society for Nuclear Cardiology gave a class I indication in patients with suspected ACS where initial serum cardiac markers and ECG are nondiagnostic. **$300**

→ **CT.** While not routinely used initially, it may be of some use in patients at low risk for ACS. Patients can also be scanned using a "triple rule-out" algorithm, which aims to assess for aortic dissection, coronary disease, pulmonary embolism, and other thoracic diseases. **$262**

Clinical Entities	Medical Knowledge

ST-Elevation Myocardial Infarction (STEMI)

Pφ Acute coronary syndrome is often due to rupture of plaques with less than 50% stenosis. Atherosclerotic plaques are typically asymptomatic until exceeding 70% to 80% stenosis. This obstructive lesion can lead to critical reduction in blood flow to the myocardium, which results in typical angina. In patients with STEMI, plaque rupture results in thrombus formation that is typically occlusive as compared to that in NSTEMI, which tends to be nonocclusive. Thrombogenesis is mainly initiated by tissue factor, which is expressed by monocytes, macrophages, endothelial cells, and smooth muscle cells. Tissue factor binds to activated factor VII. This complex then activates factors X and IX, which results in thrombosis. Within the atherosclerotic plaque, apoptotic cell death results in shedding of membrane microparticles that account for nearly all the tissue factor activity within the plaque itself.

  Instability of plaques is not completely understood, but inflammation and accelerated breakdown of collagen and matrix components are thought to have a role in weakening the fibrous caps of plaques. Inflammation is present at the site of plaque rupture where activated monocytes and macrophages are present. Infiltration by activated neutrophils also has a role in inflammation. Macrophages contribute to plaque instability by releasing metalloproteinases, which further destabilize the fibrous cap. This results in hemorrhage from the vasa vasorum or from the lumen of the artery. Macrophages also release tissue factor, which may initiate thrombus formation. Once the artery is occluded, the myocardium no longer receives blood flow, resulting in hypoxic cell injury resulting in release of cardiac enzymes.

TP Classically the patient presents with substernal chest pain or pressure radiating to the neck and left arm, with associated shortness of breath, diaphoresis, and nausea. While this is the classic presentation, there is variability in presentation, particularly in women.

Dx STEMI is defined as ST-segment elevation with serum cardiac biomarker elevation. On ECG, acute ST-elevation MI is defined as elevation at the J-point in two contiguous leads with cutoff points: ≥0.2 mV in men or ≥0.15 mV in women in leads V_2–V_3 and/or ≥0.1 mV in other leads. Initial lab tests should include complete blood count with platelet count, prothrombin time and international normalized ratio (INR), activated partial thromboplastin time (aPTT), chemistry panel, blood glucose, and serum lipid profile.

Pericarditis

Pφ Pericarditis involves disease of the pericardium, which can be the result of viral infection, tuberculosis, radiation injury, myocardial infarction, cardiac surgery, trauma, drugs and toxins, uremia, hypothyroidism, malignancy, and collagen vascular diseases.

TP Patients typically present with chest pain that is of a fairly sudden onset. Pain is located classically over the anterior chest and is described as sharp and made worse by inspiration. Pain is often decreased when the patient sits up and leans forward. Pain can radiate to the trapezius ridges.

Dx Patients may have a pericardial rub on physical exam, which may be because of friction generated by the inflamed layers of pericardium rubbing on one another. However, one may also hear a rub even with large pericardial effusions. ECG shows diffuse new ST elevations and PR depressions.

Tx The underlying cause must be addressed. Treatment involves relief of pain and inflammation. Aspirin or other nonsteroidal anti-inflammatory drugs (NSAIDs) can be administered. In patients refractory to NSAIDs, steroids may be considered. If patients have significant hemodynamic compromise from a pericardial effusion, pericardiocentesis can be done. **See Cecil Essentials 11.**

Pulmonary Embolism (PE)

Pφ Most thrombi arise from the deep venous system of the lower extremities but can originate in the pelvic, renal, upper extremity veins, or the right heart. Emboli travel to the lung and may lodge at the bifurcation of the main pulmonary artery or lobar branches causing hemodynamic compromise.

TP Symptoms include dyspnea at rest or with exertion (usually occurs acutely), pleuritic chest pain, cough, orthopnea, calf or thigh pain or swelling, and wheezing.

Dx Since many of the symptoms of a pulmonary embolism overlap with those of acute coronary syndromes, similar tests are performed to distinguish the two. ECG can be suggestive of PE; the most common ECG finding is sinus tachycardia. There may also be evidence of right ventricular strain: S wave in lead I, Q wave in lead III, and T-wave inversion in lead III. Chest radiograph is of limited use due to the nonspecific nature of findings. Imaging with ventilation/perfusion (V/Q) scan, which looks at ventilation to perfusion, as well as CT angiography, is typically diagnostic, particularly when patients have a high pretest probability based on risk factors for PE. It should be noted that a V/Q scan is of limited use in patients with severe pulmonary disease. Because of the easy availability of CT scans, this modality is very commonly used. Lower extremity ultrasound may be useful for patients suspected of having PE, since treatment for both conditions is similar. Patients at low probability for a PE may have a D-dimer test, which is very sensitive for PE and is good for ruling it out if negative. However, many comorbid conditions may elevate D-dimer, resulting in a diagnostic and management dilemma, which often results in the need for further imaging.

Tx The mainstay management of pulmonary embolism is anticoagulation. For those in whom anticoagulation is contraindicated (such as patients with a gastrointestinal hemorrhage), an inferior vena cava (IVC) filter may be used. Patients with significant hemodynamic compromise may be candidates for thrombolysis, which is associated with an increased risk of hemorrhage. **See Cecil Essentials 19.**

Pneumothorax

Pφ Air around the pleural space. Causes are classically secondary to trauma or rupture of subpleural blebs.

TP Classically patients complain of chest pain on the affected side as well as dyspnea. Patients may also exhibit decreased chest wall excursion on the affected side as well as diminished breath sounds. In a large or tension pneumothorax, patients may have tracheal deviation away from the affected side.

Dx Diagnosis is made on clinical grounds a well as imaging showing air around the pleural space. Chest radiograph is often sufficient, but in severe pulmonary disease, chest CT may be needed.

Tx Management initially involves removal of air around the pleural space via a chest tube. However, those patients with a small pneumothorax may be monitored. Further management involves treatment of the underlying disorder to prevent recurrence. **See Cecil Essentials 21.**

Gastroesophageal Reflux

Pφ Increased gastroesophageal reflux of gastric juice with impaired esophageal clearance.

TP Classically described as a retrosternal burning sensation. Burning may often be epigastric with radiation upward along the esophagus. Patients may also complain of cough or a sour taste in their mouth when they wake up in the morning.

Dx Diagnosis is most often made on clinical grounds, but in suspected complicated disease, esophageal pH monitoring and esophageal manometry can be used to assess reflux as well as impaired clearance of the regurgitant.

Tx Treatment most often is acid-suppressive medication. More complex etiologies require treatment of the underlying disorder such as *Helicobacter pylori* infection or tumor. **See Cecil Essentials 36.**

Mediastinitis

Pφ Often caused by odontogenic infections, esophageal perforation, complications of cardiac surgery, or upper gastrointestinal or airway procedures.

TP Typically patients present with chest pain, which may also be accompanied by other symptoms such as vomiting or odynophagia depending on the underlying condition. If infection is present (for instance from a sternotomy wound), there may be redness around the site or possibly purulent exudates. Patients will also have extreme tenderness around the incision site.

Dx Diagnosis is often made on clinical grounds depending on the cause, but even if a diagnosis is made, imaging may be needed to help characterize the extent of disease (for instance, the severity of a sternotomy infection). Chest radiography may be helpful as it may show an enlarged mediastinum or free peritoneal air. A CT scan can give a more precise view by showing details such as esophageal wall edema and extraesophageal air.

Tx Thoracic rupture typically requires surgical intervention. Infection may be treated with antibiotics but may also require debridement. **See Cecil Essentials 21.**

Chest Wall Pain

Pφ   May be secondary to minor or major trauma and involves some type of inflammatory response.

TP   Patients present with chest pain that can often be re-created by palpating the affected area.

Dx   After more serious causes such as acute coronary syndrome have been ruled out, diagnosis is typically made on clinical grounds. A chest radiograph may be indicated if there is some concern of a more serious process such as a rib fracture.

Tx   Treatment involves pain management and management of inflammation with NSAIDs. In patients with more severe disease or arthritis, corticosteroid injection may be helpful. In those with muscle spasm, a muscle relaxant may also be helpful. **See Cecil Essentials 4.**

ZEBRA ZONE

a. **Cardiac syndrome X:** is a condition in which patients exhibit angina or angina-like chest pain with exertion but have clean coronary arteries with no coronary-induced spasm. It is a diagnosis of exclusion.

b. **Stress-induced (takotsubo) cardiomyopathy:** is a condition that is triggered by physical or emotional stress or critical illness and closely mimics an MI. A transient akinesis or dyskinesis of the apical and midventricular segment is seen, along with the absence of an obstructive coronary lesion. Treatment is similar to that of left ventricular systolic dysfunction, and patients typically make a complete recovery.

c. **Variant angina or Prinzmetal angina:** consists of spontaneous episodes of angina associated with ST-segment elevations, which return to normal when symptoms subside. It is caused by coronary artery spasm. Medical treatment with calcium channel blockers or nitrates can be helpful.

Practice-Based Learning and Improvement: Evidence-Based Medicine

Title
Early intravenous then oral metoprolol in 45,852 patients with acute myocardial infarction: randomised placebo-controlled trial

Authors
Chen ZM, Pan HC, Chen YP, et al.

Institution
Clinical Trial Service Unit and Epidemiological Studies Unit (CTSU), Richard Doll Building, Old Road Campus, Oxford OX3 7LF, UK

Reference
Lancet 2005;366:1622–1632

Problem
Previous randomized trials on the use of early β-blocker therapy in patients with suspected MI in addition to standard interventions such as aspirin and fibrinolytic therapy remain uncertain with respect to risks and benefits.

Intervention
A total of 45,852 patients admitted to 1250 hospitals within 24 hours of suspected acute MI onset were randomly allocated to receiving metoprolol (up to 15 mg intravenously, then 200 mg orally daily; $n = 22,929$) or matching placebo ($n = 22,923$). Treatment was to continue until discharge or up to 4 weeks in hospital.

Quality of evidence
Level I

Outcome/effect
Two prespecified co-primary outcomes were (1) composite of death, reinfarction, or cardiac arrest, and (2) death from any cause during the scheduled treatment period. Neither co-primary outcome was significantly reduced by metoprolol. For death, reinfarction, or cardiac arrest, 9.4% of the metoprolol patients had an event compared with 9.9% of those allocated to placebo ($P = 0.1$). For death, this was 7.7% in the metoprolol group versus 7.8% in the placebo group ($P = 0.69$). Reinfarction for the metoprolol group was 2.0% versus 2.5% for the placebo group ($P = 0.001$). There was a reduction in occurrence of ventricular fibrillation, with 2.5% for metoprolol versus 3.0% for placebo ($P = 0.001$). However, these reductions were associated with 11 per 1000 treated patients in the metoprolol group developing cardiogenic shock (5.0% vs. 3.9%; $P < 0.00001$). This was mainly during days 0 to 1 after admission. Reductions in reinfarction and ventricular fibrillation emerged more gradually.

The trial concluded that while early β-blocker therapy in acute MI does reduce risks of reinfarction and ventricular fibrillation, it also increases risk of cardiogenic shock, especially early. Thus, it was reasoned that it may be advantageous to consider starting β-blocker therapy in the hospital after hemodynamics have been stabilized after an MI.

Historical significance/comments

This was an important trial, which was cited in the ACC/AHA 2007 STEMI Guidelines. The trial showed the potential harm in early β-blocker use, since it may result in increased risk of cardiogenic shock early despite gradual benefit in reducing ventricular fibrillation and reinfarction. The guidelines now suggest oral β-blockers be used within the first 24 hours in patients who do not have signs of heart failure, evidence of low-output state, risk for cardiogenic shock (age > 70 years, systolic blood pressure < 120 mm Hg, sinus tachycardia > 110 bpm or heart rate < 60 bpm, increased time since onset of symptoms of STEMI), or relative contraindications of β-blockade (PR interval > 0.24 seconds, second- or third-degree heart block, active asthma, or reactive airway disease).

Interpersonal and Communication Skills

Educate Patients about Risk Factor Modification

Patient education is of utmost importance in the management of CAD. Patients should be made aware of risk factors and interventions they can undertake to modify their risk, such as an appropriate diet, weight loss, and smoking cessation. Patients should also be educated on medical management of their disease and the importance of appropriate medication use in preventing adverse outcomes. From a psychosocial perspective, a diagnosis of heart disease and its implications may be a very difficult and scary prospect for many patients. Being aware of these emotions and working together supportively with the patient to arrive at a treatment plan will maximize the likelihood of patient compliance.

Professionalism

Beware of Extraneous Side Conversations

Patients undergoing a procedure such as a cardiac catheterization will be mildly sedated and draped for the procedure. It is important to remember that even under these circumstances, the patient may still be aware of extraneous conversations. Whereas open medical discussion may often be appropriate within earshot of the patient, *be mindful of extraneous side conversations.* Focus should be on the patient at hand and not how you spent your weekend or with whom you had dinner last night. Being exposed to such conversations may send a message that the patient is not your prime concern.

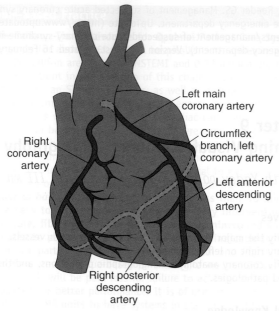

Figure 9-1 Coronary anatomy. (From Mann BD: Surgery: a competency-based companion. Philadelphia: Saunders; 2009. Fig. 59-1.)

coronary artery arises from the left aortic sinus and usually bifurcates into the left anterior descending (LAD) artery and the left circumflex (LCX) artery. Generally, the LAD artery supplies the anterior/anterolateral walls and the interventricular septum of the left ventricle (LV). The LCX artery generally supplies the lateral/posterolateral walls of the LV. The right coronary artery (RCA) arises from the right aortic sinus and supplies the right ventricle (RV) and, in 85% of the population, gives rise to the posterior descending artery (PDA), which supplies the inferior portion of the interventricular septum. Anatomically, right or left "dominance" is determined by the artery that gives off the PDA. A small segment of the population is "left dominant," indicating that the PDA originates from the LCX. Figure 9-1 is a basic schematic of the coronary anatomy.

"ANGIOGRAPHER'S" PERSPECTIVE

To effectively interpret coronary angiograms, one must understand that the heart is situated on an oblique axis in the chest cavity.

Therefore, coronary arteries are best visualized from either a right or left oblique angle. The rotation, as well as cranial and caudal angulation of the image intensifier and x-ray source, allows us to perform comprehensive imaging while eliminating overlap and foreshortening of the arteries.

Oblique views can be thought of as turning the patient's right or left shoulder toward the image intensifier. Nomenclature generally refers to the location of the image intensifier in relation to the patient's long axis. Cranial and caudal angulations can be obtained by rotating the image intensifier along the long axis of the patient.

To visualize the arteries in a way that may be more anatomically familiar, an image in the rotation of right anterior oblique (RAO) of about 30 degrees can be performed. In this angle, the interventricular septal plane and the atrioventricular plane are perpendicular to each other. Both planes meet to form the crux of the heart. An example is shown in Figure 9-2.

Here are some characteristics that can be used to identify the epicardial vessels on coronary angiography:

1. **Left main** coronary artery—easily identified as a large-caliber artery arising from below the sinotubular junction of the aorta, from the left aortic sinus. It bifurcates into the LAD and LCX. It may trifurcate, meaning it may give off a third branch called the ramus intermedius branch, supplying the high lateral wall. It may be cloacal, meaning very short. In rare cases it may be absent altogether, suggesting dual ostia of the LAD and LCX. The left main coronary artery is best seen in the anteroposterior (AP), left anterior oblique (LAO) cranial, and LAO caudal views.
2. **LAD**—best seen in the *cranial* angulation. In this angulation, the artery extends downward in its entirety to the apex. In normal circumstances, the LCX will not extend to the apex. The LAD gives off septal branches called septal perforators, which appear to be small threadlike arteries traversing toward the interventricular septum. The LAD also gives off diagonal branches that travel in a lateral direction.
3. **LCX**—best visualized in the *caudal* angulation. The LCX artery traverses posteriorly along the atrioventricular groove, giving off obtuse marginal branches. It often appears to be of large caliber as a result of its proximity to the x-ray source. Objects closer to the x-ray source appear larger on imaging.
4. **RCA**—usually a solitary artery, arising from the right aortic sinus. It is best seen in the view in which it is engaged—that is, the *LAO view*. The side branches extending from it are the right ventricular marginal branches, which supply the RV. In most of the population, as the RCA traverses posteriorly, it gives off the PDA. The PDA can be identified in the *cranial* angulation, giving off septal

4. Connect the dots to complete the PDA in the LAO cranial projection.

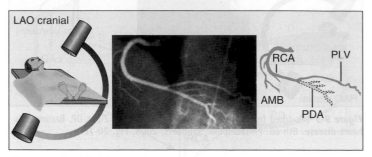

Figure 9-6 (Modified from Libby P, Bonow RO, Mann DL, Zipes DP. Braunwald's heart disease. 8th ed. Philadelphia: Saunders; 2008. Figure 20-8B.)

Helpful Clues in Angiographic Interpretation

Interpreting angiograms takes practice and repetition. Understanding which view and angulation the image is in can help the angiographer identify vessels and vessel characteristics. Here are some clues that can help identify the view and angulation.

First, the location of the spine can help distinguish which oblique angle was used. Generally, if the spine is located on the right side of the screen, it is an RAO angle. If the spine is on the left side of the screen, it is in an LAO angle. If the spine is in the center, it is generally in the AP projection.

The location of the diaphragm may help distinguish cranial and caudal angulations. Generally, if the diaphragm is prominent in the image, the view is usually caudal. In cranial views, the LAD is seen in full length, traveling in a downward fashion. The LCX appears to be traversing upward. The opposite is true of caudal views. In caudal views the LCX travels downward on the image, whereas the LAD travels upward from its origin. The LAO angle tends to splay out the thoracic aorta and is a good angle to view the origin of the great arteries.

"THINK LIKE AN INTERVENTIONAL CARDIOLOGIST"

Sizing of the vessel is of extreme importance to the interventional cardiologist. Appropriately choosing stent size further reduces the risk of perforation, vessel dissection, and other complications. One clue that angiographers use is the size of the catheter. Catheters are sized using the French scale or gauge. The conversion factor of 1 Fr is 0.33 mm. Most of the catheters used for coronary angiograms are 4, 5, or 6 Fr catheters. For example, if the lumen of the middle segment of the LAD looks similar to a 6 Fr catheter tip diameter, the diameter of the mid-LAD would be approximately 2 mm.

Interpretation Exercises

Answers are at the end of the chapter. See Figures 9-7 through 9-9.

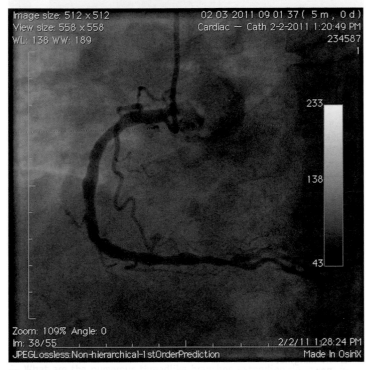

Image size: 512 x 512   02 03 2011 09 01 37 (5 m , 0 d)
View size: 558 x 558   Cardiac — Cath 2-2-2011 1:20:49 PM
WL: 138 WW: 189   234587
                                                 1

233

138

43

Zoom: 109% Angle: 0
Im: 38/55   2/2/11 1:28:24 PM
JPEGLossless:Non-hierarchical-1stOrderPrediction   Made In OsiriX

Figure 9-7

1. What artery is this?
   a. LAD
   b. LCX
   c. RCA

2. In what angle was this image taken?
   a. LAO
   b. RAO
   c. AP

Chapter 10
Congestive Heart Failure (Case 5)

Sameer Bashey MD and Michael Kim MD

Case: The patient is a 68-year-old woman with a past medical history of hypertension and rheumatoid arthritis. Her hypertension has been well controlled over the past few years with hydrochlorothiazide. She now presents to your office stating she's become progressively short of breath over the past few months, most notably with exertion. Initially she felt she was simply "out of shape," as these symptoms began upon starting an exercise regimen now that she's retired. However, over the past few months her symptoms have continued to worsen despite regular exercise. She reports having no other associated symptoms and denies chest pain, nausea, vomiting, or palpitations. When not exerting herself, she feels she is at her usual state of health and is enjoying the extra time she has to catch up on several of her interests.

On physical examination, you note a mildly diminished carotid upstroke, nondisplaced point of maximal impact, and a normal jugular venous pressure (JVP). You also note a grade 3/6 systolic murmur most notable at the apex and 1+ pitting edema in the lower extremities bilaterally.

Differential Diagnosis

Aortic stenosis	Dilated cardiomyopathy	Ischemic cardiomyopathy
Mitral regurgitation	Hypertrophic cardiomyopathy	Pulmonary hypertension
Diastolic dysfunction	Restrictive cardiomyopathy	

Speaking Intelligently

When encountering a patient presenting with shortness of breath, first try to understand what the patient is actually experiencing, as the sensation of shortness of breath can encompass a range of symptoms including difficulty with air movement, dyspnea despite adequate air movement, and generalized fatigue. These and other associated symptoms may help narrow the differential diagnosis specifically to pulmonary, cardiac, musculoskeletal, or psychiatric causes. In patients with symptoms consistent with heart failure, the next step is to determine the presence of heart failure, the underlying etiology, and the severity for both medical management and prognosis. Finally, it important to bear in mind that effective treatment of chronic heart failure requires a multimodal approach encompassing patient education, coordination of care with nurses and other midlevel providers, and a stepwise implementation of medical and device therapies aimed at improving patient morbidity and mortality.

PATIENT CARE

Clinical Thinking
- Given the broad range of possible etiologies leading to heart failure, a careful history is required to narrow the diagnosis.
- Particular attention must be paid to the chronicity of symptoms, risk factors for ischemic heart disease, and evidence of systemic diseases associated with heart failure.
- Keeping in mind the pathophysiology and subsequent differences in presentation between right-sided versus left-sided heart failure as well as systolic versus diastolic dysfunction is helpful in both establishing a diagnosis and understanding appropriate interventions.
- In patients with an established diagnosis of heart failure, the severity of disease by New York Heart Association (NYHA) classification, staging, or LV ejection fraction is important in determining appropriate therapeutic interventions.

History
- As 50% to 75% of systolic heart failure cases are secondary to ischemia, assessing CAD risk factors to form a pretest probability is an important first step in establishing a diagnosis. Ischemic cardiomyopathy is not only the most common cause of heart failure but is also somewhat reversible in a minority of patients with large proportions of "hibernating" myocardium secondary to chronic ischemia. Age is another important factor to help inform a differential diagnosis. Aortic stenosis, mitral regurgitation, and diastolic dysfunction increase with age and are oftentimes pathophysiologically related via increased pressure and thus workload, leading to various structural changes.
- Determining the chronicity of symptoms may provide a diagnostic clue. In younger patients and those with rapid onset of symptoms without prior limitation in exercise tolerance, the symptoms may be secondary to systemic diseases, most commonly an infectious myocarditis.
- A careful history including evaluating for evidence of rheumatologic, infectious, and hereditary causes of heart failure is important.

- Regardless of the etiology, patients with left-sided heart failure will predominantly present with symptoms of exercise intolerance secondary to shortness of breath, fatigue, orthopnea, or paroxysmal nocturnal dyspnea.
- In isolated right-sided heart failure, dependent edema and increased abdominal girth may predominate.

Physical Examination
- Classically, patients will present with elevated jugular vein distension, pulmonary crackles, lower extremity edema, and hypoxia.
- In more advanced disease, patients may have a laterally displaced point of maximal impact, a pulsatile liver, or extrasystolic heart sounds (S_3 or S_4).
- Additional heart sounds, murmurs, and special maneuvers to alter hemodynamic parameters may assist in diagnosing many etiologies including aortic stenosis, mitral regurgitation, hypertrophic cardiomyopathy, and pulmonary hypertension.
- Evidence of extracardiac manifestations of systemic disorders should also be evaluated.

Tests for Consideration
- **Serum troponin concentrations** are elevated in conditions associated with cardiac ischemia, such that measurement of this parameter is frequently ordered in patients presenting with an acute exacerbation of congestive heart failure (CHF) to rule out an acute MI as the cause of the new decompensation. However, interpretation can be difficult as patients with advanced heart failure frequently have ongoing myocardial cell death secondary to heart failure that is unrelated to coronary ischemia. Similarly, patients with chronic kidney disease will accumulate troponin as it is cleared by the kidneys. $14
- **Brain natriuretic peptide (BNP)** is secreted by the ventricles in response to excessive stretching and is elevated in heart failure. It is frequently used to differentiate shortness of breath secondary to heart failure versus that caused by intrinsic pulmonary disease. While BNP levels less than 100 pg/mL and greater than 500 pg/mL are generally used as cutoffs to exclude or diagnose CHF, respectively, often the results fall somewhere in between with an indeterminate significance. $45
- **ECGs** are useful in patients presenting with clinical signs and symptoms of heart failure to determine an etiology. Evidence of prior ischemia may be noted in patients with ischemic cardiomyopathy. Left ventricular hypertrophy secondary to aortic stenosis, long-standing hypertension, or hypertrophic cardiomyopathy may similarly be noted. Finally, low voltage in the precordial leads may be seen in restrictive cardiomyopathy. $27

IMAGING CONSIDERATIONS

→ **Transthoracic echocardiography (TTE)** is the single most helpful study in diagnosing heart failure and determining the etiology. By providing both qualitative and quantitative data regarding ventricular and atrial chambers, valvular function, wall thicknesses, and Doppler measurements, one is able to differentiate among most etiologies of heart failure. Additionally, wall motion abnormalities provide evidence of infarction in ischemic cardiomyopathy. $393

→ **Stress echocardiography** is a transthoracic echocardiograph done at rest followed by a dobutamine infusion to increase heart rate and contractility. It can be used to diagnose ischemic cardiomyopathy by looking for new wall motion abnormalities as well as hypertrophic cardiomyopathy by assessing the functional significance of an outflow obstruction. $580

→ **Cardiac catheterization** is divided into left and right heart catheterization. A left heart catheterization is the reference standard for diagnosing coronary disease and should be performed on patients with new-onset heart failure of unclear etiology to exclude coronary disease. A right heart catheterization can assess the severity of pulmonary hypertension and obtain myocardial tissue to diagnose the various restrictive and dilated cardiomyopathies. $2718

→ **Cardiac MRI** is relatively new imaging modality. It is mainly used to diagnose various dilated and restrictive cardiomyopathies but also can define anatomic parameters similar to echocardiography with a higher degree of accuracy. $534

Clinical Entities   Medical Knowledge

Aortic Stenosis (AS)

Pφ In industrialized countries, degenerative calcification of a congenital bicuspid valve and degenerative calcification of an anatomically normal trileaflet valve represent the two most common causes of AS. Worldwide, rheumatic disease is the most common etiology. Degenerative calcification is characterized by a process of lipid accumulation and inflammation, leading to calcification.

TP Patients most commonly present with decreased exercise tolerance and dyspnea on exertion. In more advanced disease, exertional chest pain, syncope, and symptoms of heart failure may be present and portend a poor outcome without intervention. Physical examination may be notable for a weak and delayed carotid upstroke (*parvus et tardus*), a mid- to late-peaking systolic murmur heard best in the right second intercostal space, or clinical signs of heart failure.

Dx TTE provides the most information by determining leaflet morphology and severity of AS by aortic valve area calculations, as well as evidence of any LV dysfunction. ECG and chest radiograph may demonstrate left ventricular hypertrophy (LVH) and an enlarged cardiac silhouette.

Tx Treatment is primarily limited to valve replacement in symptomatic patients with severe AS. These patients have a life expectancy of 1 year without intervention, but this is markedly improved with valve replacement. In mild to moderate AS, medical therapy is limited to symptomatic treatment, as no therapy directly targeting progression of AS has been shown to be effective. Anginal symptoms may be relieved by β-blockers, calcium channel blockers, nitrates, or revascularization, while pulmonary congestion can be improved with use of diuretics. Transcatheter aortic valve implantation (TAVI) is an exciting potential new therapy for patients with severe aortic stenosis who are at high risk for mortality or serious morbidity with aortic valve replacement (AVR) or those considered too high risk to have AVR (extreme risk). This technology has been approved in Europe and is currently being investigated in randomized controlled trials in the United States. **See Cecil Essentials 8.**

Mitral Regurgitation (MR)

Pφ Insufficiency of the mitral valve (MV) can occur acutely or chronically. Acutely, as may occur following MI or endocarditis, an increase in left atrial pressure can lead to acute pulmonary edema. Chronically, MR is most commonly seen secondary to MV prolapse, prior ischemia, or heart failure in the United States and Europe. Worldwide, rheumatic heart disease is the most common etiology. Compensatory dilation of the heart in long-standing MR can progress to heart failure.

TP As with AS, patients typically present with a progressive limitation in exercise tolerance. With acute MR, symptoms of ischemic chest pain or endocarditis may be noted. In advanced cases, patients may also present with palpitations secondary to new-onset atrial fibrillation from left atrial dilation. On exam, a laterally displaced point of maximal impact, a diminished S_1, or a wide splitting of S_2 may be noted along with a holosystolic murmur over the apex radiating to the left axilla.

Dx TTE is used both for diagnosing MR and for determining medical and surgical management. The cause of MR can be determined by looking for evidence of secondary causes including prior evidence of ischemia, heart failure, or a primary disorder of the MV apparatus including the leaflets, annulus, chordae tendineae, and papillary muscles. Severity of MR is assessed by measuring regurgitant volumes and orifice area, as well as degree of LV compensation by assessment of LV size and function.

Tx As with AS, treatment for MR is primarily limited to surgical intervention given the absence of medical therapies to limit progression of disease. Determining the appropriate time to intervene can be difficult, and surgery is generally performed in patients with severe MR before deterioration of LV function. MV repair is generally preferred over MV replacement to avoid the need for anticoagulation. Symptomatic treatment consisting of arterial vasodilators (nitroprusside, hydralazine) can improve symptoms in acute MR but have limited use chronically in nonoperative candidates. **See Cecil Essentials 8.**

Ischemic Cardiomyopathy

Pφ Ischemic cardiomyopathy describes the impairment in LV function resulting from CAD. Most commonly, this occurs following MI secondary to infarction of tissue that is no longer contractile. Less commonly, coronary disease may result in hibernating myocardium, tissue that is functionally reduced secondary to chronic ischemia that may be partially reversible with revascularization.

Dx An echocardiogram showing impaired systolic function in the absence of another etiology requires further evaluation. In addition to evaluating for CAD, testing is directed at identifying the underlying etiology and may include laboratory or imaging studies for evidence of infectious, rheumatologic, or endocrine diseases. Occasionally, an endomyocardial biopsy is required.

Tx In addition to treating the underlying cause, treatment guidelines are similar to those in ischemic heart disease and include use of β-blockers, ACE inhibitors, diuretics, and ICD placement as indicated. However, as several etiologies are reversible, judicious use of device therapies is required. **See Cecil Essentials 11.**

Hypertrophic Cardiomyopathy

Pφ Similar to dilated cardiomyopathies, HCMs are diseases of intrinsic myocardial tissue and exclude hypertrophy secondary to hypertension or valvular disease. Between 60% and 70% of cases are secondary to one of many mutations in genes encoding contractile proteins within the sarcomere and are expressed in an autosomal-dominant pattern of inheritance with a high degree of penetrance. Ventricular arrhythmias leading to sudden cardiac death (SCD) are caused by myocyte disarray, fibrosis, and ischemia secondary to obstruction of the LV outflow tract.

TP Clinical presentation is highly variable and does not correlate well with severity of outflow obstruction. Many patients are asymptomatic or have mildly limited exercise tolerance that advances with age. Others can present with ischemic chest pain or syncope related to outflow obstruction as well as SCD secondary to ventricular arrhythmias.

Dx Symptomatic patients require more aggressive evaluation, as they are at increased risk for SCD. ECG can show dramatically increased voltage, prominent Q-waves, or deep T-wave inversions. Echocardiography is used to evaluate LV wall thickness as well as severity of outlet obstruction. Additional testing to identify patients at high risk for SCD requiring ICD placement includes a Holter monitor for nonsustained ventricular tachycardia and a stress test to evaluate for an abnormal BP response.

Tx Asymptomatic patients without high-risk features (nonsustained ventricular tachycardia [NSVT] on Holter, syncope, family history of SCD, abnormal BP response on stress, or LVH > 30 mm) can be followed annually without need for further therapy. Those with two or more high-risk features or prior cardiac arrest require ICD placement. Additionally, β-blockers can improve palpitations secondary to premature ventricular beats or NSVT. First-degree relatives of patients with HCM also require periodic evaluation. **See Cecil Essentials 11.**

Restrictive Cardiomyopathy

Pφ Restrictive cardiomyopathies are characterized by impaired ventricular filling secondary to a variety of disease states affecting the myocardial substrate. These diseases can be classified as infiltrative (amyloidosis, sarcoidosis), storage (hemochromatosis, Fabry disease), endomyocardial, and noninfiltrative (idiopathic, familial) diseases. Constrictive pericarditis, while also impairing ventricular filling, is not included within this classification, as it occurs secondary to a pericardial effusion rather than as an intrinsic myopathy.

TP Clinical presentations are varied relating to other systemic manifestations of the underlying etiology. Clinical signs or symptoms of heart failure in the absence of typical risk factors should prompt further investigation.

Dx An ECG with low voltage in the precordial leads may provide an early clue. Systolic heart failure is confirmed by echocardiography, although no other structural abnormality is generally present. An endomyocardial biopsy is considered the reference standard, though cardiac magnetic resonance imaging is also helpful in establishing a diagnosis.

Tx Treatment is similar to that for other etiologies of systolic heart failure, including ACE inhibitors, β-blockers, diuretics, digoxin, spironolactone, and device therapies for advanced heart failure. **See Cecil Essentials 11.**

Pulmonary Hypertension (PH)

Pφ Defined by elevated pulmonary arterial pressures eventually leading to right heart failure, PH is classified according to etiology by World Health Organization (WHO) Group 1–5 designation corresponding to idiopathic, left heart, intrinsic pulmonary, chronic thromboembolic, or inflammatory diseases.

recommended therapies. Emphasize the significant functional and mortality benefit from optimal medical therapy. Patient and family education can improve adherence to a difficult management plan that involves dietary and lifestyle modifications, as well as initiation of multiple medications for what is perceived as a single medical condition.

Professionalism

Disclose Relationships with Drug and Device Makers

The advent of newer technologies has increasingly turned the treatment of heart failure toward invasive management and costly device therapies. Pharmaceutical companies often compete for physicians to prescribe their particular medication brands and to use their particular devices. In a time of new drugs and devices, physicians frequently have consulting relationships with commercial concerns that compensate them for their knowledge and expertise. Gifts from industry should never be accepted, and it is the professional responsibility of the physician to publicly disclose any relationships that he or she may have with a pharmaceutical or device company. The primary factor in a decision to prescribe medications or perform invasive therapy should always be made on the basis of the evidence. A physician's relationship with a particular company should never be the driving force in directing patient care.

Systems-Based Practice

Monitor Core Measures to Optimize Care

Monitoring compliance with core measures has been adopted as a way to compare the practices of individual physicians and hospitals both to inform patients and to provide a basis for pay-for-performance models. With respect to CHF, it is expected that all patients have a measured ejection fraction as an evaluation of LV systolic function and those with ejection fractions less than 40% and without contraindication will be placed on an ACE inhibitor or angiotensin II receptor blocker (ARB) on discharge from hospitalization. Patients are also to be given information at discharge to help them in managing heart failure symptoms. Core measures and their documentation are helping to standardize patient care. This is a small but important inroad into developing a more integrated model of care that improves communication between patients, doctors, and nurses.

Chapter 11
Palpitations and Arrhythmias (Case 6)

Arzhang Fallahi MD and Michael Kim MD

Case: A 75-year-old man with a history of hypertension and hyperlipidemia presents to the emergency department complaining of palpitations. He states that for the past day he has felt a strange feeling in his chest, like his heart is racing, and says he is mildly short of breath. He has had similar episodes in the past, but they went away with rest and tended to "come and go." He reports some light-headedness. He denies any chest pain, cough, or history of thyroid disease. He has never seen a cardiologist before and has never had "serious heart problems." His only medications are aspirin 81 mg, hydrochlorothiazide 25 mg, and simvastatin 40 mg, all taken once daily. There is no family history of heart disease. His pulse is 135 bpm, and his BP is 145/70 mm Hg. On exam he seems to be in no acute distress but appears anxious. He has clear lung fields bilaterally and an irregular heart rate with no obvious murmurs, rubs, or gallops and no elevated neck veins. He has trace edema in his lower extremities.

An ECG reveals a narrow complex tachycardia at 135 bpm, irregularly irregular with no P waves and no delta waves; aVL shows a QRS complex of 12 little boxes in height; no other ST elevations or depressions are noted.

decompensation. In patients with severely reduced ejection fraction, agents such as digoxin, in combination with AV nodal agents, may be of benefit.

- There are various precipitants of atrial fibrillation, but initially acute coronary syndrome must be ruled out. Monitoring for signs of angina and elevated cardiac markers is crucial. Hypo- or hypervolemia may also trigger atrial fibrillation. Use of sympathomimetic agents such as caffeine, amphetamines, and cocaine can also trigger tachycardia and must be considered.

History

- Determine when the palpitations started and what triggered them. Associated symptoms, such as chest pain, may suggest an acute coronary event. Other contributing symptoms such as shortness of breath, leg swelling, and paroxysmal nocturnal dyspnea may suggest CHF. Symptoms such as weight loss and heat intolerance may suggest an endocrine etiology such as hyperthyroidism. The time course of symptoms is also important. Is this acute, chronic, or intermittent?
- Risk stratification, such as patient age, history of CHF, diabetes, and history of stroke, will help guide subsequent management.
- Medications, diet, and social history: Has the patient taken any medications that may have contributed to tachycardia? Does the patient have a history of illicit drug use?

Physical Examination

- **Vital signs:** Assess the patient's heart rate, and check for hypertension or hypotension. The patient should also be assessed for respiratory distress and oxygen saturation. Monitor the patient's temperature to see if infection may be the cause for the underlying condition.
- **General appearance:** Examine for diaphoresis, respiratory distress, and signs of shock for potential hypotension requiring immediate intervention.
- **Respiratory exam:** Listen to breath sounds bilaterally to make sure they are symmetric, and listen for any signs of fluid accumulation from either pulmonary and/or cardiac dysfunction or other diseases. Percussion may help identify areas of consolidation.
- **Cardiac auscultation** (to determine if rate is regular or irregular): Determine whether the heart sounds appear distant, which may suggest a pericardial effusion; assess for murmurs and abnormal heart sounds, since an S_3 gallop may indicate CHF or a dilated chamber, while an S_4 gallop may indicate the stiff LV of hypertensive heart disease. Look at neck veins to see if they are elevated, which may indicate volume overload or an inability to adequately distribute blood volume.
- **Vascular auscultation** (carotid bruits): to assess atherosclerotic status.
- **Abdominal examination:** Assess that there is no evidence of an acute abdomen or possible gastrointestinal hemorrhage, which could have led to the tachycardia.

- **Neurologic examination:** Quickly assess patient's mental status to determine if there is adequate perfusion of the brain. A screening neurologic exam should be performed to see if there are any focal deficits that might preclude use of anticoagulation therapy.
- **Extremities:** Check to see if extremities are warm to assess perfusion.

Tests for Consideration
- **ECG** is critical to obtain in all patients promptly. ECG can be used to categorize the type of tachyarrhythmia, which will help guide management. $27
- **Cardiac markers** (serum troponins and/or CK-MB) are needed to determine if an acute coronary syndrome is precipitating the event. $49
- **Metabolic panel** with **thyroid-stimulating hormone (TSH)**, creatinine, and electrolytes will help determine if an underlying metabolic disturbance is resulting in cardiac dysfunction. An acute decompensation in renal function may be a sign of shock. A low TSH concentration may suggest hyperthyroidism. $39
- **Complete blood count:** to determine if the patient has an underlying infection, which may contribute to the tachyarrhythmia. Hemoglobin and hematocrit are important to determine if the patient is anemic. $11
- **Liver function tests** may be helpful to help ascertain if there is a hepatic cause of infection. $12
- **Coagulation tests** are helpful to see whether the patient is prone to thrombosis or at high risk of bleeding. They are also helpful if the patient is to have a procedure, such as ablation to treat the arrhythmia. $15
- **A urine toxicology screen** should be obtained in patients suspected of using illicit drugs as a precipitant of the arrhythmia. $21

IMAGING CONSIDERATIONS

→ **Chest radiography** is helpful to see if any pulmonary disease or process such as a pneumonia, effusion, or pneumothorax is present. Cardiomegaly can be assessed, but quality may be suboptimal with a portable chest radiograph. Radiography can also help determine if there is a widened mediastinum, which may be suggestive of an aortic dissection. $45

→ **Echocardiography** is helpful not only to assess ventricular and valvular dysfunction, but also possibly to help determine if there is a thrombus, which may embolize if the patient is cardioverted. $393

Multifocal Atrial Tachycardia (MAT)

Pφ In most cases the different P-wave morphologies seen on the ECG suggest that a pacemaker arises in different locations within the atria. Cardiac disease (coronary, valvular, and congestive heart failure) is associated with MAT. Pulmonary disease, especially COPD, is also associated with MAT. Pulmonary arterial hypertension results in increased right atrial stretch, which can result in ectopic atrial activity. Hypokalemia and hypomagnesemia can also contribute to MAT.

TP Patients may not have symptoms or may complain of palpitations. One must always consider the underlying cause that is contributing to the arrhythmia.

Dx Diagnosis is made by ECG, which reveals P waves with three different morphologies (best seen in leads II, III, and V_1), atrial rate over 100 bpm, P waves separated by isoelectric intervals, and PP, PR, and RR intervals that vary.

Tx Treatment should be focused the underlying disorder. β-Blockers and calcium channel blockers (i.e., verapamil) have been shown to be effective. Due to risk of bronchospasm in patients with pulmonary disease, verapamil is most commonly used, although in the absence of such comorbidities, agents such as metoprolol can also be effective. Repletion in those with low magnesium (and even in those with normal magnesium) may be of some benefit. Repletion of potassium may also be of benefit. Ablation may be an option in some patients with MAT. **See Cecil Essentials 10.**

Atrioventricular Nodal Reentrant Tachycardia (Junctional Reciprocating Tachycardia)

Pφ Structural heart disease is not required for AVNRT, and most times AVNRT develops in patients with otherwise normal hearts, although it can also occur in patients with organic heart disease. While there are usually no precipitating factors, AVNRT can be brought on by nicotine, alcohol, stimulants, or surges in vagal tone.

In patients with normal sinus rhythm, a normal sinus beat enters the AV node and passes down both fast and slow pathways. The fast pathway reaches the His bundle, creating a refractory wake. Consequently this blocks the impulse from the slow pathway, since the area in the final common pathway is refractory because of the fast pathway that just traveled through it. In the most common form of AVNRT, a critically timed premature beat goes down the slow pathway (which has recovered excitability), and the beat conducts down through the final common pathway to the bundle of His. Meanwhile, if the fast pathway has recovered excitability, the impulse via the slow pathway can conduct retrograde up the fast pathway. This creates a circuit, which then conducts down the slow pathway following retrograde conduction up the fast pathway, resulting in a sustained tachycardia.

TP Patients typically present with palpitations, a strange feeling in the chest, and possible dizziness. In severe cases, patients may feel dyspnea and chest pain, and possibly fatigue or syncope.

Dx Diagnosis is made by ECG. Usually the rate is between 120 and 220 bpm. In most cases, the retrograde atrial activation causes the P wave to be buried or fused with the QRS complex. If the P wave occurs shortly after the QRS complex, a fused waveform can appear as a pseudo-R' in lead V_1 and a pseudo-S wave in the inferior leads. The axis of the P wave, because of retrograde activation, is typically inverted in leads I, II, III, and aVF.

Tx In unstable patients with evidence of hemodynamic collapse, DC cardioversion is the treatment of choice. In the absence of severe symptoms or hemodynamic collapse, vagal maneuvers (carotid massage, cough, Valsalva) can be used to break the rhythm. Adenosine can be used for rapid conversion to sinus rhythm. Non-dihydropyridine calcium channel blockers or β-blockers can also be used. For chronic cases of AVNRT, patients can undergo catheter ablation. **See Cecil Essentials 10.**

Atrioventricular Reentrant (or Reciprocating) Tachycardia

Pφ In AVRT a defined circuit exists consisting of two distinct pathways: the normal AV conduction system and an AV accessory pathway, which are linked by proximal tissue (the atria) and distal tissue (the ventricles). The two major forms of this type of arrhythmia are orthodromic AVRT and antidromic AVRT.

Practice-Based Learning and Improvement: Evidence-Based Medicine

Title
A comparison of rate control and rhythm control in patients with atrial fibrillation

Authors
Van Gelder IC, Hagens VE, Bosker HA, et al.; Rate Control versus Electrical Cardioversion for Persistent Atrial Fibrillation Study Group

Institution
AFFIRM Clinical Trial Center, Axio Research, 2601 4th Avenue, Suite 200, Seattle, Washington 98121, USA

Reference
N Engl J Med 2002;347:1834–1840

Problem
The treatment of atrial fibrillation has relied on two basic strategies: rhythm and rate control. Rhythm control offers the prospect of maintaining sinus rhythm, while rate control can be achieved with drugs that are generally less toxic. A comparison of these two strategies with respect to mortality before this trial had not been performed.

Intervention
A total of 4060 patients with atrial fibrillation were randomized to receive either rate control (with β-blockers, calcium channel blockers, digoxin, or combinations of these drugs) or rhythm control (amiodarone, sotalol, propafenone, procainamide, quinidine, flecainide, disopyramide, moricizine, dofetilide, or combinations of these drugs). Average length of follow-up was 3.5 years.

Quality of evidence
Level I

Outcome/effect
The primary end point was overall mortality. The composite secondary end points were death, disabling stroke, disabling anoxic encephalopathy, major bleeding, and cardiac arrest. The overall mortality between the two groups was not statistically significant. The rates of composite end points were also similar in both groups. The rhythm control group did have higher rates of bradycardic arrest and TdP.

Historical significance/comments
This was an important trial that showed that rhythm and rate control are associated with no difference in mortality. Since the rhythm control group had more complications and used drugs with higher potential toxicity, this trial was instrumental in physicians adopting a rate control strategy initially in most patients with atrial fibrillation.

Interpersonal and Communication Skills

Assist Patients in Making Informed Decisions

In patients diagnosed with atrial fibrillation, use of anticoagulation raises many issues of balancing the benefits and risks. The patient should understand that the reason for use of anticoagulation is to prevent stroke, but must also be made to realize that with this comes a risk of bleeding and the need for careful monitoring. These concerns should be factored into the decision to choose this therapy. Patients must be given complete information to make informed decisions about this treatment modality, and their decisions must be respected.

Professionalism

Ensure Access to Care for the Medically Vulnerable

Management of cardiac arrhythmias requires long-term follow-up with either a primary-care physician or cardiologist (or both). When patients with atrial fibrillation are started on a rate control strategy, they need to be followed to determine how effectively the medication is working and how well they are tolerating it. Furthermore, with the need for anticoagulation, patients must be closely monitored to be sure they are anticoagulated at the appropriate level (INR of 2–3 if on warfarin) and to be monitored for signs of bleeding. Access to health care and to proper follow-up is an important issue in these patients and should be a major concern for physicians.

Systems-Based Practice

Anticoagulation: Coordinating Care in the Outpatient Setting to Reduce Costs and Complications

The decision to begin anticoagulation for a patient with atrial fibrillation has important considerations at the outset of therapy. Many patients are started on anticoagulation as part of an inpatient hospital admission. Traditionally, these patients had remained in the hospital until their INRs were therapeutic, at times adding multiple days to an inpatient stay without the acuity to warrant continued hospitalization. Most hospitals now have instituted pathways to bridge patients at home until they are fully anticoagulated. These programs involve the coordinated use of subcutaneous injections of a low-molecular-weight heparin in conjunction with oral warfarin. INRs

medicine rotation, one useful exercise is to pull multiple ECG tracings from the charts of patients and review them, perhaps even with the help of a resident. The more ECGs you read, the more comfortable you will be interpreting them.

P waves, T waves, and QRS complexes appear differently in each of the 12 standard ECG leads. The P waves, T waves, and QRS complexes have been labeled in lead II in Figure 12-1. Label them for leads aVR and V_6.

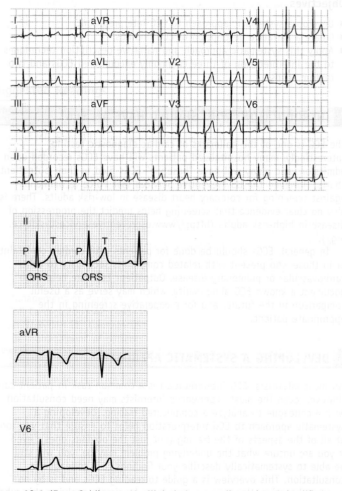

Figure 12-1 (From Goldberger AL. Clinical electrocardiography: a simplified approach. 7th ed. Philadelphia: Mosby; 2006, p. 44, question 1.)

A systematic stepwise approach includes examination in five major areas of the ECG tracing in the following order:

Step 1: Rate
Step 2: Rhythm
Step 3: Axis
Step 4: Hypertrophy/chamber size
Step 5: Ischemic changes/infarction

Step 1: Determining the Rate

To calculate the rate, find an R wave that is lined up with a heavy border of a background grid box. After this, you simply count down until your next R wave appears. The counting is specific: the distance to the next grid line is 300 bpm, to the second grid line is 150 bpm, the third is 100 bpm, the fourth is 75 bpm, the fifth is 60 bpm, and the sixth is 50 bpm. Often the next R wave will appear between two major grid lines, and in these cases you simply estimate the rate. For example, if your rate determination falls exactly between the 75 and the 60 line, you can perhaps estimate the heart rate at 68 bpm. Note: to be precise the distance between two heavy grid lines is 1/300 of a minute. Therefore, the distance between two heavy grid lines is 2/300, and three grid lines is 3/300, which can be simplified to 1/150 and 1/100, respectively. That's where these numbers come from, so committing them to memory can be helpful.

If the heart rate is normal at rest, it should fall somewhere between 60 and 100 bpm. If the heart rate is generated from the sinus node, then a slow (or bradycardic) rate is less than 60 bpm. A fast (or tachycardic) rate is greater than 100 bpm. If the sinus node (or another atrial focus) fails to set pace, a junctional automaticity focus would assume the pace; if this focus fails, a ventricular automaticity focus would pace the heart. A junctionally generated rhythm is usually between 40 and 60 bpm. A ventricular focus would generate a rate of 20 to 40 bpm. Rates slower than 50 bpm require counting how many beats occur in a 6-second time period and then multiplying that number by 10.

The rate you determine will become the first part of your systematic description; for example, *"The rate is about 75 beats per minute."* Take a moment now to determine the rate in the ECG in Figure 12-1.

Step 2: Determining the Rhythm

After finding the rate, determining the rhythm (i.e., from where the heart rate is being generated) is the next step. Some common rhythms are:

■ **Sinus rhythm:** This rhythm is described as "regular," meaning the pattern is constant and does not vary. All of the cycles are of equal

If we now refer to the first ECG tracing in this chapter (see Fig. 12-1), you can continue your description: *"The rate is approximately 75 beats per minute, the rhythm is sinus, and the axis is normal."*

Step 4: Look for Hypertrophy and Chamber Size

Corresponding waveforms can provide information about chamber size.

- **Atrial enlargement:** Leads II and V_1 are the best place to look at P-wave size. When a P wave appears diphasic (i.e., having an upward and a downward portion), there is atrial enlargement. If the upward portion is bigger than the lower portion, then the right atrium is enlarged. If the downward portion is more significant, then the left atrium is enlarged. It is also possible to have bi-atrial enlargement.
- **Ventricular hypertrophy:** Here we will look at the QRS complex. Look for right ventricular hypertrophy in lead V_1: if the S wave is smaller than the R wave, then the right ventricle is hypertrophied; the R waves in leads V_2 through V_4 will also become progressively smaller. In left ventricular hypertrophy, there will be a deep S wave in V_1 and left-axis deviation. There will also be a very tall R wave in V_5. If you add the number of smaller grid boxes from the size of the S wave in lead V_1 and the size of the R wave in V_5 and you find more than 35 boxes, there is left ventricular hypertrophy. You can also look at lead aVL; if the height of the R wave is greater than 11 small grid boxes, there is left ventricular hypertrophy. Examining these features in our original ECG (see Fig. 12-1), the description now reads: *"Rate of 75 bpm, sinus rhythm, normal axis with no hypertrophy."*

Step 5: Look for Evidence of Ischemia, Injury, or Infarction

- **Ischemia:** This means the blood supply to a section of heart is compromised and insufficient. The classic sign of ischemia on an ECG is inverted T waves. Look for this finding in every ECG you read.
- **Infarction:** Here you will need to examine the ST segments. In a normal ECG (such as in Fig. 12-1), this segment is flat, without a wave to it. When the ST segment is elevated, there is acute injury to the underlying myocardium. It is the earliest sign of a myocardial infarction on the ECG. If the ST segment is elevated without a Q wave, this may be a non–Q-wave infarction. ST segments can also be depressed. This usually happens in patients with subendocardial infarctions that do not extend through the full thickness of the heart wall and is another type of non–Q-wave infarction. Q waves form when an area of the heart becomes necrotic. A significant Q wave is at least one small grid box wide.
- The location of the above findings in particular leads helps to discern the area of the heart that is affected and even the vessel most likely involved.

- **Any patient with these findings needs immediate attention in the ER setting.**

Create a narrative description for an ECG described as follows: *"The rate is approximately 90 bpm, the rhythm is sinus, the axis is normal, there is no hypertrophy, there are ST segment depressions in leads I, II, III, aVL, aVF, and V_2 through V_6. There are no Q waves."* This is severe subendocardial ischemia (Fig. 12-6).

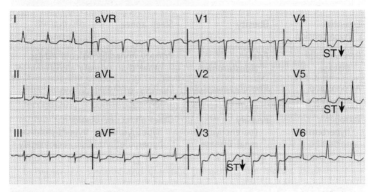

Figure 12-6 (From Goldberger AL. Clinical electrocardiography: a simplified approach. 7th ed. Philadelphia: Mosby; 2006, Figure 9-6.)

Chapter 13
Hypertension (Case 7)

Elie R. Chemaly MD, MSc *and Michael Kim* MD

Case: A 59-year-old African-American woman is referred by her primary physician. She has had a history of severe hypertension for 38 years. She complains of dizziness, occipital headaches with blurred vision, and palpitations correlated with high BP sometimes reaching 200 mm Hg systolic and 120 mm Hg diastolic. She also has claudication of the legs and thighs upon walking four street blocks. She has a history of thyroid disease and is presently hypothyroid. Her medications on presentation were valsartan/hydrochlorothiazide 320 mg/25 mg (one tablet daily in the morning), clonidine 0.3 mg (one tablet daily in the evening), verapamil SR 240 mg (one tablet twice a day), and levothyroxine 0.1 mg (one tablet daily). Although she takes her medications each day as

- Medications, diet, and social history: Drugs that may aggravate or cause hypertension include sympathomimetics, steroids, NSAIDs, and estrogens; psychiatric medications causing a serotonin syndrome; cocaine and alcohol abuse. Withdrawal syndromes and rebound effects also need to be considered: alcohol, benzodiazepines, β-blockers, and clonidine.
- Family history
- Comorbidities, especially diabetes; diseases that can be secondary causes of hypertension (e.g., kidney disease); other cardiovascular risk factors (e.g., tobacco).
- Symptoms of sleep apnea: early-morning headaches, daytime somnolence, snoring, erratic sleep.
- Symptoms of severe hypertension, end-organ damage, or volume overload: epistaxis, headache, visual disturbances, neurologic deficits, dyspnea, chest pain, syncope, claudication.
- Symptoms suggestive of a secondary cause: headaches, sweating, tremor, tachycardia/palpitations, muscle weakness, and skin symptoms.

Physical Examination
- **Proper measurement of BP:** Away from stressors, with an appropriate cuff size, use Korotkoff phase V for auscultatory DBP. Korotkoff phase V is when the sounds disappear; one can use phase IV when they muffle if they do not disappear until a BP of 0 mm Hg. SBP, measured by auscultation, can and should also be measured through the radial pulse: when the cuff is inflated above the SBP, the radial pulse disappears. This maneuver allows the assessment of auscultatory gap (a stiff artery that does not oscillate and leads to an auscultatory underestimation of SBP) and pseudo-hypertension (a stiff artery not compressed by the cuff; SBP is overestimated). In selected settings, BP should be measured in both arms (especially in the younger patient to assess for coarctation of the aorta). Measurements should be repeated at different visits, unless BP is markedly elevated, before treatment.
- **Vital signs,** in particular heart rate in relationship to BP and treatments already taken. It may be important, especially in the acute setting, to know if the patient is febrile or hypoxic. Mental status is an important vital sign in the acute setting (hypertensive emergencies and urgencies).
- **General appearance:** body fat, skin (cutaneous manifestations of endocrinopathies causing secondary hypertension).
- **Funduscopic examination** to evaluate retinal complications.
- **Thyroid examination.**
- **Cardiac auscultation** (for murmurs and abnormal sounds: An S_4 gallop may indicate the stiff left ventricle of hypertensive heart disease).
- **Vascular auscultation** (carotid bruits, renal bruits, pulses): to assess atherosclerotic status and the presence of renal artery stenosis; the

relationship between carotid artery disease, its treatment, and hypertension is not well understood.
- **Abdominal examination,** especially of the aorta and the kidneys.
- **Neurologic examination,** if applicable.

Tests for Consideration
- **ECG,** mainly to assess for complications (atrial fibrillation, myocardial ischemia, LVH). Tachycardia (or atrial fibrillation) in the setting of hypertension may point to a secondary cause as well. $27
- **Glucose finger-stick** to rule out hypoglycemia, pulse oximetry, arterial blood gas to rule out hypercapnia or hypoxia (in acute settings). $5
- **Metabolic panel:** serum creatinine and electrolytes, especially potassium and glucose. The kidney is a key organ in the pathology of hypertension (see causes and complications), renal function and electrolytes are affected by antihypertensive therapy, and some metabolic abnormalities are a clue to a secondary cause. Examples include hypokalemia (in mineralocorticoid excess) and new-onset diabetes in the setting of several causes of secondary hypertension (e.g., Cushing). $12
- **Complete blood count** including hemoglobin and hematocrit. These abnormalities can be a clue to many life-threatening illnesses, some related to the hypertension. Besides, anemia can cause hyperdynamic circulation and polycythemia can cause hyperviscosity, and, in acute settings, thrombocytopenia can point to a microangiopathic condition associated with hypertension. $11
- **Urinalysis** and **microalbumin/creatinine ratio** in urine. $10
- **Thyroid profile** and other endocrine studies as indicated in the search for a secondary cause. Hypothyroidism is common in older women, has atypical presentations, and may worsen atherosclerosis and obesity; it is listed as a secondary cause of hypertension. $24
- **Lipid profile** to assess cardiovascular risk. $19
- **Toxicology screen,** especially when substance abuse is suspected. $21
- Laboratory and imaging workup for secondary causes (see individual paragraphs).
- **Sleep studies** if applicable. $795
- **Ambulatory BP monitoring,** when white coat hypertension or masked hypertension is suspected, to diagnose paroxysmal hypertension (i.e., pheochromocytoma), and to assess resistance to treatment. $65
- **Echocardiography** to assess LVH (end-organ damage) and if cardiac dysfunction is suspected. $393

- Drug monotherapy must be initiated at 140/90 mm Hg, and initial dual therapy may be needed above 160/100 mm Hg.
- Major categories of antihypertensive medications can be simply classified according to the British AB/CD algorithm. "A" designates ACE inhibitors and ARBs, to which we can add the new renin inhibitor aliskiren. "B" designates β-adrenergic blockers. "C" designates calcium channel blockers. "D" designates diuretics.
- Regardless of BP reading, certain antihypertensive medications (mainly those in the AB category) are indicated in patients with a variety of cardiovascular and renal diseases. These compelling indications must be addressed and the appropriate therapy prescribed. Examples include the use of ACE inhibitors and ARBs in heart failure and kidney disease, and the use of β-blockers in ischemic heart disease and heart failure.
- Goal BP is generally 140/90 mm Hg. It should be 130/80 mm Hg in the setting of diabetes, chronic renal failure with proteinuria, and also in patients with cardiovascular disease. The amount of BP reduction is the most important factor in the benefit of antihypertensive therapy. In the absence of other compelling indications, and if the side effect profile is acceptable, a thiazide diuretic is the first choice of monotherapy. If dual therapy is needed, the most recommended strategy is to add an ACE inhibitor or an ARB to the diuretic. Generally, a "synergistic" combination of two antihypertensives includes one drug from the AB group and one from the CD group. β-Blockers should not be used as the initial monotherapy for isolated, essential hypertension; this recommendation is based on available clinical trials comparing them to other drugs.
- Other categories of antihypertensive medications are less commonly used; they include vasodilators (hydralazine, minoxidil), α_1-adrenergic blockers, and α_2-adrenergic agonists. Some medications combine β- and α-adrenergic blockade (labetalol). Also, diuretics can be combined with potassium-sparing diuretics (e.g., amiloride, triamterene, or spironolactone). The addition of an aldosterone antagonist may improve BP control in resistant hypertension.
- β-Blocker and centrally acting antihypertensives may cause rebound effects if discontinued abruptly.

Hypertensive Crisis

- Hypertensive urgencies represent substantial elevations in BP (DBP >120 mm Hg) with progressive end-organ damage, and perioperative hypertension. They require BP reduction within hours.
- Hypertensive emergencies include accelerated hypertension (BP > 210/130 mm Hg) with headaches, blurred vision, or focal neurologic symptoms; and malignant hypertension (with papilledema). Immediate mean BP reduction by 20% to 25% is needed to prevent end-organ complications (mean BP can be calculated grossly as ⅓ SBP + ⅔ DBP but is best measured directly by integrating the BP waveform in the arterial line; automated BP cuff machines give mean BP directly).
- In hypertensive emergencies, parenteral antihypertensive therapy is required. Intensive care unit monitoring is required, and intra-arterial BP measurement may be required. Parenteral agents include fenoldopam, sodium nitroprusside (caution: can cause thiocyanate intoxication and methemoglobinemia), labetalol (drug of choice in pregnancy), nitroglycerin (mostly in the setting of myocardial ischemia/infarction), esmolol (a β-blocker), nicardipine (approved for postoperative hypertension), enalaprilat (an ACE inhibitor that may give marked hypotension in high-renin states), and hydralazine (a good choice during pregnancy).
- In all cases of treatment, avoid precipitous drops in BP that can cause brain hypoperfusion. The goal is a mean BP reduction of 20% to 25% or a target DBP < 110 mm Hg, and should be attained over minutes to hours. In hypertensive urgencies, BP lowering can even be more progressive. BP normalization should be accomplished over several days. The circulation needs to adjust its properties to maintain flow at lower BP.
- Aortic dissection is beyond the scope of this chapter but is related to hypertensive emergencies and requires parenteral antihypertensive therapy as well. **See Cecil Essentials 13.**

Primary (Parenchymal) Renal Disease

Pφ Hypertension occurs in kidney disease, acute or chronic. It is usually seen in vascular or glomerular disease, but polycystic kidney disease also frequently results in hypertension.

In acute glomerular disease, hypertension is related to sodium and water retention.

In vascular disease, it is primarily the activation of the renin-angiotensin system in the ischemic kidney that causes hypertension.

In chronic kidney disease, hypertension is highly prevalent, and several mechanisms are involved: sodium and water retention, activation of the renin-angiotensin system, high sympathetic tone, endothelial dysfunction, high levels of parathyroid hormone, and arterial stiffening.

TP Elevation of the serum creatinine with a glomerular filtration rate below 60 mL/min and/or proteinuria. Edema is characteristic of acute glomerulonephritis.

Dx Serum BUN and creatinine with urinalysis make the positive diagnosis. Etiologies are numerous and outside the scope of this chapter. Hypertension may itself cause kidney disease (nephroangiosclerosis, which can be acute, malignant or chronic).

Tx Treatment depends on the cause. Fluid removal by diuretics and dialysis is important in acute glomerulonephritis, while inhibition of the renin-angiotensin system is important in vascular causes. Aggressive treatment of hypertension is important in chronic kidney disease to reduce disease progression and cardiovascular risk. Goal BP is 130/80 mm Hg. The treatment of proteinuria is also essential.

ACE inhibitors and ARBs specifically reduce the progression of chronic kidney disease and are indicated to reduce proteinuria but can result in further decrease in glomerular filtration and hyperkalemia; thus, they need to be used carefully. Most ACE inhibitors are eliminated by the kidneys, but fosinopril is cleared by the liver. Keep in mind that a small (~30%) and limited elevation of the serum creatinine that stabilizes over 1–2 months when treating with ACE inhibitors or ARBs does not require treatment interruption but is a sign of treatment efficacy. Hyperkalemia can be managed with diuretics and/or kayexalate. Diuretics are needed to treat volume overload, and loop diuretics are needed if the glomerular filtration rate falls below 30 mL/min. **See Cecil Essentials 13.**

Iatrogenic Hypertension

Pφ A number of prescribed or over-the-counter medications can cause or aggravate hypertension through different mechanisms.
- Oral contraceptives can elevate BP within the normal range or induce hypertension; the mechanism is poorly understood.
- NSAIDs secondary to inhibition of renal prostaglandin production, especially prostaglandin E_2 and prostaglandin I_2, with subsequent sodium and fluid retention.
- Licorice is discussed in the section on mineralocorticoid excess.
- Glucocorticoids are discussed in the section on Cushing syndrome.
- Erythropoietin-induced hypertension is multifactorial and involves not only increased blood viscosity from a rising hematocrit, but also changes in vascular reactivity.
- Cyclosporine causes renal vasoconstriction and sodium/water retention.
- Sympathomimetics and stimulants (enhance sympathetic tone).
- Certain herbal supplements (depending on the content).

TP As in essential hypertension. Malignant hypertension can occur with oral contraceptives. Edema, renal failure, and hyperkalemia can occur with NSAIDs. In the case of erythropoietin, hypertensive encephalopathy can occur with rapid rise of BP.

Dx The association is not automatic; it may be established only when discontinuation of the medication lowers the BP.

Tx Discontinuation or dose reduction of the responsible agent is usually effective. In terms of analgesics, acetaminophen may be better than NSAIDs (although acetaminophen was also associated with hypertension). In terms of oral contraceptives, hypertension is rare but may be severe. In the case of erythropoietin, slowly increasing the hematocrit along with fluid removal and antihypertensive therapy is helpful. Antiplatelet agents may reduce the risk of erythropoietin-induced hypertension. In the setting of cyclosporine-induced hypertension, calcium channel blockers are the drugs of choice; diltiazem can be used and reduces cyclosporine metabolism, but the benefit on cyclosporine nephrotoxicity is unproven. **See Cecil Essentials 13.**

Hypertension Secondary to Alcoholism and Substance Abuse

Pφ Alcohol: Reactive acute hypertension can occur during alcohol withdrawal, but chronic alcohol consumption, even if moderate, can lead to hypertension. The mechanism is not clear. Cocaine inhibits norepinephrine reuptake.

TP Alcohol can lead to hypertension that may be treatment-resistant. Cocaine raises BP but usually presents with acute cardiovascular complications (myocardial infarction, arrhythmias, stroke, and also aortic dissection among other manifestations).

Dx History, toxicology screen, other features of intoxication or abuse.

Tx Abstinence and management of the (acute) complications of the intoxication. **See Cecil Essentials 13, 135.**

Pheochromocytoma

Pφ Excess production of norepinephrine, epinephrine, or dopamine by a tumor usually located in the adrenal medulla (90%), but also anywhere along the sympathetic chain.

TP Half of the patients have paroxysmal hypertension and most of the rest have "what appears to be essential hypertension." Some patients are normotensive. There is a triad of symptoms: headache, sweating, and palpitations. Many other presentations are possible. Secondary diabetes and a cardiomyopathy may occur.

Dx Diagnosis is established by measurement of 24-hour urine metanephrines and catecholamines. Plasma free metanephrines can also be measured; some authors consider them the test of choice (they are sensitive but less specific). Urinary VMA (vanillylmandelic acid) is specific but less sensitive. CT scan or MRI of the abdomen should follow to locate the tumor (usually intra-adrenal; if not, can still be intra-abdominal). If using CT scan with contrast, keep in mind that iodine contrast agents can precipitate a hypertensive crisis in the setting of a pheochromocytoma. MIBG scintigraphy can locate tumors not seen on CT or MRI; MIBG scintigraphy is also useful to locate metastases of a malignant pheochromocytoma. ^{111}In-pentetreotide scintigraphy (Octreoscan), or total-body MRI, and PET scanning are other imaging options to locate extra-adrenal or multiple tumors.

A pheochromocytoma can occur in the setting of a multiple endocrine neoplasia (MEN) or a phacomatosis. Both types of syndromes bring associations of life-threatening diseases. Uncovering the association is a caveat when a pheochromocytoma is diagnosed.

Tx Removal of the tumor after appropriate pre-operative medical preparation. Surgery is usually delayed until hypertension is controlled by a combination of α- and β-blockade; β-blockers should not be used until appropriate α-blockade is achieved. **See Cecil Essentials 13, 67.**

Primary Aldosteronism and Other Mineralocorticoid Excess States

Pφ Aldosterone can be produced in excess by a tumor or a hyperplasia of the adrenal cortex. Less commonly, disorders of the synthesis of the steroid hormones can lead to the inappropriate accumulation of steroids (aldosterone or other metabolites or precursors of cortisol) that have mineralocorticoid effect. One situation is of interest: The deficiency in 11β-hydroxysteroid dehydrogenase type 2 (11βHSD2) that converts cortisol to cortisone in the renal tubule and prevents cortisol from having mineralocorticoid action, since this enzyme can be inhibited by the ingestion of licorice and both situations lead to apparent hypermineralocorticism.

TP Hypertension with hypokalemia and metabolic alkalosis (usually spontaneous hypokalemia). However, (severe) hypertension alone can lead to the diagnosis, and hypokalemia is thought to be a late manifestation and is often absent in patients with primary aldosteronism.

Dx Hypertension, unexplained hypokalemia, and metabolic alkalosis. Some patients have a normal serum potassium concentration. The next step is to measure plasma renin activity and serum aldosterone levels. Typically, in primary aldosteronism, renin is suppressed and aldosterone elevated with an aldosterone-to-renin ratio above 20 and often above 50. Imaging of the adrenal glands follows to search for the adenoma, and adrenal vein sampling to demonstrate asymmetric secretion of aldosterone may be needed either if imaging is equivocal or if surgical removal of an adenoma is considered. If both renin and aldosterone are suppressed, then the hypermineralocorticism is not aldosterone-dependent. Glucocorticoid-remediable aldosteronism is one of the zebras in this category, and it requires genetic testing to demonstrate the hybrid gene in which aldosterone synthase is driven by adrenocorticotropic hormone (ACTH).

Tx Removal of the tumor (especially if a carcinoma) and/or a mineralocorticoid receptor antagonist such as spironolactone or eplerenone. Dexamethasone suppression in the rare case of glucocorticoid-remediable aldosteronism. **See Cecil Essentials 13, 67.**

TP Cushingoid facies, central obesity, ecchymoses, and muscle weakness. Exogenous steroid administration is a key question to ask.

Dx History of steroid ingestion is essential, since it is most often iatrogenic. Initial testing includes a 24-hour urine cortisol or dexamethasone suppression test. If positive, more advanced testing is needed to establish if the syndrome is adrenal (ACTH-independent) or ACTH-dependent (may be pituitary or ectopic ACTH or ectopic corticotropin-releasing factor [CRF]).

Tx A mineralocorticoid receptor antagonist should be the best antihypertensive therapy. Otherwise, removal of the tumor producing ACTH or cortisol (or CRF) is the definitive treatment. **See Cecil Essentials 13, 67.**

Other Endocrine Diseases

Pφ • Hypothyroidism: increased peripheral vascular resistance.
   • Hyperthyroidism: hyperdynamic circulation (high cardiac output and oxygen consumption with decreased peripheral vascular resistance).
   • Hyperparathyroidism: The association with hypertension is not well established, but arterial stiffening is a likely complication.

TP Symptoms are variable but often subtle for all three entities that are detected on more or less routine laboratory testing. However, note that pulse pressure is narrow in the setting of hypothyroidism and wide in the setting of hyperthyroidism.

Dx Hypothyroidism is diagnosed by a typically elevated TSH and low T_4 if peripheral in origin, or low to normal TSH and low T_4 if pituitary in origin. In hyperthyroidism it is almost always peripheral in origin, so a low TSH is characteristic (other situations are very rare). Hyperparathyroidism comes with hypercalcemia, hypophosphatemia, and high parathyroid hormone concentrations. Further workup is needed to determine the etiology. Individual situations are often complex in terms of thyroid and parathyroid disease, and their discussion is beyond the scope of this chapter. MEN should be looked for in the setting of hyperparathyroidism, since hypertension may be due to an associated adrenal or pituitary tumor.

Tx Varies according to the entity. BP responds variably to the correction of the endocrine disorder. **See Cecil Essentials 66, 74.**

ZEBRA ZONE

a. This chapter focuses on hypertension in adults, but **coarctation of the aorta** is a major cause of hypertension in children. Other diseases of the aorta, such as Takayasu's arteritis, have been reported to mimic a coarctation of the aorta.

b. **Impaired autonomic reflexes** and **autonomic dysfunction** have been related to hypertension. Instances of baroreflex failure after brainstem stroke are an example of such situations. Another situation in that category is Guillain-Barré syndrome; BP may swing rapidly from hypertension to hypotension in those cases.

c. **Acromegaly** is a cause of secondary hypertension.

Practice-Based Learning and Improvement: Evidence-Based Medicine

Title
Effect of lower targets for blood pressure and LDL cholesterol on atherosclerosis in diabetes: the SANDS (Stop Atherosclerosis in Native Diabetics) randomized trial

Authors
Howard BV, Roman MJ, Devereux RB, et al.

Institution
MedStar Research Institute, 6495 New Hampshire Avenue, Suite 201, Hyattsville, MD 20783, USA

Reference
JAMA 2008;299:1678–1689

Problem
Diabetes mellitus (DM) is associated with an increased cardiovascular risk and requires aggressive management of BP and low-density lipoprotein cholesterol (LDLc). Standard targets for these parameters as recommended by the guidelines in the DM population are SBP less than 130 mm Hg and LDLc less than 100 mg/dL.

Intervention
Participants were 499 American Indian men and women aged 40 years or older with type 2 DM and no prior cardiovascular disease (CVD) events. They were randomized to aggressive ($n = 252$) versus standard ($n = 247$) treatment groups with stepped treatment algorithms defined for both. Aggressive treatment targets were SBP less than 115 mm Hg and LDLc less than 70 mg/dL.

Suggested Readings

Calhoun DA, Jones D, Textor S, et al. Resistant hypertension: diagnosis, evaluation, and treatment. A scientific statement from the American Heart Association Professional Education Committee of the Council for High Blood Pressure Research. Hypertension 2008;51:1403–1419.

Kaplan NM, Lieberman E, Neal W. Kaplan's clinical hypertension. 8th ed. Philadelphia: Lippincott Williams & Wilkins; 2002.

Morrison A, Vijayan A. Hypertension. The Washington manual of medical therapeutics. 32nd ed. Philadelphia: Lippincott Williams & Wilkins, 2007, Chapter 4, pp. 102–118.

Victor RG. Arterial hypertension. Cecil Medicine, 24th ed. Philadelphia: Saunders/Elsevier, 2012, pp. 373–389.

Thorough and continuously updated reviews on several subjects can be found on www.uptodate.com. These include an overview of hypertension in adults, hypertension in kidney disease, and the screening for renovascular hypertension.

Section IV
PULMONARY DISEASES

Section Editor
Sean M. Studer MD, MSc

Section Contents

14 **Dyspnea (Case 8)**
    Esaïe Carisma DO and Christina Migliore MD

15 **Cough (Case 9)**
    Ranjit Nair MD and Sean M. Studer MD, MSc

16 **Hemoptysis (Case 10)**
    Sudheer Nambiar MD and Pratik Patel MD

17 **Pulmonary Nodule (Case 11)**
    Smitha Gopinath Nair DO and Jennifer LaRosa MD

18 **Teaching Visual: How to Interpret a Chest Radiograph**
    Irtza Sharif MD and Sean M. Studer MD, MSc

PATIENT CARE

Clinical Thinking
- Determine the onset, duration, and severity of the symptom.
- Abrupt onset of dyspnea is usually of a cardiac or pulmonary origin that requires urgent diagnosis and treatment.
- Chronic dyspnea can generally be evaluated in an ambulatory setting.

History
A detailed history should focus on:
- The timing of the symptom
- Precipitating factors
- Associated symptoms
- Environmental irritant exposure (e.g., smoke from a building fire)
- Tobacco exposure history (active or passive smoking)
- Illicit substance abuse and use of specific medications
- Past medical, occupational, and travel history

Physical Examination
- **General appearance:** Severity of dyspnea may be evaluated by observing the patient's respiratory effort, accessory muscles use, and mental status.
- **Neck:** Inspect for stridor, vein distension, and goiter.
- **Chest and lungs:** Include observation of respiratory excursion for symmetry. Observe configuration of the chest, and palpate for tenderness and subcutaneous emphysema. Absence of breath sounds may suggest pneumothorax or pleural effusion; these conditions are distinguished by percussion, in which hyper-resonance is demonstrated in patients with pneumothorax and dullness in patients with pleural effusion. Auscultation of the lungs may reveal wheezing, crackles, or rhonchi.
- **Heart:** Auscultation of the heart may reveal cardiac murmurs and/or extra heart sounds.
- **Extremities:** Examination of the digits is important to evaluate for clubbing and cyanosis. The lower extremities should be assessed for pitting edema, which may indicate volume overload or cor pulmonale (or both).

Tests for Consideration
- **Pulse oximetry** measures the patient's level of oxygenation; however, normal values do not exclude anemia or certain hemoglobinopathies, which may limit oxygen delivery. $3
- **Complete blood count (CBC)** may reveal anemia; severe dyspnea usually occurs at a hemoglobin level of 7 g/dL or below. Erythrocytosis may be seen in patients with severe COPD. $11

- **Electrocardiogram (ECG)** may demonstrate myocardial ischemia or arrhythmia. $27
- **Peak flow meter assessment** in a patient with suspected asthma may help determine the severity of the exacerbation. $22
- **Arterial blood gas (ABG)** is useful in the hospital setting and selected outpatient situations. It assesses arterial pH and partial pressures of carbon dioxide and oxygen, and allows determination as to whether the condition is primarily respiratory or metabolic. $27
- **Brain natriuretic peptide (BNP)** concentrations measured in the serum may help differentiate cardiac from noncardiac causes of dyspnea; patients with concentrations less than 100 pg/mL are unlikely to have acute heart failure. $48
- **Thyroid function testing** may determine a systemic cause of dyspnea, such as hyperthyroidism or hypothyroidism. $24
- **D-dimer testing** in serum is useful when pulmonary embolism is suspected. It has a high sensitivity but limited specificity. A negative test will essentially exclude pulmonary embolism as a cause of dyspnea. $14
- **Spirometry** is essential in the evaluation of chronic dyspnea. It distinguishes patients with airway obstruction from those with restrictive lung disease and provides an objective measurement of lung impairment and an estimate of diffusing capacity. $52

IMAGING CONSIDERATIONS

→ **Plain chest radiographs (posteroanterior [PA] and lateral)** may help to exclude conditions such as pneumonia, pulmonary edema, pneumothorax, emphysema, and pleural effusion. $45

→ **High-resolution computed tomography (CT) scan** is recommended if interstitial lung disease is suspected and to further evaluate other abnormalities found on plain chest radiography. $334

→ **Echocardiogram** is the initial test of choice if heart failure is suspected. Elevated right ventricular pressure may suggest pulmonary embolism or pulmonary hypertension. $393

→ **Venous Doppler of the lower extremities** should be ordered to evaluate for deep vein thrombosis when pulmonary embolism is suspected. $107

| **Clinical Entities** | **Medical Knowledge** |

Pulmonary Embolism (PE)

Pφ PE is a potentially lethal condition. It commonly occurs when a deep vein thrombus fragments and travels through the vena cava to the right side of the heart, eventually becoming lodged in the pulmonary artery or one of its branches.

TP Patients usually complain of the sudden onset of dyspnea. Pleuritic chest pain, tachypnea, and hemoptysis may also be present. Syncope may be the only presenting symptom and is usually a sign of extensive compromise of cardiac output.

Dx CT angiography (CT scan with intravenous contrast) is becoming more widely used for the diagnosis of PE; filling defects within segmental or larger pulmonary arteries are specific for the diagnosis. A ventilation/perfusion (V/Q) scan will show perfusion defects without corresponding ventilation defects; it should be ordered in patients with renal insufficiency to avoid the use of contrast. If the V/Q scan is negative, it essentially rules out the diagnosis of PE. V/Q scan results often state that there is low probability for PE or that the probability of PE is indeterminate. If the suspicion for PE remains high in such cases, further testing such as venous Doppler of the lower extremities or pulmonary angiogram should be pursued.

Tx Unfractionated heparin or low-molecular-weight heparin is the treatment of choice. In patients with massive PE and hemodynamic instability, thrombolysis or thrombectomy can be considered. **See Cecil Essentials 19.**

Pulmonary Edema

Pφ Pulmonary edema is usually cardiac in nature. Typical causes of pulmonary edema include myocardial infarction, acute decompensation of chronic left ventricular failure, and valvular heart disease. However, a number of other conditions such as sepsis and blood transfusion reaction may also cause pulmonary edema.

TP Patients present with severe dyspnea, production of pink frothy sputum, and diaphoresis. Tachycardia is usually observed. A third heart sound (S_3 gallop) is often present.

Dx Chest radiograph may reveal an enlarged cardiac silhouette and diffuse vascular congestion. An echocardiogram should be ordered to determine the cardiac function.

Tx Treatment may involve supplemental oxygen, diuretics, nitroglycerin (if angina is present), and afterload reduction along with inotropic agents to increase contractility (see Chapter 10, Congestive Heart Failure). **See Cecil Essentials 6, 23.**

Asthma

Pφ Asthma is a chronic inflammatory disorder of the lung characterized by reversible airway obstruction.

TP Patients present with episodic wheezing, dyspnea, cough, and chest tightness. Symptoms may worsen with exercise, upper respiratory tract infections, and emotional stress.

Dx A pulmonary function test (PFT) usually reveals a decreased FEV_1/FVC ratio; reversibility of obstruction is indicated by improvement in FEV_1 after administration of a short-acting β_2 agonist. If PFT is nondiagnostic, a methacholine bronchial provocation test may also be ordered. A positive test is generally defined as a 20% decrease in FEV_1 induced by methacholine.

Tx Treatment includes short-acting bronchodilators to relieve acute symptoms, and inhaled corticosteroids; long-acting bronchodilators are utilized for moderate to severe symptoms. Systemic corticosteroids are often used for acute and severe exacerbations. **See Cecil Essentials 17.**

COPD or Emphysema

Pφ COPD is a disorder with progressive airway obstruction. COPD includes an overlapping spectrum of diseases including chronic bronchitis, defined as a productive cough for 3 months or more in 2 consecutive years, and emphysema (abnormal enlargement of air spaces with destruction of alveolar walls). Emphysema is characterized by loss of elastic recoil and increased airway resistance, which lead to reduced expiratory airflow.

TP Patients usually present in their sixth decade complaining of productive cough, dyspnea on exertion, and occasional wheezing.

Dx Spirometry is the recommended screening tool for COPD. FEV_1/FVC ratio less than 70% is diagnostic for obstructive lung disease. PFT reveals decreased vital capacity and expiratory flow rates with increased residual volume and total lung capacity. Chest radiographs may show hyperinflation and bronchial thickening but are nonspecific and do not reflect severity of disease.

Tx Smoking cessation is necessary to slow the progression of disease. Bronchodilators including β_2-adrenergic agonists and anticholinergic drugs are the mainstay of treatment. Corticosteroids are reserved for patients with severe disease. **See Cecil Essentials 17.**

Sleep Apnea

Pφ Sleep apnea is a disorder usually characterized by resistance to airflow in the upper airway. The patient's airway frequently collapses while sleeping, leading to hypopnea and/or apnea. These events can lead to oxygen desaturation producing cardiovascular disease and subsequent dyspnea.

TP Patients usually have a history of loud snoring associated with a choking sensation, and excessive daytime sleepiness. Patients will usually complain of morning headache, nocturia, and waking up with dry mouth and nightmares. Patients tend to be overweight with a crowded oropharynx and large neck circumference.

Dx Nocturnal polysomnography is the gold standard for the diagnosis of sleep apnea. Apnea is defined as the cessation of airflow for at least 10 seconds. It is classified as central apnea if there is neither respiratory effort nor airflow, obstructive apnea if there is continuous respiratory effort, or mixed if there is absence of effort at the beginning followed by demonstrated effort without airflow.

Tx Behavior modification is important in treating this condition; weight loss can be curative. Continuous positive airway pressure (CPAP) is the treatment of choice; it improves oxygen saturation, sleep quality, daytime alertness, and ultimately cardiac function. **See Cecil Essentials 20.**

Pleural Effusion

Pφ Pleural effusion occurs when more fluid enters the pleural space than is removed. Pleural effusions are either transudative or exudative in character.

TP Dyspnea, cough, and pleuritic chest pain are the most common presenting symptoms. Fremitus and breath sounds are decreased over the effusion.

Dx Thoracentesis should be performed for diagnosis. An effusion is exudative if any one of the following three criteria is present: (1) the ratio of pleural fluid to serum protein is >0.5, (2) the ratio of pleural fluid to serum lactate dehydrogenase (LDH) is >0.6, (3) pleural fluid LDH is greater than two thirds the upper limit of the normal serum LDH. Transudates are associated with low concentrations of protein. Transudates result from imbalances of hydrostatic and oncotic forces, and are caused by limited conditions such as congestive heart failure and cirrhosis. Exudates have higher protein concentrations and tend to be inflammatory or neoplastic in origin.

Tx Treat the underlying cause. Empyema, as a complication of pneumonia, must be drained with an appropriately sized chest tube and in a timely manner to prevent complications (i.e., need for video-assisted thorascopic surgery [VATS] or thoracotomy). **See Cecil Essentials 21.**

Pneumothorax

Pφ Pneumothorax is the accumulation of air in the pleural space. It is classified as spontaneous or traumatic. Spontaneous pneumothorax is further classified as primary in the absence of clinical lung disease or secondary in the presence of lung disease. Trauma is the most common cause of pneumothorax.

TP Pleuritic chest pain and dyspnea are the most common symptoms. Tachycardia, decreased breath sounds, and hyper-resonance are the usual physical exam findings.

Dx A visceral pleural line on chest radiograph is diagnostic. Mediastinal shift is observed if a tension pneumothorax is present.

Tx Treatment depends on the severity of the pneumothorax. A small pneumothorax does not require therapy. Chest tube placement (i.e., tube thoracostomy) is indicated for large pneumothoraces or those demonstrating tension. **See Cecil Essentials 21.**

Interstitial Lung Disease (ILD)

Pφ ILDs, or diffuse parenchymal lung diseases, are a collection of disorders that are grouped together because of their similar presenting symptoms and radiographic appearance. The pathophysiology is thought to initially center on the lung interstitium, but alveolar, pleural, and other lung structural changes may result as the disease progresses. They are classified and named primarily based on their underlying histopathology.

TP Persistent and progressive dyspnea and nonproductive cough are common initial symptoms. Crackles or "Velcro rales" are commonly auscultated with most forms of ILD but are commonly absent in granulomatous diseases including sarcoidosis.

Dx PFT will reflect a restrictive ventilatory defect. A chest radiograph may reveal diffuse reticular opacities; however, a thoracic CT scan will demonstrate interstitial changes with greater sensitivity and specificity. When the radiographic appearance is not definitive enough for diagnosis, a lung biopsy, via bronchoscopy or VATS, may be necessary.

Tx Treatment depends entirely on the histopathologic subtype. Corticosteroids are commonly prescribed as initial anti-inflammatory therapy and may be effective in sarcoidosis but are unlikely to be of any benefit for usual interstitial pneumonitis, a subtype with no known effective medical therapy. Chronic respiratory failure due to ILD is a common indication for lung transplantation. **See Cecil Essentials 18.**

Practice-Based Learning and Improvement: Evidence-Based Medicine

Title
Salmeterol and fluticasone propionate and survival in chronic obstructive pulmonary disease

Authors
Peter MA, Calverley MD, Anderson JA, et al.

Institution
Multiple institutions

Reference
N Engl J Med 2007;356:775–789

Problem
The treatment of COPD with inhaled corticosteroids and β-adrenergic receptor agonists is well established. However, to date there had not been a trial addressing the survival benefit of combination therapy.

Intervention
Randomized, double-blind trial comparing salmeterol 50 µg plus fluticasone propionate 500 µg twice daily, with placebo, salmeterol alone, or fluticasone propionate alone for 3 years

Quality of evidence
Level I

Outcome/effect
The combination therapy did not reach the predetermined level of statistical significance.

Historical significance/comments
Although the trial did not reach its primary outcome, which was a 25% reduction in mortality, it showed that subjects receiving combination therapy had significant reduction in exacerbations, use of oral steroids, and protection against deterioration of lung function.

Interpersonal and Communication Skills

Communicate the Importance of Smoking Cessation

One of the major risk factors for chronic bronchitis, COPD, asthma, and heart disease is cigarette smoking. Studies have shown that patients are more likely to be compliant with medications and lifestyle modification when their physician has properly educated them about their condition. Patients should be provided resources to assist in their own efforts to quit smoking. Their families need to be engaged to be sources of encouragement and support, and it is essential for the physician to take the time to speak personally with family members on this point. Helpful tips for the patient include setting a quit date, informing family and friends about his or her plan to quit smoking, and joining a support group such as Nicotine Anonymous or 1-800-QUITNOW. Provide patients with a list of products that can help with the feeling of nicotine withdrawal including the nicotine patch, gum, lozenges, and medications.

Professionalism

Avoid Conflicts of Interest When Accepting Gifts from Patients

In caring for patients with long-standing chronic illnesses, like COPD, physicians develop relationships with patients and families that span many years. Even early in the course of a relationship, there may be clinical moments where, in the eyes of patients, their physician has literally saved their life by getting them through a serious exacerbation of the disease or working with them to alleviate significantly uncomfortable symptoms. Occasionally patients express their gratitude in the form of gifts, especially at holiday time. Hospital systems maintain specific guidelines when it comes to accepting gifts, which may even include monetary thresholds for acceptance.

Systems-Based Practice

Hospital Reimbursement

Your patient has COPD and requires admission to the hospital. While hospitalized, his respiratory status worsens. He is transferred to the intensive care unit and requires intubation and mechanical ventilation. He later develops pneumonia and a deep venous thrombosis. How does the hospital get paid for the services provided? In the past, hospitals would assemble a list of all of the services provided, and the insurance companies would pay for them; however, this is no longer the case. Hospitals typically get paid in one of three ways. The most common is a *case payment*, in which the hospital receives a fixed amount of money for the patient's entire stay; the amount is dependent on the diagnoses of the patient and does not factor in the specifics of the individual case, unless length of stay is exceptionally long. Second, hospital reimbursement can be made by *per diem payments*, in which the hospital receives a defined amount of money for every day that the patient is in the hospital. Third, some hospitals participate in a *capitation payment* structure, in which they receive a fixed amount of money per member per month to provide care for a group of patients; the hospital receives this money whether or not the patients are actually admitted to the hospital. As a result, the hospital and the entire health system have a financial incentive to keep patients healthy and out of the hospital.

Chapter 15
Cough (Case 9)

Ranjit Nair MD and Sean M. Studer MD, MSc

Case: The patient is a 66-year-old man with a history of diet-controlled diabetes mellitus who works as a truck driver and has not seen a physician for more than 10 years. He presents to the emergency department from home in respiratory distress for the past 8 hours. He admits to having rhinorrhea for the past 2 weeks, a cough with rust-colored sputum for the past 3 days, and right-sided chest pain every time he takes a deep breath. He also reports some shaking chills and subjective fever. He has never been hospitalized and has no known drug allergies. He smokes cigarettes only when he is drinking alcohol on the weekends.

On physical exam, his vital signs are temperature of 102.1° F orally, pulse of 105 beats per minute (bpm), respiratory rate of 30 breaths per minute, and blood pressure of 135/80 mm Hg; pulse oximetry is 85% on room air and 96% on 4 L oxygen via nasal cannula. In general, he appears anxious. On lung exam, crackles are auscultated at the right base.

Differential Diagnosis

Pneumonia	Acute bronchitis	Influenza
Tuberculosis	Bronchiectasis	Cystic fibrosis

Speaking Intelligently

Cough is one of the most common respiratory complaints. Acute cough can be a symptom of a potentially life-threatening illness (e.g., pneumonia or pulmonary embolism), although most episodes are of minor consequence. Chronic cough (i.e., persisting for more than 3 weeks) is much more common and is associated with conditions such as postnasal drip, asthma, gastroesophageal reflux, chronic bronchitis, and bronchiectasis. Medications, specifically angiotensin-converting enzyme (ACE) inhibitors, may also be associated with chronic cough. Lung cancer and aspiration are less common etiologies of chronic cough.

PATIENT CARE

Clinical Thinking

- Duration may be an important clue as to etiology of cough.
- Acute cough occurs in those with upper and lower respiratory infections, inhalation of noxious gases or chemicals, and aspiration.
- Chronic cough (i.e., cough persisting for more than 3 weeks) is usually explained by a careful history and physical examination, followed by specific diagnostic tests.
- For a cough to be worrisome enough for the patient to undergo a thorough assessment, it should be present for at least 6 to 8 weeks, not just a residual effect from a preceding respiratory tract infection.

History

- Include associated symptoms of fever, chills, pleuritic chest pain, and dyspnea.
- If the cough is productive, the character of the sputum should be described, including whether or not blood is present.
- Medication history may detect current use of an ACE inhibitor.
- A history of cigarette smoking, including current use and pack-year history, should prompt counseling regarding smoking cessation.
- Risk factors for pulmonary tuberculosis should be sought.
- Multiple prior lung infections might suggest bronchiectasis.
- Cystic fibrosis should be considered in the right clinical setting.

Physical Examination

- Given the possibility that postnasal drip may trigger cough, a thorough examination of the nose, sinuses, pharynx, and larynx should be performed.
- Associated wheezing may suggest the diagnosis of asthma or obstructive lung disease, or perhaps congestive heart failure.
- In the patient with acute cough, dullness to percussion, increased tactile fremitus, and localized crackles are strongly suggestive of bacterial pneumonia.

Tests for Consideration

- **Sputum analysis** (Gram stain, acid-fast bacillus [AFB] smears, cytology) and culture may suggest a specific etiology, although fiberoptic bronchoscopy may be required if the diagnosis remains elusive. — $56
- **Blood cultures** in patients in whom bacterial pneumonia is suspected — $15

- Rapid testing of **nasopharyngeal specimens for influenza A and B antigens** in the appropriate clinical setting $34
- **Pulmonary function tests (PFTs)** if airway obstruction is considered likely $52

IMAGING CONSIDERATIONS

→ **Chest radiography** is indicated, although a radiographic image rarely identifies the etiology. $45

→ **CT imaging** may be required, depending upon the likely etiology. $334

Clinical Entities	Medical Knowledge

Pneumonia

Pφ Pneumonia is an infection of the lung parenchyma, usually occurring after aspiration of upper airway resident flora or inhalation of aerosolized material. Bacterial pneumonia is a common cause of morbidity and mortality in older adults, especially in those with comorbidities such as diabetes or congestive heart failure. A yearly influenza vaccine is important for all patients. Immunization with the 23-valent pneumococcal polysaccharide vaccine is recommended for all patients over the age of 64 years and other adults with specific risk factors. The 13-valent pneumococcal conjugate vaccine has recently been FDA approved for use in adults 50 years of age and older. The most common pathogens associated with community-acquired bacterial pneumonia are *Streptococcus pneumoniae, Mycoplasma pneumoniae, Chlamydophila pneumoniae, Legionella pneumophila, Haemophilus influenzae,* and *Moraxella catarrhalis.*

TP The patient with community-acquired bacterial pneumonia typically has fever, rigors, pleuritic chest pain, and cough productive of purulent sputum. In patients with atypical pneumonia the fever may be low grade, and patients may have nonproductive cough and no chest pain. However, there is variation in the initial symptoms and signs such that these presentations cannot reliably distinguish the specific infectious cause of the pneumonia. On physical exam there may be signs of consolidation, which can include the presence of localized dullness to percussion, increased tactile fremitus, and crackles. Examples of these sounds can be heard at this website: http://www.rale.ca/Repository.htm.

Dx Chest radiographs (PA and lateral) reveal parenchymal opacities, which will establish the diagnosis in the appropriate clinical setting (i.e., leukocytosis, fever, sputum production). A CBC with differential may help determine if there is a bacterial infection, and specifically, a differential will indicate a "left shift," or increased numbers of bands, which suggests that a bacterial etiology is likely. An ABG measurement may help determine the severity of hypoxemia and inpatient disposition (i.e., whether admission to the ICU is necessary).

Pathogen identification should be attempted before antimicrobial therapy is initiated; this is especially important whenever the result is likely to change the approach to management, especially in patients in whom drug-resistant pathogens are eventually isolated. Pretreatment blood cultures should be drawn. Sputum Gram stain and culture should be obtained in hospitalized patients, because sensitivities can help guide therapy and help tailor antibiotics toward a specific organism. Patients with severe community-acquired pneumonia should also have urinary antigen tests sent for *L. pneumophila* and *S. pneumoniae*, although the *Legionella* urinary antigen is positive only in cases caused by *L. pneumophila* serogroup I. CT of the chest is usually not necessary to establish the diagnosis but should be considered if a complicated infection is considered (e.g., post-obstructive pneumonia or empyema). HIV testing should be considered in patients who have risk factors associated with this disease. A diagnosis of HIV would be important to know so as to also consider infection caused by certain opportunistic organisms (e.g., *Pneumocystis jirovecii* or *Mycobacterium tuberculosis*).

Tx The decision concerning disposition of patients with community-acquired pneumonia is sometimes difficult; there have been a few proposed criteria to determine inpatient vs. outpatient therapy. One proposed severity of illness criterion that may help predict a complicated course is CURB-65. Scoring 1 point for each criterion, patients with a score of 0–1 can be managed as outpatients, those with a score of 2 should be admitted to a hospital ward, and those with scores of 3 or higher often require ICU care. Another model (the pneumonia severity index [PSI] from the Pneumonia Patient Outcomes Research Team) stratifies patients into five mortality risk classes. Although use of these objective criteria may decrease the number of hospitalized patients with community-acquired pneumonia, subjective factors (such as the ability of the patient to safely and reliably take oral medications) must be considered. Admission to an ICU is required for patients with community-acquired pneumonia who develop septic shock requiring vasopressors or have acute respiratory failure requiring intubation and mechanical ventilation.

Specific antimicrobial recommendations for patients with community-acquired pneumonia depend on resistance of pathogens to commonly used antimicrobial agents and local susceptibility patterns. In previously healthy outpatients with community-acquired pneumonia and no history of antimicrobial use within the past 3 months, therapy should be a macrolide (e.g., azithromycin or clarithromycin) or doxycycline. Recommended empiric antimicrobial therapy for a hospitalized non-ICU patient includes a respiratory fluoroquinolone (e.g., levofloxacin, gemifloxacin, or moxifloxacin) or a macrolide combined with a β-lactam (e.g., ceftriaxone or cefuroxime). For patients admitted to the ICU, a β-lactam plus either azithromycin or a respiratory fluoroquinolone should be used. For patients in whom infection caused by methicillin-resistant *Staphylococcus aureus* (MRSA) is also possible, vancomycin or linezolid should be added. **See Cecil Essentials 22, 99.**

Acute Bronchitis

Pφ Bronchitis is inflammation of the respiratory system, which includes the nasal passages down to the trachea and bronchi but does not include the lung parenchyma, so the chest radiograph is clear. Acute bronchitis is most commonly a result of a viral infection that may last up to 2 weeks but occasionally may be caused by bacterial pathogens similar to those that cause community-acquired pneumonia.

TP Patients with bronchitis usually present with a several-day history of symptoms such as fever, rhinorrhea, and cough, which may be purulent in nature. Patients may suffer from sore throat due to a pharyngeal irritation secondary to cough. Patients also may have been exposed to a sick contact.

Dx A patient with clinical presentation of an acute onset of fever, cough, and purulent sputum, but normal chest radiograph, is most likely suffering from acute bronchitis. The Gram stain, culture, and sensitivity of the sputum may reveal the infecting pathogen but are not usually part of routine management.

Bronchiectasis

Pφ Bronchiectasis is irreversible dilation and destruction of large bronchi secondary to chronic infection and inflammation. This destruction is facilitated by the fact that most of the causes are related to impaired mucus clearance. The most common causes are repeated infections, cystic fibrosis, and immune defects.

TP A patient who has developed bronchiectasis due to persistent infections may present with cough for many years and a history of recurrent pneumonia. A patient with bronchiectasis may have a similar presentation to that of a patient with pneumonia, but the patient with bronchiectasis has many recurring episodes associated with a longer course. Eliciting a history of copious sputum production on a daily basis also points to a possible diagnosis of bronchiectasis.

Dx A diagnosis of bronchiectasis can be made on chest radiograph, where one will find the typical tram-track appearance caused by dilated, thick-walled bronchi. High-resolution CT of the chest is the test of choice, however, for defining the extent of bronchiectasis; the test is nearly 100% sensitive and specific. The CT typically shows thickening of the airways characterized by tram-track parallel lines or ring shadows representing thickened bronchial walls when imaged in cross-section.

Tx Treatment is based on treating the underlying cause of the bronchiectasis. It is important to treat infections with appropriate antibiotics, so cultures and sensitivities should be known. Prophylactic antibiotics are considered controversial because of their implication in promoting infection caused by resistant organisms. Chest physiotherapy and postural maneuvers have been shown to improve or facilitate mucus clearance but have never been shown to improve morbidity or mortality. In some patients, surgery to remove a localized area of bronchiectasis may be an option to reduce future morbidity. **See Cecil Essentials 17.**

Cystic Fibrosis (CF)

Pφ CF is a result of a defect in the gene encoding the CFTR protein. This protein is responsible for the flow of electrolytes across cell membranes. The abnormalities in salt and water transport across the cell membrane in patients with CF lead to a change in the composition of respiratory tract secretions, resulting in impaired mucociliary clearance, predisposition to infection, and airway obstruction. This eventually progresses to end-stage lung disease in many affected patients.

TP Patients with CF typically present with recurring episodes of pneumonia throughout their lifetime. CF has several clinical manifestations in other organ systems, especially the gastrointestinal, endocrine, and reproductive systems. The gastrointestinal manifestations include fat malabsorption due to exocrine pancreatic insufficiency and distal intestinal obstruction syndrome (DIOS) due to thick mucus blocking bowel contents. Pancreatic damage also results in reduced insulin secretion and diabetes, while infertility is common in males due to congenital absence or obstruction of the vas deferens.

Dx The sweat chloride test, in combination with newborn screening and/or a sibling with a known diagnosis of CF, can establish the diagnosis. The sweat chloride test must be repeated twice to be considered abnormal; in adults, a level > 60 mEq/L and a typical clinical presentation are suggestive of CF. The criteria for diagnosis are elevated sweat chloride level on two occasions or identification of mutations known to cause CF in both CFTR genes or in vivo demonstration of characteristic abnormalities in ion transport across the nasal epithelium, plus one or more phenotypical features of CF, as follows: sino-pulmonary disease, characteristic nutritional or gastrointestinal disorders, obstructive azospermia, salt loss syndrome, a sibling with CF, or positive newborn screening.

Tx Treatment is based on treating the underlying pneumonia and using techniques that will help the patient with mucociliary clearance. Because of the increased likelihood of bacterial infection caused by *Pseudomonas aeruginosa* and *Burkholderia cepacia*, antimicrobial therapy should be directed toward these pathogens. Postural techniques have been shown to improve mucus drainage but not to improve morbidity or mortality. At this time prophylactic antibiotics are not recommended, as they may increase drug resistance yet bring about no improvement in pulmonary function or rate of infection. Dornase alfa, which selectively cleaves DNA, reduces mucus viscosity and, as a result, improves airflow in the lung. Improved pulmonary function decreases the risk of bacterial infection. Supplemental oxygen may be used in patients with exercise-induced or resting hypoxemia. In patients with end-stage lung disease, transplantation may be an option. **See Cecil Essentials 17.**

ZEBRA ZONE

a. Aspiration pneumonitis: Aspiration pneumonitis refers to the aspiration of substances that are toxic to the lower airways, independent of bacterial infection. The prototype and best-studied clinical example is chemical pneumonitis associated with aspiration of gastric acid. Aspiration pneumonitis may present similarly to bacterial pneumonia both clinically and radiologically; however, unlike pneumonia, it is not a result of an infectious etiology and therefore does not need to be treated with antibiotics.

Practice-Based Learning and Improvement: Evidence-Based Medicine

Title
A prediction rule to identify low-risk patients with community-acquired pneumonia

Authors
Fine MJ, Auble TE, Yealy DM, et al.

Institution
Department of Medicine, Graduate School of Public Health, University of Pittsburgh, PA 15213, USA

Problem
Severity of pneumonia and disposition of the pneumonia patient

Quality of evidence
Level II-1

Outcome
The prediction rule accurately identifies patients with community-acquired pneumonia who are at low risk for death and other adverse outcomes. This prediction rule may help physicians make more rational decisions about hospitalization for patients with pneumonia.

Interpersonal and Communication Skills

Preempt Future Anxieties by
Discussion of the Natural Course of Disease
Despite patients' general understanding of the diagnosis of pneumonia, you will provide reassurance and reduce anxiety if you explain the testing used to establish the diagnosis, the antimicrobial regimen you have selected, the anticipated length of hospitalization, and the expected recovery time. For example, most patients will notice improvement of their symptoms within 3 to 5 days but should expect to limit their activities for several weeks, or even longer in

older adults or those with chronic lung diseases. Some patients will inevitably develop complications such as lung abscess, hypoxemia, empyema, and respiratory failure requiring mechanical ventilation. If you have explained these potential scenarios in advance, emphasizing that you are able to treat these complications when encountered, your patient will be less frightened should one of these complications occur. Take the time to explain problems that could arise.

Professionalism

Commitment to Patient Welfare: Be Proactive in Determining Patients' Wishes Regarding Mechanical Ventilation

Older patients who develop pneumonia that leads to severe hypoxemia and/or hypercarbia may require ICU admission and mechanical ventilation. For some patients with long-standing lung disease, repeated intubation and mechanical respiratory (ventilator) support are a common occurrence. When caring for patients with severe and/or chronic pulmonary infections, it is important to discuss their wishes regarding mechanical ventilation. The discussion should include patients' families, because it is often a family member who will be the health care proxy when the patient cannot make a decision for himself or herself. A patient's autonomy must be acknowledged. Both the medical caregivers and the health care proxy must act in accordance with a patient's wishes. Some patients whose quality of life has already been permanently compromised by their pulmonary disease may opt against prolonged (and presumably futile) mechanical ventilation and may wish to establish a "Do Not Intubate" (DNI) order to avoid this situation.

Systems-Based Practice

Standardize Practice through Evidence-Based Guidelines

Many organizations have initiated processes to develop evidence-based practice guidelines to provide guidance to physicians to standardize medical practice. These guidelines are not meant to apply to the care of all patients with a specific diagnosis, but typically provide strengths of specific recommendations and quality of evidence (based on the design and outcome of clinical trials or opinions of respected authorities) leading to a specific recommendation. The Infectious Diseases Society of America and the American Thoracic Society have collaborated on guidelines for the diagnosis and management of community-acquired pneumonia.[1] These guidelines include recommendations for site-of-care decisions, diagnostic testing, antibiotic treatment, duration of therapy, and prevention (see also Chapter 6, Common Problems in Ambulatory Internal Medicine).

Reference

1. Mandell LA, Wunderink RG, Anzueto A, et al. Infectious Diseases Society of America/American Thoracic Society Consensus Guidelines on the Management of Community-Acquired Pneumonia in Adults. Clin Infect Dis 2007;44:S27–S72.

Chapter 16
Hemoptysis (Case 10)

Sudheer Nambiar MD and Pratik Patel MD

Case: The patient is a 70-year-old African-American woman who was admitted with massive hemoptysis. Seven months before this admission, she had been diagnosed with pulmonary tuberculosis based on the presence of acid-fast bacilli in her sputum. Tuberculous arthritis was confirmed by ankle cartilage biopsy. Antituberculous treatment with isoniazid, rifampin, pyrazinamide, and ethambutol was prescribed, and excision drainage and internal fixation of her right ankle was performed. One month before this admission she had presented with massive hemoptysis. At the time of that admission, coarse crackles were auscultated over her left lower chest.

Differential Diagnosis

Tuberculosis	Pulmonary embolism	Diffuse alveolar hemorrhage syndromes
Lung cancer	Aspergilloma (mycetoma)	

Speaking Intelligently

Hemoptysis, the expectoration of blood, can range from blood streaking of sputum to the presence of gross blood in the absence of any accompanying sputum. Bronchitis, neoplasms such as bronchogenic carcinoma, and bronchiectasis are the most common causes of hemoptysis depending upon the patient population studied. Bronchitis is more likely to cause blood-tinged sputum, while bronchiectasis and tuberculosis are more often associated with massive hemoptysis. Although the term hemoptysis typically refers to expectoration of blood originating from the lower respiratory tract, it must be recognized that blood from the upper respiratory tract and the upper gastrointestinal tract (i.e., pseudo-hemoptysis) can be expectorated and can mimic blood coming from the lower respiratory tract. The term massive hemoptysis is reserved for bleeding that is potentially life-threatening.

PATIENT CARE

Clinical Thinking
- Determine the amount of blood expectorated, as the differential diagnosis and urgency of the problem differ based on whether there is blood-tinged sputum or massive hemoptysis.
- Massive hemoptysis has been defined by a number of different criteria, often ranging from more than 100 mL at one time to more than 600 mL of blood over a 24-hour period.
- Massive hemoptysis is a rare but always a potentially life-threatening event.
- Death from massive hemoptysis is usually due to complications related to aspiration of blood, not to exsanguination. Thus, the initial evaluation should occur simultaneously with efforts to control the patient's airway and respiratory status.

History
- Determine whether the blood was expectorated or is more likely from an upper respiratory or gastrointestinal source.
- Question the patient regarding recent epistaxis, vomiting, or retching.
- The consistency of blood, and whether sputum is present, help to differentiate recent from past hemorrhage, and the presence of copious, purulent sputum supports an infectious source.
- The pattern of bleeding (e.g., episodic vs. monthly recurrences) and presence of constitutional symptoms should be ascertained. Symptoms such as fever, night sweats, and weight loss support lung abscess or tuberculosis as causes, whereas isolated weight loss is more consistent in patients with carcinoma.

Physical Examination
- Cachexia, Horner syndrome, unilateral supraclavicular lymphadenopathy, hoarse voice, and digital clubbing support an underlying cancer diagnosis.
- Gingival thickening and nasal septal perforation suggest Wegener granulomatosis.
- Fever and focal crackles heard during lung auscultation and corresponding dullness to percussion suggest lobar pneumonia.

Tests for Consideration

• Measurement of **hematocrit**	$4
• **Urinalysis**	$4
• **Tests of renal function**	$12
• **Coagulation profile**	$15
• **Fiberoptic bronchoscopy** may allow localization of the site of hemoptysis and visualization of endobronchial pathology causing the bleeding.	$732
• **Pulmonary angiogram** is performed when a vascular disorder is suspected, such as an arteriovenous malformation; **CT angiography** has reduced the need for formal angiograms.	$2087, $338

IMAGING CONSIDERATIONS

→ **Chest radiograph**	$45
→ **CT scan** if indicated	$334

Clinical Entities   Medical Knowledge

Tuberculosis

Pφ Following a marked decline in the incidence of TB in the United States over several decades, the incidence escalated dramatically and peaked in 1992. In the United States, important risk factors for TB infection are as follows: close contact with a person infected with TB; immigration from an endemic area (e.g., Africa, Asia, or Latin America); exposure to persons with untreated cases of TB in congregate living facilities (e.g., homeless shelters, correctional facilities, nursing homes, or other health care facilities); age; and residence in high-incidence locations (e.g., inner cities or foreign endemic areas). HIV-associated TB accounts for approximately 10% of TB cases in the United States; among TB patients between 25 and 44 years of age, 22% are known to be infected with HIV. A majority of TB cases in the United States now occur in foreign-born individuals emigrating from countries with high rates of endemic TB. The majority of cases of TB are caused by *Mycobacterium tuberculosis*, and the lungs are the major site of infection. Pulmonary manifestations of TB include primary, reactivation, endobronchial, and lower lung field infection. Reactivation TB represents 90% of adult cases in the non-HIV-infected population and results from reactivation of a previously dormant focus seeded at the time of the primary infection.

TP Low-grade fever lasting 14–21 days, chest pain, fatigue, cough, sputum production, night sweats, weight loss, arthralgias, and pharyngitis are some common symptoms. The physical examination is usually normal; pulmonary signs included pain to palpation and signs of an effusion. Complications of TB (i.e., hemoptysis, pneumothorax, bronchiectasis, and in some cases extensive pulmonary destruction) can also involve the lung. Most common sites of extrapulmonary involvement include the pleura, lymph nodes (particularly cervical and hilar), central nervous system (CNS) (as meningitis or tuberculoma), genitourinary system, blood, and bone marrow. TB can cause massive hemoptysis by sudden rupture of a Rasmussen aneurysm; this is an aneurysm of the pulmonary artery that slowly expands into an adjacent cavity because of inflammatory erosion of the external vessel wall, causing it to rupture.

Dx The most common abnormality on chest radiography is hilar adenopathy, occurring in 65% of patients. Pleural effusions, pulmonary infiltrates, nodules, and cavitations are also seen in varying frequency. The standard skin tuberculin test consists of 0.1 mL (5 tuberculin units) of purified protein derivative (PPD) administered subcutaneously, usually on the volar surface of the forearm. The reaction is read 48 to 72 hours after injection as induration, which suggests a history of infection with TB but does not mean that the patient has tuberculous disease. Similarly, positive blood tests (interferon-γ release assays that measure how the immune system reacts to the bacterium that causes TB) suggest that the patient has tuberculous infection but should not be used to diagnose active TB. Sputum samples for acid-fast bacilli smear and culture are an important diagnostic tool. If the smear is negative, bronchoscopy with brushings or bronchoalveolar lavage and transbronchial biopsy have been shown to be useful. The diagnosis of drug-resistant TB depends upon the collection and processing of adequate specimens for culture and sensitivity testing before the institution of therapy. Detection of mycobacterial growth on conventional media requires 4 to 8 weeks. Target amplification using nucleic acid amplification tests such as the polymerase chain reaction has been more sensitive than standard techniques.

Tx A four-drug antituberculous regimen is preferred, including isoniazid (INH), rifampin, pyrazinamide, and ethambutol. If the isolate is sensitive to both INH and rifampin by drug sensitivity testing, ethambutol can be discontinued; pyrazinamide, which has an early mycobactericidal effect, is usually discontinued after a total of 2 months. Massive hemoptysis from Rasmussen aneurysm, a dilated blood vessel in the vicinity of a tuberculous cavity, is a surgical emergency. **See Cecil Essentials 15, 22, 99.**

Lung Cancer

Pφ Lung cancer is the most common cause of cancer mortality worldwide for both men and women, causing approximately 1.2 million deaths per year. A number of environmental and lifestyle factors have been associated with the subsequent development of lung cancer, of which cigarette smoking is the most significant. Other risk factors include exposure to radiation therapy, asbestos, radon, metals (arsenic, chromium, and nickel), ionizing radiation, and polycyclic aromatic hydrocarbons. Lung cancers are classified as either small cell or non–small cell lung cancer (SCLC or NSCLC). This distinction is essential for staging, treatment, and prognosis. The relative incidence of adenocarcinoma has risen dramatically, and there has been a corresponding decrease in the incidence of other types of NSCLC and SCLC.

TP Common symptoms include cough, hemoptysis, chest pain, and dyspnea. Hemoptysis is reported by 25% to 50% of patients who are diagnosed with lung cancer. Lung cancers can often cause a post-obstructive pneumonia. Obstruction of the superior vena cava (SVC) causes symptoms that commonly include a sensation of fullness in the head and dyspnea. Physical findings include dilated neck veins, a prominent venous pattern on the chest, facial edema, and a plethoric appearance. Lung cancers arising in the superior sulcus cause a characteristic Pancoast syndrome manifested by pain (usually in the shoulder, and less commonly in the forearm, scapula, and fingers), Horner syndrome, bony destruction, and atrophy of hand muscles.

   The most frequent sites of distant metastasis are the liver, adrenal glands, bones, and brain. Neurologic manifestations of lung cancer include metastases and paraneoplastic syndromes. Symptoms from CNS metastasis are similar to those with other tumors and include headache, vomiting, visual field loss, hemiparesis, cranial nerve deficits, and seizures. Brain metastases are seen in 50% of patients with SCLC at autopsy.

Dx There are several options for sampling a primary tumor: imaging-guided percutaneous needle aspiration or biopsy, blind transbronchial fine-needle aspiration (TBNA), conventional flexible bronchoscopy with forceps biopsy, and endobronchial ultrasound (EBUS)–guided forceps biopsy.

In patients with pleural effusion, thoracentesis is a simple bedside procedure that permits fluid to be rapidly sampled, visualized, examined microscopically, and quantified. Malignant pleural effusions are typically exudative and may be serous, serosanguineous, or grossly bloody. The yield of pleural fluid cytology after a single thoracentesis (and examination of 50–100 mL) in patients with documented pleural involvement is about 60%.

Nonsurgical approaches, surgical approaches, or both, may be used to obtain a tissue sample from patients with suspected lymph node metastasis. Nonsurgical approaches include EBUS-guided TBNA, transesophageal endoscopic ultrasound-guided fine-needle aspiration (EUS-FNA), and conventional bronchoscopy with blind TBNA. Surgical approaches include mediastinoscopy and thoracoscopy.

Tx The mainstay of treatment for SCLC is chemotherapy and radiation therapy. For NSCLC, surgery is the choice of treatment up to stage IIIa. For stages IIIb and IV, chemotherapy and radiation therapy are the preferred treatments. **See Cecil Essentials 24, 57.**

Aspergilloma (Mycetoma)

Pφ Aspergilloma refers to the disease caused by a "ball" of fungal mycelia that can occur within a cavity, usually within the parenchyma of the lung. It is generally thought that the presence of *Aspergillus* in pulmonary cavities reflects saprophytic colonization and not actual tissue invasion. An aspergilloma usually arises in a preexisting cavity in the lungs. Any condition that causes cavitation in the lungs may subsequently be associated with the development of an aspergilloma; these include TB, sarcoidosis, neoplasms, other fungal infections such as histoplasmosis or coccidioidomycosis, cystic fibrosis, or invasive aspergillosis. The fungus ball is composed of fungal hyphae, inflammatory cells, fibrin, mucus, and amorphous debris. Within a pulmonary cavity, the mass may be free or attached to the wall of the cavity. The usual species of *Aspergillus* recovered from such lesions is *A. fumigatus*, but other species are also found.

TP Patients with pulmonary aspergilloma can be asymptomatic. The most frequent symptom directly related to the fungal mass is hemoptysis, which may occur in up to 75% of patients. Less commonly, patients can develop chest pain, dyspnea, malaise, wheezing, or fever that may be secondary to the underlying disease, bacterial superinfection of the cavity, or the aspergilloma itself.

Dx Chest radiography is useful in demonstrating the presence of a mass within a cavity. Typically, there is a solid mass surrounded by a radiolucent crescent (crescent sign, Monod sign). If the fungus ball is mobile, repeating the radiograph with the patient in the lateral decubitus position will show that the mass has moved. When chest radiography does not clearly delineate a cavity, CT scanning of the lungs can be used to demonstrate a cavity and any intracavitary structures. Cultures of the sputum may or may not be positive for the fungus. If there is no communication between the cavity and the bronchial tree, cultures will probably be negative. Sputum cultures, especially a single culture, cannot establish a diagnosis since *Aspergillus* is a common colonizer of an abnormal respiratory tract. However, the finding of a mass within a pulmonary cavity and the recovery of *Aspergillus* species, particularly from multiple sputum cultures, is strongly supportive of the diagnosis.

Tx Antifungal therapy provides limited benefit for the treatment of a single aspergilloma. The main indication for primary medical therapy with antifungals is if surgical intervention is not an option. Antifungal therapy is commonly used as adjunctive therapy following surgical resection; itraconazole, voriconazole, and possibly posaconazole have been recommended, although topical instillation of amphotericin B has been performed in some cases, either to control continued fungal growth or to try to limit the effects of the space-occupying lesion. The major mode of therapy for aspergilloma has been surgical resection of the cavity and removal of the fungal ball. Lobectomy is the most commonly employed procedure, although segmentectomy is sometimes adequate and pneumonectomy is occasionally required. The main indication for surgery is recurrent hemoptysis. **See Cecil Essentials 91, 109.**

Diffuse Alveolar Hemorrhage (DAH) Syndromes

Pφ A variety of diseases are associated with the development of DAH.

TP The onset of DAH is most often abrupt or of short duration (less than 7 days). Cough, hemoptysis, fever, and dyspnea are common initial symptoms. Some patients, however, present with acute severe respiratory distress requiring mechanical ventilation. The pulmonary examination is usually nonspecific, unless there are physical signs of an underlying systemic vasculitis or connective tissue disorder.

Dx The chest radiograph is nonspecific and most commonly shows new patchy or diffuse alveolar opacities. Recurrent episodes of DAH may lead to pulmonary fibrosis and interstitial opacities. Thoracic CT scanning confirms the presence of ground-glass or airspace-filling opacities that are usually diffuse and bilateral but may occasionally be unilateral. Laboratory findings in DAH are often nonspecific. A number of diseases that can result in the pulmonary-renal syndrome present with pulmonary hemorrhage in combination with rapidly progressive glomerulonephritis. In this setting there is an elevated serum creatinine concentration, usually with an abnormal urinalysis (containing red blood cells, white blood cells, proteinuria, and red cell and white cell casts). A positive antinuclear cytoplasmic antibody (ANCA) test can be associated with DAH due to Wegener granulomatosis or microscopic polyarteritis. Perinuclear ANCA (P-ANCA) with antimyeloperoxidase specificity enzyme-linked immunosorbent assay (anti-MPO ELISA) favors the diagnosis of microscopic polyarteritis or Churg-Strauss syndrome. The presence of antibodies specific to glomerular basement membrane (GBM) in the serum is diagnostic for anti-GBM antibody disease (Goodpasture syndrome). Antibodies directed against streptococcal antigens, including those specific to streptolysin O, DNase B, or hyaluronidase, or the documentation of positive blood cultures can suggest a diagnosis of post-streptococcal glomerulonephritis or bacterial endocarditis, respectively. Diagnostic clues can be found from the biopsy of affected tissue (usually kidney or lung).

Tx Glucocorticoids are the mainstay of therapy for the DAH syndromes associated with systemic vasculitis, connective tissue disease, Goodpasture syndrome, and isolated pulmonary capillaritis.

The decision to start additional immunosuppressive therapy for DAH (i.e., cyclophosphamide or azathioprine) is dependent upon the severity of the illness, the responsiveness to glucocorticoids, and the underlying disease. Plasma exchange is generally used in the treatment of DAH associated with Goodpasture syndrome. The possible role of intravenous immunoglobulin (IVIG) in patients with DAH due to vasculitis or other connective tissue diseases is unknown. **See Cecil Essentials 18.**

Pulmonary Embolism

Pφ PE refers to obstruction of the pulmonary artery or one of its branches by material (e.g., thrombus, tumor, air, or fat) that originated elsewhere in the body. Most emboli arise from thrombi in the deep venous system of the lower extremities. However, they may also originate in the right side of the heart or the pelvic, renal, or upper extremity veins. Most patients with acute PE have an identifiable risk factor at the time of presentation. These risk factors include immobilization, surgery within the last 3 months, stroke, paralysis, history of venous thromboembolism, malignancy, central venous instrumentation within the last 3 months, and chronic heart disease. Acute PE is a common and often fatal disease. Mortality can be reduced by prompt diagnosis and therapy. Unfortunately, the clinical presentation of PE is variable and nonspecific, making accurate diagnosis difficult. Impaired gas exchange due to PE cannot be explained solely on the basis of mechanical obstruction of the vascular bed and alterations in the ventilation-to-perfusion ratio. Gas exchange abnormalities are also related to the release of inflammatory mediators, resulting in surfactant dysfunction, atelectasis, and functional intrapulmonary shunting.

TP The most common symptoms are dyspnea at rest or with exertion, pleuritic chest pain, cough, greater than two-pillow orthopnea, hemoptysis, calf or thigh pain, calf or thigh swelling, and wheezing. The onset of dyspnea is usually within seconds or minutes. The most common signs are tachypnea, tachycardia, crackles, decreased breath sounds, an accentuated pulmonic component of the second heart sound, and jugular venous distension.

Dx Spiral (helical) CT scanning with intravenous contrast is now more commonly being utilized as the test of choice in patients with suspected PE. Other tests for consideration are lower extremity venous ultrasound, ventilation-perfusion (V/Q) scan, and echocardiography. Pulmonary angiography is the definitive diagnostic technique or "gold standard" in the diagnosis of acute PE.

Tx Anticoagulant therapy is indicated when there is a high clinical suspicion of PE or PE confirmed by CT angiography and no excess risk for bleeding. Anticoagulation prevents further clot formation but does not dissolve the existing thromboemboli or decrease the thrombus size. Thus, it should not be expected to affect mortality within the first hours of delivery. The efficacy of anticoagulant therapy depends upon achieving a therapeutic level of anticoagulation within the first 24 hours of treatment. Therapeutic options include subcutaneous low-molecular-weight heparin or intravenous unfractionated heparin. Thrombolytic therapy should be considered for patients with confirmed PE and hemodynamic instability. **See Cecil Essentials 19.**

Practice-Based Learning and Improvement

Title
Cryptogenic hemoptysis: from a benign to a life-threatening pathologic vascular condition

Authors
Savale L, Parrot A, Khalil A, et al.

Institution
Hôpital Tenon, Assistance Publique-Hôpitaux de Paris and Université Pierre et Marie Curie, Paris, France

Reference
Am J Respir Crit Care Med 2007;175:1181–1185

Problem
Data are limited regarding cause and outcome of patients with hemoptysis of unknown (cryptogenic) source.

Intervention
A cohort of 81 patients with cryptogenic hemoptysis were followed through their clinical course and for outcome following hospital discharge.

Outcome/effect
This was an observational study showing that the bleeding was controlled using nonsurgical approaches (bronchoscopy, bronchial artery embolization) in the majority of patients with cryptogenic hemoptysis.

Historical significance/comments
This was the first careful survey of cryptogenic hemoptysis and showed that Dieulafoy malformation of the bronchus may be involved in a subset of patients.

Interpersonal and Communication Skills

Different Diagnoses Mandate Different Communication Priorities

For patients with hemoptysis due to a bacterial infection of the lower respiratory tract, it is important to reassure them that the hemoptysis should resolve with antibiotic therapy. In patients who develop hemoptysis secondary to bronchogenic carcinoma, the priority of communication is to support the patient emotionally by providing detailed information regarding planned therapy and prognosis. Such communication may reduce the anxiety associated with the unknown and allow the patient to make informed decisions pertaining to surgery, chemotherapy, and radiation therapy. In patients with hemoptysis due to pulmonary tuberculosis, communication must be to both the patient and the staff regarding infection control, use of protective equipment, and meeting the reporting requirements of local public health agencies.

Professionalism

Maintain Patient Confidentiality

Open and accurate communication among members of the hospital care team for patients with hemoptysis, as for all patients, is essential to provide optimal patient care. At times, depending on the underlying etiology, patients with hemoptysis must be reported to local public health agencies. Note, however, that sharing details regarding a patient's medical condition with hospital staff *not* involved in the patient's care or with the patient's visitors or friends (without the expressed permission of the patient) is a violation of professional ethics. A breach in patient confidentiality may have legal implications under the privacy requirements of the Health Insurance Portability and Accountability Act (HIPAA). It is also important to be mindful of patient confidentiality when discussing patient information in public areas of the hospital, such as elevators and cafeterias. Information overheard by others violates confidentiality and may raise the concern of other patients and their families that *their* private medical information will not be treated confidentially.

Systems-Based Practice

Intensivists Improve Quality of Care in the ICU

The approach to the patient with hemoptysis requires an interdisciplinary approach that involves physicians, nurses, and technicians. For the patient with massive hemoptysis and a threatened or compromised airway, urgent evaluations by a pulmonologist and a thoracic surgeon are necessary; transfer to an

ICU setting is often required. Scientific evidence suggests that quality of care in an ICU is strongly influenced by whether *intensivists* are the care providers. Mortality rates seem to be significantly lower in hospitals where the ICU is exclusively managed by a board-certified intensivist. In ICUs with high-intensity staffing where intensivists manage or co-manage all patients, compared to low-intensity staffing where intensivists manage or co-manage only some or none of the patients, there is a 30% reduction in hospital mortality and a 40% reduction in ICU mortality. Based upon these data and because of the potential benefits for patients, the Leapfrog Group (an initiative driven by organizations that buy health care who are working to initiate breakthrough improvements in the safety, quality, and affordability of health care for Americans; http://www.leapfroggroup.org) has focused on ICU physician staffing as one of its safety standards.

Chapter 17
Pulmonary Nodule (Case 11)

Smitha Gopinath Nair DO *and Jennifer LaRosa* MD

Case: The patient is a 68-year-old woman with a history of hypertension and diabetes mellitus who recently moved to New York from Ohio and presents for her annual physical examination. She is noted to have a 35 pack-year history of cigarette smoking and briefly worked with her husband installing home insulation. She complains of productive cough upon awakening every morning and dyspnea with moderate activity. On physical examination she is noted to be well dressed and overweight. Her lung exam reveals mild wheezing, and she has some clubbing of her fingers. A routine chest radiograph reveals a 1-cm nodule in the right mid-lung field.

Differential Diagnosis

Primary lung cancer		Coccidioidal pulmonary nodule
Dirofilariasis	Hamartoma	*Histoplasma* pulmonary nodule

Speaking Intelligently

A solitary pulmonary nodule (SPN) is a common clinical problem. It is typically an incidental finding on chest roentgenogram or CT scan of the chest, and in one study was seen in 25% of healthy, asymptomatic individuals. The majority of nodules will have a benign etiology. However, since lung cancer is both asymptomatic and curable in its early stages, it is imperative that all nodules be considered malignant until proven otherwise. The recommendations for further testing to evaluate the pulmonary nodule vary according to the pretest probability. If the pretest probability is less than 5%, the nodule should be followed with serial CT scans at 3, 6, 12, and 24 months. If it is between 5% and 60%, options include CT scan, positron emission tomography (PET) scan, biopsy, or resection. A pulmonologist may be consulted for guidance. If the pretest probability is greater than 60%, biopsy and resection should be strongly considered. See Figure 17-1.

PATIENT CARE

Clinical Thinking
- An SPN is defined as a lesion greater than 8 mm and less than 3 cm in diameter; it is within normal lung parenchyma and causes no distortion of other structures.
- Nodules can be broadly categorized as benign or malignant, which can be determined only by a tissue biopsy.
- There are patient characteristics that can suggest one etiology as being more likely than another.
- The lesion should be inspected for shape, size, the presence and pattern of calcification, growth rate, location, and density.
- The patient should be assessed for malignancy risk factors, including advanced age, smoking, and occupational and environmental exposures, and PFTs should be performed.

History
- The presence of occupational and environmental risk factors, especially cigarette smoking, should be diligently sought. Tobacco smoking increases a patient's relative risk of lung cancer 10- to 30-fold over that of nonsmokers; this risk decreases after 5 years of smoking cessation but never falls to the level of a patient with no smoking history.
- Age is another leading risk factor. The older a person is, the greater the likelihood of malignancy. In one study, a solitary pulmonary nodule had a 65% chance of being malignant in patients over 50 years of age versus 33% in patients under 50 years of age.

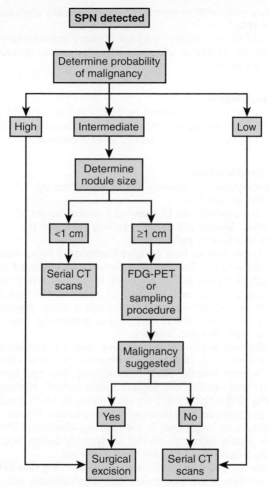

Figure 17-1 Algorithm for solitary pulmonary nodule. (Reproduced with permission from Weinberger SE. Diagnostic evaluation and initial management of the solitary pulmonary nodule. In: UptoDate, Basow, DS (Ed), UpToDate, Waltham, MA, 2011. Copyright © 2011 UptoDate, Inc. For more information visit www.uptodate.com.)

- A past medical history of malignancy raises the suspicion of metastatic lung disease. Extrapulmonary malignancies that are most likely to lead to pulmonary metastases include sarcoma, malignant melanoma, and carcinomas of breast, colon, kidney, and testicle.
- SPNs, by definition, do not affect surrounding tissue and, as such, are almost invariably asymptomatic.

- Cough is a nonspecific symptom and may accompany any potential cause of SPN.
- Weight loss can accompany malignant (primary and metastatic) causes of SPN, as well as infectious etiologies such as *Mycobacterium tuberculosis* infection.

Physical Examination

As stated earlier, an SPN is defined by its size (<3 cm) and the fact that it does not distort or affect surrounding tissues. Therefore, the SPN rarely, if ever, causes abnormal findings on physical exam.

Tests for Consideration

- **Chest radiographs** are generally the initial method by which SPNs are identified. $45
- Nodular characteristics on **CT scan**, such as size, border, calcification, density, and growth, can help to predict if a nodule is benign or malignant. $334
  - **Size:** Larger nodules have a higher likelihood of being malignant than smaller ones. The odds of malignancy are estimated at 0.2% for nodules smaller than 3 mm, 0.9% for nodules 4 to 7 mm, 18% for nodules 8 to 20 mm, and 50% for nodules larger than 20 mm.
  - **Border:** Smooth borders generally indicate a benign etiology, while irregular and spiculated borders suggest malignancy; these findings are not highly specific, however.
  - **Calcification:** Benign lesions can have "popcorn" calcifications (as with hamartomas), concentric calcifications, or central calcifications (may indicate infection-related granulomas). Eccentric, laminated, and stippled calcifications suggest a more ominous etiology.
  - **Density:** Hounsfield units (HU) are a means by which the density of a structure can be determined radiographically. Though this modality is no longer used in the routine evaluation of SPNs, higher density lesions (>164 HU) are typically benign, and lower density lesions (<147 HU) are often malignant.
  - **Growth:** Malignant lesions have a volume doubling time between 20 and 400 days. A doubling time of 100 days correlates with a 30% increase in the diameter of a SPN. Lesions that are stable in size on CT scans over a 2-year period are believed to have doubling times consistent with benign etiologies.
- **FDG-PET:** 18-fluorodeoxyglucose PET can help determine the likelihood of an SPN being malignant. It is most accurate when an SPN is greater than 1 cm. It has a high negative predictive value and a poor positive predictive value. A total of 78% of benign lung nodules will result in a normal FDG-PET, and 95% of malignant nodules will have an abnormal FDG-PET. Tumors with relatively low metabolic activity can produce false negative results; such examples include bronchoalveolar carcinoma and carcinoid. $1037

- **Nodule Sampling:** Biopsy of the SPN is imperative when malignancy is considered to be possible or likely. Biopsy techniques include transthoracic needle aspiration (TTNA), bronchoscopy with transbronchial biopsy (TBBX), and surgical resection.
  - **TTNA** is performed through the chest wall using either fluoroscopy or CT scanning to guide the biopsy needle. The overall diagnostic yield for suspected lung cancer is approximately 90%, a higher rate than that achieved with TBBX. TTNA biopsy success is increased with greater SPN size, increased number of needle passes, and the presence of an on-site histopathologist. $677
  - **Bronchoscopy** allows collection of airway cells using lavage, brushings, or direct biopsy methods such as needle or forceps. Though bronchoscopy has a high yield for central endobronchial lesions, most SPNs cannot be described as such. Therefore, bronchoscopy is the least likely maneuver to yield a positive biopsy result for the SPN. Fluoroscopy or EBUS helps localize the lesion and increase the diagnostic yield. Rates of success for nodules smaller than 2 cm vary from 10% to 50%. $732

Clinical Entities	Medical Knowledge

Primary Lung Cancer

Pφ   The pathophysiology of lung cancer is intricate and not completely understood. What is thought to influence pathogenesis are genes that produce proteins involved in cell growth and differentiation, cell cycle processes, apoptosis, angiogenesis, tumor progression, and immune regulation. When there is dysregulation between cell growth and apoptosis, this leads to malignancy. The identification of the mechanism that produces this asynchrony may lead to the development of better risk stratification, prevention, and therapy.

TP   Lung cancers that present as an SPN are typically incidental findings and have a better prognosis. Lung cancers that are found secondary to symptoms are more advanced and have a worse prognosis. Common symptoms include cough, dyspnea, hemoptysis, and weight loss. The most common cell type is adenocarcinoma, followed by squamous cell carcinoma and large cell carcinoma. Adenocarcinoma, large cell carcinoma, and the less common small cell carcinoma typically originate as a peripheral lesion, whereas squamous cell carcinoma is typically discovered as a central lesion.

Dx CT scan of the chest and PFTs are essential for all patients with a lesion potentially consistent with lung cancer. CT scan will reveal characteristics of the lesion that make it more or less likely to be malignant. Abnormal PFTs demonstrating a pattern consistent with emphysema make lung cancer a more likely diagnosis in a newly discovered SPN. All lesions with a possibility of lung cancer must be considered for biopsy or resection.

Tx Stage I lung cancer can be cured by resection. This reason alone makes appropriate workup of an SPN essential. More advanced stages of lung cancer can be treated with a combination of surgery, chemotherapy, and radiation therapy. Despite these treatment options, prognosis for advanced lung cancer remains poor.

Dirofilariasis

Pφ Pulmonary dirofilariasis is caused by *Dirofilaria immitis*, a zoonotic filarial nematode commonly carried in the gastrointestinal tracts of dogs, coyotes, wolves, and cats. Humans may become infected via the fecal-oral route through contact with these animals. The human represents a dead-end host where the filariae travel to the lungs and are consumed by the granulomatous process.

TP Human infections are usually asymptomatic. Rarely, individuals may have self-limited infection with chest pain, cough, hemoptysis, fever, and malaise.

Dx Definitive diagnosis is made only if the patient undergoes a biopsy. A peripheral eosinophilia of about 10% may also be present, but this finding is nonspecific for dirofilariasis. Serology using indirect hemagglutination or ELISA is available but not widely employed.

Tx No therapy is generally required. In rare cases, ivermectin followed by diethylcarbamazine may be necessary.

Hamartoma

Pφ Hamartomas result from an abnormal formation of normal tissue. They grow along with, and at the same rate as, the organ from whose tissue they are made. They rarely invade or compress surrounding structures. They are benign lesions usually arising from connective tissue and are generally formed of fat, cartilage, and connective tissue cells. Lung hamartomas are more common in men than in women.

TP Hamartomas are generally asymptomatic. Some lung hamartomas can compress surrounding lung tissue, but this is generally not debilitative or even noticed by the patient, especially for the more common peripheral lesions. The great majority of them form in the connective tissue on the surface of the lungs, although about 10% form deep in the linings of the bronchi.

Dx CT scan may show characteristic cartilage and fat cells. When it does not, it may be confused with a malignancy, and biopsy may become necessary.

Tx They are treated, if at all, by surgical resection. The prognosis is excellent.

Coccidioidal Pulmonary Nodule

Pφ Coccidioidomycosis is an infection caused by a dimorphic fungus, most commonly *Coccidioides immitis*. The majority of cases in the United States occur in the San Joaquin River Valley and Saguaro Desert. Infection may be acquired by inhalation of a single arthroconidium. Within the lung, the arthroconidium becomes spherical and enlarges. In several days the mature spherules rupture, releasing endospores into the infected tissue. Each endospore is capable of producing more spherules and further disseminating the disease. In most cases, however, the spherules are consumed and contained by granulomatous inflammation.

TP The majority of patients will be asymptomatic or have a self-limited illness with cough and fever.

Dx Isolation of the organism in culture establishes the diagnosis. Other options include serologic tests for antibodies and nucleic acid amplification tests such as PCR. PCR testing is 100% sensitive and 98% specific. Biopsy is an alternate way to make the diagnosis. Staining with hematoxylin and eosin, periodic acid–Schiff, or Grocott–methenamine silver stain will demonstrate the organism.

Tx Treatment is rarely necessary, as the disease is usually self-limited. However, immunocompromised hosts, such as those with malignancy or HIV infection, will need to receive antifungal therapy in the form of fluconazole or itraconazole. An amphotericin B preparation should be considered only in severe or widely disseminated cases.

Histoplasma Pulmonary Nodule

Pφ Lungs are the port of entry for *Histoplasma capsulatum*. Within the United States it is most common in the midwestern states. Macrophages initially ingest but cannot kill the fungus. Cellular immunity develops in 10–14 days after exposure in immunocompetent hosts. Sensitized T lymphocytes, tumor necrosis factor, and interferon-α are important mediators in the host defense against *Histoplasma* infection.

TP Less than 5% of patients develop symptoms. For those who do, symptoms are nonspecific and may include fever, chills, headache, myalgias, anorexia, cough, and chest pain.

Dx Serologic tests for *Histoplasma*-specific antibodies reveal the diagnosis. Histopathology using stains for fungi, culture, and antigen detection in the urine, blood, or bronchoalveolar lavage fluid may also be employed.

Tx Most infections by *Histoplasma* are self-limited, and no therapy is required. However, immunocompromised patients or those exposed to a large inoculum may require antifungal therapy. Itraconazole is used in mild to moderate histoplasmosis, and an amphotericin B preparation is used for severe infections.

ZEBRA ZONE

a. **Rheumatoid nodule:** Found in patients with rheumatoid arthritis, is benign in nature.

b. **Pseudotumor/interlobular pleural effusion:** Occurs within pulmonary fissures and is commonly associated with transudative pleural effusions such as congestive heart failure (CHF).

c. **Fibroma:** Benign tumor composed of connective tissue.

d. **Arteriovenous malformation**

e. **Bronchogenic cyst:** Rare cystic lesion, most are benign. It may transform into a sarcoma or carcinoma.

Practice-Based Learning and Improvement: Evidence-Based Medicine

Title
Early Lung Cancer Action Project (ELCAP)

Authors
Henschke C, McCauley D, Yahnkelevitz D, et al.

Institution
Cornell, Columbia, New York University medical centers, New York, NY, USA; McGill University, Montreal, PQ, Canada

Reference
Lancet 1999;354:99–105

Problem
Overall 5-year survival of lung cancer is about 12%. Five-year survival for stage I cancer is 70%. This implies that lung cancer screening would improve survival.

Intervention
A total of 1000 asymptomatic patients who had smoked the equivalent of at least 10 pack-years underwent lung cancer screening with low-dose spiral CT and chest radiograph.

Outcome/effect
CT scans detected more benign and malignant nodules compared to chest radiographs (benign, 20.6% vs. 6.1%; malignant, 2.7% vs. 0.7%). Over 95% of the nodules were benign based on radiographic stability or tissue biopsy. Of the 27 malignancies identified, 23 of them were stage I disease. This study brings two major points to light: (1) CT scan identified three to four times as many SPNs as chest radiographs, and (2) the majority of identified malignancies were stage I and curable with resection.

Historical significance/comments
This was the first screening and follow-up study that employed CT scanning for detecting lung nodules in the hopes of detecting lung cancer at an earlier stage than chest radiography.

Interpersonal and Communication Skills

Develop a Sensitive Style to Deliver Unexpected News
A solitary nodule is found incidentally on approximately 0.20% of chest radiographs and even more frequently on CT scans of the thorax. As a physician, you will frequently be called upon to deliver news of an unexpected finding. Though the initial conversation about such a finding may be one of many such conversations during the course of your career, hearing such news for the first time creates a memory for your patient that may be "replayed" frequently. It is

important that your initial contact about an unexpected finding
be informative, honest, straightforward, and sensitive. If you can
honestly be reassuring, let the patient know that the finding "may
not be important or significant, though it may require further
workup." If you believe this is a finding of great concern, you should
articulate your concerns but with terms that are as hopeful as
possible, such as "We'll define this and determine what the very best
treatment should be."

Professionalism

Recognize Personal Boundaries When Caring for Family Members
If one of your close relatives is found to have a solitary pulmonary
nodule on routine chest radiograph, how would you interact with her
or his doctor? Would you insist she or he be seen immediately by a
specialist at a high-volume center? Would your relative expect you to
set up immediate follow-up? As a basic principle, it is important to
respect the boundary between family and professional practice. Honor
the relationship that relatives may have with their physician, and
offer your opinion only when asked. If you have serious concerns
about the management, it is appropriate to ask your relative if he or
she would like you to discuss the issues with his or her physician.
Alternatively, sometimes physicians do not make necessary calls to a
relative's doctor because they think it may be easier to address the
problem on their own, or they don't want to "bother" a colleague
with more phone calls to return. It's important to recognize that
objectivity doesn't always exist when a patient is a close relative or
friend. It can be difficult to relinquish the role of physician in the
family environment, but, in general, being the family member is the
best role to take; let your relative's physician be the doctor.

Systems-Based Practice

Standardizing Follow-up for Incidentally Detected Lung Nodules
Optimizing successful outcomes for patients with pulmonary nodules
should be based on a standardized and thorough approach to each
patient. The Fleischner Society has provided recommendations for
follow-up for patients with incidental pulmonary nodules (Table
17-1). These recommendations are based on nodules smaller than
8 mm detected incidentally on nonscreening CT scans with varying
recommendations based on whether the patient is at *low risk*
(minimal or absent history of smoking and of other known risk
factors for cancer) or *high risk* (history of smoking and of other
known risk factors for cancer). These recommendations are useful in
providing guidance for management of the patient with a pulmonary
nodule.

Table 17-1 Recommendations for Follow-up and Management of Nodules Smaller Than 8 mm Detected Incidentally at Nonscreening CT

Nodule Size (mm)*	Low-Risk Patient†	High-Risk Patient‡
≤4	No follow-up needed§	Follow-up CT at 12 months; if unchanged, no further follow-up‡
>4-6	Follow-up CT at 12 months; if unchanged, no further follow-up‡	Initial follow-up CT at 6-12 months, then at 18-24 months if no change‡
>6-8	Initial follow-up CT at 6-12 months, then at 18-24 months if no change	Initial follow-up CT at 3-6 months, then at 9-12 and 24 months if no change
>8	Follow-up CT at around 3, 9, and 24 months, dynamic contrast-enhanced CT, PET, and/or biopsy	Same as for low-risk patient

Note: Newly detected indeterminate nodule in persons 35 years of age or older.
*Average of length and width.
†Minimal or absent history of smoking and of other known risk factors.
‡History of smoking or of other known risk factors.
§The risk of malignancy in this category (<1%) is substantially less than that in a baseline CT scan of an asymptomatic smoker.
‡Nonsolid (ground-glass) or partly solid nodules may require longer follow-up to exclude indolent adenocarcinoma.
From MacMahon H, Austin JH, Gamsu G, et al. Guidelines for management of small pulmonary nodules detected on CT scans: a statement from the Fleischner Society. Radiology, November 2005;237:395–400. Copyright 2005 Radiological Society of North America.

Suggested Readings

Gould MK, Maclean CC, Kuschner WG, et al. Accuracy of positron emission tomography for diagnosis of pulmonary nodules and mass lesions: a meta-analysis. JAMA 2001;285:914–924.

Henschke C, McCauley D, Yahnkelevitz D, et al. Early Lung Cancer Action Project. Lancet 1999;354:99–105.

MacMahon H, Austin JH, Gamsu G, et al. Guidelines for management of small pulmonary nodules detected on CT scans: a statement from the Fleischner Society. Radiology 2005;237:395–400.

Midthun DE, Swensen SJ, Jett JR. Approach to the solitary pulmonary nodule. Mayo Clin Proc 1993;68:378–385.

Santambrogio L, Nosotti M, Bellaviti N, Pavoni G, Radice F, Caputo V. CT guided fine needle aspiration cytology of solitary pulmonary nodules: a prospective, randomized study of immediate cytologic evaluation. Chest 1997;112:423–425.

Schreiber G, McCrory DC. Performance characteristics of different modalities for diagnosis of suspected lung cancer: summary of published evidence. Chest 2003;123(1 Suppl):115S–128S.

Siegelman SS, Zerhouni EA, Leo FP, et al. CT of the solitary pulmonary nodule. Am J Roentgenol 1980;135:1–13.

Toomes H, Delphendahl A, Manke H-G, Vogt-Moykopf I. The coin lesion of the lung. A review of 955 resected coin lesions. Cancer 1983;51:534–537.

Wallace JM, Deutsch AL. Flexible fiberoptic bronchoscopy and percutaneous needle lung aspiration for evaluating the solitary pulmonary nodule. Chest 1982;81:665–671.

Zerhouni EA, Stitik FP, Siegelman SS, et al. CT of the pulmonary nodule: a cooperative study. Radiology 1986;160:319–327.

Chapter 18
Teaching Visual: How to Interpret a Chest Radiograph

Irtza Sharif MD and Sean M. Studer MD, MSc

As with interpretation of other radiologic studies, reading chest radiographs should be approached by the novice reader in a systematic fashion. There are a few simple steps that the student may use to glean valuable information from a chest radiograph. This process begins with identifying technique, learning the features of the normal film (Fig. 18-1), and then methodically reviewing and characterizing the radiograph for apparent abnormalities.

As with all films, one must first *identify* the *type* of film and the *quality* of the study; if these are appropriate, then one must systematically review the visible anatomic structures. For a chest radiograph, this includes the **lung fields,** the **mediastinum,** surrounding **soft tissues,** and the **bony structures.** There are also nonanatomic structures such as lines and implanted devices that should be reviewed. Keep in mind that the radiograph compresses three dimensions down to two, so there is loss of detail for which you need to account. Also, remember that the radiodensities of different structures in the chest may be the same, so the viewer often cannot differentiate between soft tissues. In fact, it is best to think of structures in terms of three densities: **(1) air, (2) soft tissue and fluid,** and **(3) bone.**

When interpreting the film, note the positioning of the patient and consider the direction of the radiation beam. Typically, radiographs are taken in one of three directions: **AP, PA, and lateral.**

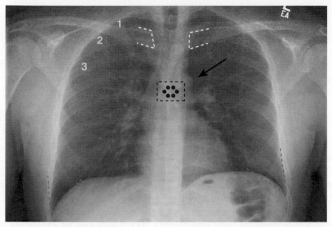

Figure 18-1 Normal chest radiograph (aka plain chest radiograph).

- **AP:** the x-ray beam enters the front of the chest and hits the film, which is **posterior** to the patient (the portable chest radiograph is an AP study).
- **PA:** the x-ray beam enters the patient's back and penetrates the chest before the film, which is placed along the patient's anterior chest wall. **The PA film is the preferred method of obtaining a chest radiograph, as it more accurately reflects the size of the cardiac and mediastinal silhouettes.**
- **Lateral** view (often combined with the PA view): the radiation beam usually enters the right side of the patient, with the patient's left side against the film.
- Additional views (or variations in above styles) are also possible if you need to evaluate particular findings. An example is a **decubitus** view, which might be obtained so as to differentiate a pleural effusion from consolidation.

Regarding the quality of the film, it is important to consider *penetration, rotation, and inspiration.* Penetration refers to the adequacy of the radiation dose given to expose the film. This dose is variable, since patients' body sizes (i.e., amounts of subcutaneous soft tissue) are variable. An inadequate radiation dose will make it difficult to evaluate denser tissues such as bone and soft tissue. A high dose may overexpose the less-dense lung tissue, making it difficult to differentiate subtle patterns. An easy way to determine if a film is properly penetrated is by looking at the mediastinum; the vertebrae and the spinous processes should be easily visible (note the red dots on Figure 18-1). Rotation of the film can be determined by looking at the distance of the medial head of the clavicles from the spinous processes; they should be equidistant if there is no rotation (note the white dashes on Figure 18-1). Examining adequacy of inspiration is a fundamental part of deciding if a chest radiograph is adequate. A good inspiration will allow you to see 6 or more anterior ribs, or 10 or more posterior ribs, above the right hemidiaphragm (note the yellow numbers on the right anterior ribs on Figure 18-1). We have started the count for you. How many anterior ribs do you count above the right hemidiaphragm?

When evaluating the lung fields, there are numerous pathologic abnormalities that may be present; however, many of these abnormalities might appear the same on a chest radiograph. For this reason it's best to think of the findings in terms of their *radiographic appearance*, which may help the reader arrive at a proper differential diagnosis. Things to note are the *location* of a finding, *symmetry* (i.e., does it appear on the contralateral side?), and whether a finding is associated with a *previously known diagnosis*.

For example, the appearance of a nodule (or small opacity) on a radiograph within the lung parenchyma (Fig. 18-2) can be caused by a number of entities such as *neoplasm, granuloma, focal pneumonia, vascular phenomena* (such as vessels on end), or an *infarct*. Knowing if the opacity was present previously can help you assess it for growth; increased growth over time often suggests *malignancy*. There are also particular properties that can help differentiate a benign from a malignant lesion, but they are not completely reliable; these are discussed in Chapter 17, Pulmonary Nodule.

Another important lung finding is a *cavity* (Fig. 18-3A and B). A cavity is an opacity that may appear to have a different density within it (i.e., the center may be more radiolucent). The interior of the cavity may contain fluid (see Fig. 18-3B) or other radio-opaque substance.

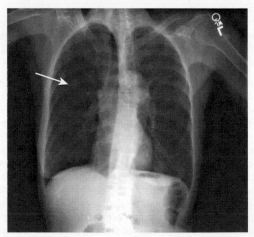

Figure 18-2 A solitary pulmonary nodule in the right chest (*arrow*).

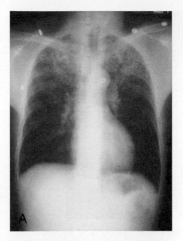

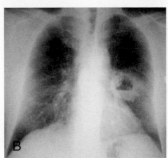

Figure 18-3 **A**, Radiolucent area in the left lung apex indicative of a lung cavity. **B**, A large, thick-walled cavitary lesion noted in the left chest with a horizontal opacity located within the cavity suggesting an air-fluid level.

Cavities may be ***malignant,*** may be ***caused by an infectious agent,*** or may result from an ***infarct.***

More diffuse findings can be subtle and pose difficult diagnostic challenges. Generally, such **diffuse findings** should be described based on the **pattern** noted. Common patterns are **consolidation, reticular, nodular,** and **cystic.**

- A ***consolidation*** is generally a large single opacity in which the bronchial tree is visualized within the consolidation, so-called air bronchograms. **The position of the opacity may give a hint as to its location.** For example, if the right- or left-side heart borders are not preserved, the blurred border may indicate that there is a (contiguous) pneumonia affecting the right middle lobe (Fig. 18-4) or lingula, respectively. Consolidation patterns are typical of pneumonia.
- A ***reticular pattern*** is one in which the opacity consists of multiple lines that often appear to be crisscrossing. Reticular patterns are

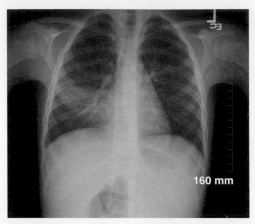

Figure 18-4 Consolidation of the right middle lobe. (Courtesy of Richard Ruchman, MD)

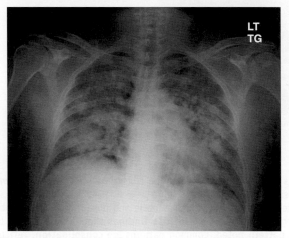

Figure 18-5 Diffuse nodular opacities affecting the lung bilaterally with relative sparing of the lung periphery.

often seen in connective tissue and fibrosing (interstitial scarring) diseases such as systemic lupus erythematosus and idiopathic pulmonary fibrosis. A reticular pattern may also be seen in specific types of pneumonia, such as pneumonia caused by *Pneumocystis jirovecii*.

■ A ***nodular pattern*** is one in which the opacity consists of many distinct, small opacities as may be seen in patients with ***metastatic disease, sarcoidosis, miliary tuberculosis, or Langerhans cell histiocytosis*** (Fig. 18-5).

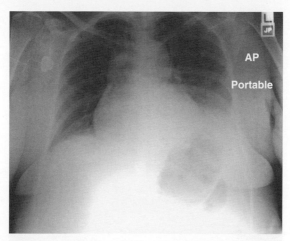

Figure 18-6 Dense opacification affecting the left hemithorax and obscuring the costophrenic angle suggestive of left pleural effusion.

- A ***cystic pattern*** is one in which numerous ring shapes are identified as may be seen in patients with bronchogenic cysts and pulmonary sequestrations.

The radiograph should be evaluated for effusion and proper diaphragmatic function. The costophrenic angles (note blue dashes on Fig. 18-1) are usually sharp, acute angles. Blunting of this angle is a sign of probable pleural effusion (Fig. 18-6).

The right and left hemidiaphragms should be visualized domes with the liver under the right hemidiaphragm and usually a gastric air bubble below the left side. Air immediately under the right hemidiaphragm implies free air in the abdomen, which may be seen with rupture of an intra-abdominal viscus or (normally) after laparotomy.

The heart silhouette is a two-dimensional representation of a three-dimensional organ. As the chest radiograph does not differentiate ventricular content from ventricular muscle, it is not a good measure of cardiac function; nonetheless, a heart that is more than 50% the width of the intrathoracic cavity on a PA film is highly suggestive of cardiomegaly (Fig. 18-7).

A symmetrically enlarged heart (often termed the "water bottle" appearance) may be indicative of a pericardial effusion. Widening of the superior portion of the heart on the left may be evidence of left atrial enlargement.

Superior to the heart is the aorta. Usually the ascending and descending portions can be identified as well as the aortic notch (see arrow in Fig. 18-1). Widening of the mediastinum may be seen in patients with ascending aortic dissection, although it is not a specific phenomenon; for example, although an uncommon disease, inhalational

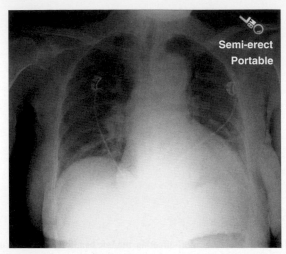

Semi-erect
Portable

Figure 18-7 Cardiac silouhette encompassing more than 50% of the width of the intrathoracic cavity on a PA film.

anthrax can result in a widened mediastinum. On a nonrotated film, widening of the mediastinum often implies mediastinal pathology, so further investigation is warranted even if aortic dissection is not high on the pretest differential diagnosis.

Soft tissue is often overlooked by inexperienced readers of chest films, since examination of the soft tissues is generally not the reason for which the study was ordered. However, the soft tissues should always be carefully examined and incidental findings should be noted and appropriately addressed. When something visualized on the chest film appears abnormal, always check for symmetry. Generally, if a similar structure in the soft tissues cannot be identified on the contralateral side, it is more likely to be an abnormal finding. Soft-tissue edema or masses may often appear as simple areas of asymmetry.

Bones that appear on a chest radiograph include cervical through upper lumbar vertebrae, the ribs, the scapulae, and the right humerus and left humerus. Search for periosteal elevation and thickening along the edge of these bones, and look for fracture lines within the bones. Such bony findings are often subtle and easy to miss. Cystic structures within the bones may also be visible. Although these are rare findings, it is important to review these structures for completeness.

One additional issue to consider when looking at a chest radiograph is the multitude of radio-opaque foreign bodies that may be visible. Such radio-opaque bodies commonly include catheters, pacemakers, and defibrillators, as well as endotracheal and nasogastric tubes. It is important to note the position of these objects and to ensure that they terminate at anatomically appropriate positions. For example, typically the tip of an endotracheal tube should be 3 to 5 cm from the carina; the tip of a central line catheter should be in the superior vena cava just above the right atrium.

By using a systematic approach to interpreting the chest radiograph, even the novice reader may gain important information about the patient.

Consider the resources listed below for further learning regarding chest radiograph interpretation.

Suggested Readings

http://www.learningradiology.com
   A detailed slide-based overview of basic chest radiograph interpretation (click on "Chest" from home page).
http://www.med-ed.virginia.edu/courses/rad/cxr/index.html
   A nice overview focusing on ICU chest films.

Section V
RENAL DISEASES AND ELECTROLYTE DISORDERS

Section Editor
Michael Gitman MD

Section Contents

19 **Acute Kidney Injury (Case 12)**
    Isai Gopalakrishnan Bowline MD *and Akhtar Ashfaq* MD

20 **Edema (Case 13)**
    Ellena Linden MD *and Dennis Finkielstein* MD

21 **Acid-Base Disorders (Case 14)**
    Kavita Ahuja DO *and Ilene Miller* MD

22 **Abnormal Electrolytes (Case 15)**
    Rabeena Fazal MD *and Alessandro Bellucci* MD

23 **Hematuria (Case 16)**
    Spirithoula Vasilopoulos MD *and Michael Gitman* MD

24 **Dysuria (Case 17)**
    Cindy Baskin MD *and Michael Gitman* MD

25 **Renal Mass (Case 18)**
    Azzour Hazzan MD

Chapter 19
Acute Kidney Injury (Case 12)

Isai Gopalakrishnan Bowline MD and Akhtar Ashfaq MD

Case: The patient is a 77-year-old man with diabetes, hypertension, and benign prostatic hypertrophy who was admitted with nausea, vomiting, and altered mental status. He was well until 2 weeks ago when he developed cough and myalgias. He was seen in a walk-in clinic and prescribed antibiotics for an upper respiratory infection (URI). Although his URI symptoms subsided, he subsequently developed loose stools and anorexia. For the past 2 days he has been unable to keep down any food, and the morning of presentation he became confused and disoriented. His family has noticed that he has not been urinating much but states that he has not been drinking much either. On exam he is hypotensive and tachycardic. Initial admission lab tests show a blood urea nitrogen (BUN) of 43 mg/dL and a creatinine (Cr) of 3.5 mg/dL.

Differential Diagnosis

Prerenal	Renal	Postrenal
Volume depletion	Vascular • Thrombotic thrombocytopenic purpura (TTP); hemolytic uremic syndrome (HUS)	Urinary tract obstruction • Ureteral obstruction • Bladder neck obstruction
Decreased effective circulation • Sepsis • Heart failure • Cirrhosis	Glomerulonephritis Acute interstitial nephritis (AIN) Acute tubular necrosis (ATN)	

Speaking Intelligently

Acute kidney injury (AKI) is defined by a sudden decline in kidney function as manifested by a decrease in glomerular filtration rate (GFR). The etiologies of AKI can be divided into three categories:

prerenal azotemia, postrenal azotemia, and intrinsic renal disease. Prerenal azotemia is a physiologic response to volume depletion or renal hypoperfusion. Postrenal azotemia is due to an obstruction of the urine flow from the kidney. Intrinsic azotemia is due to dysfunction of the renal parenchyma.

PATIENT CARE

Clinical Thinking
- Evaluate AKI with a systematic approach to reverse any potential causes, minimize any further injury, and initiate appropriate therapy.
- Determine whether the elevated serum creatinine is due to an acute insult or whether the creatinine is chronically elevated; our patients are often unaware of any previous disease, and it is helpful to look at their past creatinine values.
- Classify the patient based on urine output.
- Anuria is defined as a urine output less than 100 mL/day; anuria is rare and suggests complete obstruction, ATN, or a vascular event.
- Oliguria is defined as urine output less than 400 mL/day; oliguria is commonly seen with AKI, and patients with oliguria should be evaluated closely because fluid overload and electrolyte abnormalities can occur rapidly.

History
- When evaluating for prerenal azotemia, it is important to inquire about volume loss.
  - Has the patient had any diarrhea, vomiting, or burns, or is he or she taking diuretics?
  - Hypovolemia can cause profound renal failure especially in the setting of certain medications (nonsteroidal anti-inflammatory drugs [NSAIDs], angiotensin-converting enzyme [ACE] inhibitors or angiotensin II receptor blockers [ARBs]) and conditions (renal artery stenosis) that limit the kidneys' ability to compensate for hypovolemia.
  - Evaluate for any signs of infection that may also result in hypovolemia. Has the patient had any cough, congestion, diarrhea, dysuria, fevers, or chills?
  - Review the patient's medical history for any cardiac conditions that may reduce cardiac output and forward flow to the kidneys.
  - Inquire about liver disease, which may result in decreased renal perfusion as a consequence of arterial vasodilation in the splanchnic circulation.

- Eliminating postrenal etiologies involves assessing urine output.
  - Ask the patient about urgency, hesitancy, incontinence, and frequency of urination; each of these can be a symptom of incomplete bladder emptying.
  - Inquire about hematuria; gross hematuria can be a sign of stone disease or malignancy, and blood clots can lead to obstruction.
  - Review medications for use of anticholinergic medications that may cause urinary retention.
- Consider etiologies that precipitate intrinsic renal disease.
  - Review the patient's medical history for systemic diseases that affect the kidney, such as systemic lupus erythematosus (SLE), diabetes, hypertension, HIV infection, or hepatitis C.
  - Inquire about recent trauma, which can precipitate rhabdomyolysis.
  - Consider atheroembolic disease in patients with recent endovascular procedures.
  - Inquire about symptoms of fever, rash, and arthralgias to support the diagnosis of interstitial nephritis.
  - Review medications that may potentially cause ATN, such as the aminoglycosides.

Physical Examination

- Physical assessment of volume status is very important in evaluating the cause of AKI.
- Vital signs are crucial; look for hypotension and tachycardia to support the diagnosis of prerenal azotemia.
- Central venous pressure (CVP) tracings and wedge pressures can give a more definitive assessment of volume status.
- Dry mucous membranes and hyperthermia support hypovolemia as a diagnosis.
- Distended neck veins, S_3 gallop, bibasilar crackles, and edema support the diagnosis of heart failure with resultant renal hypoperfusion.
- Stigmata of cirrhosis may support the diagnosis of hepatorenal syndrome. Periorbital, sacral, and lower extremity edema can be signs of glomerular diseases.
- Examine the skin thoroughly to evaluate for any rash that may hint at an allergic interstitial nephritis.
- Blue toes with palpable pulses and livedo reticularis support the diagnosis of atheroembolic disease.
- Be mindful of physical exam findings associated with the systemic diseases that have renal manifestations, such as the malar rash of SLE. A palpable bladder, enlarged prostate, or palpable pelvic masses are suggestive of obstruction.

Tests for Consideration

- **Serum chemistries:** Chemistries are essential to determine the existence and extent of AKI and the presence of associated electrolyte abnormalities. The BUN/Cr ratio is often greater than 20:1 in prerenal azotemia. This occurs as a result of low urinary flow allowing increased reabsorption of urea. ATN usually results in a BUN/Cr ratio less than 20:1.　　　　　　　　　　　　　　　　　　$12

- **Urine sodium (UNa)** can be used to differentiate between prerenal azotemia and ATN. UNa less than 20 mmol/L is a good indicator of prerenal azotemia; maximal sodium retention is an attempt to conserve volume in the setting of hypoperfusion. ATN is usually associated with UNa greater than 40 mmol/L.　　　　　　　　　　　　　　　　　$7

- The **fractional excretion of sodium** (FE_{Na}) helps to differentiate between prerenal azotemia and ATN in the setting of oliguric AKI. FE_{Na} is calculated by: (UNa)(plasma Cr) / (plasma Na)(urine Cr). FE_{Na} less than 1% is observed with prerenal azotemia, while a FE_{Na} greater than 1% is seen in ATN. FE_{Na} is variable in postrenal etiologies. It is difficult to interpret FE_{Na} in the setting of diuretic use; in these cases, the fractional excretion of urea would be more helpful.　　$26

- **Urinalysis** is important in determining which part of the kidney is damaged. Significant proteinuria is often a sign of glomerular pathology. Isosthenuric urine is often a sign of ATN. The presence of absence of hematuria alters the differential of AKI.　　　　　　　　　　　　　　　$4

- **Microscopic examination of the urine sediment** can be very useful in diagnosing AKI. The urine sediment is usually normal in prerenal and postrenal azotemia. Renal tubular epithelial cells and muddy-brown granular casts may be visualized with ATN. Red blood cell casts exemplify glomerular injury. White blood cell (WBC) casts suggest interstitial nephritis or pyelonephritis.　　　　　　　　　　　　　　　　$3

- **Urine eosinophils** are often present in the setting of allergic interstitial nephritis.　　　　　　　　　　　　　　　　　　$4

IMAGING CONSIDERATIONS

→ **Renal sonography** is the imaging test of choice. It is used to determine kidney size and symmetry as well as to look for evidence of obstruction. When bladder outlet obstruction is suspected, a bladder sonogram with post-void measurements can be added onto the study. A post-void residual of greater than 100 mL supports the diagnosis of obstruction.　　　　　　　$96

Clinical Entities	Medical Knowledge

Volume Depletion

Pφ Volume depletion activates central baroreceptors, which results in activation of the renin-angiotensin-aldosterone system, release of antidiuretic hormone (ADH), and activation of the sympathetic nervous system. These mechanisms result in systemic vasoconstriction and sodium and water retention, which maintains renal blood flow. Within the kidney, renal hypoperfusion causes dilatation of the afferent arterioles and constriction of the efferent arterioles, maintaining GFR. In cases of prolonged hypoperfusion, these mechanisms are overwhelmed and decompensation develops, resulting in decreased GFR and resultant AKI.

TP Patients present with a history of volume loss (i.e., vomiting, diarrhea, diuretic use, bleeding). On exam they are often hypotensive, tachycardic, and orthostatic.

Dx Expected laboratory findings include an elevated BUN and creatinine with a BUN/Cr ratio > 20 : 1, $Fe_{Na} < 1\%$, and UNa < 20 mmol/L. Urine sediment is bland.

Tx Restore renal blood flow. Intravenous fluids aid in returning perfusion pressures to the normal range. Crystalloids are preferred for resuscitation. Colloids such as packed-red-cell transfusions are indicated if the patient is bleeding. **See Cecil Essentials 28, 32.**

Heart Failure

Pφ Even though circulatory volume is overloaded on exam, decreased cardiac output results in a decreased effective circulation. The central baroreceptors become activated, resulting in the same neurohumoral response the body has to volume depletion. Initially the body compensates by systemic vasoconstriction with sodium and water retention, but if these mechanisms are overwhelmed, decreased GFR and AKI will develop.

TP Patients may have extensive cardiac histories with low ejection fractions. They usually present with decompensated heart failure with jugular venous distension, pulmonary edema, and lower extremity swelling.

Dx Expected laboratory findings include an elevated BUN and creatinine with a BUN/Cr ratio $> 20:1$, $FE_{Na} < 1\%$, and UNa < 20 mmol/L. Urine sediment is bland.

Tx Restore renal blood flow by improving cardiac function. Administer diuretics to assist in decreasing the work load on the heart. Inotropic support may be necessary to augment renal perfusion in refractory cases. **See Cecil Essentials 6, 28, 32.**

Thrombotic Thrombocytopenic Purpura/Hemolytic Uremic Syndrome (TTP/HUS)

Pφ TTP and HUS are characterized by fibrin and platelet thrombi in the microvasculature of various organs, primarily affecting the kidneys and brain. The inciting event appears to be injury to the endothelium, resulting in dysregulation of the coagulation/complement system and unchecked thrombosis. In typical HUS, the mechanism is associated with exotoxins found in certain bacteria that bind microvascular endothelium, leading to vascular damage and thrombi formation. With TTP and atypical forms of HUS, the underlying mechanism results from defects in proteinases or other factors that are crucial to the coagulation system.

TP The classic findings associated with both TTP and HUS consist of thrombocytopenia, microangiopathic hemolytic anemia, renal failure, neurologic symptoms, and fevers. The degree of renal failure varies between these two entities; HUS more commonly presents with overt renal failure. Neurologic symptoms include confusion, headaches, seizures, and even coma. In typical HUS, additional symptoms may include abdominal pain and bloody diarrhea.

Dx Diagnosis is primarily based on clinical assessment of the above constellation of symptoms. The microangiopathic anemia demonstrates signs of hemolysis (i.e., elevated lactate dehydrogenase [LDH], low haptoglobin, elevated bilirubin). Schistocytes can be seen on examination of the peripheral smear.

Tx Although the pathology is similar for both of these disorders, distinguishing between them is crucial to management. Plasmapheresis/plasma exchange is considered first-line therapy in patients with TTP and atypical HUS. Additional treatment modalities include intravenous immunoglobulin (IVIG), plasma infusion, and steroids. Patients with typical Shiga toxin–induced HUS fare well with supportive management. **See Cecil Essentials 29, 31, 32.**

Glomerulonephritis

Pφ Acute glomerulonephritis (GN) occurs as a result of glomerular inflammation. When the inflammation is so profound that it causes renal failure in days to weeks, the syndrome is called rapidly progressive GN. The pathologic finding in acute GN is cellular proliferation around the glomerular tuft, which is termed crescent formation. Crescent formation occurs when glomerular injury results in breaks in the glomerular basement membrane, allowing deposition of fibrin in Bowman space. The fibrin deposition causes epithelial cell proliferation and macrophage infiltration, which results in crescent formation. The etiologies of acute GN are varied and include both vasculitides (e.g., Wegener granulomatosis, microscopic polyangiitis) and immune complex diseases (e.g., SLE, post-streptococcal GN, endocarditis, IgA nephropathy).

TP Patients with acute GN typically present with hypertension, proteinuria, microscopic hematuria, and acute renal failure (ARF). The ARF can be oliguric or nonoliguric. If the acute GN is part of a systemic illness such as lupus or endocarditis, the patient will have additional symptoms suggestive of those clinical entities.

Dx Expected laboratory findings include an elevated BUN and creatinine. The urinalysis reveals an active urine sediment with microscopic hematuria, proteinuria, and red blood cell casts. A serologic evaluation and a kidney biopsy are often necessary to determine the cause of the acute GN.

Tx The treatment of an acute GN depends on the underlying cause. When acute GN is due to a systemic illness, such as endocarditis or streptococcal infection, the underlying condition should be treated. When the acute GN is the result of an autoimmune disease, such as lupus or Wegener granulomatosis, the treatment often requires immunosuppressive medications. **See Cecil Essentials 29, 32.**

Acute Interstitial Nephritis

Pφ The histologic finding in AIN is an inflammatory cell infiltrate within the renal interstitium in response to a medication or infection. The inflammatory cell infiltrate, which is made up primarily of lymphocytes, leads to interstitial edema and tubular damage. Although the provoking factor varies, animal studies have shown that both cellular and humoral mechanisms are important in its pathogenesis.

TP Patients with drug-induced AIN present with ARF occurring days to weeks after starting a new medication. The ARF can range from mild elevations in creatinine to oliguric renal failure requiring dialysis. Affected individuals may report associated fevers, rash, arthralgias, or flank pain.

Dx Expected laboratory findings include an elevated BUN and creatinine. Urinary sediment typically reveals microscopic hematuria, non-nephritic–range proteinuria, pyuria, and WBC casts. Eosinophiluria is a hallmark of this disease but also can be seen with other renal injuries. Definitive diagnosis can be made only through renal biopsy.

Tx Management is primarily supportive, requiring discontinuation of the offending agent. Corticosteroid therapy has been employed in more severe cases of AIN and may hasten recovery. Often a renal biopsy definitively diagnosing AIN is mandated before beginning therapy. **See Cecil Essentials 27, 30, 32.**

Acute Tubular Necrosis

Pφ ATN can be caused by prolonged hypoperfusion, exogenous nephrotoxins (medications, contrast agents), or endogenous nephrotoxins (myoglobin, hemoglobin, or uric acid), resulting in direct tubular damage and irreversible cellular injury. ATN commonly occurs within a hospital setting.

TP Ischemia is the most common cause of ATN, and affected patients may present with hypotension and marked volume depletion. When ATN is the result of a nephrotoxic injury, the patient will often have a history of a recent contrast study, evidence of trauma, or a history of tumor lysis syndrome.

Dx Laboratory studies show an elevated BUN and creatinine with a BUN/Cr ratio < 20:1. In addition, high UNa and an FE_{Na} >1% characterize ATN. The urine sediment shows tubular epithelial cells and granular casts. A definitive diagnosis can be made with renal biopsy but is rarely necessary.

Tx Most cases of ATN resolve once the offending agent is removed. In the setting of rhabdomyolysis and tumor lysis syndrome, intravenous hydration may prevent the tubular damage. Depending on the severity of tubular damage and level of preexisting renal function, hemodialysis may have to be initiated. **See Cecil Essentials 32.**

Urinary Tract Obstruction

Pφ Obstruction at any level of the urinary tract, irrespective of the etiology, will increase pressure in the collecting systems resulting in compensatory dilatation proximal to the lesion. If left untreated, this will result in a decreased net glomerular filtration pressure and overall decline in GFR. The extent of injury is determined by the severity and duration of the obstruction.

TP Presentations may vary widely. Patients may give a history of flank or suprapubic tenderness depending on the etiology and site of obstruction. If obstruction is complete, anuria may be reported. Patients with partial obstruction may complain of urgency or frequency. Obstruction is commonly seen in patients with enlarged prostates, history of stones, or neurogenic bladders.

Dx Laboratory findings include an elevated creatinine. Chemistries may reveal hyperkalemia and suggest type IV renal tubular acidosis (RTA). Sonography of the kidneys and bladder will show the site of obstruction.

Tx For bladder outlet obstruction, placement of a urinary catheter is usually sufficient. If a catheter cannot be placed, a suprapubic cystostomy can be employed. Ureteral obstruction is treated with cystoscopy and stent placement, or placement of percutaneous nephrostomy tubes. **See Cecil Essentials 30, 32.**

ZEBRA ZONE

Many medications have been associated with renal failure through a variety of mechanisms. It is important to be aware of the common culprits when evaluating patients with AKI. In addition to reviewing medication lists with patients, always inquire about over-the-counter medications, herbal preparations, and vitamins. Often patients do not divulge this information without being prompted. Below is a list of common drugs implicated in renal failure.*

- ACE inhibitors or ARBs
- Cyclosporine
- Tacrolimus
- Cisplatin
- Lithium
- Methotrexate
- Indinavir
- Tenofovir
- NSAIDs
- Amphotericin B
- Aminoglycosides
- Fluoroquinolones

*There are many more agents associated with renal injury; this list is not comprehensive.

Practice-Based Learning and Improvement: Evidence-Based Medicine

Title
Mortality after acute renal failure: models for prognostic stratification and risk adjustment

Authors
Chertow GM, Soroko SH, Paganini EP, et al.

Institution
Multiple centers

Reference
Kidney Int 2006;70:1120–1126. ©2006 Nature Publishing Group

Problem
Acute renal failure in critically ill patients

Intervention
Identifying clinical predictors of mortality in acute renal failure

Quality of evidence
Level II

Outcome/effect
PICARD study is a comprehensive analysis of demographic and clinical factors associated with mortality in 618 patients in ARF evaluated at three discrete time points. On the day of ARF diagnosis, advanced age, liver failure, and high BUN were associated with increased mortality; however, these factors were not statistically significant early in the course. On the day of consultation, advanced age, liver failure, high BUN, Cr less than 2 mg/dL, low urine output, acute respiratory distress syndrome (ARDS), sepsis, and thrombocytopenia were all associated with poor outcomes. On the day of dialysis initiation, advanced age, liver failure, high BUN, and Cr less than 2 mg/dL were significant predictors of death. Of note, low urine output did not correlate with mortality.

Historical significance/comments
Ability to predict mortality in patients with ARF will enable physicians, patients, and family members to more appropriately make management decisions.

Interpersonal and Communication Skills

Communicate Clearly about Risks and Benefits of Hemodialysis

Given the varied clinical manifestations and outcomes in patients with AKI, it is imperative that physicians communicate effectively regarding the specific disease process, prognosis, and treatment options. Such knowledge allows patients to make informed decisions regarding their management, specifically when the initiation of hemodialysis is a consideration. The physician must ensure that patients understand the risks of dialysis, such as hemodynamic instability, rapid fluid/electrolyte shifts, and infections, as well as the potential permanence of the treatment. All risks and benefits should be thoroughly reviewed and all questions clearly addressed. In cases of critically ill patients who are unable to participate in the decision-making process, physicians should educate the appropriate family members.

Professionalism

Demonstrate Societal Responsibility with Respect to Allocation of Finite Resources

Physicians are under constant pressure to not only meet the individual needs of patient care but also provide cost-effective management in a setting of limited resources. Nephrologists are often asked to evaluate terminally ill patients for hemodialysis. In these cases it may be evident that hemodialysis will only prolong the dying process. It is the physician's professional responsibility to consider appropriate allocation of resources. This prevents any unnecessary treatment that not only exposes patients to avoidable harm and expense, but also diminishes the resources available for others. In these cases it is imperative that the physician has a clear and honest discussion with the patient regarding his or her overall prognosis.

Systems-Based Practice

Contrast-induced Nephropathy (CIN): Know the Benefits and Risks of Diagnostic Testing

CIN has become a significant source of hospital morbidity and mortality. With the increasing use of contrast dye in diagnostic imaging and interventional procedures, CIN has become a common cause of hospital-acquired AKI. Researchers have explored prophylactic measures to prevent onset of CIN, such as the use of N-acetylcysteine, sodium bicarbonate, and IV fluids. In addition, as a quality improvement initiative, much investigation has focused on identifying patients most at risk for developing CIN. It has been noted that patients with preexisting kidney disease, age over 75 years, and diabetes appear to be at highest risk of renal injury. Other notable risk factors include congestive heart failure, left ventricular dysfunction (ejection fraction < 40%), hypertension, use of an ACE inhibitor, and periprocedural hypotension. With this knowledge, nephrologists and radiologists are able to minimize risk in these individuals.

Chapter 20
Edema (Case 13)

Ellena Linden MD and Dennis Finkielstein MD

Case: A 55-year-old man presents with complaints of increasing lower extremity swelling over the past several months. He otherwise feels well and has no other complaints. He does not have chest pain but does become short of breath when climbing stairs; he attributes this to lack of exercise and deconditioning. He has no dyspnea at rest. His past medical history is unremarkable. He does not take any medications on a regular basis. This man does not smoke or use alcohol currently, although he admits to having been an alcoholic in the past. He does not use recreational drugs. On physical exam he appears well. Blood pressure is 110/60 mm Hg, and heart rate is 80 beats per minute. His weight is 80 kg, up from 72 kg a few months ago. Cardiovascular, pulmonary, and abdominal exams are unremarkable. There is significant pitting edema of both lower extremities.

Differential Diagnosis

Cardiac disease/ right-sided heart failure	Liver disease/ cirrhosis	Kidney disease/ nephrotic syndrome	Thyroid disease (see Chapter 48)

Speaking Intelligently

Nephrotic syndrome is a constellation of findings, which includes nephrotic-range proteinuria (defined as urinary protein excretion of greater than 3.5 g in a 24-hour period), edema, hypoalbuminemia, and dyslipidemia. Proteinuria in nephrotic syndrome might be the only sign of renal disease; these patients often have normal creatinine levels, lack of hematuria, and normal-appearing kidneys on radiologic imaging. Patients with nephrotic syndrome are predisposed to thromboembolic disease.

PATIENT CARE

Clinical Thinking
   Attempt to identify the cause.
• Determine whether nephrotic syndrome is part of a systemic disease (such as diabetes mellitus or SLE) or an isolated renal disease.

- Look for evidence of systemic disease; if one is not found, it is likely that the nephrotic syndrome is due to a purely renal disease.
- Establishing that nephrotic syndrome represents a purely renal disease is the beginning of the next level of investigation as to the exact cause; this step usually requires a percutaneous renal biopsy.

History

- **Cardiac dysfunction:** Does the patient have orthopnea or paroxysmal nocturnal dyspnea?
- **Thyroid disease:** Is the patient fatigued? Is there constipation? Cold intolerance? Weight gain?
- **Liver disease:** Is there history of hepatitis, cirrhosis, or jaundice?
- **Kidney disease:** Is there hematuria?
- Certain **medications** (most notably calcium channel blockers) can cause lower extremity edema; therefore, a medication history should also be obtained.

Physical Examination

- Is the **edema** localized or generalized, pitting or nonpitting, bilateral or unilateral?
- **Cardiac function:** Is there jugular venous distension? Are there murmurs? Is there pulmonary edema?
- **Liver function:** Is there ascites? Are the liver and spleen palpable? Is the patient jaundiced? Are there any signs of cirrhosis and portal hypertension (caput medusae, telangiectasia, gynecomastia)?
- **Venous obstruction:** Is the edema unilateral, increasing the suspicion of deep venous thrombosis?
- **Thyroid disease:** Is there unexplained weight gain? Alopecia? Bradycardia? Generalized slowing such as slow movement and speech?
- **Renal function:** Unfortunately, there are often no specific physical findings of kidney disease. However, signs of systemic diseases involving the kidneys can often be identified. For example, a patient with renal involvement from lupus will have systemic signs of lupus such as rash or arthritis.

Tests for Consideration

- **Liver function tests** to assess for cirrhosis $12
- **Thyroid-stimulating hormone (TSH) levels**, especially if the edema is nonpitting $24
- **Urinalysis** to look for proteinuria and microscopic hematuria $4
- **Serum creatinine** to look for renal disease $12
- Quantify the amount of proteinuria by obtaining either a **24-hour urine** collection or a spot urine protein-to-creatinine ratio. $12
- Check **lipid panel** and **serum albumin,** $19, $7

- Once the diagnosis of nephrotic syndrome is established, the next step is to determine the cause. There are many diseases that can cause nephrotic syndrome. We start with looking for systemic causes:
  - Does the patient have diabetes? Check **fasting glucose**. $7
  - Are there any signs of **lupus**? Check **antinuclear antibodies (ANA)**, and **complements C3 and C4**. $16, $34
  - Are there any signs of **amyloid or multiple myeloma**? Check **serum** and **urine protein electrophoresis** and immunofixation. $40
  - Does the patient have **HIV**? Check **HIV antibody**. $13
  - Does the patient have **hepatitis B or C**? Check the respective **antigens and antibodies**. $54

IMAGING CONSIDERATIONS

As part of workup of lower extremity edema, obtain cardiac echocardiogram, liver ultrasound, renal ultrasound, and lower extremity Dopplers, tailoring the sequence to the level of clinical suspicion of each based on the history and physical exam.

→ **Echocardiogram** to evaluate cardiac function $393
→ Obtain a **renal ultrasound** to evaluate the size of the kidneys. Large kidneys on the ultrasound can be a clue to certain kidney diseases, most notably diabetic nephropathy and HIV-associated nephropathy. $96
→ **Liver ultrasound** $96
→ **Lower extremity Doppler**, especially if the edema is unilateral $107

Clinical Entities   Medical Knowledge

Minimal-Change Disease

Pφ Another name for minimal-change disease is nil disease. The reason for the name is that the kidney biopsy looks normal when viewed under light microscopy. However, on electron microscopy, patients with minimal-change disease have diffuse fusion, or effacement, of epithelial cell foot processes.

TP Minimal-change disease is generally thought of as a childhood disease. While it is more common in children, it can occur at any age. The typical presentation is that of a sudden onset of classic nephrotic syndrome: nephrotic-range proteinuria, hypoalbuminemia, edema, and dyslipidemia. Serum creatinine is usually normal.

Dx In a child who presents with classic nephrotic syndrome, the diagnosis of minimal-change disease is presumed because of its high prevalence in this age group. Kidney biopsy is usually not done, and empirical therapy is initiated. In an adult presenting with nephrotic syndrome, however, a biopsy is obtained and the diagnosis of minimal-change disease is based on the biopsy findings. Minimal-change disease is usually idiopathic but can be associated with medications (e.g., NSAIDs) and certain malignancies.

Tx Glucocorticoids are the mainstay of therapy in both children and adults. **See Cecil Essentials 29.**

Focal Segmental Glomerulosclerosis (FSGS)

Pφ FSGS is characterized by scarring of some of the glomeruli (focal) in some parts of the glomerulus (segmental). This scarring can be seen by light microscopy. Electron microscopy shows effacement of epithelial foot processes (similar to that found in minimal-change disease) in addition to the scarring already seen on the light microscopy.

TP FSGS usually presents as an abrupt onset of nephrotic syndrome. Unlike the typical nephrotic syndrome, these patients often have hypertension and sometimes microscopic hematuria. FSGS is more common in adults. It is also more common in African-American patients.

Dx Diagnosis is based on typical presentation followed by kidney biopsy that shows the typical lesion. Once the diagnosis of FSGS is made, it is important to look for secondary causes such as HIV and reflux nephropathy.

Tx Treatment of primary FSGS involves steroids and, in some cases, cyclosporine. Antiproteinuric therapy with an ACE inhibitor or ARB is advised for all proteinuric diseases. **See Cecil Essentials 29.**

Membranous Nephropathy

Pφ The typical finding on light microscopy is diffuse thickening of the glomerular basement membrane. Special stains can illustrate that this thickening is due to "spikes" caused by the subepithelial deposits of IgG and possibly complement. Electron microscopy confirms the presence of subepithelial deposits.

TP Patients usually present with nephrotic syndrome with variable degrees of proteinuria. Patients are frequently hypercoagulable and can present with renal vein thrombosis or deep vein thrombosis, occasionally complicated by a pulmonary embolism.

Dx Diagnosis can be made only by examining tissue obtained by a kidney biopsy. Once the diagnosis is established, secondary causes such as lupus and hepatitis B need to be excluded. Membranous nephropathy can also be associated with malignancy. Patients should undergo age-appropriate cancer screening.

Tx About one third of patients undergo spontaneous remission, one third remain unchanged, and one third continue to progress, eventually developing end-stage renal disease. Because of the high rate of spontaneous remission, most nephrologists will wait approximately 6 months before initiating treatment with steroids and either cyclophosphamide or chlorambucil. **See Cecil Essentials 29.**

Amyloidosis

Pφ Amyloid fibrils cause disease by being deposited extracellularly in various organs and interfering with that organ's function. Amyloid can involve virtually any organ including heart, liver, kidneys, central nervous system, and blood vessels. On light microscopy of renal tissue, amyloid can be seen as amorphous hyaline material. Electron microscopy, however, will show randomly organized amyloid fibrils.

TP Typical presentation depends on the organs involved. When limited to the kidney, amyloid presents as classic nephrotic syndrome.

Dx Diagnosis relies on obtaining tissue biopsy of the most easily accessible involved organ, which often is the kidney. Once tissue is obtained, the type of amyloid can be determined. Some types of amyloid are primary, some are hereditary, and some are acquired secondary to systemic diseases, such as rheumatoid arthritis.

Tx Treatment of secondary amyloid is aimed at the underlying disease. Treatment of primary amyloid can involve hematopoietic cell transplantation, melphalan (an alkylating agent), and steroids. **See Cecil Essentials 29, 51, 90.**

Diabetic Nephropathy

Pφ Diabetic nephropathy is the end result of various pathogenic insults occurring as a result of diabetes mellitus, including intraglomerular hypertension, formation of advanced glycation end products, and proliferation of various cytokines and vascular growth factors. Microscopically, kidney biopsy shows thickening of basement membrane, expansion of the mesangial matrix, and glomerular sclerosis, which often has a nodular appearance (known as Kimmelstiel-Wilson lesions).

TP In patients with onset of heavy proteinuria with long-standing diabetes and a prior history of microalbuminuria, it usually takes longer than 15 years from the development of diabetes to the development of diabetic nephropathy. Patients with both type 1 and type 2 diabetes are affected.

Dx Diagnosis is made based on the typical presentation. Biopsy is usually not necessary unless some features of the presentation are atypical or inconsistent with diabetic nephropathy. Keep in mind that type 2 diabetics are often diagnosed many years after the onset of diabetes and may develop diabetic nephropathy shortly after diagnosis of diabetes.

Tx The mainstay of treatment is achieving excellent glycemic as well as blood pressure and lipid control. ACE inhibitors and ARBs both have renoprotective effects that are independent of their antihypertensive effect. **See Cecil Essentials 29.**

ZEBRA ZONE

a. **Systemic lupus erythematosus, membranous subtype:** This is one of the subtypes of lupus nephritis that, unlike the other subtypes, presents with nephrotic syndrome. Biopsy findings are essentially those of idiopathic membranous nephropathy with occasional subtle findings (e.g., tubuloreticular structures in endothelial cells or concurrent subendothelial or mesangial deposits) that point to underlying lupus. Progression of renal disease in the membranous subtype of lupus is generally slower than in other subtypes of lupus nephritis.

b. **Light-chain deposition disease:** Plasma cell dyscrasia in which monoclonal light chains are deposited in the glomeruli, causing distortion of glomerular architecture and therefore nephrotic-range proteinuria.

Practice-Based Learning and Improvement: Evidence-Based Medicine

Title
Development and progression of nephropathy in type 2 diabetes: the United Kingdom Prospective Diabetes Study

Authors
Adler AI, Stevens RJ, Manley SE, et al.

Institution
Diabetes Trials Unit, Oxford Centre for Diabetes, Endocrinology and Metabolism, University of Oxford, Oxford, and South Cleveland Hospital, Cleveland, United Kingdom

Reference
Kidney Int 2003;63:225–232

Problem
The goal is to prospectively study the progression of nephropathy in patients with type 2 diabetes from stage to stage.

Intervention
None, this was an observational part of the large United Kingdom Prospective Diabetes Study (UKPDS). UKPDS was designed to compare efficacy of different treatment regimens on glycemic control and complications of diabetes in newly diagnosed patients with type 2 diabetes mellitus.

Quality of evidence
Level II-3

Outcome/effect
Substantial numbers of patients with type 2 diabetes develop microalbuminuria, with 25% of patients affected by 10 years from diagnosis. Relatively fewer patients develop macroalbuminuria, but in those who do, the death rate exceeds the rate of progression to worse nephropathy.

Historical significance/comments
Largest study to date of progression of diabetic nephropathy in patients with type 2 diabetes

Interpersonal and Communication Skills

Communicate Effectively in the Face of Patient or Family Demands for Unnecessary Procedures
A patient under your care in the ICU has metastatic colon cancer and presents with hypotension and AKI. His prognosis is extremely poor, but his family is insisting on urgent dialysis. What do you do? Easy access to health care information is usually helpful, but

direct-to-consumer information may not be evidence-based. Patients are also surrounded by conflicting information from friends and family. When your patient or family demands specific procedures that are unlikely to be effective, it is often difficult to say "No" in a caring, responsible way. The best approach is to validate their fears and then to present your reasons why a particular procedure is not warranted at this time. It may be difficult to reassure the family when the outcome may not be optimal. However, these discussions are important to ensure compassionate care.

Professionalism

Demonstrate Commitment to Self-Care

It is important not to overcommit to a patient. For example, suppose your patient underwent a recent kidney biopsy, which was later complicated and required admission to the hospital to treat an infection at the biopsy site. This patient is emergently admitted to the hospital on a Friday evening as you are about to leave town for a previously scheduled weekend away with your family. One can see how easy it would be to cancel your plans and follow through with this case. However, a commitment to your personal self-care, which includes time off, vacations, and stress reduction, is extremely important. Physicians have a high rate of burnout, divorce, and stress-related illness. Having protected time goes a long way in the care of your patients. Explain to the patient that your colleague will be on call while you are away and that you have shared all of the important information needed for care, and that you will, of course, follow up on your return.

Systems-Based Practice

Permitting and Restricting Patient Care: Be Aware of Societal Implications

The treatment of many renal diseases, especially in the advanced stage, can be expensive. These treatments often include costly medications and long-term dialysis therapy. At present, dialysis is offered to everyone who needs it as part of the Medicare entitlement for end-stage renal disease that has been in effect since 1972; by the end of 2008, there were about 382,000 patients undergoing dialysis in the United States. There are data showing that in some elderly patients with multiple co-morbidities, dialysis does not increase survival, suggesting that further discussion about resource allocation is needed. Given the limited health care resources and the ever increasing demand for them, it is likely that we, as a society, will have to face restricting resources or allocating them based on some predetermined criteria.

Chapter 21
Acid-Base Disorders (Case 14)

Kavita Ahuja DO and Ilene Miller MD

Case: A 46-year-old man is found unconscious on the bathroom floor by his family. The family states the patient has a medical history significant only for depression and gastroesophageal reflux disease (GERD). His medications include escitalopram and omeprazole. Upon arrival to the emergency department the patient is more responsive but still confused and drowsy. A few episodes of vomiting are noted. On exam, the patient is afebrile with a blood pressure (BP) of 90/50 mm Hg, respiratory rate (RR) of 24 breaths per minute, and heart rate (HR) of 120 beats per minute (bpm). His pupils are reactive to light with a nonfocal neurologic exam. He has dry mucous membranes and mild diffuse abdominal tenderness to palpation. No alcoholic fetor is noted. Laboratory studies are as follows: Na 132 mEq/L, K 3.4 mEq/L, Cl 90 mEq/L, serum bicarbonate (HCO_3) 10 mEq/L, BUN 60 mg/dL, Cr 1.6 mg/dL, and glucose 80 mg/dL. Arterial blood gas (ABG) reveals a pH of 7.2 and P_{CO_2} of 25 mm Hg. Serum ethanol, acetone, and serum β-hydroxybutyrate are negative. The measured serum lactate is 1.6 mmol/L. Urinalysis reveals 4+ calcium oxalate crystals.

Differential Diagnosis

Increased Anion Gap Metabolic Acidosis	Normal Anion Gap Metabolic Acidosis	Metabolic Alkalosis
Methanol and ethylene glycol poisoning	Gastrointestinal (GI) bicarbonate loss	Contraction alkalosis
Ketoacidosis	RTA	Milk alkali syndrome
Lactic acidosis		
Uremia		
Salicylate intoxication		

Speaking Intelligently

When encountering a patient whose workup reveals a significant acid-base disorder, a thorough history and physical exam, along with appropriate lab data, will help identify the underlying diagnosis. These patients may require immediate attention (i.e., hemodynamic stabilization, volume resuscitation, and optimization of oxygenation). An ABG is the best test to assess the presence of an acid-base disorder. If a toxic ingestion is suspected, a toxicology screen should be performed to aid in identifying the agent, and a poison control center should be contacted for additional guidance.

PATIENT CARE

Clinical Thinking

- An acid is a substance that donates H^+ ions, while a base is a substance that accepts H^+ ions. pH is inversely related to $[H^+]$. In other words, an increase in $[H^+]$ reduces the pH, while a decrease in $[H^+]$ increases the pH. The normal pH of extracellular blood is 7.40, correlating to an extracellular $[H^+]$ of 40 nmol/L. A pH of less than 7.35 is considered to be acidemic, while a pH of above 7.45 is alkalemic.
- **Metabolic acidosis** is associated with a low pH and low HCO_3 concentration.
- **Respiratory acidosis** is associated with a low pH and a high P_{CO_2} concentration, indicating retention of CO_2.
- **Metabolic alkalosis** consists of a high pH with an increased HCO_3 concentration.
- **Respiratory alkalosis** is associated with a high pH and a low P_{CO_2}.
- The approach to identifying and managing acid-base disturbances should be a stepwise approach, as follows (also see Table 21-1):
  1. First, identify the primary disturbance based on the pH of arterial blood to determine if it is acidemic or alkalemic. In this case, the pH of 7.2 indicates an acidemia.
  2. Next, determine whether the acidemia is secondary to a metabolic or respiratory cause by interpreting the P_{CO_2} and HCO_3. If the P_{CO_2} is elevated, the disturbance is primarily a respiratory acidosis. If the HCO_3 is low, the disturbance is primarily a metabolic acidosis. In this case the low serum HCO_3 (10 mEq/L) indicates a primary metabolic acidosis.
  3. To determine if the disorder is a simple disorder or a mixed acid-base disorder, you must next determine compensation. In metabolic acidosis, the expected compensation or expected P_{CO_2} can be calculated using Winter's formula in which expected P_{CO_2} = 1.5 [serum HCO_3] + 8 ± 2. The expected P_{CO_2} for this patient is 23 mm Hg.
  4. Next, calculate the anion gap to aid in your differential diagnosis. It is helpful to classify the metabolic acidosis into increased anion gap versus normal anion gap. The anion gap is the difference between measured serum cations and anions and can be calculated

Table 21-1 Expected Changes in Primary Acid-Base Disorders

Disorder	pH	HCO$_3^-$	Pco$_2$	Calculation for Compensation
Normal	7.40	24	40	
Metabolic acidosis	Decreased	Decreased	Decreased	Expected Pco$_2$ = 1.5 (serum HCO$_3$) + 8 ± 2
Metabolic alkalosis	Increased	Increased	Increased	ΔPco$_2$ = 0.7 × ΔHCO$_3$ or Pco$_2$ = HCO$_3$ + 15
Respiratory acidosis	Decreased	Increased	Increased	Acute: ΔHCO$_3$ = 0.1 × ΔPco$_2$ Chronic: ΔHCO$_3$ = 0.3 × ΔPco$_2$
Respiratory alkalosis	Increased	Decreased	Decreased	Acute: ΔHCO$_3$ = 0.2 × ΔPco$_2$ Chronic: ΔHCO$_3$ = 0.4 × ΔPco$_2$

as Na$^+$ − (Cl$^-$ + HCO$_3^-$). A normal anion gap is 12 ± 4. An increase in anion gap is most often caused by an increase in unmeasured anions, such as lactate or ketones. The anion gap in this patient is 32. Therefore, this patient has a high–anion gap metabolic acidosis with appropriate respiratory compensation.

5. Finally, determine the etiology of the acid-base disorder by formulating a differential diagnosis, which will guide further management. Management should focus on identifying and correcting the underlying disorder and restoring normal extracellular pH.

History

- History will provide key information and should be obtained from the patient, relatives, friends, and/or co-workers.
- Collect information regarding a history of alcoholism or drug abuse, depression, and/or previous suicide attempts, which would prompt an evaluation for possible ingestion or intoxication.
- Determine whether the patient has a history of diabetes mellitus, renal disease, recent infection, diarrhea, or vomiting, as all of these conditions can predispose to acid-base imbalances.
- Review the patient's medications, as various medications are known to cause acid-base disturbances (e.g., salicylates).

Physical Examination

- Vital signs, including BP and HR, along with assessment of skin turgor, will help to determine the volume status of the patient.

- Determine if the patient is altering his or her respiratory rate in an attempt to compensate for alterations in serum HCO_3.
- A complete neurologic exam, including assessment of mental status and pupil reactivity, should be performed. Methanol intoxication can cause an afferent papillary defect. Ethylene glycol intoxication can cause cranial nerve palsies.
- Look for signs of inebriation.
- Look for signs of malnutrition, as they may raise suspicion of alcoholic ketoacidosis.

Tests for Consideration

- **ABG:** The ABG is the best test to assess acid-base balance. The respiratory component of acid-base balance is PCO_2, and it changes through alterations in ventilation. Hypoventilation will cause retention of CO_2 and result in respiratory acidosis. Hyperventilation will cause loss of CO_2 and result in respiratory alkalosis. The metabolic component of acid-base balance is HCO_3^- and is regulated by the kidney. $27
- **Serum chemistry and calcium:** The serum chemistry will allow for calculation of the anion gap and detection of abnormalities in electrolyte concentrations and renal function. $12
- **Urine electrolytes:** The measurement of urine Na^+, K^+, and Cl^- allows for calculation of the urine anion gap (UAG). The UAG is calculated as $UAG = [Na^+] + [K^+] - [Cl^-]$. It is useful in normal anion gap, hyperchloremic metabolic acidosis to determine if acidosis is secondary to GI HCO_3 loss or renal HCO_3^- loss. A negative UAG suggests that the HCO_3 loss is via the bowel, while a positive UAG suggests that the acidosis is of renal etiology (RTA). The urine electrolytes are also helpful when evaluating metabolic alkalosis. $7
- **Serum and urine ketones:** Ketones should be measured in patients with an elevated anion gap. Ketones are produced when the body metabolizes adipose tissue for energy and the liberated fatty acids are metabolized to ketoacids (β-hydroxybutyric and acetoacetic acid), which can be detected in serum and urine. $12
- **Toxicology screen:** A toxicology screen will allow for detection of acetaminophen, salicylate, alcohol, and/or opioid ingestion. It is necessary to measure in patients who present with altered mental status or an increased osmolar gap. $21
- **Serum osmolality:** Measurement of the serum osmolality and calculation of serum osmolality allow for the detection of an osmolar gap. The osmolar gap is defined as the difference between the measured serum osmolality and the calculated osmolality. Serum osmolality is calculated

as $2[Na^+]$ + [glucose]/18 + [BUN]/2.8. If the osmolar gap is greater than 15 mOsm/kg, ingestion of a toxic substance should be suspected. $9

• **Urinalysis and examination for crystalluria:** Urine sediment, when viewed under polarized light, can allow for detection of crystalluria. Ethylene glycol toxicity can lead to formation of needle- or dumbbell-shaped calcium oxalate monohydrate crystals or envelope-shaped calcium oxalate dihydrate crystals. $12

Clinical Entities	Medical Knowledge

Methanol and Ethylene Glycol Poisoning

Pφ Two toxic alcohol ingestions that lead to a severe anion-gap acidosis are methanol and ethylene glycol. The low molecular weight of these substances allows for entry into cells. Methanol and ethylene glycol are metabolized to formic acid and glycolic acid, respectively, and this metabolism generates H^+ ions, resulting in a high–anion gap acidosis. These substances are found in automotive antifreeze and de-icing solutions, windshield wiper fluid, solvents, and cleaners, and are ingested accidentally or as a suicide attempt.

TP Patients with methanol ingestion present with GI symptoms (abdominal pain, vomiting), central nervous system (CNS) symptoms (inebriation, headache, lethargy, coma), and an anion gap metabolic acidosis usually 12–24 hours after ingestion. No alcoholic fetor is present. An additional clue to the diagnosis of methanol ingestion is the presence of visual disturbances, as formic acid causes retinal injury. Ethylene glycol is found in antifreeze, and its ingestion has a similar clinical presentation but does not produce visual disturbances. The toxic metabolite of ethylene glycol causes kidney damage, and these patients often present with renal failure. Ethylene glycol, in addition to being metabolized to glycolic acid, is metabolized to oxalate, causing precipitation of calcium oxalate crystals, which can cause flank pain and further deterioration in renal function. Calcium oxalate crystals can be detected in the urine and may be seen in the form of calcium oxalate dihydrate (envelope-shaped crystals) or, more commonly, calcium oxalate monohydrate (needle-shaped or dumbbell-shaped crystals). Additionally, the urine will be fluorescent under a Wood lamp.

Dx Recognition of these ingestions should be made early, as prompt therapy is associated with significant decrease in morbidity and mortality. An increased osmolar gap is an early clue to diagnosis. The osmolar gap is defined as the difference between the measured serum osmolality and the calculated osmolality. An osmolar gap >15 mOsm/kg indicates that a toxic ingestion is the likely diagnosis. Of note, an osmolar gap can also be present in other conditions that are not associated with a high–anion gap metabolic acidosis, such as ethanol or isopropyl alcohol ingestion. Ethylene glycol poisoning can also cause hypocalcemia.

Tx Because the toxicity of methanol and ethylene glycol is due to the metabolites, therapy is directed at inhibiting metabolism of these substances. Fomepizole is an agent that blocks the metabolism of these agents by inhibiting alcohol dehydrogenase. Intravenous ethanol has also been used to competitively inhibit alcohol dehydrogenase and prevent formation of glycolic acid. Sodium bicarbonate can be used to correct acidosis. Hemodialysis, which allows for removal of toxic metabolites, is another modality that can be instituted if severe metabolic derangement or end-organ damage is present. **See Cecil Essentials 28.**

Lactic Acidosis

Pφ Lactic acidosis is a frequent cause of increased anion gap in hospitalized patients. Lactate is the end product of anaerobic metabolism of glucose, and, under normal conditions, its production is minimal. When lactate production increases faster than lactate can be metabolized, lactic acidosis ensues. Lactic acid exists in two forms, called isomers: L-lactate and D-lactate. L-lactate is produced in human metabolism and increases with impairments in tissue oxygenation secondary to increased anaerobic metabolism. D-lactate is produced by bacteria and is therefore primarily seen in patients with colonic bacterial overgrowth such as those with short-gut syndrome, gastric bypass, or small bowel resection.

TP Patients with lactic acidosis can present with abdominal pain, nausea, vomiting, CNS symptoms, and alterations in respiration. The severity of symptoms varies with the cause and degree of acidosis. L-lactic acidosis can be classified as type A or type B lactic acidosis. Type A lactic acidosis occurs in the setting of tissue hypoperfusion and is usually seen in shock, cardiopulmonary arrest, and/or hypoxemia. A transient lactic acidosis may be seen with seizures or excessive exercise. Type B lactic acidosis is found in patients without symptoms of hypoperfusion and often results from medications that interfere with lactate or pyruvate metabolism, such as metformin or reverse transcriptase inhibitors.

Dx The diagnosis of lactic acidosis should be considered in all cases of anion gap metabolic acidosis. In lactic acidosis, the anion lactate accounts for the increase in anion gap. Lactic acidosis is diagnosed when elevated levels of serum lactate are demonstrated. Routine serum lactate assays measure the L-lactate isomer but do not detect the D-lactate isomer. If D-lactic acidosis is suspected, the appropriate assay should be ordered.

Tx Treatment of lactic acidosis is aimed at treatment of the underlying disorder. For example, in septic shock, treatment should include restoring adequate tissue perfusion with the use of IV fluids and vasopressor support. The role of HCO_3 in lactic acidosis is controversial, as HCO_3 therapy may worsen intracellular acidosis. **See Cecil Essentials 28.**

Ketoacidosis

Pφ Ketones are produced when the body metabolizes adipose tissue for energy and the liberated fatty acids are metabolized to ketoacids (β-hydroxybutyric and acetoacetic acid), which can be detected in serum and urine. The two most common types of ketoacidosis are diabetic ketoacidosis (DKA) and alcoholic ketoacidosis (AKA). In both situations a decrease in the insulin-to-glucagon ratio leads to fatty acid mobilization and ketoacid accumulation.

TP Patients with DKA typically present with hyperglycemia, polyuria, polydipsia, nausea, vomiting, abdominal pain, and hyperventilation. Physical exam may reveal signs of volume depletion resulting from a combination of an osmotic diuresis from hyperglycemia along with vomiting and poor oral intake. Fruity odor and hyperventilation may also be noted.

AKA should be suspected in a patient with a history of alcohol abuse with recent binge drinking and poor oral intake. These patients, in contrast to those with DKA, may be hypoglycemic on presentation.

Dx The diagnosis of DKA is made in a hyperglycemic patient with a high–anion gap acidosis and detection of serum or urine ketones. AKA is diagnosed in a patient with a history of alcohol abuse and high–anion gap acidosis with positive serum or urine ketones. The predominant ketone in AKA is β-hydroxybutyrate.

Tx Therapy for DKA consists of administration of insulin, as well as volume and electrolyte repletion. Close monitoring of glucose levels and serum chemistries is essential. The treatment of AKA similarly consists of volume resuscitation and electrolyte repletion. Additionally, these patients require glucose and thiamine administration. Glucose administration stimulates insulin release and stops fatty acid generation. **See Cecil Essentials 28, 69.**

Uremia

Pφ Early in the course of renal failure, a non–anion gap, hyperchloremic metabolic acidosis may be present due to impaired ammonium excretion. However, as the GFR decreases further, the kidney becomes unable to excrete organic and inorganic anions, causing a high–anion gap metabolic acidosis.

TP Patients generally present with symptoms secondary to renal failure and the resulting metabolic acidosis. These symptoms include anorexia, nausea, vomiting, hyperventilation, congestive heart failure, muscle weakness, and changes in mental status.

Dx The presence of an elevated BUN and creatinine with acidosis suggests that renal failure is the cause of metabolic acidosis.

Tx Treatment of metabolic acidosis secondary to uremia consists of HCO_3 supplementation to restore normal blood pH and alleviate symptoms. Diuretics are often used in cases of volume overload. Refractory cases of metabolic acidosis may warrant initiation of dialysis. **See Cecil Essentials 33.**

Salicylate Intoxication

Pφ Salicylate (aspirin) intoxication is another cause of elevated anion gap metabolic acidosis. At toxic concentrations, salicylate uncouples oxidative phosphorylation and leads to increased production of organic acids. Aspirin is widely available, and therefore salicylate intoxication is a common poisoning.

TP The symptoms of salicylate intoxication are dose-dependent, with most patients showing signs of toxicity at plasma concentrations >40–50 mg/dL. Common clinical manifestations include nausea, vomiting, tinnitus, pulmonary edema, altered mental status, and coma. Adults may present with a mixed disorder of high–anion gap acidosis with respiratory alkalosis, as salicylate stimulates the respiratory center, causing increased ventilation. Severe intoxication can lead to death from CNS toxicity and cardiorespiratory depression.

Dx The diagnosis is made in the setting of an increased anion gap acidosis in combination with a respiratory alkalosis in a patient with an elevated plasma salicylate concentration.

Tx Treatment includes GI decontamination with activated charcoal, correction of fluid and electrolyte disorders, and facilitating excretion of the drug. HCO_3 infusion will cause alkalemia and alkalinization of the urine and therefore inhibit diffusion of salicylate into brain tissue while promoting renal excretion. Hemodialysis should be considered in patients with extremely high salicylate levels (usually >100 mg/dL), severe neurologic disturbances, renal failure, or refractory acidosis. **See Cecil Essentials 28.**

GI Loss of HCO_3

Pφ Intestinal fluid distal to the stomach has a high concentration of HCO_3, and GI HCO_3 loss is a common cause of metabolic acidosis. The HCO_3 loss most commonly occurs with diarrhea but can also be seen with excessive biliary and/or pancreatic fluid loss. The excessive volume loss causes the kidneys to reabsorb NaCl, resulting in a normal anion gap hyperchloremic acidosis. The kidneys, in response to acidosis, will increase urinary excretion of NH_4^+, which will lead to a negative urine anion gap.

TP Patients typically present with a history of diarrhea and serum chemistries showing both a normal anion gap acidosis and hypokalemia. With excessive volume loss, they can present with hypotension and tachycardia.

Dx The diagnosis of GI HCO_3 loss as the etiology of metabolic acidosis is made by detection of a normal anion gap metabolic acidosis with a negative urine anion gap and a clinical history suggestive of GI HCO_3 loss.

Tx Treatment is aimed at treating the cause of GI HCO_3 loss. Those with severe acidosis or prolonged acidosis require HCO_3 repletion. Hypokalemic patients require potassium repletion. **See Cecil Essentials 28.**

Renal Tubular Acidosis

Pφ RTA refers to a group of disorders characterized by hyperchloremic, normal anion gap metabolic acidosis as a result of impaired renal HCO_3 absorption or H^+ secretion in the setting of a normal GFR. RTA may be a primary disorder or secondary to a number of systemic diseases such as diabetes mellitus, multiple myeloma, or autoimmune diseases. Medications and toxins have also been known to cause RTA.

TP Patients are generally asymptomatic but may present with nonspecific symptoms related to the underlying cause of RTA. Patients with type I RTA often develop nephrolithiasis. Patients with type IV RTA are often hyperkalemic. However, often RTA may be incidentally discovered on routine blood screening.

Dx RTA is suspected in the presence of a normal anion gap, hyperchloremic metabolic acidosis in conjunction with a positive urine anion gap. This indicates an inability of the kidney to excrete NH_4.

Tx Treatment of RTA includes identifying the underlying cause along with administration of alkali (i.e., sodium bicarbonate) to correct the acidosis. Potassium supplementation is often necessary. Thiazide diuretics may also be used in some instances to increase proximal tubule HCO_3 reabsorption. **See Cecil Essentials 28.**

Contraction Alkalosis

Pφ Contraction alkalosis is a term used to describe a combined presentation of volume contraction and primary metabolic alkalosis. It is seen in patients with vomiting and diuretic use and results from the loss of HCO_3-free fluid. The alkalosis is then maintained by chloride depletion. Specific cells in the distal tubule exchange chloride for HCO_3, and thus chloride depletion will not allow HCO_3 excretion and correction of the alkalosis.

TP Metabolic alkalosis is generally well tolerated and is only discovered on routine laboratory testing. However, patients with serum HCO_3 concentrations > 50 mmol/L may manifest with neurologic symptoms such as seizures, delirium, or stupor. Other symptoms may be related to other associated abnormalities such as hypokalemia and volume depletion.

Dx The diagnosis requires a history suggesting volume depletion and Cl^- loss such as vomiting, nasogastric suctioning, and/or diuretic use. Laboratory data reveal increased serum HCO_3, hypokalemia, and an elevated arterial pH. Urine electrolytes show a urine Cl^- < 20 mmol/L.

Tx Treatment involves correction of the underlying disorder and volume expansion with NaCl. The distal tubular cells exchange HCO_3 for Cl^- and correct the alkalosis. Electrolytes such as K^+ and Mg^{2+} may need to be supplemented. **See Cecil Essentials 28.**

Milk-Alkali Syndrome

Pφ Milk-alkali syndrome is characterized by metabolic alkalosis, hypercalcemia, and renal insufficiency. It occurs in the setting of continuous alkali (sodium bicarbonate) ingestion along with excess calcium intake (milk or $CaCO_3$). The hypercalcemia produces a reduction in GFR. This reduction in GFR does not allow the kidneys to excrete HCO_3, and metabolic alkalosis develops.

TP Approximately 50% of these patients are asymptomatic. The remaining 50% present with symptomatic hypercalcemia, including nausea, vomiting, weakness, muscle aches, polyuria, polydipsia, nephrolithiasis, and mental status changes.

Dx A history of calcium and alkali ingestion (often in the form of calcium carbonate), along with laboratory data indicating hypercalcemia and metabolic alkalosis, suggests milk-alkali syndrome.

Tx Treatment consists of withdrawal of the offending agent, which generally leads to rapid improvement. Symptomatic patients can be treated with isotonic saline and loop diuretics. Renal insufficiency is reversible and improves with correction of hypercalcemia. **See Cecil Essentials 28, 74.**

ZEBRA ZONE

a. **Ureteral diversion:** refers to surgical diversion of the ureters into the bowel, usually into the sigmoid colon or ileum. This is generally seen in patients with abnormalities or cancer of the bladder. These patients often have a resultant hyperchloremic, normal anion gap metabolic acidosis. Urinary chloride is reabsorbed by the intestine and exchanged for HCO_3, resulting in HCO_3 loss and metabolic acidosis. Metabolic acidosis is much more common with uretero-sigmoidostomy, as contact time between urine and intestinal surface is much shorter with uretero-ileostomy, limiting exchange of metabolic products. However, if a metabolic acidosis is detected in a patient with an uretero-sigmoidostomy, obstruction of the ileal loop should be ruled out, as the obstruction would increase contact time between urine and intestine.

Practice-Based Learning and Improvement: Evidence-Based Medicine

Title
Fomepizole for the treatment of methanol poisoning

Authors
Brent J, McMartin K, Phillips S, et al.

Institution
University of Colorado Health Sciences Center, Denver, CO, USA

Reference
N Engl J Med 2001;344:424–429

Problem
Treatment of patients with methanol poisoning

Intervention
Eleven consecutive patients with methanol poisoning were treated with fomepizole, an inhibitor of alcohol dehydrogenase.

Quality of evidence
Level II-1

Outcome/effect
Plasma formic acid levels fell and metabolic abnormalities resolved in response to fomepizole. Fomepizole was well tolerated and appears to be safe and effective in the treatment of methanol poisoning.

Historical significance/comments
Fomepizole is now considered a reasonable treatment option in patients with methanol poisoning.

Interpersonal and Communication Skills

Identify the Proper Decision Makers and Anticipate Disagreements among Family Members

Patients with severe metabolic acid-base disturbances often present to the acute setting with a change in mental status. In this situation, physicians may need to obtain informed consent from the patient's family members regarding emergent diagnostic and treatment procedures. As most people do not have a living will or health care proxy, physicians often find (unfortunately) that there may be disagreement regarding care plan decisions among members of the same family. Such disagreement is usually related to prior medical experiences and the emotional state of the parties. It is important for the physician to understand the chain of decision making when there is no health care proxy and, to the extent possible, to help the family reach consensus. The physician must clearly, calmly, and patiently explain all management options and consequences to family members, preferably in a family meeting that takes place away from the bedside. In some instances it may be prudent for the physician to consult other health care team members, such as the social worker and hospital ethicist.

Professionalism

Commitment to Improve Access to Care for the Community

All too often patients present to the acute care setting with severe metabolic acid-base disturbances that could have been prevented. Diabetic ketoacidosis and uremia, for example, are conditions whose frequency can be reduced and can sometimes be avoided with good medical follow-up, education, and preventive care. Unfortunately, in communities where access to the health care system is suboptimal, fairly simple and inexpensive medical interventions, such as BP control and weight loss counseling, are not available. As part of their professional responsibility, physicians must do their part to support improvement in access to care and community outreach programs.

Systems-Based Practice

The Patient-Centered Medical Home

Prevention and management of renal failure and DKA require care not only by a capable physician but also by a team of nurses, nutritionists, case workers, and social workers. Patients with renal failure, heart failure, and diabetes, all of whom are susceptible to metabolic disturbances, need frequent contact with medical health professionals. Preferably, in the future care will be delivered to such patients in the form of the "patient-centered medical home," in which the primary physician delivers high-quality, patient-centered, and evidence-based care and integrates the care of the other team members in a way that enables patients to navigate easily as more complex treatments and diagnostic modalities are required. Effective primary care has been shown to improve quality and reduce cost by emphasizing preventive care and early interventions to reduce the need for higher cost tertiary care.

Chapter 22
Abnormal Electrolytes (Case 15)

Rabeena Fazal MD and Alessandro Bellucci MD

Case: A 76-year-old woman with a history of hypertension and coronary artery disease presents to the ED with complaints of weakness, nausea, and muscle cramps. Her daughter states that she has been mildly confused over the past 2 days. She reports that her primary-care physician prescribed hydrochlorothiazide for elevated BP 2 weeks ago. The patient claims to be more thirsty than usual and, as a result, has been drinking more water. She denies any fevers, chills, vomiting, or diarrhea. Her other medications include metoprolol, aspirin, and simvastatin. On physical examination, the patient appears mildly lethargic and is oriented to name and place, but not to date. Her BP is 149/65 mm Hg without orthostatic changes, with a HR of 68 bpm. The cardiac and chest examinations are normal. No lower extremity edema is present. Neurologic examination reveals no focal deficits. Laboratory studies reveal a serum sodium 118 mEq/L, serum potassium 2.8 mEq/L, serum chloride 80 mEq/L, serum bicarbonate 29 mEq/L, BUN 34 mg/dL, serum creatinine 0.9 mg/dL, and serum calcium 11.2 mg/dL.

Differential Diagnosis

Hyponatremia	Hypokalemia	Hypocalcemia
Hypernatremia	Hyperkalemia	Hypercalcemia

Speaking Intelligently

Electrolyte disorders are common clinical problems, especially among hospitalized patients. Fluids and electrolytes are normally very carefully maintained within narrow parameters to allow the cells of the body to function normally. Electrolyte abnormalities can affect the resting membrane potential, resulting in cardiac, neurologic, and musculoskeletal symptoms. Serum sodium concentration is a major determinant of extracellular osmolality, and abnormalities in sodium concentration lead to changes in intracranial pressure. The severity of the symptoms usually depends on how quickly the electrolyte disturbance occurs. The electrolytes that may be affected include sodium, potassium, and calcium. Since these disorders are accompanied by significant morbidity and mortality, appropriate diagnosis and treatment are essential.

PATIENT CARE

Clinical Thinking

- Electrolyte disturbances represent an imbalance between ingestion and excretion, a shift between the intracellular and extracellular environment, or fluid loss or gain.
- Increased concentration of an electrolyte occurs as a result of excess total body amount, shift from intracellular to extracellular environment, or an absolute or relative water deficit.
- Decreased concentrations are a result of depleted total body amount, shift among compartments, or an absolute or relative water excess.

History

- For **dysnatremias:**
  - Search for causes of volume depletion, such as vomiting, diarrhea, GI bleeding, and decreased oral intake, or conditions associated with a low effective arterial blood volume, such as congestive heart failure (CHF), renal failure, and cirrhosis.
  - Review the patient's medications and their side effect profile, as many medications can cause sodium disturbance. For example, thiazide diuretics can cause hyponatremia by interfering with the ability of the kidneys to dilute the urine.
  - Check the type of intravenous fluids being given in a hospital setting.
  - Assess whether the patient has neurologic symptoms related to hyponatremia, such as nausea, vomiting, headaches, mental status changes, or seizures. These symptoms are related to brain swelling and require immediate treatment.

- For **potassium disorders:**
  - Perform a careful review of the patient's diet and medications.
  - Question the patient about GI disorders such as diarrhea or vomiting that can result in potassium losses.
  - Search for the presence of renal dysfunction, as this can result in an inability to excrete potassium.
  - Surreptitious vomiting or laxative abuse may be difficult to identify but should be excluded.
  - The family history is important, because there can be rare cases of hereditary potassium disorders.
- For **calcium disorders:**
  - Ask about water intake and urinary habits.
  - Polyuria and polydipsia are common in patients with hypercalcemia and hypokalemia, as these disturbances interfere with the action of ADH in the distal tubule, resulting in nephrogenic diabetes insipidus.
  - Ask about a history of renal disease, because hypocalcemia and hyperphosphatemia are common in patients with advanced renal dysfunction and secondary hyperparathyroidism.
  - Hypercalcemia incidentally found on an outpatient basis is most commonly related to primary hyperparathyroidism, and affected individuals may give a history of nephrolithiasis.
  - Malignancy can cause hypercalcemia; when it is the cause, the underlying malignancy is usually readily apparent.

Physical Examination
- Focus on signs of volume depletion or volume overload.
- Evaluate for mental status changes and other neurologic findings.
- The presence of Trousseau or Chvostek sign can point to a diagnosis of hypocalcemia.

Tests for Consideration
The diagnosis and treatment of fluid and electrolyte disorders are based on serum electrolyte concentrations, urine electrolyte concentrations, and serum and urine osmolality. Once the specific electrolyte abnormality has been diagnosed, additional tests can be done to aid in determining the etiology.

- **TSH** and **cortisol levels** can exclude hypothyroidism and adrenal insufficiency, respectively, as causes of hyponatremia. $24, $23
- In potassium disorders, determination of **acid-base status** can aid in the workup.
- **Radiologic tests** (e.g., **chest radiograph**, **CT scan of the chest**, **neuroimaging**) can provide evidence of malignancy, which can be a cause of hyponatremia or hypercalcemia. $45, $334, $334

Clinical Entities	Medical Knowledge

Hyponatremia

Pφ Hyponatremia is defined as a serum sodium concentration < 135 mEq/L. Hyponatremia may be hypertonic, hypotonic, or isotonic, associated with a high, low, or normal serum osmolality, respectively. Isotonic hyponatremia is the result of laboratory artifact due to a decreased aqueous component of plasma such as may be seen in patients with hyperlipidemia and hyperproteinemia. Hypertonic hyponatremia results from the presence of solutes, such as mannitol and glucose, which do not freely cross cell membranes, and represents a hyperosmolar state. Most hyponatremia is hypotonic, representing an excess of total-body water relative to total-body sodium, and is caused by impaired renal water excretion combined with continued water intake. Reasons for impaired water excretion include renal failure, volume depletion, high-ADH states, hypothyroidism, adrenal insufficiency, and low osmolar intake. Thiazides impair the ability of the kidneys to excrete free water, and, if the patient maintains a high water intake, as in the case illustrated above, a positive water balance ensues and hyponatremia results.

TP The symptoms of hyponatremia reflect cerebral edema and range from headache, nausea, vomiting, and mental status changes to seizures, coma, brainstem herniation, and death. The majority of patients present with mild symptoms such as nausea, weakness, and confusion. On exam they may have signs of hypovolemia, hypervolemia, or euvolemia.

Dx Most patients with hyponatremia will have a low serum osmolality and a urine osmolality > 100 mOsm/kg, reflecting an impaired renal diluting ability (the normal renal response should be to dilute the urine to 60 mOsm/kg). The urine sodium concentration will vary depending on the source of volume loss (renal or nonrenal) and the amount of sodium intake.

Tx The urgency of treatment is dictated by the severity of symptoms and the time course of development of the hyponatremia. In the presence of severe, symptomatic hyponatremia, an infusion of hypertonic 3% saline solution is the standard approach. For asymptomatic patients the treatment depends on the cause of hyponatremia. Hypovolemic hyponatremia should be corrected with isotonic saline. Syndrome of inappropriate antidiuretic hormone secretion (SIADH), renal failure, and psychogenic polydipsia are treated primarily with fluid restriction. In cases of low osmolar intake, increase dietary solute and decrease water intake. Edematous states require water and sodium restriction. In addition, loop diuretics (e.g., furosemide) can be added to promote water loss in excess of sodium loss. The rate of correction should not exceed 0.5 mEq/L/hr to avoid osmotic demyelination (central pontine myelinolysis), the most feared consequence of overly rapid correction. **See Cecil Essentials 28.**

Hypernatremia

Pφ Hypernatremia is defined as serum sodium > 145 mEq/L and generally results from loss of water combined with a failure to adequately replace the water deficit. The causes of hypernatremia can be divided into three categories: (1) increased water loss, which may be renal losses (diabetes insipidus, osmotic diuresis, diuretic use) or extrarenal losses (diarrhea, vomiting, excessive sweating, burns), (2) decreased water intake due to impaired thirst mechanism or altered mental status, and (3) iatrogenic causes such as administration of hypertonic saline.

Diabetes insipidus (DI) results from the inability of the kidneys to concentrate the urine due to either a deficiency of ADH or lack of response to ADH. Central DI is characterized by decreased secretion of ADH and is most often due to brain tumors, head injuries, CNS infections, or inherited disorders. Nephrogenic DI is due to unresponsiveness of the kidney to the effects of ADH; it can be congenital or caused by certain medications such as lithium.

TP Patients typically present with neurologic symptoms such as altered mental status and lethargy, and occasionally seizures or coma if the hypernatremia is severe. They may complain of polyuria or excessive thirst. On exam, patients are usually volume depleted, but in certain instances they can be hypervolemic or euvolemic.

Dx In most cases the etiology of the hypernatremia can be determined based on history and physical. Laboratory tests such as urine osmolality, urine sodium concentration, and blood glucose can provide further diagnostic clues. Hypovolemia with a urine sodium concentration < 20 mEq/L is consistent with extrarenal losses. The hallmark of DI is polyuria with low urine osmolality, whereas osmotic diuresis—as can be seen with hyperglycemia—is associated with polyuria and a daily solute excretion (urine volume × urine osmolality) in excess of 900 mOsm/kg.

Tx The goals of treatment are (1) to stop ongoing loss of water and (2) to replace the water deficit. The water deficit can be estimated as follows:

Water deficit = $0.6 \times$ body weight (kg) $\times [(Na/140) - 1]$

In hypovolemic patients, especially those with hemodynamic compromise, replacement of volume with 0.9% saline is a first priority. Subsequently, free-water deficit can be replaced using hypotonic fluids. Using the oral or gastric route to replace free water is preferred; however, if not possible, IV fluids such as D5W or 0.45% saline can be used. The major complication of overly rapid correction is cerebral edema. To avoid this, the rate of increase of sodium should not exceed 0.5 mEq/L/hr. **See Cecil Essentials 28.**

Hypokalemia

Pφ Hypokalemia is defined as a serum potassium concentration <3.5 mEq/L. Hypokalemia is caused by decreased intake, increased excretion, or intracellular shifts. A typical American diet is rich in potassium, and the kidney is efficient at conserving potassium; thus, it is rare to see hypokalemia on the basis of low potassium intake. Intracellular shift of potassium can be stimulated in patients with metabolic alkalosis, insulin, and certain drugs such as theophylline and β-agonists. A strong clue for this mechanism is the lack of an associated acid-base abnormality. Increased potassium excretion occurs via the GI tract or the kidney. GI losses can occur in patients with diarrhea, as a result of loss of potassium in the stool, or with vomiting. Vomiting also leads to potassium loss in the urine through volume depletion and secondary hyperaldosteronism. Potassium loss via the kidneys can be further classified based on the associated acid-base abnormality and the presence of hypertension. Metabolic alkalosis accompanies vomiting, diuretic use (as in the case illustrated above), and distal tubular defects such as Bartter and Gitelman syndrome. Metabolic alkalosis with hypertension is associated with hypokalemia from primary mineralocorticoid excess, such as in patients with adrenal adenomas. Hypokalemia from RTA is associated with metabolic acidosis. Another cause of hypokalemia without acid-base disturbances, but with hypocalcemia, is hypomagnesemia.

TP Weakness, fatigue, and muscle cramps are the most frequent complaints in patients with mild to moderate hypokalemia. Smooth muscle involvement may result in constipation or ileus. Electrocardiographic (ECG) changes can occur and include flattening or inversion of T waves, prominent U waves, and ST-segment depression and arrhythmias. Severe hypokalemia can lead to flaccid paralysis, respiratory failure, arrhythmias, rhabdomyolysis, and nephrogenic DI.

Dx The source of potassium loss is very often evident upon careful history. When the cause is not apparent, the 24-hour urinary potassium can help distinguish between renal and extrarenal losses. Potassium excretion >20 mEq in 24 hours in the presence of hypokalemia implies renal potassium loss. Alternatively, measurement of the transtubular potassium gradient can be used. Assessment of the patient's volume status, BP, and acid-base status provides additional diagnostic clues.

Tx Each 1-mEq/L decrement in serum potassium concentration below a level of 4 mEq/L may represent a total-body deficit of 200–400 mEq. Mild to moderate deficiency (3.0–3.5 mEq/L) may best be treated with oral potassium chloride (KCl). Severe hypokalemia (<3.0 mEq/L) requires IV replacement with KCl. The maximum rate of KCl administration is 10 mEq/L/hr via a peripheral IV line and 20 mEq/L/hr via a central line. The latter requires continuous ECG monitoring. Serum potassium levels should be checked frequently during correction. When present, magnesium deficiency must be corrected to allow potassium correction. **See Cecil Essentials 28.**

Hyperkalemia

Pφ Severe hyperkalemia is a life-threatening emergency, requiring immediate treatment. Hyperkalemia can be caused by increased intake, transcellular shift, decreased excretion, or some or all of these. Transcellular shift involves transient movement of potassium out of cells and into the extracellular space. This can be triggered by acidosis, hypertonic states, and insulin deficiency, as well as with drugs such as β-blockers and digoxin. Release of potassium from cells can also be caused by tissue breakdown as seen in patients with rhabdomyolysis and tumor lysis syndrome. Decreased renal excretion is the most common mechanism of hyperkalemia, due to (1) decreased renal function, (2) aldosterone deficiency or tubular unresponsiveness to aldosterone, or (3) decreased delivery of sodium to the distal tubule. Aldosterone acts on the principal cells of the collecting duct, where it causes increased sodium reabsorption and potassium excretion. Causes of true or functional hypoaldosterone states leading to hyperkalemia include adrenal insufficiency and drugs such as ACE inhibitors, ARBs, NSAIDs, aldosterone receptor blockers, and potassium-sparing diuretics. Conditions associated with low urinary sodium and decreased urine output, such as advanced liver cirrhosis or CHF, severely limit the ability of the kidneys to excrete potassium. Pseudo-hyperkalemia is a factitious elevation of serum potassium often seen in patients with hemolysis, thrombocytosis (platelet count > 1 million/μL), or leukocytosis (WBC count over 100,000/μL). In these instances the ECG is normal, and the patient has no apparent clinical reasons to be hyperkalemic.

TP Most patients with hyperkalemia are asymptomatic. When present, symptoms include muscle weakness, ascending paralysis, respiratory failure, and cardiac arrhythmias. ECG changes in patients with hyperkalemia are progressive and include peaked T waves, flattened P waves, prolonged PR interval, widened QRS complex, and, finally, a sine wave pattern.

Dx The ECG is the most important tool to evaluate the severity of the hyperkalemia and to guide the therapeutic approach. If the ECG is normal and the patient has no clinical reason to be hyperkalemic, pseudo-hyperkalemia should be excluded. Careful venipuncture without using a tourniquet and measuring plasma instead of serum potassium usually clarifies the diagnosis. Hyperkalemia is often multifactorial, and the diagnostic approach is to systematically address the possible mechanism. Often an iatrogenic intervention such as the initiation of an ACE inhibitor or an aldosterone receptor antagonist will precipitate hyperkalemia in a predisposed patient. Heparin inhibits aldosterone synthesis and can cause hyperkalemia in hospitalized patients.

Tx Severe hyperkalemia with ECG changes is a medical emergency and requires immediate treatment. The initial treatment is aimed at stabilizing the cardiac cell membrane to prevent cardiac death by giving intravenous calcium gluconate. Further measures aim to shift potassium intracellularly by administering insulin, D50W, sodium bicarbonate, and nebulized β_2-adrenergic agonists. Finally patients are treated with diuretics, cation exchange resins, or even dialysis to decrease potassium. Dialysis should be reserved for patients with renal failure and those with severe life-threatening hyperkalemia unresponsive to more conservative measures. **See Cecil Essentials 28.**

Hypocalcemia

Pφ Calcium homeostasis is maintained through the actions of parathyroid hormone (PTH) and vitamin D. PTH acts directly upon the bone to mobilize calcium and upon the kidneys to reabsorb calcium. PTH acts indirectly upon the GI tract by increasing the amount of active vitamin D. Vitamin D acts directly upon the GI tract to facilitate calcium absorption. Hypocalcemia is defined as a reduction in serum ionized calcium concentration and can be caused by decreased entry of calcium into the circulation or loss of calcium from the circulation. Conditions that result in a decreased entry of calcium into the circulation include vitamin D deficiency and hypoparathyroidism. Vitamin D deficiency is not uncommon in the elderly and is usually the result of malabsorption or poor oral intake. True hypoparathyroidism is rare and is usually the result of surgical removal, while a functional hypoparathyroid state can result from hypomagnesemia or bisphosphonate therapy. Loss of calcium from the circulation can be seen in patients with acute pancreatitis, rhabdomyolysis, or massive transfusions.

TP Hypocalcemia increases excitation of nerve and muscle cells, primarily affecting the neuromuscular and cardiovascular systems. Patients with significant deficiency may complain of muscle cramps, tetany, and paresthesias of the lips and extremities. Severe hypocalcemia may cause lethargy, confusion, laryngospasm, or seizures. Prolongation of the QT interval may be present and predisposes to the development of ventricular arrhythmias.

Dx Patients with hypocalcemia may exhibit Chvostek sign and Trousseau sign. The diagnosis is confirmed, however, by a low serum ionized calcium. Once hypocalcemia has been confirmed, further testing for PTH, vitamin D, magnesium, phosphorus, and creatinine should be performed. Additional testing for pancreatitis or rhabdomyolysis should be performed if clinically warranted.

Tx Severe, symptomatic hypocalcemia should be corrected with IV calcium. Chronic treatment of hypocalcemia requires oral calcium supplementation of 1–2 g of elemental calcium daily, given with vitamin D. In patients with hypoparathyroidism, calcium should be supplemented to maintain serum calcium at the lower limit of normal (8.0 mg/dL) so as to minimize hypercalciuria and precipitation of renal stones. Hypomagnesemia should be corrected when it is present. **See Cecil Essentials 74.**

Hypercalcemia

Pφ Together, primary hyperparathyroidism and malignancy account for the vast majority of cases of hypercalcemia. Primary hyperparathyroidism is the most common cause of hypercalcemia in ambulatory patients, whereas malignancy is the most common cause of hypercalcemia in hospitalized patients. Primary hyperparathyroidism causes hypercalcemia through two distinct mechanisms: PTH acts directly on the kidney resulting in calcium reabsorption, and PTH increases vitamin D synthesis, which results in increased calcium absorption through the GI tract. Hypercalcemia associated with malignancy is commonly caused by increased osteoclastic activity. Other causes of hypercalcemia include exogenous vitamin D intake, granulomatous disorders such as sarcoidosis and tuberculosis, milk-alkali syndrome, and immobilization. Thiazide diuretics increase renal calcium reabsorption; however, hypercalcemia rarely results from thiazide use alone and should raise the suspicion of the presence of an underlying hyperparathyroidism.

TP Hypercalcemia may affect GI, renal, and neurologic function. Mild hypercalcemia is often asymptomatic. Symptoms usually occur if the serum calcium is above 12 mg/dL and tend to be more severe if hypercalcemia develops acutely. Even mild elevation of calcium can induce symptoms in hypoalbuminemic patients, as less calcium is bound and more is free. Neurologic manifestations may range from mild drowsiness to weakness, lethargy, confusion, and coma. GI symptoms may include constipation, nausea, vomiting, anorexia, and peptic ulcer disease. The ECG shows a shortened QT interval. Hypercalcemia induces nephrogenic DI and polyuria. The ensuing dehydration has an important role in decreasing renal calcium excretion and increasing the serum calcium.

Dx The serum calcium level should be corrected for serum albumin, or serum ionized calcium should be measured. Once hypercalcemia is confirmed, measurements of PTH, PTH-related protein (PTHrP), and vitamin D should be ordered. Hyperparathyroidism is diagnosed by finding a high PTH level. Patients with malignancy-induced hypercalcemia usually have a known malignancy and may have an elevated PTHrP. The vitamin D level will be high in patients taking exogenous vitamin D, as well in those with hypercalcemia from granulomatous disease.

Tx Until the primary disease can be brought under control, acute treatment of hypercalcemia is directed at increasing calcium excretion and decreasing resorption of calcium from bone. The first step is volume repletion with 0.9% saline. After extracellular volume has been restored, a loop diuretic (such as furosemide) is added to increase calcium excretion and prevent volume overload. Thiazides should not be used because they will worsen hypercalcemia. Bisphosphonates and calcitonin can also be used to inhibit bone resorption, although may be required up to 3 days before the effect of bisphosphonates is seen. In certain cases, such as patients with CHF or renal failure, dialysis with low-calcium dialysate may be needed. **See Cecil Essentials 74.**

ZEBRA ZONE

a. Familial hypokalemic periodic paralysis: This is an autosomal-dominant disorder that causes hypokalemia due to a transcellular shift of potassium. This disorder is associated with recurrent episodes of flaccid paralysis that begin in childhood. Episodes are usually triggered by high-carbohydrate meals (increased insulin) or after a period of exercise (catecholamine excess).

Practice-Based Learning and Improvement: Evidence-Based Medicine

Title
Association between rise in serum sodium and central pontine myelinolysis

Authors
Norenberg MD, Leslie KO, Robertson AS

Institution
Veterans Administration Medical Center, Denver, CO, USA; University of Colorado Health Sciences Center, Denver, CO, USA

Reference
Ann Neurol 1982;11:128–135

Problem
What is the association between central pontine myelinolysis and hyponatremia?

Intervention
The study reviewed two groups of hyponatremic patients with and without central pontine myelinolysis (CPM), and their associated rate of rise of sodium during correction.

Quality of evidence
Level II-2

Outcome/effect
The analysis suggested that CPM can be caused by a rapid rate of correction of serum sodium in hyponatremic patients.

Historical significance/comments
This is one of the initial studies that established an association between CPM and the rate of correction of hyponatremia. Subsequent studies established that the maximum rate of correction should not exceed 0.5 mEq/L/hr so as to limit the risk of CPM.

Interpersonal and Communication Skills

Discuss Issues of Diet and Nutrition with Both Patients and Families

Most electrolyte abnormalities occur in the acute-care setting and resolve once the underlying etiology has been diagnosed and corrected. In some cases, however, the underlying disorder is not correctable, and management of the electrolyte abnormality remains a chronic issue (e.g., hyperkalemia in patients with chronic kidney disease). In such instances it is often necessary to obtain the assistance of family members involved in meal preparation and grocery shopping, in addition to educating the patient on the importance of dietary compliance. These family members should meet with the dietitian to be provided with the knowledge necessary to assist the patient in the recommended dietary restrictions.

Professionalism

Improve Access to Care for the Individual

Chronic management of electrolyte disorders requires frequent monitoring of serum electrolyte levels. In those with chronic illness and social vulnerabilities (e.g., lack of family support or low socioeconomic status), it can be difficult for the patient to make frequent trips to an outpatient lab for blood work. Many programs have recently started to address this issue with home phlebotomy. It is important for the physician to be aware of which patients will need special services and how to access these services for them. In some programs, for example, the physician faxes a prescription with orders for blood work to an agency that then sends a phlebotomist to the patient's home to collect the specimen and transport it to the lab. The results are sent to the physician, who can then adjust the patient's treatment regimen accordingly. This type of access to care can make a big difference in patients' compliance and reduce the necessity for recurrent ED visits or hospital readmission.

Systems-Based Practice

Nutrition Support Services
One of the main tools in the management of electrolyte disorders is dietary intervention, which can be frustrating for patients. Engaging the services of a dietitian in the management of these patients can be invaluable. A dietitian can arrange meetings with the patient and family members to educate them on the nutritional contents of foods, so they can differentiate between foods that are acceptable and foods that contain substances they need to limit or avoid. The dietitian can also provide Internet-based resources that the patient can use for guidance in daily meal preparations. Many large medical offices have a dietitian on staff or available for consultation. These services are covered by most health insurance companies with a doctor's referral.

Chapter 23
Hematuria (Case 16)

Spirithoula Vasilopoulos MD *and Michael Gitman* MD

Case: The patient is a 60-year-old male who, during an annual physician visit, was found to have hematuria. His medical history is significant for emphysema from years of smoking, as well as an episode of right-sided nephrolithiasis approximately 1 year ago. At that time he passed the stone spontaneously, and subsequently his urinalysis had been normal. His medications include albuterol and ibuprofen. After hearing of the hematuria, he states that he has never seen any blood in his urine and he certainly does not have any pain. Other than complaints of his chronically poor urinary stream, he feels great. After some discussion, he agrees to complete any evaluation that is necessary.

Differential Diagnosis

Glomerular Hematuria	Nonglomerular Renal Hematuria	Urologic Hematuria
IgA nephropathy Alport syndrome	Polycystic kidney disease Chronic tubulointerstitial nephritis (CTIN)	Nephrolithiasis Transitional cell carcinoma (TCC) Cystitis Papillary necrosis

Speaking Intelligently

Hematuria is a common clinical problem, occurring in 10% to 20% of adult men and postmenopausal women. It can originate from anywhere within the genitourinary tract including the kidneys, ureters, bladder, and urethra. Its clinical significance varies dramatically from innocuous diseases such as cystitis to a life-altering diagnosis, such as renal failure or malignancy. A thorough history, physical exam, and urine evaluation will help to identify the cause of hematuria and the extent of clinical evaluation that is necessary.

PATIENT CARE

Clinical Thinking

- Determine the context in which the sample was taken. A urinalysis done in the setting of urinary tract infection (UTI), catheter trauma, significant coagulopathy, menstruation, after sexual intercourse, or after vigorous exercise may need to be repeated.
- If the hematuria is evaluated in the appropriate setting, determine whether the red blood cells originated in the kidney or in the lower urinary tract.
- Red blood cells originating in the kidney will be dysmorphic, while red blood cells that originate in the lower urinary tract will retain their usual morphology on visual exam. If the red blood cells originated in the glomerulus, you may see red blood cell casts.
- Hematuria accompanied by proteinuria is often of glomerular origin.
- Categorize the hematuria as gross or microscopic, and glomerular or nonglomerular. Deciding on the origin will help narrow the differential and assist in ordering the appropriate diagnostic tests and referring the patient to the appropriate specialist.

History

- Determine the **degree of hematuria**: Is it microscopic or macroscopic? Although macroscopic hematuria can be seen with glomerular diseases, it is much more often a sign of lower urinary tract pathology and is often the initial symptom of genitourinary cancer.
- Look for **associated symptoms**, which are extremely important. Unintentional weight loss, fevers of unclear origin, or night sweats suggest neoplasm. Colicky flank pain radiating to the groin associated with nausea or vomiting suggests nephrolithiasis. Difficulty initiating urination, poor urinary stream, and nocturia suggest benign prostatic hypertrophy (BPH). Dysuria, frequency, urgency, and suprapubic pain suggest cystitis.
- Ask about **recent skin infections or URIs**, and the timing of the infections relative to the onset of hematuria. Post-streptococcal glomerulonephritis occurs over a week after an infection, whereas hematuria from IgA nephropathy can be seen concurrent with the URI.
- A **family history** of males with kidney disease and hearing deficit suggests Alport syndrome, whereas a family history of renal failure and stroke suggests polycystic kidney disease.
- Review **cigarette smoking history and toxin** exposures. Exposure to aromatic amines, aniline dyes, benzidine, or cyclophosphamide, as well as analgesic abuse, are risk factors for urothelial carcinoma.

Physical Examination

- Hypertension and edema are common in glomerular diseases, but they are not specific findings. Large, polycystic kidneys can often be palpated during the abdominal exam.
- Suprapubic tenderness can be seen with cystitis.
- Costovertebral tenderness can be seen with pyelonephritis or nephrolithiasis.
- Prostatic enlargement and tenderness can be seen with BPH or prostatitis.

Tests for Consideration

- **Urinalysis** can confirm the presence of hematuria and determine if there is concomitant proteinuria. It will show if there is pyuria and bacteriuria, which are often present in the setting of infection. $4
- **Urine microscopic examination** will show whether there are dysmorphic red blood cells and red blood cell casts, which can be seen with glomerular diseases. WBC casts are often present in patients with interstitial nephritis. $6
- **Urine culture** confirms the presence of infection and guides antibiotic therapy. $15

- **Serum chemistries** will determine if the patient has renal dysfunction or metabolic abnormalities such as hypercalcemia or hyperuricemia, which can lead to hematuria. $12
- **Urine cytology** is a screening test for bladder cancer. $58
- **Cystoscopy** can be used to rule out anatomic bladder or urethral pathology, as well as to search for urothelial malignancies. $473
- **Renal biopsy** is performed if the hematuria is suspected to be of renal origin; it is performed when a definitive diagnosis is necessary. $676

IMAGING CONSIDERATIONS

A **renal sonogram** is an excellent screening tool to rule out anatomic abnormalities of the kidney or to diagnose obstruction of the urinary tract. It is noninvasive and does not carry the risk of contrast. When stones are suspected, a **CT scan without contrast** is the test of choice, while **IVP** is the test of choice to look for papillary necrosis or for subtle lesions in the urinary tract.

→ **Ultrasound** of the kidneys, ureters, and bladder can detect structural abnormalities of the urinary tract, obstruction, renal abscesses, and stones. $96
→ **Intravenous pyelogram (IVP)** is the test of choice to look for papillary necrosis or subtle lesions in the urinary tract. $183
→ **Abdominal radiography** can be used to diagnose calcium-containing renal stones. $45
→ **CT scan** of the abdomen and/or pelvis can detect masses or stones within the urinary tract and can evaluate renal parenchyma. $334

Clinical Entities	Medical Knowledge

IgA Nephropathy

Pφ IgA nephropathy is caused by the production of abnormal immunoglobulin A molecules that cannot be effectively cleared from the circulation. These IgA complexes deposit in the mesangial portion of the glomeruli and cause an inflammatory reaction that leads to renal damage. It is usually a slowly progressive disease, but more than 25% of those affected will eventually progress to end-stage renal disease.

TP Patients with IgA nephropathy can present with several different clinical syndromes: recurrent synpharyngitic macroscopic hematuria in the setting of an upper respiratory illness; nephrotic-range proteinuria and microscopic hematuria; acute renal failure due to crescentic glomerulonephritis; or microscopic hematuria and non–nephrotic-range proteinuria with normal or slowly worsening renal function.

Dx The diagnosis is made by renal biopsy showing mesangial deposits of IgA and complement.

Tx The treatment of IgA nephropathy depends on the clinical presentation. Patients with recurrent macroscopic hematuria and normal renal function, and patients with microscopic hematuria and normal renal function, have an excellent prognosis and usually require no treatment. Patients with crescentic glomerulonephritis have a poor prognosis and are treated aggressively with immunosuppressive agents. Patients with nephrotic-range proteinuria are often treated with corticosteroids. Patients with microscopic hematuria and non–nephrotic-range proteinuria with progressive renal failure are treated with antiproteinuric therapy and possibly immunosuppressive medications. **See Cecil Essentials 29.**

Alport Syndrome

Pφ Alport syndrome is a type of hereditary nephritis resulting in renal failure and deafness in some affected individuals. The inheritance in most cases is X-linked, and the majority of cases result from mutations in the gene that codes for the $\alpha 5$ chain of type IV collagen. Since type IV collagen is integral to the basement membrane of the kidney, cochlea, and eye, affected individuals manifest abnormalities of these organs.

TP Males often present with persistent microscopic hematuria from an early age. As the disease progresses, they often develop proteinuria and hypertension. The majority will go on to develop renal failure and require renal replacement therapy. Many will also develop sensorineural deafness. Females will often have intermittent microscopic hematuria but are much less likely to develop significant renal failure.

Dx The diagnosis is made by observing a typical presentation in a patient with a strong family history of Alport syndrome. On kidney biopsy, electron microscopy shows typical ultrastructural changes in the basement membranes.

Tx There is no specific therapy for Alport syndrome. Hypertension and proteinuria are treated with ACE inhibitors. If a patient develops end-stage renal disease, he or she is started on dialysis or given a renal transplant. **See Cecil Essentials 29.**

Chronic Tubulointerstitial Nephritis

Pφ CTIN results from chronic inflammation of the renal tubules and interstitium. Histologically, the kidney shows interstitial scarring and fibrosis. There are many reported causes of CTIN. Exposure to drugs, including analgesics, and exposure to heavy metals, including lead, have been implicated. Rheumatologic conditions such as SLE and Sjögren syndrome can cause CTIN. Persistent hypokalemia, hypercalcemia, and reflux nephropathy can also cause CTIN.

TP CTIN is often discovered incidentally during a routine physical exam when laboratory abnormalities are discovered. In the early stages, patients are found to have microscopic hematuria and non–nephrotic-range proteinuria. When the disease is discovered late in its course, patients can present with hypertension and renal failure.

Dx The diagnosis is often made presumptively in patients who give a history of exposures or conditions associated with the development of CTIN and are found to have hematuria and non–nephrotic-range proteinuria. Renal biopsy is often necessary to confirm the diagnosis.

Tx Treatment is often supportive and includes BP control and electrolyte management. Implicated drugs should be stopped, and metabolic and rheumatologic diseases should be treated aggressively. **See Cecil Essentials 27, 30.**

Polycystic Kidney Disease

Pφ There are two major types of autosomal-dominant polycystic kidney disease. Type 1 is the most common and most severe, with approximately 50% of affected individuals requiring dialysis by the age of 60 years; it is linked to an abnormal gene on chromosome 16, named *PKD1*. Type 2 is less common and less severe, and is linked to an abnormal gene on chromosome 4, named *PKD2*. *PKD1* and *PKD2* encode proteins named polycystin-1 and polycystin-2, respectively. These proteins are involved in cell-cell and cell-matrix interactions, and mutations in these genes lead to cyst formation through an as-yet-undefined mechanism.

TP Patients often present with flank pain resulting from an infected cyst, hemorrhagic cyst, or nephrolithiasis. Other patients present with renal insufficiency and hypertension. Many patients present with extrarenal cystic manifestations; hepatic cysts can be detected in over one half of cases and are more commonly seen in women and elderly patients. Still others present with either gross or microscopic hematuria. Additional manifestations include intracranial aneurysms, which tend to cluster in families.

Dx For patients who are older than 15 years and at risk for the disease, the diagnosis is made by demonstrating multiple cysts on sonography. The number of cysts necessary to make a diagnosis depends on the patient's age. Genetic testing can be considered for patients with equivocal results on sonography or in patients who are younger than 30 years and need a definite diagnosis.

Tx Aggressive treatment of high BP may slow the progression to renal failure. ACE inhibitors are frequently used to lower BP and control proteinuria, if present. If the patient develops complications of chronic kidney disease such as anemia, acidosis, or bone disease, these manifestations should be treated. If these patients progress to end-stage renal disease, they can either receive a renal transplant or be placed on dialysis. After they are on renal replacement therapy, some patients require nephrectomy for recurrent urinary cyst infection or hemorrhage. **See Cecil Essentials 30.**

Transitional Cell Carcinoma

Pφ TCC is a common malignancy, resulting from neoplastic transformation of transitional cells lining the bladder, ureters, or renal pelvis. Risk factors for the development of TCC include environmental exposure to chemical carcinogens. These carcinogens include tobacco, analgesics, cyclophosphamide, aromatic amines, textile dyes, and chemicals used in rubber and plastic manufacturing. The exposure is theorized to cause chronic irritation and subsequent neoplastic changes.

TP Patients will typically present with macroscopic or microscopic hematuria. Additionally, patients with TCC involving the upper urinary tract may present with a palpable abdominal mass and renal colic, while patients with TCC involving the bladder may present with dysuria and frequency.

Dx The diagnosis of TCC is often difficult to establish. The difficulty stems from the limited accessibility of the ureters and renal pelvic anatomy, and from the broad differential diagnoses that must be considered in the evaluation of hematuria. Urine cytology is a good screening test, but cystoscopy and biopsy are necessary to confirm the diagnosis of TCC.

Tx Treatment depends on the cancer staging. Superficial lesions are treated with resection with or without intravesical chemotherapy. Deeply invasive tumor is usually treated with cystectomy and urinary diversion. Metastatic disease is often treated with chemotherapy. Many clinical trials are currently ongoing, evaluating the effectiveness of adjuvant chemotherapy. **See Cecil Essentials 57.**

Nephrolithiasis

Pφ Risk factors for kidney stones include Caucasian race, male gender, older age, obesity, and a history of polycystic kidney disease, hyperparathyroidism, or RTA. Kidney stones arise when the urine becomes supersaturated with calcium, oxalate, or uric acid, resulting in nidus formation. Ions from supersaturated urine will collect around the nidus to form stones. The most common type of kidney stones is calcium stones, followed by struvite stones, and uric acid stones. Cystine stones are rare. Calcium stones are more likely to form when there is excess calcium or oxalate in the urine, or when there is a deficiency of citrate in the urine. Struvite stones almost always occur in the setting of chronic or recurrent UTIs. Uric acid stones occur in the setting of excess uric acid secondary to malignancies or disorders of uric acid metabolism.

TP Kidney stones may be asymptomatic and found incidentally on abdominal imaging or in a workup for hematuria. Patients with large stones that cause obstruction or infection present with symptoms. The most common symptom is intense, colicky pain in the back, flank, lower abdomen, groin, and/or genitals. Patients often complain that they cannot find a position to alleviate the pain. Urinalysis usually shows microscopic hematuria.

Dx When the history suggests kidney stones, the diagnosis is made through imaging tests. Potential tests include abdominal radiography, ultrasound, IVP, retrograde pyelogram, and noncontrast spiral CT scan. Currently, noncontrast spiral CT scan is the test of choice. When a stone is obtained, its composition should be determined by stone analysis. Patients with recurrent stones should have a 24-hour urine stone risk profile performed. This evaluation can detect metabolic abnormalities of calcium, citrate, oxalate, and uric acid that make stone formation more likely.

Tx Treatment depends on the type and size of the kidney stone. Options include conservative management with hydration and pain control, extracorporeal shock wave lithotripsy (ESWL), and surgical removal. Prevention of stone formation includes high fluid and low sodium intake in all affected individuals. Additional therapy depends on the type of stone and associated metabolic abnormality but may include thiazide diuretics for individuals with hypercalciuria, dietary modification for individuals with hyperoxaluria, and urine alkalization and allopurinol for patients with uric acid stones. Complicated cases require nephrology and urology referrals. **See Cecil Essentials 30.**

Cystitis

Pφ Cystitis is caused when microorganisms that are capable of infecting bladder cells such as *Escherichia coli*, *Staphylococcus saphrophyticus*, *Proteus mirabilis*, *Enterococcus* spp., or *Klebsiella* spp. gain access to the bladder. Most commonly this occurs when microorganisms of the rectal and vaginal flora gain access to the bladder by first entering the distal urethra. Less commonly, cystitis can occur after urethral instrumentation. In men, isolated infectious cystitis is quite uncommon. When it does occur, it is often seen in the setting of anatomic or functional urinary tract obstruction.

TP Patients with cystitis present with dysuria, which is often associated with frequency and urgency. The location of the pain is typically suprapubic. The presence of fever, nausea, vomiting, or flank pain suggests pyelonephritis. Urinalysis will typically show microscopic hematuria, WBCs, and bacteriuria.

Dx The diagnostic approach to cystitis depends on the clinical scenario. To make a proper diagnosis a clinician must first categorize the cystitis. Uncomplicated cystitis occurs in young, healthy women. Complicated cystitis occurs in patients who are male, elderly, pregnant, diabetic, immunocompromised, after instrumentation, or in the presence of urolithiasis, urinary tract malignancy, foreign body, or functional or structural urinary tract abnormalities. The diagnosis of cystitis in a young, healthy woman can initially be a clinical one. A female with dysuria, frequency, and urgency can be presumptively diagnosed and treated for uncomplicated cystitis. On the other hand, patients with complicated cystitis should undergo formal diagnosis with urinalysis, culture, and sensitivity testing. The degree of pyuria and bacteriuria required to make a diagnosis of UTI will differ depending upon the clinical scenario.

Tx Cystitis is treated with antimicrobial agents. In uncomplicated cystitis in young, healthy females, empirical treatment with trimethoprim-sulfamethoxazole or a fluoroquinolone (e.g., ciprofloxacin) for a short 3-day course is acceptable. A clinician should be aware of geographic antimicrobial resistance patterns in his or her area. Treatment of cystitis in patients other than young, healthy females should be case-specific and guided by the urine culture and sensitivity. **See Cecil Essentials 105.**

Papillary Necrosis

Pφ Papillary necrosis results from ischemia to the renal medulla. The papillae, which are located in the medulla, are vulnerable to ischemic injury due to their limited blood supply and the surrounding hypertonic environment. Conditions associated with papillary necrosis include analgesic use, diabetes mellitus, sickle cell disease, and UTIs.

TP Affected individuals often present with hematuria, which can be microscopic or macroscopic, and dysuria. If the sloughed papillae cause obstruction, patients can present with renal colic. Patients with multiple sloughed papillae or solitary kidneys can present with acute renal failure. When there is an associated infection, patients will have fever and leukocytosis.

Dx The most sensitive test to diagnose papillary necrosis is an IVP. This test will show irregular calyces with central contrast defects representing the necrosed papillae. Sloughed papillae can cause filling defects in the ureters.

Tx Treatment is supportive. If patients are hypotensive, they should be given IV fluids. If the hematuria is significant, patients may need to be transfused. Offending analgesics should be stopped. UTIs must be treated with antibiotics. If the sloughed papillae are obstructing the ureters, they may have to be removed by interventional means.

ZEBRA ZONE

a. **Sickle cell disease:** Patients with sickle cell anemia commonly have microscopic hematuria that is thought to result from microthrombotic infarction of the renal medulla caused by sickling of red blood cells in the vasa recta. Affected patients can also develop papillary necrosis and have resultant microscopic or macroscopic hematuria.

b. **Hyperuricosuria and hypercalciuria:** The presence of both hyperuricosuria and hypercalcuria has been associated with microscopic hematuria. The correlation is found more commonly in children than adults. Hyperuricosuria can be treated with allopurinol, while hypercalciuria can be treated with hydrochlorothiazide.

Practice-Based Learning and Improvement: Evidence-Based Medicine

Title
A prospective analysis of 1930 patients with hematuria to evaluate current diagnostic practice

Authors
Khadra MH, Pickard RS, Charlton M, Powell PH, Neal DE

Institution
Freeman Hospital, University of Newcastle upon Tyne, United Kingdom

Reference
J Urol 2000;163:524–527

Problem
To determine guidelines for the evaluation of hematuria

Intervention
A total of 1930 consecutive cases of hematuria were prospectively evaluated. Every patient underwent IVP, abdominal sonogram, and cystoscopy.

Quality of evidence
Level II-2

Outcome/effect
In 61% of the subjects no basis of hematuria was found; 12% had bladder cancer, 13% had UTI, 4% had stones, and 10% had nephrologic causes.

Historical significance/comments
Most evidence-based recommendations for the urologic evaluation and follow-up of hematuria

Interpersonal and Communication Skills

Balance Concern with Reassurance in Patients with an Unexpected Finding

When discussing asymptomatic microscopic hematuria, the clinician needs to balance a patient's awareness of the potential diagnoses, which can include malignancy, with the reassurance that hematuria is usually related to a benign process. If you allow patients to ask questions and ensure timely follow-up, patients will become more at ease with the evaluation and the uncertainty. Early in the evaluation, patients should also understand that the cause of hematuria is often not discovered, and periodic (and even prolonged) follow-up may be necessary.

Professionalism

Honor Patient Autonomy

Patient autonomy often becomes an issue when a clinician recommends an invasive diagnostic test such as renal biopsy. When a patient refuses a test that a clinician feels is important to the patient's well-being, the clinician must ensure that the refusal is made in a properly informed setting. Physicians should offer a comfortable environment free of time restraints to discuss such matters, allowing patients to voice their fears and questions. If the patient refuses a procedure after thorough education and discussion, the patient's decision must be honored and the patient should also be assured that the clinician's care will continue.

Systems-Based Practice

Process Improvement

Popular business models are beginning to be used to reengineer the health care system. *Six Sigma*, a business model of process improvement, consists of specific steps—"define, measure, analyze, improve, and control"—that can be applied to health care process improvement. In the case of a patient with massive hematuria, processes must be in place to ensure appropriate initial management and ongoing care. In this case, one could *define* the problem, *measure* any process issues that may lead to a delay in diagnosis or management, *analyze* methods to ensure mobilization of appropriate team members, *improve* coordination of care, and *control* the process to ensure a better outcome (e.g., by defining measures to determine the problem and ensure timely intervention). To improve on patient care, there must be a commitment to process reengineering and to customer service.

Chapter 24
Dysuria (Case 17)

Cindy Baskin MD *and Michael Gitman* MD

Case: The patient is a 68-year-old woman with a past medical history of hypercholesterolemia controlled with simvastatin. Her husband is a 72-year-old man with a past medical history of BPH; his symptoms are controlled with tamsulosin. They are both retired and have a very healthy and active lifestyle. She is seeing you today for her annual checkup. She feels generally well but for the past 3 weeks has noticed an uncomfortable feeling when she urinates. She remembers when her husband had complained of similar symptoms 3 years ago and was diagnosed with BPH. She jokes and states she knows her problem must not be related to the prostate.

Differential Diagnosis

Infection and Inflammation of Urinary Tract Organs	Infection and Inflammation of Non-Urinary Tract Organs	Obstructive and Structural Abnormalities
Urethritis	Vulvovaginitis	BPH
Cystitis	Prostatitis	Urethral stricture
Pyelonephritis	Epididymo-orchitis	Urethral diverticula
		Nephrolithiasis

Speaking Intelligently

Dysuria is a very common complaint in adults. Etiologies differ according to gender. Infection of the urinary tract organs is the most common cause in women, but vaginal infections and inflammation can also cause dysuria. In men isolated bladder infections are rare, but urethritis and disorders of the prostate often present with dysuria.

PATIENT CARE

Clinical Thinking
- History and physical exam frequently reveal the etiology of dysuria.
- In patients who present with dysuria, and a history and physical exam consistent with an uncomplicated UTI, empirical

antibiotics can usually be prescribed without further diagnostic testing.
- Further diagnostic testing is required for patients with symptoms or signs suggestive of complicated UTIs, noninfectious urinary tract disorders, or non–urinary tract disorders.

History
- Ask about the duration and location of the pain, as well as the presence of frequency or hematuria; chronic symptoms are less likely to be infectious.
- Internal or suprapubic pain is more likely to be secondary to cystitis, while external pain is more likely to be due to urethritis, or vaginal infection or inflammation.
- Back pain is suggestive of pyelonephritis or nephrolithiasis.
- Frequency and hematuria are often symptoms of a UTI.
- Co-morbid conditions that predispose patients to UTIs, such as prior UTIs or recent urinary tract instrumentation, should be sought out.
- All patients should be asked if they are sexually active, as sexual activity is a risk factor for urethritis, cystitis, vaginitis, and cervicitis.
- Women should be asked about the timing of the pain during urination and the presence of vaginal discharge, lesions, or dryness.
- Pain during urination often suggests urethritis or vaginitis, while pain directly after urinating suggests cystitis.
- Vaginal discharge is often a symptom of vaginitis or cervicitis, while vaginal lesions suggest vaginal infections and/or inflammation. Vaginal dryness, postmenopausal status, and dyspareunia suggest hypoestrogenemia or atrophic vaginitis (or both).
- Sexually active women are at increased risk for vaginal, cervical, or urinary tract infection.
- Men should be asked about the duration of pain and the presence of associated symptoms. Chronic symptoms suggest chronic prostatitis. Fever, chills, malaise, myalgias, obstructive symptoms, and cloudy urine suggest acute bacterial prostatitis. Testicular pain suggests acute epididymitis or orchitis. Pruritus, genital lesions, or discharge at the urethral meatus suggests urethritis secondary to a sexually transmitted disease.

Physical Examination
- In women, the physical exam should include vital signs, a thorough abdominal exam, and assessment for costovertebral tenderness. A pelvic exam should be performed if signs and symptoms are not suggestive of a UTI. The exam should evaluate for vaginal, urethral, and/or cervical discharge as well as for cervical motion tenderness.

- In men, the physical exam should include vital signs, a thorough abdominal exam with assessment for costovertebral tenderness, and inspection and palpation of the testes, penis, and epididymides. Additionally, the prostate should be palpated for size, nodules, swelling, and tenderness. The urethra should be inspected for the presence of urethral discharge.

Tests for Consideration

- **Urinalysis** can screen for the presence of hematuria, pyuria, and bacteriuria, which are often present in the setting of infection. $4
- **Urine culture** confirms the presence of infection and guides antibiotic therapy; culture is not required if the patient does not have pyuria. $15
- **Vaginal/urethral smears and cultures** can detect *Trichomonas vaginalis*, *Candida* spp., *Neisseria gonorrhoeae*, and *Chlamydia trachomatis*. $27
- **Cystoscopy** can be used to rule out anatomic bladder or urethral pathology. $473
- **Urine cytology** is a screening test for bladder cancer. $58

IMAGING CONSIDERATIONS

→ In men with UTIs, as well as women with complicated UTI, **ultrasound** of the bladder, ureters, kidneys, and prostate can detect structural abnormalities of the urinary tract, obstruction, renal abscesses, and stones. It can also be used to measure prostate size. $96

→ **CT scan of the abdomen** can detect masses or stones within the urinary tract and can evaluate the renal parenchyma. When a ureteral stone is suspected, a CT scan of the abdomen without contrast is the imaging study of choice. $334

→ **MRI** of the abdomen can detect masses or stones within the urinary tract and evaluate the renal parenchyma. $534

| Clinical Entities | Medical Knowledge |

Urethritis

Pφ Urethritis can be infectious or noninfectious. In women, infectious urethritis can be secondary to typical urinary tract organisms such as *Escherichia coli*, *Staphylococcus saprophyticus*, *Proteus mirabilis*, *Enterococcus* spp., or *Klebsiella* spp. Additionally, infectious urethritis can be due to sexually transmitted organisms such as *N. gonorrhoeae* or *C. trachomatis*, or organisms associated with vaginitis, such as *T. vaginalis*, *Candida* spp., herpes simplex virus, and bacterial vaginosis.

In males, urethritis is most commonly secondary to sexually transmitted organisms including *N. gonorrhoeae*, *C. trachomatis*, *Trichomonas*, *Candida*, and herpes simplex virus. In both males and females, irritants, such as spermicides, lubricants, perfumes, and soaps, can cause a chemical urethritis.

TP Painful urination, which is often associated with frequency and urgency, is the main presenting symptom of urethritis. Hematuria may be present when the cause is infection with typical urinary tract organisms but is often absent in urethritis due to *C. trachomatis*. Purulent discharge may be seen in urethritis secondary to *N. gonorrhoeae*. Patients with genital herpes may present with vesicular lesions.

Dx Urinalysis reveals pyuria in urethritis secondary to typical urinary tract organisms and *N. gonorrhoeae* or *C. trachomatis*, but bacteriuria is often absent in *N. gonorrhoeae* or *C. trachomatis* urethritis. In urethritis secondary to typical urinary tract organisms, urine culture often reveals the causative organism. Urethritis secondary to *N. gonorrhoeae* or *C. trachomatis* is best diagnosed by DNA amplification of the urethral discharge. Urethritis caused by typical vaginal organisms is best diagnosed by examination of the discharge on smear and wet mount, assessment of the pH, and culture of the discharge. For patients who present with typical vesicular lesions, culture for herpesvirus can confirm the diagnosis. In patients with irritant urethritis, a temporal relationship between product use and symptoms suggests the diagnosis.

Tx Treatment of infectious urethritis is antibiotics aimed at the offending organism. For typical urinary tract urethritis, empirical antibiotic therapy without isolation of a specific organism may be appropriate. Treatment of noninfectious urethritis is aimed at removing the irritant. **See Cecil Essentials 105, 107.**

Cystitis

Pφ Cystitis may be infectious or noninfectious. Infectious cystitis is caused by typical urinary tract organisms, such as *E. coli*, *S. saprophyticus*, *P. mirabilis*, *Enterococcus* spp., or *Klebsiella* spp. Unlike urethritis, sexually transmitted organisms and organisms associated with vaginitis do not typically cause infectious cystitis. In men, isolated infectious cystitis is quite uncommon. When it does occur, it is often seen in the setting of anatomic or functional urinary tract obstruction.

Interstitial cystitis is a cause of noninfectious cystitis. The pathogenesis is not clearly defined but may be due to an abnormality in the growth of cells that line the bladder. This disorder most commonly affects young women.

TP Cystitis presents with painful urination, which is often associated with frequency and urgency. The location of the pain is typically suprapubic.

Dx In infectious cystitis, urinalysis reveals pyuria and bacteriuria, and urine culture reveals a colony count >100,000 colony-forming units (CFU)/mL. Interstitial cystitis is diagnosed by typical symptoms and the absence of other etiologies. Pain and urgency symptoms elicited by filling of the bladder during cystoscopy may support the diagnosis.

Tx Treatment of infectious cystitis is antibiotics aimed at the offending organism. Treatment of interstitial cystitis is aimed at pain relief with oral pain relievers as well as local instillation of anesthetics. Additionally, pentosan polysulfate is approved for the treatment of interstitial cystitis. **See Cecil Essentials 105.**

Pyelonephritis

Pφ Acute pyelonephritis most commonly results from lower urinary tract organisms that ascend and invade the renal parenchyma. Anatomic abnormalities, such as vesicoureteral reflux, or obstruction at any level of the urinary tract, are risk factors for pyelonephritis. Additionally, host factors including the P1 blood group phenotype, which is associated with the presence of antigens that allow bacterial attachment to the urinary tract epithelium, are important to the development of pyelonephritis. Specific bacterial adhesion molecules, including the P-fimbriae family, are commonly found in pyelonephritis-producing *E. coli*.

TP Patients with acute pyelonephritis present with lower urinary tract symptoms of dysuria and frequency as well as upper urinary tract symptoms of flank pain and costovertebral angle tenderness. Patients often have systemic symptoms including fever, chills, nausea, and vomiting.

Dx The diagnosis of acute pyelonephritis is made by its typical clinical presentation, in conjunction with pyuria and isolation of a typical urinary tract pathogen. Other laboratory results, such as leukocytosis, may reveal signs of systemic infection. Urinalysis may reveal WBC casts. Imaging may not be necessary in otherwise healthy patients who respond to antibiotic therapy within 72 hours of treatment initiation. Pre- and post-contrast CT scan is the test of choice to reveal signs of complicated pyelonephritis, such as a perinephric abscess.

Tx Treatment of acute, uncomplicated pyelonephritis can often be achieved in the outpatient setting. For severe infections and in immunocompromised hosts, hospitalization may be necessary. Empirical treatment of acute pyelonephritis should be aimed at the likely offending organism, followed by targeted therapy once an organism has been isolated by urine or blood culture. If no organism is isolated, initiation of empirical broad-spectrum antibiotic therapy to cover gram-negative organisms (e.g., ceftriaxone or ciprofloxacin) is appropriate. **See Cecil Essentials 105.**

Vulvovaginitis

Pφ The etiology of vulvovaginitis can be infectious or noninfectious. Infections with agents causing vulvovaginitis can be sexually transmitted, such as *T. vaginalis* or herpes simplex virus, due to *Candida albicans*, which may be exacerbated by antibiotic use, or a result of bacterial vaginosis, which is caused by an overgrowth of certain bacterial organisms. Noninfectious etiologies of vulvovaginitis include irritants, including soaps, sprays, and perfumes, and hypoestrogenemia in postmenopausal women.

TP Patients with infectious vulvovaginitis typically present with external dysuria, vaginal discharge, odor, itch, irritation, and erythema. Hypoestrogenemia and atrophic vaginitis present with vaginal dryness, dyspareunia, and thinning of the vaginal mucosal lining.

Dx The diagnosis of infectious vulvovaginitis is often made by vaginal culture and smear. On wet mount, the presence of branching hyphae and buds is typical of *Candida,* while mobile trichomonads are found in patients infected with *T. vaginalis.* Bacterial vaginosis is diagnosed by a positive whiff test and the presence of clue cells on wet mount. The diagnosis of noninfectious vulvovaginitis requires a careful history for use of irritants, sexual activity, and menopausal status in conjunction with a physical exam lacking vaginal discharge and perhaps significant for vaginal dryness and mucosal thinning.

Tx Treatment of vulvovaginitis is aimed at removing the offending agent, treating the underlying causative infection, and restoring vaginal hormonal balance as applicable. **See Cecil Essentials 107.**

Prostatitis

Pφ Acute prostatitis is usually infectious in origin and is caused by typical gram-negative urinary tract organisms as well as the agents of sexually transmitted infections. The infection is believed to result from reflux of infected urine into the prostatic ducts. Hematogenous, lymphatic, or contiguous spread from local infections can also occur. Acute prostatitis can occur after instrumentation of the urinary tract or prostate. It occurs most frequently in men with obstructive uropathy.

Chronic prostatitis is less well understood. Chronic prostatitis may be infectious or noninfectious. Infectious chronic prostatitis is caused by bacterial infections similar to those that cause acute prostatitis, but they recur or persist. Noninfectious chronic prostatitis is associated with a chronic pelvic pain syndrome in men that may not even involve infection or inflammation of the prostate gland.

TP Acute prostatitis presents with symptoms of dysuria, as well as perineal, back, penile, and/or testicular pain. Patients often have associated urinary frequency, hesitancy, and incomplete bladder emptying. At times, systemic symptoms of fevers, myalgias, nausea, and vomiting are present.

Chronic bacterial prostatitis presents with recurrent symptoms similar to those of acute prostatitis. Chronic noninfectious prostatitis–chronic pelvic pain syndrome presents with symptoms of pain, including pain with ejaculation, urinary hesitancy, and frequency.

Dx The diagnosis is made by a typical historical presentation in conjunction with a tender and swollen prostate on exam. Urinalysis and culture before and after prostatic massage can confirm the diagnosis and identify a causative organism. Prostatic massage is often deferred in the setting of acute prostatitis to avoid hematogenous spread of the infection.

Tx Antibiotics are used to treat acute bacterial prostatitis. The choice of antibiotic is aimed at the suspected or confirmed offending organism. When empirical treatment is required, the choice of antibiotic will depend upon the history and will be directed at either typical urinary tract organisms or sexually transmitted organisms. Mild infections can be managed on an outpatient basis, while severe infections with systemic symptoms will require hospitalization. The treatment of chronic bacterial prostatitis is the same as that for acute bacterial prostatitis, but longer courses of antibiotics are often necessary. α-Blockers and pain relievers may also be prescribed to lessen the urinary symptoms. Chronic noninfectious prostatitis is more difficult to manage. NSAIDs may be beneficial. **See Cecil Essentials 72, 105.**

Epididymo-Orchitis

Pφ Epididymo-orchitis most often results from retrograde extension of bacteria from the vas deferens. Causative organisms include both typical urinary tract organisms and sexually transmitted infections. Rarely, epididymitis is caused by nonbacterial organisms, such as *Candida*, or chemical irritants, such as reflux of sterile urine.

TP Patients with epididymo-orchitis present with dysuria, hesitancy, and frequency, as well as urethral discharge and a painful, edematous scrotum. Patients may also complain of abdominal pain and systemic symptoms.

Dx The diagnosis is made by careful history and physical exam revealing a tender, erythematous, swollen scrotum. Early in the course of disease, before testicular involvement, tenderness may be localized to the epididymis. Gram stain and culture of the urethral discharge, and/or DNA amplification, can confirm the causative agent. The most important diagnosis to exclude when a patient presents with such symptoms is testicular torsion; imaging with Doppler ultrasound is often necessary to exclude this serious condition.

Tx Treatment consists of antibiotics aimed at the causative agent. **See Cecil Essentials 72.**

Benign Prostatic Hypertrophy

Pφ BPH refers to the enlargement of the prostate gland, not from hypertrophy, but from hyperplasia of the stromal and epithelial cells of the prostate. This hyperplasia often occurs in the periurethral portion of the prostate. The pathogenesis is not completely understood, but it is clear that androgens, particularly dihydrotestosterone (DHT), are necessary but not sufficient to cause BPH. Further research shows that high estrogen levels accompanied by lower levels of free testosterone probably have a role in the development of BPH.

TP Men with BPH present with obstructive and irritative urinary symptoms such as hesitancy, frequency, straining, and weakened stream. Men may be asymptomatic and be diagnosed by physical exam alone.

Dx Diagnosis is made by finding an enlarged prostate on physical exam and possibly by a history of typical symptoms.

Tx Treatment is indicated only for symptomatic patients. Lifestyle modifications, such as decreasing night-time fluids, should be initiated in all symptomatic men. α-Blockers may decrease urinary symptoms by relaxing the smooth muscles in the bladder neck and prostate, thereby improving urine flow. 5α-Reductase inhibitors decrease the levels of circulating DHT. Multiple herbal supplements that have demonstrated varied efficacy also exist. If medication fails to sufficiently control symptoms, invasive and minimally invasive surgical options are available. **See Cecil Essentials 72.**

Urethral Stricture

Pφ Urethral strictures usually occur in patients with inflammation or scarring of the urethra resulting from recurrent urethritis or urethral instrumentation (most commonly by a urinary catheter or cystoscope). It is less common in women than men due to the short length of the female urethra. Rarely, external compression by a tumor can cause urethral stricture.

TP Dysuria, difficulty urinating, spraying of urine, and slow urine stream are all symptoms of a stricture.

Dx A suggestive history should prompt the clinician to obtain a retrograde urethrogram and/or a cystoscopy, which can definitively diagnose the disease.

Tx There are no medical treatments for urethral stricture. A temporary suprapubic catheter may be necessary in the acute setting. Urethral dilation, urethroplasty, and/or urethrotomy can be performed depending on the severity, length, and location of the stricture.

Urethral Diverticulum

Pφ Urethral diverticulum is a condition seen in women who have an outpouching of a localized area of the urethra into the anterior vaginal wall. The etiology of the diverticulum is believed to be repeated infection of the periurethral glands, which leads to inflammation, fibrosis, and the formation of a cavity. This process ultimately leads to the development of a urethral diverticulum.

TP The classic triad of symptoms includes post-void dribbling, dysuria, and dyspareunia. Frequency, urgency, incontinence, and recurrent infections are also common.

Dx Typical symptoms, along with detection of an anterior vaginal wall mass that expresses urine when palpated, is highly suggestive of a urinary diverticulum. A voiding cystourethrography and MRI exam confirm the diagnosis and localize the pathologic area.

Tx Treatment options include both open and endoscopic surgeries.

Nephrolithiasis

Pφ Risk factors for kidney stones (i.e., nephrolithiasis) include Caucasian race, male gender, older age, obesity, a history of polycystic kidney disease, hyperparathyroidism, and RTA. Kidney stones arise when the urine becomes too concentrated and urinary minerals develop crystals that combine to form stones. The most common type of kidney stone is calcium stones, followed by struvite stones and uric acid stones. Cystine stones are rare. Calcium stones are more likely to form when there is excess calcium or oxalate in the urine or when there is a deficiency of citrate in the urine. Struvite stones almost always occur in the setting of chronic or recurrent UTIs. Uric acid stones occur in the setting of excess uric acid secondary to malignancies or disorders of uric acid metabolism.

TP Kidney stones may be asymptomatic and found incidentally on abdominal imaging or in a workup for hematuria. Patients with large stones that cause obstruction or infection present with symptoms. The most common symptom is intense, colicky pain in the back, flank, lower abdomen, groin, and/or genitals. Other signs and symptoms may include hematuria, frequency, nausea, vomiting, fever, and chills.

Dx When the history suggests kidney stones, the diagnosis is made through imaging tests. Potential tests including abdominal radiography, ultrasound, IVP, retrograde pyelogram, and noncontrast spiral CT scan. Currently noncontrast spiral CT scan is the test of choice. When a stone is obtained, its composition should be determined by stone analysis. Patients with recurrent stones should have a 24-hour urine stone risk profile performed. This evaluation can detect metabolic abnormalities of calcium, citrate, oxalate, and uric acid that make stone formation more likely.

Tx Treatment depends on the type and size of the kidney stone. Options include conservative management with hydration and pain control, ESWL, and surgical removal. Prevention of stone formation includes high fluid and low sodium intake in all affected individuals. Additional therapy depends on the type of stone and associated metabolic abnormality but may include thiazide diuretics, dietary modification, urine alkalization, allopurinol, and treatment and prevention of urinary infections. **See Cecil Essentials 30.**

ZEBRA ZONE

a. **Behcet syndrome:** is a multisystem inflammatory disorder. Patients present with recurrent painful oral ulcers, ocular disease, CNS disease, a nondestructive arthritis, as well as penile, scrotal, or vulvar ulcerations. Affected patients often develop dysuria. The diagnosis is a one of exclusion, and the treatment often requires symptomatic therapy and corticosteroids.

Practice-Based Learning and Improvement: Evidence-Based Medicine

Title
Randomized study of single-dose, three-day, and seven-day treatment of cystitis in women

Authors
Greenberg RN, Reilly PM, Luppen KL, Weinandt WJ, Ellington LL, Bollinger MR

Reference
J Infect Dis 1986;153:277–282

Problem
How long should we treat women with uncomplicated cystitis with antibiotics?

Intervention
Women with uncomplicated cystitis were randomized to receive either cefadroxil or trimethoprim-sulfamethoxazole for a 1, 3-, or 7-day course.

Quality of evidence
Level 1

Outcome/effect
The results indicated that 3-day treatment might improve cure rates and reduce relapse over single-dose, and that 3-day may be as effective as 7-day therapy.

Historical significance/comments
Physicians generally treat uncomplicated cystitis in women with 3-day courses of antibiotics.

Interpersonal and Communication Skills

Sensitivity in Obtaining a Sexual History Applies to All Age Groups
Sexually transmitted diseases are not only problems of teenagers and young adults, but affect all populations and all age groups. An appropriate sexual history is therefore part of a complete history in all patients. Elderly men and women often find new partners and remain sexually active. Though asking older patients about their sexual activity may be uncomfortable for the physician and elicit unease in the patient, it is very necessary. As in younger patients, a sexual history should be obtained in a gentle, nonjudgmental manner. Patients should be interviewed in private. This may at times be difficult in situations in which one partner is the caregiver for the

other. In this situation it may be necessary to utilize the help of office staff to ensure a safe, confidential conversation. Sexual relations occur outside of marriage and do occur in long-term care, nursing homes, and assisted-living facilities. While elderly patients no longer require birth control, it is important to ask and counsel about condom use for prevention of sexually transmitted infections.

Professionalism

Commitment to the Health of the Community

When physicians diagnose patients with sexually transmitted infections, they must remember that their professional commitment requires not only notification and treatment of the patient but a responsibility to ensure effective infection control strategies for their patients' partners and their community. Many options exist for ensuring infection control, but unfortunately they are not always utilized. Physicians should advise their patients to abstain from sexual activity during treatment, use condoms, and inform their partners of their diagnosis. Additionally, physicians should make a follow-up inquiry as to whether or not their patients notified their partners and if their partners received treatment. Physicians can ask their patients for their partner contact information and notify partners personally, or report their patients' contact information to the state health department. Some states allow physicians to give medications to their patients for their partners to use. Whatever method is employed, physicians have a responsibility to treat their individual patients and to control infections in their community.

Systems-Based Practice

Be Attentive to Psychological Care in Patients with Chronic Problems

Conditions that cause dysuria and associated symptoms are often chronic in nature, including interstitial cystitis, atrophic vaginitis, and chronic noninfectious prostatitis. Management of these conditions is often best achieved by a multidisciplinary care team that includes a primary-care physician, urologist or gynecologist (or both), a pain management team, and a therapist. Because of the chronic pain and symptoms that may restrict normal activities, patients often become depressed. Effective management must address both the pain and psychological symptoms in order to help the patient maintain the highest level of functioning despite the frequently incomplete resolution of symptoms.

Chapter 25
Renal Mass (Case 18)

Azzour Hazzan MD

Case: A 46-year-old woman presents for an evaluation of hematuria and flank pain over the past few days. Her pain is dull without radiation, and she has no associated nausea or vomiting. She denies dysuria or frothy urine. Her father died at age 50 years from an intracranial aneurysm. Her exam is remarkable for elevated BP, distended flanks, and left flank tenderness to palpation.

Differential Diagnosis

Polycystic kidney disease (PCKD)	Renal cancer
Acquired cystic kidney disease	Renal manifestations of tuberous sclerosis and renal angiomyolipoma
Medullary sponge kidney (MSK) disease	

Speaking Intelligently

Certain factors should be considered when evaluating a patient with a renal mass or renal masses. These include the ultrasonographic characteristics of the mass, the presence of patient-specific risk factors for renal malignancy, and systemic signs and symptoms that suggest specific diseases. For example, a 2-cm renal mass that is cystic in nature on ultrasound with no septations in a 30-year-old patient who is otherwise healthy is most likely a benign cyst and needs no further workup. Conversely, a 5-cm mass with complex features such as calcifications or septations in a 60-year-old patient with a history of anemia, fever, and weight loss is very suggestive of renal cell carcinoma.

PATIENT CARE

Clinical Thinking
- Renal lesions are most often discovered incidentally during abdominal imaging.

- Patients with PCKD usually have a family history of renal insufficiency and are hypertensive.
- Patients with acquired cystic kidney disease usually have a known history of renal disease, often requiring dialysis.
- Patients with MSK often give a history of nephrolithiasis and UTIs.
- Renal cancers are usually larger than 4 cm and often are associated with weight loss, fever, or hematuria.
- Hamartomas or angiomyolipomas can be part of a systemic syndrome such as tuberous sclerosis.

History
- Patients with PCKD often have a family history of PCKD with relatives requiring dialysis, as well as a family history of intracranial aneurysms. The patients often carry a diagnosis of hypertension and chronic kidney disease but may not have been diagnosed with PCKD. They can present with UTIs, kidney stones, or hematuria, but often they are asymptomatic and only diagnosed when multiple renal cysts are discovered on unrelated imaging.
- Patients with acquired cystic kidney disease usually have a known history of long-standing advanced chronic kidney disease. These cysts are more common in African-American men. They can present with painful hematuria but more commonly are asymptomatic and only discovered on unrelated imaging.
- The medullary cysts found as part of medullary sponge kidney disease can be diagnosed as part of the workup of the associated nephrolithiasis but are often found incidentally.
- Patients with renal neoplasm can present with fever and weight loss as well as hematuria and flank pain.
- Renal angiomyolipomas can be seen as part of tuberous sclerosis complex or von Hippel-Lindau (VHL) disease. When they are part of tuberous sclerosis complex, patients can have a history of seizures and mental retardation. When associated with VHL disease, they can be associated with retinal angiomas, and spinal and cerebellar hemangioblastomas.

Physical Examination
- Accurate BP measurement is essential. Although hypertension is not specific to any particular cystic entity, it is almost always seen in advanced PCKD and it is a target of treatment for all renal diseases.
- The abdominal exam ranges from unremarkable in cases of small cysts, to palpable masses with flank tenderness in cases of large cysts or renal masses.
- Hypomelanotic skin lesions, called ash-leaf spots, can be seen in tuberous sclerosis.

- Rarely, when a renal cancer invades and obstructs the left renal vein, this can result in a left testicular varicocele.

Tests for Consideration
- **Basic metabolic panel** to assess kidney function. Serum creatinine can be abnormal in PCKD and acquired cystic disease. It is usually normal in medullary sponge kidney disease and renal cancer. $12
- **Renal biopsy:** Biopsy samples of indeterminate lesions can help to determine a histologic diagnosis; biopsies are usually *not* done for cystic disease. $676
- **Genetic testing** for polycystic kidney disease: Can be done if sonographic diagnosis is questionable or the patient is considering kidney donation. $5275

IMAGING CONSIDERATIONS

→ **Ultrasound** is inexpensive and has an acceptable sensitivity for most diseases. It can readily distinguish solid from cystic lesions; however, it is operator dependent and is unable to distinguish vascular from nonvascular lesions. Ultrasound is a good initial test, because it can differentiate benign cysts from potentially malignant lesions. If the criteria for a simple cyst by ultrasonography are not satisfied, the patient should undergo CT scanning before and after injection of iodinated contrast. $96

→ **CT**, with and without contrast, is helpful in evaluating cysts with complex components. **CT urography** allows imaging of both the renal parenchyma and the collecting system. Cysts or masses that enhance with contrast are concerning for malignancy. $334

→ **MRI** may be useful when ultrasonography and CT are nondiagnostic or when radiographic contrast cannot be administered because of allergy or poor renal function (or both). MRI, like CT, is helpful in evaluating cysts with complex components or solid masses. Cysts or masses that enhance with contrast are concerning for malignancy. MRI may be particularly valuable if a tumor is present to identify the presence and/or extent of involvement of the collecting system and/or inferior vena cava. $534

Clinical Entities	Medical Knowledge

Polycystic Kidney Disease

Pφ There are two major types of autosomal-dominant PCKD. Autosomal-dominant PCKD type 1 is the most common and most severe, with approximately 50% of affected individuals requiring dialysis by the age of 60 years. It is linked to an abnormal gene on chromosome 16, named *PKD1*. Autosomal-dominant PCKD type 2 is less common and less severe, and is linked to an abnormal gene on chromosome 4, named *PKD2*. *PKD1* and *PKD2* encode the proteins polycystin-1 and polycystin-2, respectively. These proteins are involved in cell-cell and cell-matrix interactions. Mutations in these genes lead to cyst formation through an as-yet-undefined mechanism.

TP Often affected patients present with flank pain, resulting from an infected cyst, hemorrhagic cyst, or nephrolithiasis. Other patients present with renal insufficiency and hypertension. Still others present with extrarenal cystic manifestations. Hepatic cysts can be detected in over one half of cases and are more commonly seen in women and in patients over the age of 40 years. An additional manifestation includes intracranial aneurysms, which tend to cluster in families.

Dx For patients who are older than 15 years and at risk for the disease, the diagnosis is made by demonstrating multiple cysts on sonography. The number of cysts necessary to make a diagnosis depends on the patient's age. Genetic testing can be considered for patients with equivocal results on sonography or in patients who are younger than 30 years and need a definite diagnosis.

Tx Aggressive treatment of high BP may slow the progression to renal failure. ACE inhibitors are frequently used to lower BP and control proteinuria. If the patient develops complications of chronic kidney disease such as anemia, acidosis, or bone disease, these manifestations should be treated. If these patients reach end-stage renal disease, they can either receive a renal transplant or be placed on dialysis. After they are on renal replacement therapy, some patients require nephrectomy for recurrent urinary cyst infection or hemorrhage. **See Cecil Essentials 30.**

Acquired Cystic Kidney Disease

Pφ Acquired cystic kidney disease is a specific disorder in which renal cysts develop in the kidneys of patients with advanced kidney disease. These cysts have an increased risk of malignant transformation. In acquired cystic kidney disease the cysts are limited to the kidney and not dependent upon the underlying cause of kidney failure, which suggests a local rather than systemic cause of cyst development. The cysts likely develop as a result of progressive nephron loss and compensatory hypertrophy and hyperplasia in the remaining nephrons. When the tubular segment of these hyperplastic nephrons becomes obstructed, cyst development occurs. Activation of proto-oncogenes may lead to malignant transformation.

TP Typically acquired cystic kidney disease is asymptomatic and found incidentally on unrelated imaging. Occasionally patients present with flank pain and fever suggestive of cyst infection, hematuria due to cyst hemorrhage, or systemic signs of malignancy after the development of renal cell carcinoma.

Dx Diagnosis is established through imaging studies. Ultrasound, CT scan, and MRI are all sensitive tests. At the time of diagnosis, patients often have multiple bilateral renal cysts. The cysts are usually <0.5 cm in diameter.

Tx No treatment is necessary for asymptomatic cysts. Nephrectomy is the treatment of choice if these cysts have potential malignant features such as septations or calcifications. Nephrectomy is also indicated if the patient develops recurrent cyst infections, kidney stones, or painful cyst hemorrhage. **See Cecil Essentials 30.**

Medullary Sponge Kidney Disease

Pφ MSK is caused by a developmental abnormality in the terminal collecting ducts of the kidney. This developmental error is associated with the formation of renal cysts involving the renal medulla, but not the renal cortex. The mechanism of cyst development is not well understood. Although some families seem to have an autosomal-dominant inheritance, there is no evidence of hereditary transmission.

TP Patients with MSK are usually asymptomatic, and their condition is only discovered incidentally during unrelated radiographic testing. When symptoms do occur they can be related to kidney stones, which are more common in this population.

Dx The diagnosis has historically been made by IVP, but CT scan with contrast has recently proven to be a sensitive alternative. The appearance of a "brush" radiating from the renal calyx is the typical finding. Calcium stones, resulting from urinary stasis, can appear in the renal calyces. Ultrasonography is less specific than IVP but typically reveals a uniformly echogenic corticomedullary junction due to calcium deposits in the affected regions.

Tx Treatment is indicated only for UTI and for recurrent stone formation. UTIs are treated with antibiotics directed at the cultured organism. Nephrolithiasis is treated with increased water intake and specific therapy targeted at the underlying metabolic abnormality.

Renal Cancer

Pφ Renal cell carcinoma is a common malignancy arising from the renal tubular epithelium. There are several distinct histologic types. Clear cell is the most common type, accounting for the majority of tumors. It originates from the proximal tubule and is specifically associated with VHL disease. Chromophilic or papillary cell carcinoma is the second most common type, and also originates from the proximal tubule. Chromophobic tumors are less common than clear cell or chromophilic carcinoma, and are thought to arise from the cortical collecting duct. Oncocytomas constitute approximately 5% of renal neoplasms; they are believed to originate from the distal collecting tubule and rarely metastasize.

TP The classic triad of flank pain, abdominal mass, and hematuria is rarely present at the time of diagnosis. Other patients present with fever, weakness, and weight loss, or paraneoplastic syndromes (hypercalcemia or polycythemia). Systemic symptoms at the time of diagnosis are often a sign of advanced disease.

Dx CT scan is the preferred method to evaluate potentially malignant renal masses. It can determine the size of the mass, as well as any possible spread, which will allow staging. Tissue diagnosis is required.

Tx Treatment of renal cell cancer depends on the stage of the disease. A surgical approach is advised for localized cancers. For patients with a resectable stage I, II, or III tumor, surgery offers the best chance of cure. As opposed to the surgical approach, which is considered curative, systemic therapy with molecularly targeted therapy and immunotherapy are the primary approaches for patients with unresectable or recurrent disease. **See Cecil Essentials 30, 57.**

Renal Manifestations of Tuberous Sclerosis and Renal Angiomyolipoma

Pφ Renal angiomyolipomas are benign neoplasms. They can occur sporadically or as part of the tuberous sclerosis complex. They are composed of adipose tissue, smooth muscle cells, and blood vessels. When they are found as part of tuberous sclerosis they are usually bilateral and larger, while when they occur sporadically they are usually unilateral and small.

TP Small angiomyolipomas are usually asymptomatic. Larger lesions can rupture and cause flank pain and life-threatening retroperitoneal hemorrhage. Some lesions can become large and impinge upon normal renal tissue, resulting in hypertension and renal failure.

Dx The diagnosis is most often made by CT scan, which shows that the lesion has the density of fat. Patients with angiomyolipomas should be evaluated for undiagnosed tuberous sclerosis.

Tx Treatment is dependent upon the size of the mass. If the lesion is smaller than 4 cm, it can be monitored closely and only resected if the growth rate is rapid, or symptoms such as flank pain or hematuria develop. Surgical resection is divided into renal-sparing surgery and complete nephrectomy. The former includes partial nephrectomy and transcatheter embolization. Complete nephrectomies are performed if the tumor invades local tissues or the renal vein. **See Cecil Essentials 30.**

ZEBRA ZONE

a. **Metanephric adenomas:** are rare benign renal lesions, developing from remnants of the metanephric blasterma. They are usually clinically silent but can present as large masses or with hematuria. A definitive diagnosis is usually made only after surgical resection.

b. **VHL disease:** is an autosomal-dominant syndrome resulting from loss of function of a tumor suppressor gene on the short arm of chromosome 3. Patients present with benign as well as malignant tumors. The tumors include renal cell carcinoma, retinal hemangioblastoma, and pheochromocytoma. Patients with VHL should also be referred to a VHL center that offers a multidisciplinary approach to patient care.

Practice-Based Learning and Improvement: Evidence-Based Medicine

Title
Effect of antihypertensive therapy on renal function and urinary albumin excretion in hypertensive patients with autosomal-dominant polycystic kidney disease

Authors
Ecder T, Chapman AB, Brosnahan GM, et al.

Institution
University of Colorado School of Medicine

Reference
Am J Kidney Dis 2000;35:427–432

Problem
To determine the optimal medication to use to control hypertension in patients with PCKD

Intervention
Patients with PCKD were randomized to BP control with amlodipine or enalapril.

Quality of evidence
Level I

Outcome/effect
BP control was similar in the two groups, but enalapril significantly reduced the albumin-to-creatinine ratio.

Historical significance/comments
In many forms of renal disease, suppression of proteinuria is a surrogate for improved renal survival. Although further studies are necessary, this gives evidence that ACE inhibitors or ARBs may be the hypertensive medication of choice for patients with PCKD.

Interpersonal and Communication Skills

Demonstrate Empathy When Discussing the Impact of an Inheritable Disease

PCKD is a chronic progressive disease with multiple potential complications. Patients often have affected first-degree relatives who may be on dialysis or who may have died prematurely from cerebral aneurysms. Therefore, it is very important to have a discussion that allows and encourages a patient to openly discuss his or her personal experiences and fears. Such discussions should be conducted privately with the patient, as close family members may not be aware that they are at risk of having PCKD. Parents often do not want their children to know that they are at risk until they are old enough to understand the diagnosis and management.

Professionalism

Assess the Impact on the Individual When Considering Screening

Patients with PCKD commonly ask their nephrologists for recommendations about screening their children for PCKD. Being diagnosed with PCKD at an early age before the development of complications is not medically necessary and may cause the individual unwarranted difficulties. Patients with PCKD have difficulty obtaining life insurance and have to deal with the emotional hardship of being diagnosed with a chronic progressive medical illness. The current recommendation is to not screen asymptomatic children younger than 18 years of age. Individuals older than 18 years who would like to donate a kidney should be screened to avoid transplanting a diseased kidney. In all other asymptomatic individuals at risk, it is advisable to address risk as well as benefits and make an informed decision with the patient. Issues such as insurability and employment must be addressed.

Systems-Based Practice

Assessing the Cost-Effectiveness of Screening

Although patients with PCKD are at risk for cerebral aneurysm, it is not cost-effective to screen all patients with PCKD for aneurysms. Aneurysms cluster in families, so it is recommended to screen only those patients with a family history of aneurysm, as well as those individuals who would endanger others if they were to incur the complication of cerebral aneurysm rupture. An individual employed as an airplane pilot would be such an example.

Section VI
GASTROINTESTINAL AND LIVER DISEASES

Section Editors
Giancarlo Mercogliano MD, MBA, AGA
and Barry D. Mann MD

Section Contents

26 **Abdominal Pain (Case 19)**
Shamina Dhillon MD, Henry Schoonyoung MD, and Jessica L. Israel MD

27 **Nausea and Vomiting (Case 20)**
Owen Tully MD and Bob Etemad MD

28 **Esophageal Dysphagia (Case 21)**
Benjamin Ngo MD and John Abramson MD

29 **Gastrointestinal Bleeding (Case 22)**
Melissa Morgan DO, Michael Share MD, and Marc Zitin MD

30 **Constipation (Case 23)**
Christopher P. Farrell DO and Gary Newman MD

31 **Diarrhea (Case 24)**
David Rudolph DO and James Thornton MD

32 **Jaundice (Case 25)**
Austin Hwang MD and Giancarlo Mercogliano MD, MBA, AGA

Chapter 26
Abdominal Pain (Case 19)

Shamina Dhillon MD, Henry Schoonyoung MD, and Jessica L. Israel MD

Case: A 54-year-old man with a history of hypertension, diabetes mellitus, and hyperlipidemia presents to the emergency department (ED) complaining of progressive epigastric pain for the last 2 days. The pain initially woke him from a deep sleep. He describes his discomfort as "sharp" and states it has worsened in intensity over the last few hours. He also complains of nausea and has had two episodes of clear vomiting. He has been unable to tolerate any solid food since the onset of the pain. He is passing gas and recalls his last bowel movement was earlier in the day. He has never had symptoms like this before. He denies any fevers or chills. He has had no sick contacts. He is not a heavy drinker and reports only drinking one glass of wine with dinner 5 days ago. He quit smoking several years ago.

On physical exam, his temperature is 100.4° F. His heart rate is 110 beats per minute (bpm) and blood pressure (BP) is 151/92 mm Hg. The patient's sclerae are mildly icteric, but there is no overall evidence of jaundice. His abdomen is soft with mild distension. He has significant tenderness in the epigastrium and right upper quadrant (RUQ) to palpation but without any guarding or rebound.

Differential Diagnosis

Perforated viscus	Cholecystitis	Acute mesenteric ischemia
Diverticulitis	Appendicitis	
Pancreatitis	Choledocholithiasis	

Speaking Intelligently

When evaluating a patient with abdominal pain, a detailed history about the character, duration, and quality of pain is imperative. It is important to discern exactly how and when the pain started and inquire about its location; this can give you important clues as to the underlying diagnosis. A nocturnal component to the pain often suggests an organic or serious cause. It is also important to inquire about exacerbating and alleviating factors, as well as any association of the pain with nausea, vomiting, fevers, or chills, and if ingestion of food worsens the pain.

PATIENT CARE

Clinical Thinking
- When evaluating a patient with abdominal pain, it is important to determine if the symptom is acute or chronic.
- A patient with a 6-month history of pain is less likely to have an acute abdomen.
- A good clinician must always be on the lookout for the possibility of an abdominal disorder requiring surgery, which would require urgent intervention; time may be critically important in these cases.

History
- Pain that is sudden in onset or wakes a person from sleep usually signifies an acute abdominal process. It is thus important to ask the patient what he or she was doing when the pain began.
- It is also imperative to determine if the pain was mild and progressively worsened, or if it was severe at onset.
- Ask patients to rate their pain on a scale of 1 to 10.
- Pain associated with nausea and vomiting can be seen in patients with pancreatitis.
- Fever and chills are associated with cholecystitis.

Physical Examination
- The most urgent assessment during a physical exam is to determine if there are signs of **peritonitis**, including a careful assessment for rebound tenderness and guarding.
- **Absent bowel sounds** may also signify a more critical intra-abdominal pathology.
- The location of tenderness can be important to elucidate a particular etiology for the patient's symptoms. For example, right lower quadrant (RLQ) pain is often seen in patients with **appendicitis**, and left lower quadrant (LLQ) tenderness is closely associated with **diverticulitis**.
- **Tachycardia** and **hypotension** can be signs of both pain and volume depletion.

Tests for Consideration
- **White blood cell (WBC) count:** This can signify either infection or an intense inflammatory response. $11
- **Liver function tests:** Aspartate aminotransferase (AST), alanine transaminase (ALT), alkaline phosphatase, prothrombin time (PT), partial thromboplastin time (PTT), amylase, and lipase $12

IMAGING CONSIDERATIONS

→ **Plain abdominal radiographs:** This is most important
for evaluating for free air in the abdomen, which
implies perforation and the need for urgent surgery. $45
→ **CT scan:** This is best done with both oral and
IV contrast. If perforation is suspected,
a water-soluble oral contrast agent is often used. $334

Clinical Entities	Medical Knowledge

Perforated Viscus

Pφ This is a transmural injury of an organ resulting in perforation
through the serosa. Common etiologies of perforation include
ulcer disease in the duodenum or stomach, intestinal ischemia,
and diverticular transmural inflammation.

TP Patients present with sudden onset of acute pain. On physical
examination, most patients will have signs of peritonitis such as
rebound or guarding. It is important to recognize these findings,
as some patients will require emergent surgical intervention.

Dx The abdominal exam is often the most telling. Patients are
extremely uncomfortable and lying still. They will often have pain
when going over bumps in the stretcher or ambulance. Abdominal
imaging will show free air. If a CT scan is done, it can show
extravasation of contrast at the point of perforation.

Tx The treatment is surgical repair. These patients also require
antibiotics (targeted principally against gram-negative bacilli and
anaerobes) as well as fluid resuscitation. **See Cecil Essentials
34, 37.**

Cholecystitis

Pφ The hallmark of this disease is gallbladder inflammation, most
often secondary to gallstones. Acute cholecystitis can be
associated with cystic duct obstruction. On a pathologic
spectrum, the disease can manifest as mild edema, acute
inflammation, or necrosis and gangrene of the gallbladder.
The clinician should be aware of the possibility of acalculous
cholecystitis. This entity is clinically similar to acute cholecystitis
but is not associated with gallstones. Acalculous cholecystitis is
usually found in the critically ill patient.

TP Acute cholecystitis presents as steady RUQ pain with fever and leukocytosis. The pain can also be located in the epigastrium, and it can radiate to the patient's right shoulder or back. The pain may be associated with nausea, vomiting, and anorexia. On exam, patients are usually ill-appearing and tachycardic. A Murphy sign may be positive.

Dx Patients with uncomplicated cholecystitis do not always have elevated bilirubin, because the common bile duct is not obstructed. Mild elevation in serum aminotransferases can be seen. An ultrasound often shows gallbladder wall thickening >4 mm, along with gallstones and pericholecystic fluid. A hepatobiliary iminodiacetic acid (HIDA) scan may be helpful to rule out choledocholithiasis; a positive test will show no visualization of the gallbladder after IV injection of the isotope due to obstruction of the cystic duct.

Tx The treatment of acute cholecystitis consists of IV hydration, correction of electrolyte abnormalities, and analgesia. IV antibiotics should target common biliary pathogens including *Klebsiella*, *Enterococcus*, *Enterobacter*, *Escherichia coli*, and anaerobes. Early cholecystectomy (now almost always performed laparoscopically) is ideal, and surgical consultation should be obtained. **See Cecil Essentials 46.**

Choledocholithiasis

Pφ Pain secondary to gallstones is referred to as biliary colic. It is caused by gallbladder contraction in response to hormonal or neural stimulation. Often this contraction forces a stone against the gallbladder outlet or the opening of the cystic duct, resulting in pain. The stone will often fall back from the cystic duct as the gallbladder relaxes.

TP The typical pattern of pain in patients with biliary colic is one of constant epigastric or RUQ discomfort that progresses over an hour and then slowly diminishes over the next several hours. The pain may radiate to the back and the right shoulder, and may be associated with nausea and vomiting. Unlike individuals with acute cholecystitis, most people with biliary colic are not ill-appearing and have no fever or leukocytosis.

Dx The first step in diagnosis is obtaining a typical history paired with an ultrasound showing the presence of cholelithiasis. There is usually no gallbladder wall thickening or pericholecystic fluid. Elevations of serum transaminases can be seen during an acute attack.

Tx Patients with typical biliary colic and gallstones are advised to undergo prophylactic cholecystectomy so as to avoid more serious complications such as cholangitis, pancreatitis, or Mirizzi syndrome, which is obstruction of the common bile duct caused by chronic cholecystitis and large gallstones resulting in compression of the common bile duct. The risk of further symptoms and complications in patients with biliary colic and gallstones is approximately 70% within 2 years of initial presentation. **See Cecil Essentials 46.**

Diverticulitis

Pφ Diverticulitis is inflammation of colonic diverticula. Diverticula form at certain points of weakness in the bowel wall. The cause is thought to be a microscopic or macroscopic perforation of a diverticulum. Erosion of the diverticular wall occurs because of increased intraluminal pressure leading to inflammation, followed by focal necrosis and eventually perforation.

TP The most common symptom is LLQ pain that can occur several days before presentation. The severity of symptoms is often based on the underlying inflammatory process. Pain is often accompanied by fever and elevated WBC count. Diarrhea or constipation can be seen in at least 30% of patients. Patients present with tenderness in the LLQ. A macroscopic perforation may lead to localized peritoneal signs.

Dx In addition to the history and physical exam, the diagnosis of acute diverticulitis is established with a CT scan of the abdomen with IV and oral contrast. Findings include soft-tissue density within the pericolic fat around an area of colonic diverticula and bowel wall thickening. CT scan is also helpful in identifying the complications of diverticulitis, such as a localized abscess formation or a fistulous connection to the urinary bladder, vagina, or the abdominal wall.

Tx For patients with uncomplicated diverticulitis, bowel rest and antibiotics are the mainstays of therapy. The antibiotic coverage is targeted at colonic anaerobic and aerobic gram-negative flora. Abscess occurs in 16% of patients with acute diverticulitis and can be managed with percutaneous drainage performed by an interventional radiologist. If there is peritonitis or perforation, surgical therapy with a two-stage procedure is recommended. **See Cecil Essentials 34.**

Appendicitis

Pφ The most common physiologic mechanism for the development of appendicitis is obstruction of the appendiceal lumen. The obstruction may be secondary to follicular hyperplasia in the young, or possibly malignancy, such as carcinoid or adenocarcinoma, in the older population. A superimposed inflammatory process of the appendiceal wall then leads to ischemia, perforation, or the development of an abscess.

TP Many patients present with nonspecific signs and symptoms such as generalized malaise or indigestion. Pain can be produced on abdominal examination over the McBurney point, which is located one third of the distance along a line from the anterior superior iliac spine to the umbilicus. The Rovsing sign is the development of pain in the RLQ upon palpation in the LLQ. The initial pain can also be dull and constant in the epigastric or periumbilical region. Eventually the pain localizes to the RLQ once the parietal peritoneum is involved. The pain is associated with nausea and vomiting. A low-grade fever may also be present.

Dx In addition to a thorough history and physical, a CT scan of the abdomen and pelvis may be performed if there is doubt of the clinical picture. Notable findings include thickened appendiceal walls, free fluid, and fat stranding in the RLQ. The presence of contrast or air in the appendix actually helps to exclude the diagnosis.

Tx The definitive treatment is an appendectomy. Preoperative treatment includes hydration and perioperative antibiotics. If, however, CT scanning reveals an abscess, percutaneous drainage is needed before surgery. **See Cecil Essentials 34.**

Pancreatitis

Pφ Acute pancreatitis is an inflammatory condition of the pancreas characterized by abdominal pain and elevated levels of the pancreatic enzymes amylase and lipase. While there are clear etiologic conditions associated with the disease, the exact cellular pathogenesis of the disorder is not fully understood. It is thought that intra-acinar activation of pancreatic proteolytic enzymes leads to an autodigestive injury to the gland. In general, acute pancreatitis can be divided into two broad categories: edematous or mild acute pancreatitis, and necrotizing or severe acute pancreatitis. Patients with severe acute pancreatitis can develop systemic complications including acute respiratory distress syndrome, fever, renal failure, and shock.

The most common cause of acute pancreatitis in the world is gallstones—specifically, the mechanical obstruction by the stone of the pancreatic ampulla. Alcohol is another common cause of acute pancreatitis. A serum triglyceride concentration above 1000 mg/dL can also precipitate acute pancreatitis. A medication history is imperative when evaluating a patient with pancreatitis, as many medications are associated with pancreatitis, such as metronidazole, tetracycline, furosemide, thiazide diuretics, tamoxifen, valproic acid, didanosine, and pentamidine. Less common etiologies include hypercalcemia, infection (mumps, coxsackievirus), vasculitis, and, rarely, pancreatic cancer. Pancreatitis is seen in 3% of patients undergoing diagnostic endoscopic retrograde cholangiopancreatography (ERCP). A full 30% of patients with acute pancreatitis fall into the idiopathic category.

TP Patients typically present with acute upper abdominal pain that is in the mid-epigastrium or RUQ. Pain can also be diffuse in nature. Patients commonly describe a pain that radiates to the back in a "bandlike" fashion. The pain may improve upon bending forward. Nausea and vomiting are commonly associated symptoms. On physical exam, patients have significant tenderness in the epigastric region. Ecchymotic discoloration of the costovertebral angle (Turner sign) or the periumbilical region (Cullen sign) is seen in 1% of cases and is associated with intra-abdominal hemorrhage.

Dx An elevation in serum amylase and lipase in the appropriate clinical setting strongly suggests a diagnosis of pancreatitis. In gallstone pancreatitis, a concomitant rise in ALT is also seen. A CT of the abdomen and pelvis is not necessary on the first day of admission if the history and biochemical markers suggest pancreatitis but should be done if the diagnosis is questionable. It is important to remember that many patients present with significant hypovolemia, and an IV contrast CT could worsen renal function. Some experts advocate a CT scan with contrast in 2–3 days after presentation following appropriate volume repletion to assess for pancreatic necrosis.

Tx All patients should receive supportive care including vigorous fluid resuscitation, correction of electrolyte abnormalities, and adequate pain control. The use of aggressive fluid therapy cannot be stressed enough. Patients with severe pancreatitis can sequester large amounts of fluid in the injured pancreatic bed, and rates of 250 mL of IV fluids per hour may be required for the first 24–48 hours if the cardiac status permits. Inadequate fluid replacement can be evidenced by persistent hemoconcentration. Thus, the hematocrit should be measured on admission, 12 hours after admission, and 24 hours after admission to assess the adequacy of fluid resuscitation. Transfer to the intensive care unit (ICU) is warranted in patients with evidence of sustained organ failure. In mild pancreatitis, the patient can be fed orally in 3–5 days upon cessation of abdominal pain, with diets advancing from clear liquids to a more regular, but low-fat, diet. In those with severe pancreatitis, enteral feeding with a jejunal tube distal to the ligament of Treitz is preferred over total parenteral nutrition. The use of prophylactic antibiotics is recommended only in those with severe necrotizing pancreatitis. **See Cecil Essentials 40, 46.**

Acute Mesenteric Ischemia

Pφ Acute mesenteric ischemia is caused by a reduction in intestinal blood flow secondary to occlusion, vasospasm, or hypoperfusion of the mesenteric vasculature. Chronic mesenteric ischemia is referred to as intestinal angina and is a separate clinical entity that will not be discussed here. The intestinal blood supply consists of the celiac artery, superior mesenteric artery, inferior mesenteric artery, and an extensive network of collateral blood vessels known as the splanchnic circulation. The four major causes of acute mesenteric ischemia are superior mesenteric artery embolism, superior mesenteric artery thrombosis, mesenteric venous thrombosis, and nonocclusive ischemia. Risk factors for mesenteric arterial disease include advanced age, atherosclerosis, states of low cardiac output, cardiac arrhythmias, recent myocardial infarction (MI), and intra-abdominal malignancy. Risk factors for mesenteric venous thrombosis include hypercoagulable states, portal hypertension, abdominal infections, pancreatitis, splenectomy, and malignancy in the portal region.

TP Patients with acute arterial embolism have rapid onset of severe periumbilical pain that may be out of proportion to the findings on the physical exam. Arterial thrombosis or mesenteric vein thrombosis will present in a more insidious fashion, with vague abdominal pain that can be present for days to weeks before the diagnosis.

Dx After appropriate resuscitation and supportive measures, a CT scan with IV contrast should be done to evaluate the mesenteric arterial and venous vasculature as well as assess for bowel wall ischemia and injury, which can be seen as bowel wall thickening or intestinal pneumatosis with portal vein gas. Mesenteric angiography is the gold standard diagnostic study for acute arterial ischemia and has both diagnostic and therapeutic importance. CT angiography and MR angiography are noninvasive alternatives. Laboratory evaluation may reveal an elevated serum lactate concentration.

Tx The ultimate goal of treatment is the rapid restoration of intestinal blood flow, which requires aggressive hemodynamic monitoring and support, correction of acidosis, antibiotics, and placement of a nasogastric (NG) tube. Immediate surgery is required in those suspected of having perforation or intestinal gangrene. In those for whom surgery is not emergent, mesenteric angiography not only can be diagnostic but also can offer therapeutic options with the administration of intra-arterial vasodilators, thrombolytic agents, angioplasty, vascular stenting, or embolectomy. In acute mesenteric venous thrombosis, treatment includes anticoagulation and resection of necrotic bowel. **See Cecil Essentials 35.**

ZEBRA ZONE

a. **Celiac artery compression syndrome** is a rare condition that occurs in healthy young and middle-aged individuals, and presents as chronic epigastric abdominal pain that occurs after eating and may be associated with an epigastric bruit and weight loss.

b. **Hereditary angioedema** is a disease that results from defects in the C1 inhibitor of the classical complement pathway. Patients have recurrent episodes of colicky abdominal pain associated with nausea, vomiting, and diarrhea. Diagnosis is made with blood tests that show a low C4 level and low C1 inhibitor antigen levels.

c. **Acute intermittent porphyria (AIP)** is an autosomal-dominant disorder resulting from a partial deficiency of porphobilinogen deaminase, previously called the third enzyme in the heme biosynthetic pathway. Abdominal pain is the most common symptom in AIP. It is usually severe, steady, and poorly localized.

Practice-Based Learning and Improvement: Evidence-Based Medicine

Title
Nutrition support in acute pancreatitis: a systematic review of the literature

Authors
McClave SA, Chang WK, Dhaliwal R, Heyland DK

Institution
University of Louisville School of Medicine

Reference
JPEN J Parenter Enteral Nutr 2006;30:143–156

Problem
To determine the optimum route for nutrition support in acute pancreatitis

Intervention
Literature review of prospective randomized trials that evaluated nutrition therapy

Quality of evidence
Level II

Outcome/effect
Patients with acute severe pancreatitis should begin enteral nutrition, as this therapy modulates stress response and promotes more rapid resolution of the disease process.

Historical significance/comments
Before studies evaluating enteral nutrition using the gastrointestinal (GI) tract, IV parenteral nutrition was often the mainstay of nutritional support. Enteral nutrition has now been shown to be the preferred route for nutritional support and has eclipsed parenteral nutrition as the new gold standard of care.

Interpersonal and Communication Skills

Specificity, Even If Uncomfortable, Is Valuable When Discussing Bowel Habits
When treating issues of the GI tract, discussing the patient's bowel movements is a necessity. It is important to obtain an accurate history from the patient on this topic so as to provide adequate treatment. The words *constipation* and *diarrhea*, for example, may mean very different things to the patient from what they mean to a

physician. While this discussion may at times feel awkward, it is important to be specific about what these words mean to your patient to ensure that you do not initiate unnecessary treatment. Specificity may at times allow the physician to reassure a patient that his or her "symptoms" may actually be within the spectrum of normal.

Professionalism

Patient Welfare in Those Who Are Psychologically Vulnerable

Not all patients who present with acute abdominal pain have an organic cause for their symptom. It is important to be aware of functional abdominal pain disorders such as irritable bowel syndrome, functional dyspepsia, and chronic abdominal pain syndrome. Patients with functional bowel disease can have intermittent episodes of severe abdominal pain in the absence of any abnormal physical, laboratory, and radiologic findings. In some of these patients, psychosocial stress can exacerbate their pain. If no clear etiology of the pain is identified, it is important to ask about possible stressors such as domestic abuse or familial illness. While these patients may not need surgical intervention or hospitalization, it is important to identify appropriate medical and psychological services that can help them deal with their problem.

Systems-Based Practice

An Algorithmic Evaluation of Abdominal Pain Is Time- and Cost-Effective

RUQ Pain: Ultrasound → (if ultrasound nondiagnostic, yet clinically suspicious for acute cholecystitis) → HIDA scan → CT scan.

Ultrasound
The initial imaging test of choice in a patient with abdominal pain is the transabdominal ultrasound, which is noninvasive, widely available, and inexpensive; it can rule in or exclude multiple disease entities. Ultrasound is sensitive and specific (88% and 80%, respectively) for diagnosing acute cholecystitis by visualizing cholelithiasis, gallbladder wall thickening (>4 mm), and pericholecystic fluid, and by eliciting a sonographic Murphy sign (tenderness and/or painful arrest of inspiration upon sonographic pressure and localization of the gallbladder). Sonography can also assess bile duct dilatation, which suggests bile duct obstruction caused by a common bile duct (CBD) stone (choledocholithiasis), an extrinsic mass such as a pancreatic tumor, or an intraluminal mass such as cholangiocarcinoma.

HIDA Scan

If the sonogram is negative or equivocal, and the clinical suspicion is still high for cholecystitis, cholescintigraphy (HIDA scan) will be helpful. This test visualizes bile flow through the use of a radioactively tagged acid that is taken up and excreted by the liver. If the agent flows down the bile duct into the intestine but fails to visualize the gallbladder, this indicates presumed cystic duct obstruction and is considered diagnostic of acute cholecystitis (97% sensitive, 90% specific). This test is especially helpful when sonography cannot identify small stones that are blocking the cystic duct. False positives can occur with processes such as hepatic congestion from heart failure.

CT Abdomen

If gallbladder disease has been excluded in a patient with RUQ pain and no diagnosis has been established, a CT with IV and oral contrast is the most appropriate study. A CT visualizes the "solid organs" such as liver, pancreas, mesentery, lymph nodes, and gastric/duodenal wall, and can add definitive information regarding any abnormal findings noted on previous testing (e.g., CBD dilatation without evidence of stones on ultrasound), and may identify other causes of the patient's pain.

RLQ Pain: CT scan; ultrasound first in the pregnant patient.

CT Abdomen and Pelvis

In a **nonpregnant adult** with RLQ pain and suspected appendicitis, a CT scan with oral and IV contrast has become the imaging modality of choice. Before the advent of CT, the negative appendectomy rate could be as high as 20% to 35%, which was considered acceptable because removing a normal appendix was less likely to cause morbidity than removing a perforated one. CT scan has dramatically reduced the negative appendectomy rate and is the study of choice with a sensitivity of 92% to 97% and a specificity of 88% to 94%. It also allows the clinician to differentiate other structures and possibly establish an alternate diagnosis when there is no appendicitis.

Ultrasound

When approaching a **pregnant patient** with RLQ pain, it is important to consider studies that will minimize radiation exposure to the fetus. As such, *ultrasound* with graded compression is the first study of choice. This is highly operator-dependent, and in experienced hands it can have a sensitivity of 85% and a specificity of 90%. Some sources advocate MRI as the next study of choice for less radiation exposure and better accuracy, but this has not been sufficiently studied. CT scan with IV and oral contrast is an excellent tool even in the pregnant patient, as the cumulative radiation dose is below that which is considered dangerous for fetal exposure.

Suggested Readings

Birnbaum BA, Jeffrey RB Jr. CT and sonographic evaluation of acute right lower quadrant abdominal pain. Am J Radiol 1998;170:361–371.
Shea JA, Berlin JA, Escarce JJ, et al. Revised estimates of diagnostic test sensitivity and specificity in suspected biliary tract disease. Arch Intern Med 1994;154:2573–2581.

Chapter 27
Nausea and Vomiting (Case 20)

Owen Tully MD *and Bob Etemad* MD

Case: A 65-year-old woman presents with nausea and vomiting. She has a past medical history of hypertension, hyperlipidemia, type 2 diabetes mellitus, mild obesity, and a recent diagnosis of a herniated lumbar disk; her surgical history includes a hysterectomy for fibroid disease. She states the nausea and vomiting has been worsening for 3 days, usually after meals, and is associated with crampy abdominal pain before these episodes. She was recently seen by her primary physician, who added glipizide to her medical regimen because her hemoglobin A_{1c} (HgbA$_{1c}$) was not well controlled. She has also recently been started on a fentanyl patch for worsening pain in her cervical spine secondary to her herniated disk.

Differential Diagnosis

Gastroenteritis	Diabetes Related	Medication Related	Acid-Peptic Disease
Most cases are infectious (viral more common than bacterial).	Neuropathic diabetic gastroparesis Hyperglycemia Hypoglycemia	Fentanyl patch, glipizide, other medications	Erosive esophagitis Gastritis/gastric ulcer Duodenitis/duodenal ulcer

Ileus	Other GI Disorders	Mechanical Obstruction	Miscellaneous
Related to diabetes, narcotics, obstipation	Including cholecystitis, pancreatitis, appendicitis, and mesenteric ischemia; obstipation/ constipation	Gastric outlet obstruction related to ulcer/ inflammation Partial small bowel obstruction (SBO) related to previous surgery	Psychogenic/ anxiety/ depression Neurologic (increased intracranial pressure) Labyrinthine disorders Cardiac related (MI) Adnexal/gynecologic related

Speaking Intelligently

When a patient presents with symptoms of nausea and vomiting, it is important to consider that some patients may vomit and have minimal nausea, whereas others present with long durations of nausea punctuated with a rare episode of vomiting that does not relieve the nausea. Among the more important factors to consider are the following:

- Are the symptoms acute or chronic? Acute nausea or vomiting usually suggests a more urgent issue.
- Does the patient have a chronic medical condition in which nausea or vomiting may be a manifestation of a life-threatening complication of that condition (cardiovascular disease, diabetes, neurologic disorder, active malignancy)?
- What is the relationship between the patient's nausea and his or her vomiting? Timing, duration, exacerbating factors, associated symptoms, and new medications must be considered.
- Is there any possibility of pregnancy?
- Are there other signs or symptoms that the patient is significantly ill?

PATIENT CARE

Clinical Thinking
- Initially rule out potentially catastrophic causes for the symptoms; consider intestinal infarction, perforated viscus, volvulus, cerebral edema, hypoglycemia, and cardiac disease.
- In any woman of childbearing age, be sure to exclude pregnancy.
- Determine the time frame of symptoms. If the symptoms are roughly 1 month or less, an acute cause of the symptoms should be

considered, as catastrophic and more dangerous etiologies tend to manifest acutely.
- Asking about associated abdominal pain is often helpful in determining the etiology, especially for acute intraperitoneal conditions such as pancreatitis and appendicitis. Be aware that post-emetic abdominal pain may be related to worsening acid reflux secondary to the vomiting itself.
- Consider extraintestinal conditions causing nausea and vomiting, including electrolyte and glucose imbalance, neurologic disorders, renal colic, biliary colic, and ovarian or testicular torsion.
- While pursuing the underlying etiology, monitor and correct potential complications of nausea and vomiting, including metabolic and electrolyte abnormalities, and volume depletion.

History
- Clarify whether nausea or vomiting is the predominant symptom, and detail each symptom separately: onset, frequency, duration, associated symptoms, and medication use.
- Clarify the relationship between nausea and vomiting (which came first, which is predominant, and does vomiting relieve nausea).
- In considering **infectious causes**, ask whether close contacts have similar symptoms; ask about obvious new food exposure, diarrhea, change in bowel habits, and fever.
- **Review medication history:** New medications, missed medications, medications recently discontinued, wrong medications taken, or incorrect dose.
- In patients with diabetes, review recent glucose and HgbA$_{1c}$ levels, and any changes in diet, medications, and activity.
- In considering mechanical causes, ask about change in bowel habits, abdominal distension, more vomiting than nausea, abdominal pain, previous episodes, and previous history of mechanical bowel obstruction. Establish if any previous surgeries were performed, and consider reviewing the operative notes for any unusual circumstances surrounding the surgery.
- In considering neurologic causes, ask about vertigo, changes in vision, unilateral weakness, and headaches.
- Perform a detailed review of systems to consider the multitude of other etiologies.

Physical Examination
- **Vital signs:** Patients with more severe symptoms may have orthostatic hypotension, tachycardia, or fever. Fever is common in patients with gastroenteritis, especially of bacterial etiology, but can also be seen with inflammatory conditions and drug reactions.
- **Abnormal vital signs** suggest a more concerning process needing more urgent attention.

- **General appearance:** Is the patient "miserable" or comfortable? Is there something obvious that strikes you as concerning (distended abdomen, lying in fetal position, abnormally quiet, not moving a particular extremity)? Does the patient appear ill?
- Check for **signs of volume depletion** by examining the oral mucous membranes, eyes, and skin.
- **Lymphadenopathy** could suggest either infectious causes or malignancy.
- **Abdominal tenderness** to palpation is a clue to potential inflammatory conditions of the abdomen, such as appendicitis, cholecystitis, colitis, and diverticulitis. Rebound and guarding are important clues regarding complications (e.g., perforation). A distended, tympanitic abdomen suggests ileus or bowel obstruction. Rectal exam may demonstrate an empty rectal vault. There may be an absence of bowel sounds.
- Signs of **muscle atrophy**, **cachexia**, and **temporal wasting** could suggest malignancy.
- **Peripheral neuropathy** can be seen in patients with or without diabetic gastroparesis.
- **New neurologic abnormalities** on physical exam (e.g., unilateral weakness, paresis, numbness, facial droop, or ptosis) could suggest central nervous system (CNS) processes causing nausea and vomiting.

Tests for Consideration

- **Complete blood count (CBC):** Leukocytosis is very nonspecific. A normal CBC is somewhat reassuring but never an "all clear" in these patients. New significant anemia could be an actual cause of symptoms or suggest intra-abdominal/retroperitoneal bleeding. $11
- **Comprehensive metabolic panel (CMP):** Look for acidosis and increased blood urea nitrogen-to-creatinine (BUN/Cr) ratio as suggestive of volume depletion. An anion gap acidosis could suggest ischemia or iatrogenic etiologies. $12
- **Human chorionic gonadotropin (HCG):** If premenopausal female, to exclude pregnancy and related issues $9
- **Urinalysis:** Look for pyuria and bacteriuria; urine is concentrated in patients with infection or volume depletion. $4
- **Amylase/Lipase:** For consideration of pancreatitis $19
- **Esophagogastroduodenoscopy (EGD):** Evaluate for gastritis, esophagitis, peptic ulcer disease (PUD). $600
- **Electrocardiography (ECG):** Assess for acute ischemia as a contributing cause of symptoms or secondary effect. $27

IMAGING CONSIDERATIONS

→ **Obstruction series:** At least two views and erect/lateral view to evaluate for pneumoperitoneum. A large gastric air bubble or gastric outline suggests gastroparesis/gastric outlet obstruction. Small-bowel air-fluid levels suggest ileus. Distended loops of bowel suggest obstruction. Large amount of stool suggests constipation/obstipation. $75

→ **CT scan or ultrasound** should be considered if the patient has abdominal tenderness or features suggestive of acute cholecystitis or appendicitis. $334, $96

→ **Other:** Upper GI (UGI) series, gastric emptying study, **upper endoscopy** should be considered depending on how the differential diagnosis is evolving based on previous studies. **UGI series** may be difficult in patients with nausea and vomiting. **Gastric emptying** for gastroparesis is usually performed later in the evaluation when other causes for symptoms have been excluded. $600, $142, $244

Clinical Entities	Medical Knowledge

Gastroenteritis

Pφ Gastroenteritis is inflammation of the lining of the stomach and small and large intestines, most often caused by invasion of the GI tract by infectious agents (viral, bacterial, or parasitic). Viruses including noroviruses, rotavirus, and enteric adenoviruses are the most common etiologies. Fecal-oral spread of these viruses is the most common route of transmission. Infants and young children are particularly at risk, as are people who work in health care settings, day care, and schools. Immunosuppressed patients are at increased risk.

TP Patients often present with nausea and vomiting, and/or diarrhea. Signs of volume depletion are commonly noted. Diarrhea is more common with bacterial etiologies, while vomiting is especially common with viral etiologies. Fever and chills are present in 40% to 60% of cases.

Dx Laboratory studies are generally nonspecific. Mild elevations of liver enzymes may be seen in some bacterial and viral infections. Stool leukocytes are more often demonstrated in "invasive" bacterial infections such as that caused by *Salmonella*, *Shigella*, *Yersinia*, *Campylobacter*, and with certain *Escherichia coli* strains. Stool testing for rotavirus and other viruses is available, but only used for epidemiologic purposes and not for routine clinical care.

Tx The treatment is generally supportive. Antibiotics, including fluoroquinolones, should be reserved for patients with a high suspicion of bacterial pathogens, evidence of systemic toxicity, or immunosuppression. Prevention is one of the most important aspects of management, including aggressive hand washing, separating diaper-changing areas from dining areas in day care settings, and vaccination for specific pathogens (i.e., rotavirus). **See Cecil Essentials 37.**

Small-Bowel Obstruction

Pφ SBO is due to a physical blockage of the normal flow of intestinal contents in the small bowel. The majority of cases are caused by adhesions from prior surgeries, although cancers, incarcerated hernias, and small-bowel strictures are other causes.

TP Patients typically present with nausea, vomiting, and abdominal distension, and often have abdominal pain that is diffuse and crampy. Absence of flatus is another common presenting symptom. Inspect for scars from previous surgery; listen for bowel sounds, which may be high-pitched, hypoactive, or absent. Tympany to percussion is usually present with distension; if guarding and/or rebound is elicited, consider peritonitis complicating the obstruction. Rectal exam typically reveals an empty rectal vault.

Dx Upright abdominal radiographs should be ordered to first evaluate for free air. SBO will classically demonstrate multiple air-fluid levels in the small intestine with distended loops of bowel. CT scan, with water-soluble oral contrast, can be used if plain radiographs are equivocal. A transition point at the obstruction can often be identified. Lack of air or contrast in the distal small intestine or colon is suggestive of a complete obstruction.

Tx Initial management is supportive, with nasogastric (NG) suction, having the patient ingest nothing by mouth (NPO), and IV fluid repletion. If postoperative patients do not show signs of improvement within 12–24 hours, surgical exploration is recommended to evaluate for strangulation. Administration of water-soluble contrast (diatriozate [Gastrografin]) via NG tube can be diagnostic and, at times, therapeutic. Lysis of adhesions is often indicated, especially in patients with mild distension and proximal obstruction, and who are expected to have a single band of adhesions. **See Cecil Essentials 35, 38.**

Postoperative Ileus

Pφ Ileus refers to a nonmechanical insult that disrupts the normal peristalsis of the small intestine. It is most common in the postoperative setting, usually up to 5 days. The pathogenesis is multifactorial, including inflammation of the bowel from surgical manipulation, neural inhibitory sympathetic reflexes and local neuroinhibitory peptides acting in response to the surgical insult to the bowel, and narcotic-related delay in bowel transit from systemic opioid use. Other potential etiologies for ileus include metabolic abnormalities, pancreatitis, and other inflammatory states, sepsis, medication reactions, ischemia, and neurologic processes.

TP In addition to nausea and vomiting, patients typically present with abdominal distension, bloating, pain, absence of flatus, and/or inability to tolerate oral intake. On physical exam, patients often have abdominal distension and tympany, decreased or absent bowel sounds, and sometimes mild tenderness. The presentation is often very similar to that of an SBO.

Dx Abdominal radiographs will show distended loops of bowel with air-fluid levels. CT scan with water-soluble contrast will show these findings as well, yet unlike with SBO, there is no transition point of obstruction. Laboratory studies may demonstrate hypokalemia or hypomagnesemia.

Tx Treatment is largely supportive and very similar to that for SBO. Patients are kept NPO and are repleted with IV fluids; electrolyte imbalances are corrected, and NG tubes are sometimes placed for symptomatic relief. Minimization of narcotics is helpful; ambulation is probably beneficial. No medication has yet been proven to be effective in the treatment of ileus. Postoperative ileus appears to be less profound following laparoscopic surgeries and with the use of epidural instead of general anesthesia. Medications that may be beneficial in the *prevention* of ileus in the postoperative setting include Cox-2 inhibitors, peripheral-acting μ-opioid receptor antagonists, and magnesium oxide laxatives. **See Cecil Essentials 35.**

Gastroparesis

Pφ Gastroparesis refers to delayed gastric emptying. Its pathophysiology probably includes disordered motility related to neurologic, hormonal, and smooth muscle factors. By definition, there are no structural abnormalities contributing to the gastric delay. The most common etiology is diabetes mellitus, with autonomic neural injury the proposed mechanism. Other less common causes include medications, infection, acidosis, metabolic disorders, pregnancy, and collagen vascular disorders. In many cases the specific cause is not clearly identified.

TP Patients typically present with nausea, vomiting, bloating, and early satiety. Diabetics typically have poorly controlled glucose levels and evidence of end-organ damage including retinopathy and neuropathy. Abdominal exam may show tenderness to palpation, without guarding or rebound. A succussion splash may often be demonstrated.

Dx Structural diseases, including gastric outlet obstruction related to malignancy and peptic ulcer disease, should first be excluded with either upper endoscopy or upper GI barium studies. Upper endoscopy will often show retained food debris in the stomach, even after an overnight fast. A thorough review of medications is necessary to rule out possible triggers. Once these steps have been completed, gastric emptying scintigraphy remains the gold standard for diagnosis. Retention of >10% of the ingested meal at 4 hours or >70% at 2 hours is considered diagnostic. Medications that can either delay or increase gastric emptying should be withheld 48 hours prior to scintigraphy. Blood glucose should also be optimized, as hyperglycemia can affect scintigraphy results.

Tx Treatment includes both symptomatic therapy and prokinetic agents. Dietary modifications may help lessen symptoms and include eating small, frequent meals, avoidance of fat, avoidance of fiber to prevent bezoar formation, and avoidance of carbonated beverages, alcohol, and tobacco. Severe cases may require jejunal tube feedings or even total parenteral nutrition (TPN). The use of antinausea medications such as ondansetron is common but without definitive data to support efficacy. Beyond symptom control, promoting motility may be helpful. The use of prokinetic agents, including metoclopramide, domperidone, and erythromycin, is often helpful. Optimization of blood glucose in diabetics is also recommended. The use of botulinum toxin injected into the pylorus has been tried in refractory cases, but results are mixed. Implantation of a gastric neurostimulator has shown benefit for some refractory cases in uncontrolled trials.
See Cecil Essentials 37.

ZEBRA ZONE

a. Superior mesenteric artery (SMA) syndrome: Compression of the distal duodenum by the SMA and associated mesenteric attachments, often after prolonged periods of malnutrition and bed rest. Normally, a fat pad exists between the aorta and SMA, and weight loss predisposes to loss of this fat pad with compression of the duodenum between the aorta and SMA.

b. Bezoars: Collections of ingested foreign material in the stomach, such as vegetable matter, hair, and medications. These patients often have had previous gastric surgery, and the bezoar forms from continued ingestion of indigestible products.

c. Cyclic vomiting syndrome: A disorder characterized by recurrent episodes of intractable vomiting in the absence of an organic cause, between periods of completely normal health.

d. Gallstone ileus: A rare cause of mechanical obstruction caused by passage through a biliary-enteric fistula of a gallstone, which lodges in the terminal ileum.

e. Intussusception: A cause of SBO common in children but also presents in adults, in which the intestine telescopes onto itself.

f. Zenker's diverticulum: A diverticulum of the mucosa, just above the cricopharyngeal muscle, appearing as a "pouch" posteriorly demonstrated radiologically or on endoscopy. Patients can present with regurgitation, halitosis, and/or dysphagia.

Practice-Based Learning and Improvement: Evidence-Based Medicine

Title
Systematic review and meta-analysis of the diagnostic and therapeutic role of water-soluble contrast agent in adhesive small bowel obstruction

Authors
Branco BC, Barmparas G, Schnuriger B, et al.

Institution
University of Southern California

Reference
Br J Surg 2010;97:470–478

Problem
Diagnosis and therapeutic role of water-soluble contrast with adhesive small-bowel obstruction

Intervention
Administration of water-soluble contrast via NG tube in patients with suspected adhesive SBO

Comparison/control (quality of evidence)
Meta-analysis of 14 prospective studies that aimed to predict the need for surgery in adhesive SBO. Pooled estimates of sensitivity, specificity, positive and negative predictive values, and likelihood ratios were derived to predict the need for surgery. For the therapeutic role of water-soluble contrast agents (WSCAs), weighted odds ratio (OR) and weighted mean difference (WMD) were obtained.

Outcome/effect
Fourteen prospective studies were included. The appearance of contrast in the colon within 4 to 24 hours after administration had a sensitivity of 96% and specificity of 98% in predicting resolution of SBO. WSCA administration was effective in reducing the need for surgery (OR 0.62; $P = 0.007$) and shortening hospital stay (WMD -1.87 days; $P < 0.001$) compared with conventional treatment.

Historical significance/comments
Administration of water-soluble contrast for adhesive SBO has been found to be a viable strategy in diagnosis and therapy.

Interpersonal and Communication Skills

Be Sensitive to the Barriers Posed by Cultural Differences
As the country grows more ethnically diverse, physicians must remain ever mindful of cultural differences among patient populations. Barriers posed by language and ethnic traditions can result in negative health consequences, including:

- Failure to recognize and respond to health problems
- Inadequate informed consent
- Misinterpretation of physician instructions
- Poor compliance with treatment plans
- Missed appointments
- Inaccuracies in medical histories

Studies conducted over an 8-year period indicate that language barriers alone may be responsible for:

- Fewer clinical visits
- Lengthier clinical visits
- More laboratory tests
- More ED visits
- Limited follow-up
- Dissatisfaction with health care services

From Mann BD: Surgery: a competency-based companion. Philadelphia: Saunders/Elsevier; 2009, p. 314.

Professionalism

Demonstrate Compassion
For many etiologies of nausea and vomiting, including SBO and ileus, treatment involves placement of an NG tube. While NG tubes can offer symptomatic relief in terms of gastric decompression, they are quite uncomfortable for the patient and have been described as one of the most unpleasant experiences in the inpatient setting. Discussing uncomfortable procedures with professionalism involves acknowledging the anticipated discomfort while describing the potential benefit in realistic terms.

Systems-Based Practice

Limit Medical Waste and Unnecessary Care
A 77-year-old woman was admitted because of 3 days of nausea and vomiting; she is unable to keep down any liquids or solids. Upon admission, the severity of her state of volume depletion was not appreciated, and because she had a past history of congestive heart

failure, her IV rate was written for only 50 mL/hr. After 24 hours she is oliguric and has acute kidney injury; she now requires dialysis at an obvious cost to her quality of life and at a significant financial cost. It is estimated that billions of dollars are wasted every year in the United States on unnecessary care.

Unnecessary care falls into four categories:

- Inefficiencies in the system, such as the lack of electronic medical records leading to tests and imaging studies being needlessly repeated.
- Patient safety problems causing patients to spend additional days in the hospital or be readmitted shortly after discharge.
- The risk for malpractice suits leading to the practice of "defensive medicine"—the overuse of diagnostics in an effort to prevent potential litigation.
- Failure to effectively communicate with patients and their families resulting in futile efforts to prolong a patient's life.

Physicians can reduce unnecessary health care costs by identifying sources of wasteful spending, and by making careful and prudent efforts to reduce them.

Suggested Readings

Abell TL, Camilleri M, Donohoe K, et al. Consensus recommendations for gastric emptying scintigraphy: a joint report of the American Neurogastroenterology and Motility Society and the Society of Nuclear Medicine. Am J Gastroenterol 2008;103:753–763.

Abell TL, Lou J, Tabbaa M, et al. Gastric electrical stimulation for gastroparesis improves nutritional parameters at short, intermediate, and long-term follow-up. JPEN J Parenter Enteral Nutr 2003; 27:277–281.

Abell TL, Van Cutsem E, Abrahaamsson H, et al. Gastric electrical stimulation in intractable symptomatic gastroparesis. Digestion 2002;66:204–212.

Abraham NS, Young JM, Solomon MJ. Meta-analysis of short-term outcomes after laparoscopic resection for colorectal cancer. Br J Surg 2004;91:1111–1124.

Arts J, Holvoet L, Caenepeel P, et al. Clinical trial: a randomized-controlled crossover study of intrapyloric injection of botulinum toxin in gastroparesis. Aliment Pharmacol Ther 2007;26:1251–1258.

Böhm B, Milsom JW, Fazio VW. Postoperative intestinal motility following conventional and laparoscopic intestinal surgery. Arch Surg 1995;130:415–419.

Forster J, Sarosiek I, Lin Z, et al. Further experience with gastric stimulation to treat drug refractory gastroparesis. Am J Surg 2003;186:690–695.

Friedenberg FK, Palit A, Parkman HP, et al. Botulinum toxin A for the treatment of delayed gastric emptying. Am J Gastroenterol 2008;103:416–423.

Hansen CT, Sørensen M, Møller C, et al. Effect of laxatives on gastrointestinal functional recovery in fast-track hysterectomy: a double-blind, placebo-controlled randomized study. Am J Obstet Gynecol 2007;196:311.e1–7.

Kovacs A, Chan L, Hotrakitya C, et al. Rotavirus gastroenteritis. Clinical and laboratory features and use of the Rotazyme test. Am J Dis Child 1987;141:161–166.

Liu SS, Wu CL. Effect of postoperative analgesia on major postoperative complications: a systematic update of the evidence. Anesth Analg 2007;104:689–702.

Rodriguez WJ, Kim HW, Brandt CD, et al. Longitudinal study of rotavirus infection and gastroenteritis in families served by a pediatric medical practice: clinical and epidemiologic observations. Pediatr Infect Dis J 1987;6:170–176.

Sim R, Cheong DM, Wong KS, et al. Prospective randomized, double-blind, placebo-controlled study of pre- and postoperative administration of a COX-2-specific inhibitor as opioid-sparing analgesia in major colorectal surgery. Colorectal Dis 2007;9:52–60.

Traut U, Brügger L, Kunz R, et al. Systemic prokinetic pharmacologic treatment for postoperative adynamic ileus following abdominal surgery in adults. Cochrane Database Syst Rev 2008;1:CD004930.

Chapter 28
Esophageal Dysphagia (Case 21)

Benjamin Ngo MD and John Abramson MD

Case: A 50-year-old man is encouraged by his wife to present for an evaluation of difficulty swallowing solid food that has progressively worsened over several months. He complains of occasional heartburn and is otherwise without significant medical problems. He has had an associated 15-lb weight loss.

Differential Diagnosis

Achalasia (motility disorders)	Esophageal cancer	Eosinophilic esophagitis
Peptic stricture	Schatzki ring (esophageal ring)	

Speaking Intelligently

We consider dysphagia and weight loss in this patient as "red flags" that should cause concern. Additional diagnostic testing is necessary. Certainly there are many causes of difficulty swallowing, but in this situation dysphagia and weight loss indicate that esophageal carcinoma must first be considered. This is not a patient with nonspecific upper GI symptoms who should simply be placed on a proton pump inhibitor (PPI) and followed.

PATIENT CARE

Clinical Thinking
- Determine the onset and acuity of symptoms. Persistent dysphagia with the inability to swallow secretions suggests a foreign body or food bolus impaction. This represents a GI emergency that must be dealt with expeditiously.
- Establish if the swallowing problem is with solids, liquids, or both.
- Determine associated symptoms.

History
- A focused history should include timing of onset and duration of symptoms.
- Characterize whether symptoms are intermittent or progressive. Does the swallowing difficulty occur with solids, liquids, or both?
- Inquire about symptoms of heartburn, current or past use of over-the-counter antacids, and use of alcohol and tobacco.

Physical Examination
- There are no specific physical examination findings.
- Assess whether there has been significant weight loss, and assess nutritional status.
- Whenever we entertain a diagnosis of esophageal carcinoma, we always palpate for supraclavicular adenopathy.

Tests for Consideration
- **Barium swallow** can define many causes of dysphagia. $85
- **Upper endoscopy** has the ability to both define and potentially treat dysphagia (i.e., a peptic stricture can be dilated at the time of diagnosis) $600
- **Plain chest radiographs** may show a mediastinal mass compressing the esophagus. $45
- **Esophageal manometry** is used for the diagnosis of motility disorders. As a bolus of food or liquid passes down the esophagus, abnormal pressure wave progressions will be recorded in diseased states. $285

- **Endoscopic ultrasound**, when appropriate, can stage esophageal and periesophageal masses, and offer prognostic information to help guide future therapeutic plans. $885

Clinical Entities · Medical Knowledge

Achalasia

Pφ Achalasia results from the inability of the lower esophageal sphincter (LES) to relax, as a result of a defect in the inhibitory motor neurons. The cause of primary achalasia is unknown. It affects about 1 in 100,000 persons. Chagas disease is an uncommon form of secondary achalasia and is acquired via infection with *Trypanosoma cruzi*.

TP Patients complain at first of progressive dysphagia to solids, and then to both solids and liquids. Regurgitation can occur (usually at night) in the reclining or recumbent position. Chest pain is frequently a symptom.

Dx Barium swallow will demonstrate a classic "bird's beak" appearance of the closed LES with proximal esophageal dilation. Esophageal manometry is used to definitively diagnose achalasia. Endoscopy is typically used to rule out cancer, which can cause a syndrome of "pseudoachalasia."

Tx Medications such as calcium channel blockers (e.g., nifedipine), which relax the LES, can be used but have limited effectiveness. Botox injections via endoscopy can provide temporary relief. Pneumatic dilatation to break the sphincter muscle is another option, although perforation is a risk. A Heller myotomy (esophagocardiomyotomy) is a definitive surgical option and is effective in 90% of patients. **See Cecil Essentials 36.**

Esophageal Cancer

Pφ Esophageal cancer arises from the mucosal lining of the esophagus. It can be either a squamous cell carcinoma or adenocarcinoma. Risk factors include smoking, alcohol consumption, and obesity. In the United States, esophageal cancer is the seventh most common cancer, and adenocarcinoma is more common. Barrett esophagus is an important risk factor for developing adenocarcinoma of the esophagus.

TP Dysphagia is the most common presenting symptom. It is rapidly progressive. Weight loss is often an associated finding. Late complications include bleeding, perforation, and hoarseness caused by invasion of the recurrent laryngeal nerve.

Dx Barium studies will show strictures and intraluminal masses. Endoscopy offers direct visual inspection and the ability to perform a biopsy to make a definitive diagnosis. Endoscopic ultrasound will determine depth of invasion and staging information.

Tx Treatment depends on the stage of the cancer. Early cancers can be treated with surgical resection. There are several surgical approaches including a combined thoracic and abdominal approach (Ivor-Lewis), transhiatal esophagectomy using an abdominal and neck incision, and a "minimally invasive approach" using a laparoscopic and thoracoscopic approach combined with a neck incision. Neoadjuvant chemotherapy is often used in advanced-stage tumors before resection. When tumors are not considered resectable, chemotherapy and radiation are used. Advanced cancers are treated with palliative efforts and can include chemotherapy, radiation, and stenting procedures. **See Cecil Essentials 36, 39, 57.**

Eosinophilic Esophagitis

Pφ Eosinophilic esophagitis is becoming a more recognized and prevalent cause of dysphagia. It occurs from the infiltration of the esophageal mucosa with eosinophils that bring about inflammation of the mucosa. Some authorities consider eosinophilic esophagitis to be the result of environmental allergen exposure.

TP Patients are more commonly male. There is an association with asthma. They will typical present with intermittent dysphagia to solids. An acute food bolus impaction may be the initial presenting event.

Dx Barium study will classically show a "feline esophagus," which has the appearance of multiple rings. Endoscopy findings include mucosal tears, furrows, rings, and whitish plaques that represent eosinophilic abscesses. Biopsy confirms a high eosinophil count. Strictures can also occur.

Tx A trial of PPIs is sometimes given, as eosinophils can be seen in patients with reflux disease. Oral fluticasone is prescribed, and patients are occasionally referred to an allergist for allergy testing. Strictures can be mechanically dilated; when doing so, care must be taken to avoid perforation. **See Cecil Essentials 36.**

Peptic Stricture

Pφ Inflammation of the esophagus as a result of gastroesophageal reflux can lead to stricture formation. In untreated gastroesophageal reflux disease (GERD), up to one fourth of patients will develop strictures.

TP Patients will present with difficulty swallowing food. A history of reflux disease and heartburn is consistent with the diagnosis.

Dx Barium swallow will show intraluminal narrowing. Endoscopy offers direct visualization of the stricture. Biopsies are performed to rule out underlying malignancy.

Tx Narrow strictures are treated with dilation. This can be achieved by passing a mechanical dilator down the patient's throat or a balloon passed through an endoscope. PPIs are recommended post procedure to prevent recurrence. **See Cecil Essentials 36.**

Schatzki's Ring (Esophageal Ring)

Pφ A Schatzki ring is a thin ring of tissue that is formed by mucosa. It is typically located a few centimeters above the gastroesophageal junction and is usually associated with a hiatal hernia. These rings are benign.

TP Schatzki rings are usually found incidentally and infrequently cause symptoms. When symptoms occur they are intermittent. Patients usually are able pass the food bolus or regurgitate food, and continue their meal. "Steakhouse syndrome" occurs when a piece of meat becomes lodged proximal to a ring.

Dx Schatzki rings can be found on barium swallows and by upper endoscopy.

Tx If symptomatic, the ring is broken by dilation. After treatment, symptoms can occur months to years later. **See Cecil Essentials 36.**

Practice-Based Learning and Improvement: Evidence-Based Medicine

Title
Combined chemotherapy and radiotherapy compared with radiotherapy alone in patients with cancer of the esophagus

Authors
Herskovic A, Martz K, al-Sarraf M, et al.

Institution
Radiation Oncology Department, Oakwood Hospital, Dearborn, MI, USA

Reference
N Engl J Med 1992;326:1593–1598

Problem
Esophageal cancer is associated with a dismal 5-year survival approaching zero.

Intervention
A cisplatin-based chemotherapy regimen was added to the standard of radiation therapy.

Quality of evidence
Level I

Outcome/effect
Combined chemoradiation therapy is superior to radiation therapy alone.

Historical significance/comments
Based on the results of this trial, the standard of care for the treatment of esophageal carcinoma continues to be combined chemotherapy and radiation therapy.

Interpersonal and Communication Skills

"Doc, How Much Time Do I Have?"

You have just placed an esophageal stent in a 77-year-old man with an unresectable mid-esophageal tumor and liver metastases. Following the procedure, he asks, "Doc, how much time do you think I have?" Answering this question is not easy. It may be appropriate to determine first if the patient really wants a *numerical* answer; indeed, some patients do wish to know, but it is often difficult to give a specific time frame. Studies suggest that patients with advanced esophageal cancers can expect a median survival of 8 to 12 months before they succumb to a complication such as infection, bleeding, or tumor infiltration. In such circumstances it is important to provide an honest, but broad, range of time. Though you can broaden the time to extend hope, it is often wise in such a circumstance to suggest gently that the patient may want to "put his affairs in order." Take such a cue from your patient as an opportunity to address any fears he may have, and to reassure him that every attempt will be made to help him with his disease and to provide all comfort measures that may be necessary.

Professionalism

Maintain Patient Confidentiality

A patient with esophageal cancer is accompanied by his wife to your endoscopy suite because a barium swallow has shown an esophageal mass. Your intent is to perform a biopsy. The patient has specifically asked that you **not** inform his wife about the biopsy results, even if the lesion appears to be cancer. Such a scenario presents a difficult dilemma for the physician. The physician-patient relationship mandates the highest degree of confidentiality. Information discovered by a physician during testing and treatment must be kept in confidence and divulged to others only with the patient's approval. Physicians are bound to this ethical standard. As in the above scenario, a diagnosis of esophageal cancer cannot be discussed with the patient's wife unless the patient consents (given that the patient is competent). The only circumstance in which physician-patient confidentiality can be breached is in a situation in which patients threaten to harm themselves or others.

Systems-Based Practice

COBRA

A patient under your treatment for Barrett esophagus needs a follow-up endoscopy. She explains to your office manager that she was recently laid off from her job and therefore has lost her health insurance. Your office manager spends time educating her about **"COBRA"** insurance, the temporary continuation of a health plan for a worker and/or her family at their own cost. COBRA stands for **Consolidated Omnibus Budget Reconciliation Act** and refers to legislation passed by the U.S. Congress in 1986 to create a solution for workers who had lost their jobs and became ineligible for employer-sponsored health insurance benefits for themselves and/or their families. COBRA provides that workers and their families are eligible to apply for continued health insurance coverage under their existing employer-sponsored plan, except that the worker must now pay for that coverage in full, plus a surcharge to cover the cost of administering the plan. Coverage through COBRA continues for up to 18 months but may be extended up to 36 months under some circumstances.

Chapter 29
Gastrointestinal Bleeding (Case 22)

Melissa Morgan DO, Michael Share MD,
and Marc Zitin MD

Case: A 70-year-old woman with a past medical history of coronary artery disease, hypertension, and hyperlipidemia presents to the ED complaining of rectal bleeding that has been present all day. Earlier in the day she had a bowel movement and noted bright red blood mixed in with her stool. She complains of dizziness and light-headedness. Her outpatient daily medications include aspirin, simvastatin, and metoprolol. She also admits to taking ibuprofen twice daily for the past week for pain in her knees. She admits to "occasional" drinking and one cocktail each night after dinner.

Differential Diagnosis

Peptic ulcer disease	Arteriovenous malformation	Colon cancer
Hemorrhoids	Esophagogastric varices	
Gastric cancer	Diverticulosis	

Speaking Intelligently

When asked to see a patient with GI bleeding, it is important to remember to first stabilize the patient. It is also important to know whether the bleeding is coming from the upper or lower GI tract; this will affect both acute management and treatment. Upper GI bleeding commonly presents with hematemesis and/or melena. In comparison, lower GI bleeding presents with hematochezia. However, these distinctions are not absolute. A massive upper GI hemorrhage can also present with hematochezia, and a proximal lower GI bleed can present with melena.

PATIENT CARE

Clinical Thinking
- A thorough history and physical exam are the most important steps in differentiating the cause of GI bleeding.

- As stated previously, the management of the patient strongly depends on the cause of bleeding. Patients who are having a massive upper GI hemorrhage will most likely require intubation and observation in the ICU.
- Stabilizing the patient is the first priority, to enable him or her to sustain an intervention to control bleeding, such as endoscopy, an interventional radiology procedure, or surgery.

History
- Has this ever happened before, and if so, does the patient know what the cause of the bleeding was previously?
- Has the patient ever had an endoscopic procedure such as colonoscopy or upper endoscopy?
- **Current medications?** This includes over-the-counter medications such as nonsteroidal anti-inflammatory drugs (NSAIDs), including ibuprofen, aspirin, and naproxen.
- **Define underlying medical conditions:** risk factors for chronic liver disease, injection drug use, hepatitis B or C infection, or chronic alcohol use.
- Did the patient have **bloody vomitus** or **coffee-grounds** emesis?
- How much blood was present?
- Was there blood only on the toilet paper or in the toilet bowl as well?
- Does the patient have **abdominal pain**? If so, determine duration.

Physical Examination
- **Check the vital signs:** Tachycardia and/or hypotension indicates an active or ongoing hemorrhage.
- Look for **stigmata of chronic liver disease**, including telangiectasias of the abdomen and chest, jaundice, scleral icterus, ascites, and palmar erythema.
- **Do a thorough abdominal exam:** Epigastric tenderness may suggest PUD. Lower abdominal tenderness may suggest colitis.
- The **rectal exam** is important: black tarry stools (melena) will most likely mean an upper GI source of bleeding; bright red blood usually indicates a lower GI source. Are there masses or hemorrhoids present?
- **Placement of an NG tube** can be helpful when there is concern for an upper GI source of bleeding. Keep in mind that if the fluid aspirated from the tube is clear, this does not exclude an upper GI source. It is important to have bilious return to rule out a duodenal source. If the return is bloody, this indicates an upper GI hemorrhage.

Tests for Consideration
- **Hemoglobin and hematocrit** will help in determining the extent of the blood loss, although acute blood loss may not be evident right away, as equilibration takes time. $7

- **Prothrombin time–international normalized ratio (PT/INR)** will provide information as to whether the patient has a coagulopathy—possibly related to a medication, liver disease, or malnutrition. $6
- **CMP:** A BUN elevated in greater than a 20:1 proportion to the Cr is consistent with an upper GI hemorrhage. $12
- **Type and cross-type for packed red blood cells (RBCs).** $14
- **EGD** will aid in visualization of the esophagus, stomach, and first and second portions of the duodenum to identify and treat the source of bleeding. $600
- **Colonoscopy** can help in finding the cause of bleeding in the colon such as diverticulosis, arteriovenous malformations (AVMs), polyps, or tumors. $655
- **Video capsule endoscopy** is mostly used in the outpatient setting to look for occult GI blood loss in the small intestine. This test consists of swallowing a capsule that contains a camera. As the capsule moves through the GI tract, numerous pictures are taken. The patient wears a recording device for 8 hours and then returns the device to his or her gastroenterologist. The physician reviews the images to look for a source of bleeding. $723

IMAGING CONSIDERATIONS

→ A **tagged RBC scan** can detect blood loss at a rate of 0.1 to 0.5 mL/min and is more sensitive than angiography. This is mostly used for lower GI hemorrhages but can occasionally be used for an upper GI hemorrhage when the source is not located by EGD. $239

→ **Angiography** requires active blood loss at a rate of 1.0 to 1.5 mL/min for a bleeding site to be visualized. This is usually done after a tagged RBC scan is positive. $338

Clinical Entities	Medical Knowledge

Peptic Ulcer Disease

Pφ PUD occurs when the caustic effects of acid and pepsin in the GI lumen overwhelm the ability of the mucosa to resist their effects. Most ulcers occur when the process of mucosal protection is disrupted by *Helicobacter pylori* infection or use of NSAIDs.

TP Although gastric and duodenal ulcers are associated with epigastric pain 66% of the time, often the diagnosis is not made until complications such as hemorrhage or perforation occur. Hemorrhage will be evident by melena, hematemesis, or coffee-grounds emesis. Perforation will cause severe abdominal pain and usually presents as an acute abdomen with peritonitis, requiring surgery.

Dx Endoscopy is the most accurate diagnostic test for PUD and is the appropriate first diagnostic test for GI bleeding. Mucosal biopsies should also be obtained for rapid urease tests to determine whether *Helicobacter pylori* is present; histologic staining should be done for patients with a negative rapid urease test or for instances when the urease test is not available. However, if the concern is for a perforated ulcer presenting with free intraperitoneal air, endoscopy should not be performed and the treatment is surgical.

Tx The majority of upper GI bleeds due to PUD will stop spontaneously, but certain findings on endoscopy will predict the risk of repeat hemorrhage and should prompt early intervention: (1) a visible vessel in the ulcer bed, (2) an adherent clot, and (3) active bleeding. EGD is not only a diagnostic procedure but a therapeutic one as well; bleeding is often stopped by injection of epinephrine, use of electrocautery, and/or clips placed endoscopically. It is recommended that at least two of the above therapies be used to fully control and prevent repeat bleeding. The use of a proton pump inhibitor (PPI) infusion is helpful during an upper GI hemorrhage secondary to PUD. Raising the pH in the stomach enhances stabilization of clot formation. In patients with demonstrated infection with *H. pylori*, appropriate antimicrobial therapy should also be added. **See Cecil Essentials 37.**

Arteriovenous Malformation

Pφ Also called angiodysplasia, these abnormalities consist of ectatic, dilated, thin-walled vessels that are composed of either endothelium alone or endothelium with a small component of smooth muscle. Although the pathogenesis is not completely understood, one theory is that development occurs because of intermittent obstruction of submucosal veins in the muscularis propria, which causes dilation. AVMs can occur anywhere throughout the GI tract. They are seen in patients with numerous conditions, including end-stage renal disease, von Willebrand disease, and aortic stenosis.

TP Presentation varies based on the location of the AVM. AVMs in the stomach can cause melena or hematemesis. Those located in the small intestine or right side of the colon can cause melena, bright red blood per rectum, or even anemia with occult bleeding. Presentation depends on how extensively they bleed. Coagulopathy or platelet dysfunction can lead to more overt bleeding.

Dx Diagnosis can be made during upper endoscopy or colonoscopy if the lesions are within reach of the endoscope or colonoscope. If a cause of bleeding cannot be found, patients will undergo a video capsule study or double-balloon enteroscopy (DBE), to visualize the entire small bowel, including the jejunum and ileum.

Tx AVMs can be treated endoscopically using electrocautery or argon plasma coagulation. The choice of treatment varies on location of the lesion as well as the preference of the endoscopist. The right side of the colon is extremely thin-walled and more likely to perforate during treatment compared to other parts of the GI tract. If a hemorrhage is particularly aggressive, other options for treatment include surgery and angiography with embolization. **See Cecil Essentials 34.**

Diverticulosis

Pφ A diverticulum is a saclike protrusion of the colonic wall that does not contain all of the layers of the wall; the mucosa and submucosa herniate through the muscle layer. Diverticula develop at four points along the circumference of the colon, where the blood vessels (vasa recta) penetrate the circular muscle layer. The blood vessel can become irritated and rupture into the diverticulum, causing a brisk hemorrhage. These account for 30% to 50% of brisk rectal bleeding. A diet low in fiber can predispose a patient to diverticular disease. A low-fiber diet can cause increased intraluminal pressure in the colon, and this can lead to the formation of diverticula.

TP Painless rectal bleeding is the main presentation. This most commonly occurs in those >60 years of age but can occur in younger patients as well. As many as 50% may have had a previous episode.

Dx Diagnosis can be made via colonoscopy. If the patient has had a previous colonoscopy with documented diverticulosis and presents with a brisk lower GI hemorrhage, the bleeding will most likely be diverticular in nature. To diagnose the exact site of bleeding, colonoscopy can again be useful. However, if a significant amount of blood is present, it may be difficult to localize the bleeding. A tagged-RBC scan can aid in localization.

Tx Bleeding will cease spontaneously in 75% of episodes. If bleeding does not stop, a colonoscopy can be performed to try to localize the diverticulum involved, and a clip can be placed. However, if the bleeding cannot be localized via colonoscopy, a tagged-RBC scan followed by angiography and embolization is necessary. If the patient continues to bleed despite these efforts, surgical intervention may be necessary. **See Cecil Essentials 34.**

Hemorrhoids

Pφ Hemorrhoids arise from a plexus of dilated veins located in the submucosal layer of the rectum and are classified as internal or external based on their location from the pectinate line. Those that are above the pectinate line are considered internal, and those below are external. A patient may have both. Hemorrhoids are classically associated with advanced age, chronic constipation, pregnancy, prolonged sitting, and diarrhea.

TP Internal hemorrhoids can cause painless bleeding that can be described most often as either a slow drip into the toilet or blood that is seen solely on the toilet paper. External hemorrhoids generally lead to pruritus and the formation of skin tags, and they cause acute rectal pain when they become thrombosed.

Dx Diagnosis of external hemorrhoids is made by visual inspection of the anus. At times internal hemorrhoids can be palpated on rectal examination; they are best visualized by performing anoscopy or sigmoidoscopy.

Tx Conservative measures to treat hemorrhoids include adding fiber to the diet to add bulk to the stools, thereby lessening constipation and minimizing bleeding. Hydrocortisone suppositories and sitz baths can help with symptoms of pain and pruritus. If symptoms persist despite conservative treatment, more invasive measures may be required. Most external hemorrhoids require no further intervention. When acute thrombosis occurs, the patient may benefit from surgical evacuation of the clot and excision of the hemorrhoid within the first 48 hours. Internal hemorrhoids that persistently bleed can be treated with rubber-band ligation; if this is unsuccessful, hemorrhoidectomy becomes appropriate. **See Cecil Essentials 34.**

Esophagogastric Varices

Pφ Varices develop as a consequence of portal hypertension, usually from cirrhosis. Normal portal pressure is approximately 9 mm Hg compared to an inferior vena cava pressure of 2–6 mm Hg. Therefore, a normal portal→caval gradient is 3–7 mm Hg. At gradients >10 mm Hg, blood flow through the hepatic portal system is redirected from the liver to areas with lower venous pressures. This causes extremely dilated submucosal veins that can be present in the stomach or esophagus. Isolated gastric varices can be present from obstruction of the splenic vein.

TP Varices result in massive hematemesis, which is usually painless. Patients often demonstrate signs of systemic shock with hypotension and tachycardia on initial presentation due to the large amount of blood loss. Only 50% of patients with an acute variceal hemorrhage will stop bleeding spontaneously; 30% of patients will die during their first acute hemorrhage.

Dx Diagnosis is based on clinical history as well as endoscopic findings. If a patient is a known cirrhotic (although they can certainly develop other disease entities such as PUD), it is important to treat aggressively, as their mortality from a variceal hemorrhage is high.

Tx Treatment varies from pharmacologic, endoscopic, Blakemore tube placement (a tube with multiple balloons designed to accomplish tamponade of proximal gastric and/or esophageal varices), or transjugular intrahepatic portosystemic shunt (TIPS). All variceal hemorrhage patients should be intubated for airway protection before any intervention. A somatostatin analogue can be infused to induce splanchnic vasoconstriction and decrease portal inflow. Endoscopy should be performed as soon as possible. Therapy consists of band ligation or sclerotherapy, which consists of injecting a sclerosant solution into the bleeding varix. Blakemore tube placement is a temporizing measure, and the tube can be left in place for 24–48 hours before complications such as esophageal necrosis occur. TIPS is used as a last resort to decompress the portal system for bleeding that cannot be controlled with any of the aforementioned therapies. **See Cecil Essentials 34, 45.**

Colon Cancer

Pφ Environmental and genetic factors increase the likelihood of developing colorectal cancer. The proposed mechanism is that most cancers arise from adenomatous polyps in the colon. Polyps can progress to dysplastic polyps and ultimately to adenocarcinoma. The lifetime risk of colorectal cancer in an average-risk person is 5%. More than 90% of colorectal cancers occur in persons over the age of 50 years.

TP The majority of patients who are symptomatic from colorectal cancer present with hematochezia, abdominal pain, change in bowel habits, or unexplained iron deficiency anemia. Hematochezia is more commonly caused by a rectal rather than a colon cancer.

Dx Colonoscopy is the single best test to diagnose colon cancer. Although barium enema combined with flexible sigmoidoscopy can be used for colorectal cancer screening, the yield is much lower than with colonoscopy. Colonoscopy is considered the gold standard for the symptomatic patient.

Tx Once the diagnosis of colon cancer is made, treatment such as chemotherapy, surgery, or radiation therapy varies based on the stage of the disease. If a patient is experiencing symptoms such as hematochezia, interventions such as electrocautery can be utilized for pure palliation of bleeding. However, most lesions are friable, and definitive treatment would consist of surgical intervention. **See Cecil Essentials 39, 57.**

Gastric Cancer

Pφ Gastric cancer is the second leading cause of cancer deaths in the world. Risk factors include smoking, obesity, infection with *Helicobacter pylori*, and diet consisting of high-salt and high-nitrosamine compounds.

TP The most common presenting symptoms are weight loss and abdominal pain. Tumors located at the gastroesophageal junction, or cardia of the stomach, will present with dysphagia. Those that are located more distally in the antrum can cause gastric outlet obstructive symptoms, such as nausea and vomiting.

Dx Large tumors can be seen during an upper GI series or on CT scan. Definitive diagnosis is made endoscopically with biopsy.

Tx Treatment options are based on stage of disease. Surgery may be curative if there are no lymph nodes involved. Often patients have advanced disease at the time of diagnosis. For patients who undergo surgery and prove to have positive lymph nodes, adjuvant postoperative therapy with combination chemotherapy and radiation therapy may be of benefit. **See Cecil Essentials 39, 57.**

ZEBRA ZONE

a. **Dieulafoy lesion:** A dilated, aberrant submucosal vessel that erodes the underlying epithelium in the absence of an ulcer. It accounts for less than 1% of severe upper GI hemorrhages. Both diagnosis and treatment can be done endoscopically. The vessel most likely requires dual therapy with injection and electrocautery or clipping.

b. **Mallory-Weiss tear:** Longitudinal mucosal tears at the distal esophagus and proximal stomach usually caused by retching. Retching increases the intra-abdominal pressure and causes the tear. Diagnosis is made by endoscopy. Most tears heal spontaneously. If a tear is actively bleeding, the usual modes of endoscopic treatment can be utilized.

c. **Gastric antral vascular ectasia (GAVE) syndrome:** This disorder is also known as watermelon stomach. The term comes from the endoscopic appearance of the stomach with longitudinal flat red stripes that radiate from the pylorus into the antrum and resemble the stripes on a watermelon. Most cases are idiopathic. Treatment consists of endoscopic ablation with argon plasma coagulation. Multiple treatments are usually necessary.

Practice-Based Learning and Improvement: Evidence-Based Medicine

Title
Effect of intravenous omeprazole on recurrent bleeding after endoscopic treatment of bleeding peptic ulcers

Authors
Lau JY, Sung JJ, Lee KK, et al.

Institution
Chinese University of Hong Kong

Reference
N Engl J Med 2000;343:310–316

Problem
After endoscopic treatment of bleeding peptic ulcers, bleeding recurs in 15% to 20% of patients.

Intervention
Endoscopic therapy of bleeding peptic ulcers and then randomization to continuous infusion of omeprazole vs. placebo

Quality of evidence
Level I.
Prospective randomized trial of 240 patients with 120 patients in each group of treatment and placebo.

Outcome/effect
Bleeding recurred within 30 days in 8 patients (6.7%) in the omeprazole group, as compared with 27 (22.5%) in the placebo group.

Historical significance/comments
This information has helped clinicians substantially in treating bleeding PUD. A constant infusion of a proton pump inhibitor significantly decreases the risk of recurrent bleeding and leads to decreased morbidity and mortality from bleeding PUD. This has become one of the mainstays of treatment presently.

Interpersonal and Communication Skills

Communication Is the Cornerstone of Multidisciplinary Care
When managing a patient with GI bleeding, all specialties must work together. It may be the job of the medicine service or the ED team to stabilize the patient, while the gastroenterologist attempts to identify the cause of the bleeding. In patients with significant hypotension, endoscopy cannot be performed; therefore, the surgical team should be involved should there be a need to operate urgently. If the BP can be stabilized, upper endoscopy can be performed. If the gastroenterologist cannot find the source of bleeding, he or she needs to discuss options with the surgeon and the interventional radiologist. If the patient's condition is unstable, the team should determine whether an emergent operation or emergent angiogram for embolization is most appropriate under the particular circumstances. Good communication among the various specialties is essential to provide the best possible care.

Professionalism

Remain Nonjudgmental and Treat All Patients with Respect

When approaching a patient with a history of alcohol use who is actively bleeding and suspected of having cirrhosis, it is important to remain nonjudgmental. As much as possible, make the patient feel at ease, particularly as you inquire about social habits such as alcohol consumption and use of injection drugs. If patients feel they cannot trust you, they may not be forthcoming with the information required to treat them, and they may also refuse treatment. Variceal hemorrhage can be deadly and thus has to be treated quickly and aggressively; treatment requires a cooperative patient. Placing patients at ease and showing genuine concern will make them comfortable and more likely to agree to treatment.

Systems-Based Practice

GI Bleeding: Develop a Time-Efficient, Systems-Based Approach to Diagnosis

When we see a patient with GI bleeding in the Emergency Department, we try to keep in mind which areas of the hospital system will need to be mobilized in order to achieve expeditious diagnosis and treatment. Our initial focus is on localizing the source to either the upper or lower GI tract (i.e., proximal or distal to the ligament of Treitz). If the patient's history (e.g., hematemesis, melenic stool) and physical exam (e.g., hemodynamic instability, NG lavage with copious blood) are strongly suggestive of an upper GI hemorrhage, proceed with EGD, which can be both diagnostic and therapeutic.

NG lavage can be useful in a patient with an upper GI bleed, as return of blood or coffee-grounds–like material confirms the diagnosis of upper GI bleeding and predicts whether bleeding is caused by a high-risk lesion. However, a negative lavage does not exclude an upper GI hemorrhage, as a duodenal lesion may not cause duodenal-gastric reflux. If the EGD is unable to localize a source, proceed with colonoscopy to look for a lower tract source.

In a similar fashion, when a patient presents with a history consistent with lower GI bleeding, it is important to first rule out upper GI bleeding, as 10% to 15% of upper GI hemorrhages present with signs and symptoms of a lower GI hemorrhage. In a stable patient, after excluding an upper source with EGD (with or without NG lavage), proceed with colonoscopy.

Because many patients with lower GI bleeding will stop bleeding spontaneously (recurrent bleeding occurs in only 10% to 40% of patients), diagnosis can often be quite challenging. When the diagnosis cannot be made with endoscopic measures, radiologic imaging studies such as **radionuclide scintigraphy** and **angiography** serve their greatest purpose. In scintigraphy, the patient's RBCs are tagged with technetium-99m (^{99m}Tc), and then a gamma camera follows flow and looks for signs of RBC leakage. Scintigraphy is very sensitive to bleeding, recognizing rates as low as 0.1 mL/min, and the radionuclide tag persists for 6 hours, allowing prolonged or repeat imaging. However, *scintigraphy does not promote specific anatomic localization of lesions*. In the past, scintigraphy has been used as a screening test for angiography, but inconsistent and inaccurate localization of bleeding sites, as well as recent promulgation of wireless capsule enteroscopy (WCE) and DBE, have dramatically decreased its use. Currently, its most appropriate use is in the patient who has intermittent, recurrent bleeding in which we can take advantage of the 6-hour duration of the tag to get a rough idea of lesion location.

Angiography is less sensitive, able to recognize bleeding rates of 0.5 mL/min. However, angiography is not only able to define exact anatomy of a lesion, but can also be therapeutic with localized vasopressin injection or vessel embolization. A patient must be actively bleeding at the time of this study, so it should be used accordingly in a patient with an active bleeding source whose hemodynamic stability is threatened.

The majority of diagnoses and therapies in patients with GI bleeding are achieved with endoscopy, but there is still a role for radiologic imaging to be used in specific situations.

Suggested Readings

Aljebreen AM, Fallone CA, Barkun AN. Nasogastric aspirate predicts high-risk endoscopic lesions in patients with acute upper-GI bleeding. Gastrointest Endosc 2004;59:172–178.

Strate LL. Lower GI bleeding: epidemiology and diagnosis. Gastroenterol Clin North Am 2005;34:643–664.

Westerhof J, Weersma RK, Koornstra JJ. Investigating obscure gastrointestinal bleeding: capsule endoscopy or double balloon enteroscopy? Neth J Med 2009;67:260–265.

Chapter 30
Constipation (Case 23)

Christopher P. Farrell DO and Gary Newman MD

Case: A 67-year-old woman presents to the ED complaining of abdominal discomfort, decreased frequency of her bowel movements, and mild abdominal distension. She is clearly distressed in the ED, unable to find a comfortable position on the stretcher, and wincing with abdominal pain.

Differential Diagnosis

Irritable bowel syndrome (IBS)	Impaction
Colon cancer	Medication-related
Volvulus	Acute colonic pseudo-obstruction (Ogilvie syndrome)

Speaking Intelligently

When asked to see a patient for constipation, we first want to find out the patient's definition of constipation. Has she not been able to move her bowels in days or is it just not as frequently or as comfortable as she would like? Most cases of constipation aren't critical; however, a bowel obstruction or volvulus requires more urgent care. If she has not been able to move her bowels or pass any gas for days, she may need more immediate treatment. A thorough history is important, concentrating on alarm symptoms such as unintentional weight loss, rectal bleeding, or a recent or sudden change in bowel habits. Any surgical history should be reviewed, along with the patient's medications, followed by a dedicated abdominal and rectal exam.

PATIENT CARE

Clinical Thinking
- First, rule out any urgent condition that needs more immediate care that you can potentially help resolve, even if temporarily.

- A sigmoid volvulus, while rare, requires an urgent endoscopic decompression with flexible sigmoidoscopy; if untreated, it can lead to colonic ischemia and irreversible damage.
- A fecal impaction can be diagnosed and treated quickly with a simple rectal exam and disimpaction.
- Most causes of constipation are not emergent.

History
- Establish the patient's definition of constipation.
- Ask about the quality of the patient's bowel movements and frequency.
- Is there associated bleeding or abdominal pain?
- Determine whether or not the patient ever had a colonoscopy and, if so, when it was performed and what it showed.
- Ask about family history of GI disorders, most importantly colon cancer.
- Perform a thorough review of the patient's medications.

Physical Examination
- Assess vital signs and hemodynamic stability.
- **Abdominal exam:** Evaluate for tenderness (in all quadrants), distension, and tympany; auscultate first for the presence and quality of bowel sounds.
- If abdominal tenderness is noted, check for signs of peritonitis: rebound and/or involuntary guarding.
- **Rectal exam:** Check for masses, strictures, presence and/or quality of stool, presence of gross blood; test for occult blood.

Tests for Consideration
- **Basic metabolic panel (BMP):** Check for electrolyte abnormalities that can cause an ileus. $12
- **CBC:** Look for iron deficiency anemia, possibly unmasking an undiagnosed colon cancer. $11
- **Thyroid function studies:** Look for evidence of hypothyroidism as an underlying cause for constipation. $24
- **Flexible sigmoidoscopy or colonoscopy:** Rule out masses or mechanical reasons for obstruction in the colon or rectum. $436, $655

IMAGING CONSIDERATIONS

→ **Abdominal radiograph or obstruction series:** Usually the first examination to be performed, this may demonstrate dilated loops of bowel, excessive stool throughout the colon, or fecal impaction. A sigmoid volvulus will be noted as a greatly dilated sigmoid colon and a "coffee bean" sign or "bird's beak" sign. $45, $75

→ **CT scan of abdomen and pelvis:** Illustrates cross-sectional images of the abdomen and pelvis allowing for radiographic examination of the bowel wall and its contents. Thickening, narrowing, and masses will be noted. Oral contrast allows the visualization of the inside of the colon, while intravenous contrast allows determination of abnormalities in the bowel wall and surrounding vasculature. $334

→ **Barium enema:** Although this test is no longer performed regularly, it still does hold some value. The study can display inflammatory changes of the rectum or colon, can detect masses, and is the treatment for intussusception in children. $142

Clinical Entities	Medical Knowledge

Irritable Bowel Syndrome

Pφ IBS is a very common disorder characterized by abdominal pain, bloating, and altered bowel habits. The condition can affect both sexes at any age but is prominent in young females. Patients regularly experience abdominal cramping that is relieved with a bowel movement. The bowel habits can be either constipation-predominant or diarrhea-predominant in nature. Constipation-predominant patients usually experience chronic constipation with intermittent diarrhea or regular bowel movements. The pathophysiology of IBS remains unknown; however, hereditary and environmental factors probably play a role. Psychosocial dysfunction also contributes to IBS and its fluctuating symptoms.

TP Crampy abdominal pain, incomplete evacuation of bowels, bloating, gas (flatulence or belching), hard or lumpy stools, relief of abdominal discomfort with defecation.

Dx The main diagnostic tool is the Rome III diagnostic criteria. This includes recurrent abdominal pain or discomfort at least 3 days a month for the last 3 months associated with two of the following: improvement with defecation, onset associated with a change in frequency of stool, or onset associated with a change in form (appearance) of stool.

Tx Initially, constipation-predominant patients can be treated with fiber supplementation and psychosocial therapies, if emotional stress is a contributing factor. A bowel regimen in the form of a laxative, suppository, or enema may be needed if symptoms persist. Finally, specific medications that activate chloride channels or stimulate the release of serotonin can be used in refractory cases. **See Cecil Essentials 34.**

Colon Cancer

Pφ Colon cancer is a malignancy that usually arises from a long-standing polyp. The disease can be localized to the colon or can metastasize to other organs, most frequently the liver. Cancers in the proximal colon may present as iron deficiency anemia from a slow occult hemorrhage, while cancers in the distal colon can present with obstructive symptoms or with gross bleeding.

TP Symptomatic iron deficiency anemia, gross or occult blood in the stool, change in bowel habits (obstruction, diarrhea), unintentional weight loss, abdominal pain.

Dx CT scans can sometimes demonstrate lesions in the colon and are necessary to evaluate for metastatic disease. Colonoscopy is the best diagnostic test to assess for colon cancer, and allows for definitive biopsy samples to be taken and examination of the entire colon; flexible sigmoidoscopy permits examination of only the rectum and distal colon.

Tx Resection of polyps can usually be achieved endoscopically. Cancer resections generally require surgery, which can be performed by open or laparoscopic techniques. Radiation therapy is now used routinely for preoperative treatment of rectal cancer. When colon cancer is metastatic, chemotherapy is the treatment of choice. **See Cecil Essentials 39, 57.**

Impaction

Pφ An impaction results from an accumulation of hardened stool, most frequently occurring in the rectum. This prevents the evacuation of stool, resulting in pain and constipation. This condition occurs more commonly in the elderly and those with chronic neuropathic disorders, from immobility, and in those on medications that alter colonic motility.

TP Inability to move bowels with straining, rectal pain, and pressure. Overflow diarrhea (encopresis) may occur; rectal ulcers may develop.

Dx A fecal impaction can usually be diagnosed very easily with just a simple digital rectal exam. If the impaction is beyond the reach of a rectal exam, an obstruction series or abdominal radiograph will often demonstrate a mass of hardened stool. A CT scan can visualize and localize an area of impaction.

Tx Manual digital disimpaction can be performed at the bedside or under general anesthesia, if necessary. Enemas, suppositories, and laxatives can be used to help break up and resolve an impaction. Following the resolution of an impaction, the patient should be given a fiber supplement and a bowel regimen containing a stool softener and possibly a stimulant or osmotic laxative to prevent further episodes. Narcotics and other medications possibly contributing to the problem should be eliminated to avoid repeat episodes.

Medication-Related Symptoms

Pφ Medications are an extremely common cause of constipation. Narcotics, calcium channel blockers, and anticholinergics are frequent culprits. The chronic use of these medicines requires an adequate bowel regimen and daily fiber supplementation to avoid recurrent issues with constipation.

TP Difficulty moving bowels, infrequent bowel movements, painful bowel movements, localized rectal bleeding from straining.

Dx A thorough history is essential for diagnosing constipation due to medication administration. A complete review of the patient's medication list is required. A detailed physical exam, along with appropriate radiologic testing, is essential to rule out any other etiology for the patient's symptom of constipation.

Tx   The treatment of medication-related constipation can be as
simple as removing the offending agent. The patient should at
least temporarily be placed on a bowel regimen in the form of a
fiber supplementation, stool softener, or laxative, depending on
the severity of symptoms.

Volvulus

Pφ   A volvulus is a twisting of the bowel upon itself, causing an
obstruction, most commonly occurring in the sigmoid colon and
cecum. Alterations in anatomic features have a role in this
pathology. Left untreated, this condition can progress to ischemia
and necrosis due to compromised blood supply.

TP   Progressive abdominal distension and pain, nausea, inability to
move bowels, and the absence of flatus.

Dx   An obstruction series or abdominal radiograph is a good initial
test to evaluate for an obstruction, and a "coffee bean" or "bird's
beak" sign can be seen with a sigmoid volvulus. A CT scan of the
abdomen and pelvis helps distinguish findings such as a volvulus
and isolates the exact area of concern. A barium enema can also
diagnose this condition but is used less often and is not as
immediate or easily available.

Tx   If a patient presents with a sigmoid volvulus, an emergent
endoscopic decompression should be performed, if possible, with
a flexible sigmoidoscopy. Occasionally, a decompressive tube
is left in place beyond the area of previous torsion. Following
decompression, most patients need a sigmoidectomy to prevent a
recurrent volvulus. **See Cecil Essentials 35.**

Acute Colonic Pseudo-obstruction (Ogilvie Syndrome)

Pφ   Acute colonic pseudo-obstruction, also known as Ogilvie
syndrome, presents as gross dilatation of the cecum and right
hemicolon in the absence of an anatomic lesion causing an
obstruction that can present as constipation. Trauma, neurologic
conditions, surgery (abdominal/obstetric, cardiovascular,
orthopedic), severe medical illness, metabolic imbalance
(hypokalemia, hypocalcemia, hypomagnesemia), malignancy, and
medications (narcotics, calcium channel blockers) all can
predispose patients to this condition. Ogilvie's is more commonly
found in men over 60 years of age and is thought to be due to
impairment in the autonomic nervous system.

TP Abdominal pain, nausea, vomiting, constipation and/or diarrhea, and significant abdominal distension.

Dx On physical exam, the abdomen is distended and tympanitic, usually with bowel sounds present. An obstruction series or abdominal radiograph shows a dilated colon, more commonly from the cecum to the splenic flexure. This finding is also seen on a CT scan or barium enema, without evidence of distal obstruction.

Tx Initial treatment involves supportive care with the correction of metabolic imbalances and the removal of precipitating factors, such as medications. An NG tube and/or rectal tube can be inserted for further symptomatic relief. Gentle enemas and stimulating suppositories can be utilized to help induce colonic motility. More aggressive pharmacologic therapy can be given with neostigmine or erythromycin; however, their efficacy is questionable, and each possesses its own side effects. Finally, endoscopic decompression is sometimes warranted if symptoms are severe or colonic dilation increases (11–13 cm). A decompressive tube can be left in the transverse colon to allow for continued treatment.

ZEBRA ZONE

a. **Intussusception:** Occurs as a result of bowel telescoping into itself causing an obstruction and abdominal pain.

b. **Hirschsprung disease:** Congenital disorder of the colon where ganglion cells are absent in a section of bowel, causing chronic constipation. More commonly diagnosed in infants and children.

Practice-Based Learning and Improvement: Evidence-Based Medicine

Title
Prevention of colorectal cancer by colonoscopic polypectomy. The National Polyp Study Workgroup.

Authors
Winawer SJ, Zauber AG, Ho MN, et al.

Institution
Gastroenterology and Nutrition Service, Memorial Sloan-Kettering Cancer Center, New York, New York

Reference
N Engl J Med 1993;329:1977–1981

Problem
This study was performed to evaluate the utility of removing adenomatous polyps from the colon and rectum as a form of colorectal cancer prevention.

Intervention
Patients who underwent colonoscopies with removal of adenomatous polyps were followed with periodic surveillance colonoscopies to examine for any evidence of colorectal cancer.

Comparison/control (quality of evidence)
The incidence rate of colorectal cancer was compared with that in three reference groups—two cohorts in which polyps were not removed and one general-population registry, after adjustment for sex, age, and polyp size.

Outcome/effect
Removal of adenomatous polyps with colonoscopic polypectomies resulted in a lower than expected incidence of colorectal cancer.

Historical significance/comments
The findings from this study support the hypothesis that colorectal adenomatous polyps progress to adenocarcinoma and should be screened for and removed with colonoscopies.

Interpersonal and Communication Skills

Teaching Visual: Physician and Patient Perspectives on Procedural Preparation
Melissa Morgan DO, Michael D. Share MD, Deena Roemer, Edward Share MD

The Physician's Perspective
When I obtain consent from a patient for colonoscopy, I review the following issues:

- She will be given at least two laxative doses the day before and/or the day of the procedure. I explain that this is important to clear the colon of any stool, so that I can visualize the entire colon.
- She will lie on her left side and be given sedation.
- A rectal examination will be performed to feel for any internal rectal masses as well as to relax the anal sphincter.
- The colonoscope is then inserted into the rectum. I emphasize that it is a small, flexible tube with a light and a camera on the end; using my diagram (Fig. 30-1), I emphasize that it will be advanced all the way to the beginning of the colon.

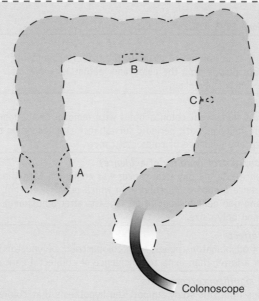

Figure 30-1 Colonoscopy

- Connect the large dashes to draw a colon for your patient.
- Demonstrate how the colonoscope will navigate to the cecum.
- Connect the small dashes, indicating how you might perform a biopsy on a tumor in the cecum (A) or sessile polyp (B) in the transverse colon, or snare a polyp on a stalk (C) in the left colon.

- Once the colonoscope is at the beginning of the colon (cecum), the scope will be slowly withdrawn, paying careful attention to the lining of the colon.
- If any abnormalities are seen, biopsy samples can be obtained with small graspers and sent to pathology. I use my diagram to show that if a **colon polyp** is seen, it can be removed using a grasper or wire snare. I usually draw a **sessile polyp** to demonstrate that some polyps have to be lifted up with saline injection to be safely removed though the colonoscope. I usually draw a **tumor** to illustrate that if I can't remove it, I will be able to obtain a definitive biopsy. See Figure 30-1.
- I discuss the possible complications, including bleeding, perforation, and the risks of sedation.
- I discuss the possibility of an incomplete exam due to technical problems. I let the patient know that proper visualization of the colon can be obscured if the prep isn't excellent and stool is still

present, and that some patients may have a tortuous colon, making it difficult to completely visualize the entire colon. I prepare the patient that if this is the case, the procedure will be terminated and the patient may be sent for a completion virtual colonoscopy (CT colonography) or barium enema.

■ I inform the patient that the risk of a perforation is in the range of 1 in 5000 to 10,000 and would require surgery for repair.

■ I also prepare her for the possibility that after the procedure she may feel bloated or have some abdominal distension. This is secondary to the air that is used to expand the lumen of the colon for proper visualization, although it may be reduced by the use of CO_2 instead of air.

The Patient's Perspective
From a patient's point of view, preparation for colonoscopy requires the following:

■ To review the step-by-step preparation instructions for the procedure with a health professional a few days before the procedure so as to ensure that the prep is done properly. Though a routine procedure, it is probably a new and uncomfortable experience for the patient. To reduce anxiety about prep error, a "walk-through" of the prep is an opportunity to address any concerns or questions.

■ To have face-to-face contact with the physician who will be performing the colonoscopy. A caring encounter on the day of the procedure, blending confidence and compassion, goes a long way to add to the security a patient craves in preparing for the discomfort of the unknown.

■ To have a clear understanding of what to expect. The fewer surprises, the better. Compassionate description of the anticipated experience will allay most anxieties.

Discuss proper follow-up. Explain what the patient should and can expect to feel after the procedure, and be sure to explain what symptoms should prompt a telephone call. Discuss how you will inform the patient regarding procedure findings and possible pathology reports. Determine whether this will be over the phone or during a follow-up office visit.

Professionalism

Demonstrate a Professional Image in Behavior
Patients who present with a fecal impaction are uncomfortable and seeking relief. Evacuating a fecal impaction is one of the least desired maneuvers a physician, resident, or medical student endures; however, it can also be one of the most rewarding. Successful

disimpaction can result in significant relief for the patient, and the patient's appreciation will be forthcoming. Whether this procedure is performed at the bedside or in the operating room under sedation, one must remain compassionate and professional throughout the process. Even though it is a topic that can provoke joking and laughter, all in attendance must remain courteous and respectful.

Systems-Based Practice

Screening Family Members for Disease

First-degree relatives of patients diagnosed with colon cancer are at an increased risk of developing colon cancer. If their family member was diagnosed over the age of 50 years, they should undergo their first colonoscopy at age 40 years. If the relative was diagnosed younger than age 50 years, they should be screened 10 years earlier than the age of diagnosis. Surveillance colonoscopies should be performed following the initial evaluation at set intervals dependent upon polyp detection and pathology results. However, repeat studies should be carried out at no longer than 5-year intervals, even if the exam is normal. This importance should be stressed to patients who have had colon cancer, so that they can inform their family members. Therefore, systems are set up in most office practices with reminder letters being sent out automatically to patients who are due for surveillance procedures.

Chapter 31
Diarrhea (Case 24)

David Rudolph DO and James Thornton MD

Case: A 22-year-old man was referred to gastroenterology with intractable bloody diarrhea. His past medical history was unremarkable until last month, when he first noted the development of crampy abdominal pain, multiple daily bloody, mucus-filled stools, rectal urgency, and tenesmus. He also reported progressive fatigue, intermittent light-headedness, diminished appetite, and a subsequent 7-lb weight loss since symptom onset. He initially didn't seek medical attention, because he thought the symptoms would just go away and, frankly, "just didn't want to describe it to anyone." He denied any recent travel, antibiotic use, close sick contacts, or high-risk sexual behaviors. On physical examination, he was somewhat ill-appearing with conjunctival pallor. Left lower quadrant abdominal tenderness was elicited with deep palpation, but no rebound or guarding was detected. The remainder of his physical examination was unremarkable.

Differential Diagnosis

Infectious diarrhea	Inflammatory bowel disease (IBD)	IBS, functional diarrhea
Malabsorption	Ischemic colitis	

Speaking Intelligently

When we encounter a patient with diarrhea, our investigation always begins with a thorough history and physical examination. The differential diagnosis for diarrhea is extremely broad, but by asking appropriate questions we can usually narrow the differential considerably. In addition, a complete physical examination helps differentiate which patients are currently stable and which patients are in need of more urgent medical attention. Volume depletion, a common sequela of secretory diarrhea, will be manifested by dry mucous membranes, poor skin turgor, and, if severe, tachycardia and hypotension. Anemia, a potential consequence of inflammatory diarrhea, should be suspected in the patient with diffuse pallor, fatigue, light-headedness, and exertional dyspnea.

PATIENT CARE

Clinical Thinking
- Determine the duration of the diarrhea. Acute diarrhea is typically defined as lasting ≤14 days and is often due to infections with viruses or bacteria. Chronic diarrhea is a decrease in fecal consistency and an increase in frequency lasting for 4 or more weeks and has a much broader differential diagnosis.
- Patients with sudden onset of *watery* diarrhea who provide a history of recent travel, close sick contacts, or ingestion of suspicious foods can be presumed to have acute infectious diarrhea, which is usually self-limited and often (in the absence of clinical volume depletion) requires no further workup or treatment.
- Pus or blood in the stools should alert the clinician to an invasive infectious or inflammatory etiology, which necessitates further

workup. In this instance, initial evaluation should include checking stools for routine culture, leukocytes, and occult blood and, in the appropriate clinical setting, performing a *Clostridium difficile* assay and examination for ova and parasites.

- Oily, foul-smelling stools that float are suggestive of steatorrhea. Workup for disorders of malabsorption or maldigestion should be undertaken in patients who present with steatorrhea.
- Patients with clinical evidence of volume depletion and/or symptomatic anemia should be admitted to the hospital for IV fluid resuscitation and/or transfusion of packed RBCs.
- Factitious diarrhea, often secondary to surreptitious laxative use, should be considered in patients with chronic diarrhea with no identifiable etiology after extensive workup.

History
- A detailed history should include the duration of the diarrhea, the frequency and volume of stools, as well as associated symptoms (abdominal pain, vomiting, fever, myalgias, arthralgias, rash, diminished appetite, weight loss).
- Ask patients about any recent travel history, close sick contacts, day care exposures, or ingestion of undercooked foods. Recent antibiotic use is suggestive of *C. difficile* infection.
- Diarrhea that awakens a patient from sleep is worrisome for a pathologic etiology. Patients with IBS are much less likely to report a history of nocturnal symptoms.
- The presence of blood or mucus in stools suggests an inflammatory or invasive infectious etiology. Large-volume watery stools are consistent with secretory diarrhea. Oily, foul-smelling stools that float are suggestive of fat malabsorption or maldigestion.
- Ask patients about a family history of IBD, lactose intolerance, celiac disease, or other malabsorption syndromes.
- Inquire about any other significant medical history. Disordered motility can result from uncontrolled hyperthyroidism or long-standing diabetes mellitus.
- Review current prescribed and over-the-counter medications. Diarrhea can be precipitated by a multitude of commonly used medications including selective serotonin re-uptake inhibitors, colchicine, metoclopramide, antibiotics, laxatives, magnesium-containing antacids, NSAIDs, antiarrhythmics, and antihypertensive agents.
- Review surgical history. Short-bowel syndrome can result in patients who have undergone previous bowel resections. Bile salt diarrhea can occur in patients who have undergone ileal resection.

Physical Examination
- Dry mucous membranes, sunken eyes, poor skin turgor, tachycardia, and orthostatic hypotension are signs concerning for volume depletion. Pallor is suggestive of anemia.

- Oral aphthous ulcers or episcleritis may be seen in patients with IBD.
- Close attention should be paid to the dermatologic examination. Erythema nodosum or pyoderma gangrenosum suggests underlying IBD. Dermatitis herpetiformis is suggestive of celiac disease.
- Abdominal examination should include inspection for surgical scars, palpation to assess for tenderness, masses, and/or hepatosplenomegaly, and auscultation for bowel sounds and abdominal bruits.
- Perianal fissures, fistulas, or abscesses provide support for a diagnosis of Crohn disease.
- Visible blood or pus on digital rectal examination (DRE) suggests an inflammatory or invasive infectious etiology.
- Palpable mass on DRE should raise suspicion for rectal neoplasm or fecal impaction.
- Fecal incontinence should be excluded with evaluation of anal sphincter tone to assess sphincter competence.
- Thyromegaly, exophthalmos, fine resting tremor, and hyperactive reflexes suggest uncontrolled hyperthyroidism.

Tests for Consideration
- **Diagnostic testing** is NOT indicated for most patients with acute diarrhea, as the disease process is usually self-limited. Diagnostic evaluation is indicated when any of the following are present: profound volume depletion, fever (temperature ≥ 38.5° C), blood or pus in stools, severe abdominal pain, and/or symptoms lasting ≥48 hours. Those patients who are hospitalized, 70 years of age or older, immunosuppressed, or who have recently used antibiotics also warrant further evaluation.
- **CBC with differential** should be obtained. Leukocytosis is suggestive of an infectious or inflammatory etiology. Anemia may be present in patients with chronic inflammatory diarrhea or a colonic neoplasm. $11
- **CMP** may reveal electrolyte derangements, azotemia, or hypoalbuminemia. $12
- Elevated **erythrocyte sedimentation** rate and **C-reactive protein** levels are suggestive of inflammation. $11
- **Thyroid function tests** may detect hyperthyroidism. $24
- **Fecal leukocytes and occult blood** help differentiate inflammatory vs. noninflammatory diarrhea. $11
- **Routine stool cultures** identify the most common pathogens, including *Salmonella*, *Shigella*, and *Campylobacter*. Clinical history often dictates the need for testing for less common pathogens. $13
- **_C. difficile_ toxin assay**, or another test to evaluate for *C. difficile* infection, should be checked in those patients who report a history of antibiotic use within the past 3 months. $16

- **Ova and parasites** should be checked in immunocompromised patients, travelers, men who have sex with men, or in patients with exposure to day care facilities. $13
- **Endoscopic evaluation** (**flexible sigmoidoscopy** or **colonoscopy**) is warranted in patients with refractory diarrhea and negative stool cultures. Mucosal biopsies help to differentiate acute infectious diarrhea from IBD or ischemic colitis. $436, $655
- **Qualitative fecal fat** (Sudan stain) should be checked if malabsorption or maldigestion is suspected. If qualitative testing is negative or equivocal, quantitative fecal fat can be checked with a 72-hour stool collection. $24
- **Stool electrolytes** (Na^+, K^+, Cl^-) can be obtained to help differentiate osmotic vs. secretory diarrhea. Fecal osmotic gap (FOG) (calculated by $290 - 2 \times$ [stool Na^+ + stool K^+]) greater than 50 mOsm/kg suggests osmotic diarrhea, while FOG less than 50 mOsm/kg suggests secretory diarrhea. $10

Clinical Entities   Medical Knowledge

Infectious Diarrhea

Pφ Infectious diarrhea can be caused by viral, bacterial, fungal, or protozoal organisms. Most cases of acute infectious diarrhea are secondary to viruses, commonly rotavirus and noroviruses. The most common bacteria isolated include *Campylobacter*, *Salmonella*, *Shigella*, and *Escherichia coli* 0157:H7. Protozoal organisms, such as *Giardia lamblia*, *Entamoeba histolytica*, *Cyclospora* spp., *Cryptosporidium*, and *Microsporidia* spp., may be detected in patients who experience protracted diarrhea, especially after travel to endemic areas. Immunocompromised patients are at increased risk of infection by opportunistic pathogens including cytomegalovirus, *Mycobacterium avium* complex, *Cryptosporidium*, *Isospora belli*, and *Microsporidium*.

TP Patients with infectious diarrhea due to enterotoxin-producing organisms, such as *Vibrio cholerae* or enterotoxigenic *E. coli*, often present with voluminous watery diarrhea. These patients can develop severe volume depletion as evidenced by dry mucous membranes, poor skin turgor, tachycardia, and hypotension on examination. Infectious diarrhea due to invasive pathogens, such as *Salmonella*, *Shigella*, *Campylobacter*, *C. difficile*, and enterohemorrhagic *E. coli*, often results in dysentery. Systemic symptoms are more prevalent when diarrhea is secondary to invasive pathogens.

Dx Acute infectious diarrhea is often self-limited. If the diarrhea is without blood or pus and the patient has no signs of systemic toxicity, additional evaluation is generally not warranted. Patients with bloody or mucus-filled diarrhea should have their stools checked for leukocytes (or lactoferrin) and bacterial culture. The need for additional testing should be based upon the patient's clinical history.

Tx Initial management of patients with acute diarrhea should focus on fluid and electrolyte replacement. In most instances, antibiotic therapy is unnecessary. However, in patients with severe diarrhea, dysentery, or signs of systemic toxicity, empirical antibiotic therapy, often with a fluoroquinolone, should be considered. Antimicrobial therapy should be modified once the results of cultures are available. **See Cecil Essentials 34, 103.**

Inflammatory Bowel Disease

Pφ IBD generally refers to two idiopathic diseases, Crohn disease and ulcerative colitis, that cause chronic inflammation of the GI tract. While similar in many respects, the two diseases have distinct characteristics. Transmucosal inflammation is present in patients with Crohn disease, while inflammation from ulcerative colitis is confined to the mucosa and submucosa. Crohn disease can involve any portion of the GI tract, while ulcerative colitis is confined to the large bowel. Ulcerative colitis has nearly universal rectal involvement with continuous proximal expansion. Crohn disease often spares the rectum, and "skip lesions" can be detected indicating regions of uninvolved mucosa in between areas of active disease.

TP The typical patient with ulcerative colitis presents with bloody, mucus-filled diarrhea, crampy abdominal pain, rectal urgency, and tenesmus. Depending upon the severity of disease, patients may also present with fevers, decreased appetite, weight loss, and anemia. Patients with Crohn disease, like ulcerative colitis, also present with abdominal pain and diarrhea; however, bloody diarrhea is usually not as prominent in Crohn disease. Fissures, fistulas, strictures, and abscesses are more commonly seen in patients with Crohn disease, and patients often present with symptoms related to these complications. Extraintestinal manifestations, such as aphthous ulcers, erythema nodosum, pyoderma gangrenosum, episcleritis, uveitis, and primary sclerosing cholangitis may be present with both diseases.

Dx Endoscopic evaluation with intestinal biopsies is necessary to confirm the diagnosis of IBD. In most instances, colonoscopy with intubation of the terminal ileum should be pursued. Stool cultures should also be obtained to exclude an infectious etiology.

Tx Treatment of Crohn disease and ulcerative colitis is similar and predicated on disease severity. Mild disease is often treated with 5-aminosalicylates. Antibiotic therapy may also be instituted for patients with Crohn disease with perianal involvement. Moderate disease often necessitates short-term corticosteroid therapy followed by maintenance therapy with immunomodulators (azathioprine, 6-mercaptopurine, methotrexate). Severe disease is often managed with anti–tumor necrosis factor-α drugs (infliximab, adalimumab, certolizumab). Surgery is indicated for disease refractory to medical management and for complications of the disease such as perforation and obstruction. **See Cecil Essentials 34, 38.**

Irritable Bowel Syndrome, Functional Diarrhea

Pφ IBS is a functional disorder characterized by abdominal pain or cramping and altered bowel habits, either diarrhea or constipation, in the absence of discernible bowel pathology. The etiology remains unknown, but both hereditary and environmental factors are believed to have a role. Proposed risk factors for the development of IBS include previous GI infection, young age, female gender, anxiety, depression, and a family history of IBS. Upon questioning, patients with IBS often relate a history of anxiety, depression, or other psychological disorder.

TP Patients with IBS complain of abdominal pain or cramping along with altered frequency and consistency of stools. Bloating sensation, flatulence, nausea, and heartburn are also common complaints. Temporary relief of symptoms with defecation is a hallmark of IBS.

Dx Rome III criteria are widely used to identify patients with IBS. Recurrent abdominal pain or discomfort must be present at least 3 days per month for the last 3 months with any two of the following: temporary relief of symptoms with defecation, onset of pain associated with a change in the appearance of stools, onset of pain associated with a change in the frequency of stools.

Tx Patients should be instructed to avoid foods that can trigger or exacerbate their symptoms. Fiber supplementation is generally recommended but should be used with caution initially, as patients can experience exacerbation of symptoms. Adjunctive therapy for treatment of IBS includes antispasmodics, antidiarrheal agents, antidepressants, and psychotherapy. **See Cecil Essentials 34.**

Malabsorption

Pφ Malabsorption refers to the impaired digestion or uptake of nutrients including carbohydrates, protein, fat, vitamins, and minerals. Malabsorption can occur as a result of inadequate intraluminal digestion, defective transport across the small intestinal mucosa, or impaired postabsorptive transport of nutrients into the circulation. Lactose intolerance, the most common form of carbohydrate malabsorption, results from an inherited or acquired deficiency of lactase. Fat malabsorption may result from celiac disease, short-bowel syndrome, postresection diarrhea, small-bowel bacterial overgrowth, mesenteric ischemia, pancreatic exocrine insufficiency, or inadequate luminal bile acid concentration.

TP Patients with global malabsorption will often present with diarrhea associated with weight loss, anorexia, and fatigue. Patients with lactose intolerance often present with crampy abdominal pain, bloating, flatulence, nausea, and watery diarrhea with symptom manifestation soon after ingestion of foods containing lactose. Patients with fat malabsorption report the passage of oily, foul-smelling stools that float, also known as steatorrhea. Malabsorption of fat-soluble vitamins may result in night blindness (vitamin A), osteopenia or osteomalacia (vitamin D), and bleeding (vitamin K). Iron deficiency anemia is commonly seen in patients with celiac disease. Peripheral edema and ascites may be a manifestation of protein malabsorption with resultant hypoalbuminemia.

Dx The gold standard for diagnosis of fat malabsorption is a 72-hour quantitative measurement of fecal fat. Alternatively, qualitative testing of stool with Sudan stain can be performed if quantitative testing is deemed too burdensome. Lactose intolerance can be assessed with a hydrogen breath test, with high levels of expelled hydrogen suggestive of carbohydrate malabsorption. Malabsorption from celiac disease, Whipple disease, Crohn disease, amyloidosis, or lymphoma can be established with upper endoscopy and small-bowel mucosal biopsies. Pancreatic exocrine insufficiency should be considered in patients with fat malabsorption and histologically normal small-bowel mucosa.

Tx Celiac disease is treated with a gluten-free diet. Lactose intolerance is treated with avoidance of lactose-containing foods or with the ingestion of capsules containing lactase enzyme before meals. Fat malabsorption due to pancreatic exocrine insufficiency can be treated with ingestion of pancreatic enzyme supplements before meals. **See Cecil Essentials 34, 38, 40.**

Ischemic Colitis

Pφ Ischemic colitis results from the sudden loss, or reduction, of blood flow to the colon. Common etiologies of colonic ischemia include decreased perfusion (acute MI, congestive heart failure, cardiac arrhythmias, sepsis), vascular occlusion (secondary to thromboembolism), acute vasospasm, medications (cocaine, digoxin, alosetron, estrogens), vasculitis, and hypercoagulable states.

TP The typical presentation of ischemic colitis is an elderly patient with a history significant for cardiac or peripheral vascular disease who develops acute, often left-sided, abdominal pain followed shortly thereafter by the passage of bloody stools. Fever, nausea, and vomiting may also be present.

Dx Laboratory studies, while nondiagnostic, may reveal a leukocytosis and increased lactate; metabolic acidosis may also be present. Segmental bowel wall thickening will often be seen on radiographic imaging, but this finding is nonspecific, as it can also be seen in infectious colitis, IBD, and radiation colitis. Angiography is usually not indicated, as thromboembolic disease is rarely believed to be the cause of acute colonic ischemia. Definitive diagnosis is made with colonoscopy, which, depending upon the severity of inflammation, will often demonstrate inflamed mucosa, petechial hemorrhages, and, in severe cases, hemorrhagic ulcerations.

Tx Management of ischemic colitis is generally supportive. Intravenous fluids should be administered to maintain appropriate hydration. Patients should initially be kept on a regimen of nothing by mouth to allow for bowel rest. Antimicrobial therapy is recommended for moderate to severe cases. Surgery, while uncommon, is necessitated when there is evidence of bowel necrosis, gangrene, or perforation. **See Cecil Essentials 34.**

ZEBRA ZONE

a. **Carcinoid syndrome:** GI carcinoid tumors that metastasize to the liver give rise to an array of findings mediated by excess serotonin and bradykinin production, including secretory diarrhea, cutaneous flushing, bronchospasm, tricuspid regurgitation, and pulmonic stenosis. Patients who present with this constellation of symptoms should have a 24-hour urinary excretion of 5-hydroxyindoleacetic acid measurement. If positive, an Octreoscan should be performed to localize the primary tumor.

b. **Microscopic colitis:** refers to both collagenous colitis and lymphocytic colitis. Both diseases have similar features including watery diarrhea and normal colonic mucosa on macroscopic examination. Colonic biopsies are necessary to establish a definitive diagnosis. Microscopic colitis typically affects middle-aged patients, with collagenous colitis being more prevalent among women (female-to-male ratio ~15 : 1). Medications used to treat microscopic colitis include budesonide, mesalamine, sulfasalazine, and cholestyramine. Prednisone can be used for severe cases.

c. **Factitious diarrhea:** Surreptitious laxative abuse is the most common cause of factitious diarrhea. This diagnosis should be considered when the etiology for chronic diarrhea remains unknown despite extensive evaluation. Factitious diarrhea is much more common in women. Evaluation for surreptitious laxative abuse should consist of checking a stool osmolal gap. Osmotic laxatives containing sorbitol, polyethylene glycol, lactose, or magnesium will cause an elevated stool osmolal gap. Direct examination of stool or urine can also be used to detect chemical laxatives.

d. **Diabetic diarrhea:** Autonomic neuropathy from long-standing uncontrolled diabetes can result in diarrhea. Patients with diabetic enteropathy report chronic nocturnal diarrhea, often associated with abdominal cramps and fecal incontinence. The mainstay of treatment is tight glycemic control. Antimotility agents (loperamide, diphenoxylate) can be used to treat increased intestinal transit, while antimicrobial therapy is indicated for diabetic enteropathy in patients with bacterial overgrowth.

Practice-Based Learning and Improvement: Evidence-Based Medicine

Title
Maintenance infliximab for Crohn's disease: the ACCENT I randomized trial

Authors
Hanauer SB, Feagan BG, Lichtenstein GR, et al.; ACCENT I Study Group

Institution
Department of Gastroenterology and Nutrition, University of Chicago Medical Center

Reference
Lancet 2002; 359:1541–1549

Problem
Does maintenance infliximab therapy confer benefit in patients with active Crohn disease who respond to a single infusion of infliximab?

Intervention
Patients with moderately to severely active Crohn disease who responded favorably to an initial infusion of infliximab were randomized to one of three maintenance treatment groups: group 1: placebo at weeks 2 and 6, and then placebo every 8 weeks; group 2: infliximab 5 mg/kg at weeks 2 and 6, and then 5 mg/kg every 8 weeks; group 3: infliximab 5 mg/kg at weeks 2 and 6, and then 10 mg/kg every 8 weeks

Quality of evidence
Level I

Outcome/effect
Patients with Crohn disease who respond to an initial dose of infliximab are more likely to be in remission at weeks 30 and 54, to discontinue corticosteroids, and to maintain their response for a longer period of time, if infliximab treatment is maintained every 8 weeks.

Historical significance/comments
The results of the ACCENT I trial led to US Food and Drug Administration approval of infliximab as maintenance therapy for patients with moderately to severely active Crohn disease.

Interpersonal and Communication Skills

Have a Low Threshold to Screening for Abuse

When taking a medical history from a patient with a history of multiple GI complaints over a long period of time and no clearly established diagnosis, it becomes important to consider a psychosocial etiology for the patient's symptoms. This is particularly true in patients with prolonged GI, genitourinary, or gynecologic complaints where an exhaustive workup has been negative. Often, these symptoms are manifestations of physical, sexual, or emotional abuse, and physicians need to elicit this history to recommend effective interventions. Asking patients if they "feel safe in their home" or if there has "ever been a time where they have not felt safe at home" is a good place to start. Even if the patient is not initially forthcoming, you may have effectively opened the door for future conversations. Establishing an environment of safety, confidentiality, and support is paramount. When appropriate, use this as an opportunity to include other members of the interdisciplinary team (e.g., social worker, counselor, or even a psychiatrist) to assist in the patient's care.

Professionalism

Show Commitment to Professional Competence Informed by Medical Evidence

As *C. difficile* infection has become a prominent cause of diarrhea in both the outpatient and hospital setting, physicians have begun to recognize the increase in morbidity and mortality from antibiotic-associated diarrhea, particularly in older patients with significant comorbid conditions. The indiscriminate use of antibiotics has a prominent role in the high prevalence of this disease. Recognize that patients often feel the need to initiate therapy for treatment of nonspecific upper respiratory or genitourinary symptoms even when antibiotics are not clinically indicated. Not uncommonly, patients will "self-medicate" without first seeking the counsel of their primary-care physician. It is important for clinicians to take the time necessary to convey to patients that antibiotics are not innocuous medications and that they can, in fact, lead to the development of other disease states, such as *C. difficile* infection.

Chapter 32
Jaundice (Case 25)

Austin Hwang MD and
Giancarlo Mercogliano MD, MBA, AGA

Case: A 60-year-old man presents with jaundice, 20-pound weight loss, intermittent nausea, and decreased appetite over the last month. He has a history of hypertension, hyperlipidemia, and diabetes. There is no past surgical history. He takes hydrochlorothiazide, simvastatin, and metformin. His BP, cholesterol, and diabetes are under good control. He has drunk three beers each day and smoked half a pack of cigarettes per day for the last 40 years. He has no abdominal pain, but he has noticed that his stools have become lighter in color and his urine has become tea-colored. He presents in the outpatient office accompanied by his wife and three of his children, who have urged him to seek medical attention.

Differential Diagnosis

Hepatocellular Causes	Extrahepatic/Obstructive Causes
Viral hepatitis	Choledocholithiasis
Alcoholic hepatitis	Cholangitis
Drug-induced hepatitis	Benign stricture
Cirrhosis	Pancreatic adenocarcinoma

Speaking Intelligently

When asked to see an older patient with jaundice, we worry about cancer. A helpful start in patients with this clinical presentation is to decide whether the cause is hepatocellular or obstructive. These two categories serve as a useful framework to think about elevated serum bilirubin levels. Treatment of hepatocellular causes is generally supportive, while treatment of obstructive causes is with endoscopy or surgery. History taking allows me to create a diagnostic hypothesis. Laboratory values and imaging help me to corroborate this hypothesis. Liver function tests (LFTs) are crucial. Ultrasonography evaluates the hepatic parenchyma and biliary ducts.

PATIENT CARE

Clinical Thinking
- Use the framework mentioned above to focus history taking and to come up with a working differential diagnosis.
- **Use LFTs and imaging** (ultrasound, CT, MRI) to help corroborate your hypothesis.
- Pattern recognition of LFTs aids in diagnosis. *Please see below*.

History
- **History of associated pain** or lack of pain is important.
- If an elderly patient presents with **painless jaundice**, think malignancy. This presentation will be associated with weight loss, fatigue, and poor appetite.
- If **abdominal pain** is present, the differential diagnosis is broad. Choledocholithiasis causes intermittent RUQ abdominal pain followed by more constant pain. Acute hepatitis can cause distension of the liver capsule and subsequent vague RUQ pain. Chronic abdominal pain that is dull in nature can be related to invasion of pancreatic cancer into adjacent tissues.

- **Past medical history is important:** History of gallstones (choledocholithiasis), colon cancer (liver metastases), or chronic pancreatitis (bile duct strictures).
- **Take a good social history**, including the following: travel, food ingestions, multiple sexual partners, alcohol use, cigarette use, injection drug use, tattoos, herbal medications, and new medications.
- **Family history:** Between 5% and 10% of patients with pancreatic cancer have a family history of pancreatic cancer.

Physical Examination

- **Jaundice** appears as yellowing of the skin, yellowing under the tongue, or scleral icterus (yellowing of the sclerae). This usually occurs with total serum bilirubin levels greater than 3.5 mg/dL.
- **Fractionate the bilirubin:** If indirect bilirubin is predominant, hemolysis and **Gilbert syndrome** (hereditary condition caused by the decreased ability of glucuronyltransferase to conjugate bilirubin) are the top two diagnoses. If direct bilirubin is predominant, the differential includes intrahepatic dysfunction vs. biliary duct obstruction.
- In the presence of **fever**, think cholangitis.
- **Asterixis** (flapping of hands with arms extended; "stopping traffic") and **encephalopathy** are signs of hepatocellular dysfunction.
- **Signs of chronic liver disease:** spider angiomas, palmar erythema, caput medusae, and gynecomastia and testicular atrophy in men.
- **Abdominal exam:** Inspect the abdomen for ascites (think malignancy or cirrhosis); listen for bowel sounds; assess hepatic size and palpate for hepatosplenomegaly and tenderness in RUQ (choledocholithiasis or acute hepatitis).

Tests for Consideration

- **Albumin and PT/INR** are markers of liver function (prothrombin and albumin are synthesized in the liver). $12, $6
- **Interpretation of LFTs**
  - A **hepatocellular pattern of injury** is indicated by transaminases that are elevated out of proportion to the bilirubin and alkaline phosphatase. This is seen commonly in intrinsic liver disease, such as viral hepatitis.
  - A **cholestatic pattern of injury** is indicated by bilirubin and alkaline phosphatase levels that are elevated out of proportion to transaminase levels. A typical example of this pattern would be choledocholithiasis. In patients with an

Table 32-1 Typical Laboratory Values*					
	Total Bilirubin	Alkaline Phosphatase	AST	ALT	AST/ALT Ratio
Hepatocellular Problem					
Cirrhosis	≥2		90	75	≥1
Alcoholic liver disease	1–6		200	100	2:1
Acute hepatitis	5	270	1400	1900	
Extrahepatic or Obstructive Problem					
Choledocholithiasis or cholangitis	6	400	150	150	
Malignant CBD obstruction (pancreatic cancer)	>15	400			

*For clarity, we have chosen typical values that are representative of each condition. Those fields that are empty are either too variable to quantify or not useful as diagnostic guides.
CBD, common bile duct.

isolated elevation of alkaline phosphatase, a γ-glutamyl transpeptidase level should be obtained; levels are elevated in patients with hepatobiliary disease but not if the elevated alkaline phosphatase is the result of a bone disorder.
- The **ratio of AST to ALT** can point toward the etiology of liver disease. See Table 32-1.
- **Amylase/lipase:** Can help to assess involvement of the pancreas. $19
- **PT/INR:** These values evaluate the liver's synthetic function. An elevated PT/INR can also occur if the patient is malnourished secondary to vitamin K deficiency. $6
- **Chem 7:** Electrolyte derangements occur secondary to underlying pathology. With decreased oral intake, many of these patients can be quite volume depleted, so the serum creatinine is important to know. Severe liver dysfunction can cause chronic hypoglycemia. $12
- **CBC:** Reduced platelet counts and anemia are common in cirrhotic patients. Leukocytosis is nonspecific, but a marked elevation may suggest cholangitis. $11
- **CA 19-9:** Marker for pancreatic cancer. $30
- **α-fetoprotein:** Marker for hepatocellular carcinoma. $24

IMAGING CONSIDERATIONS

→ **Abdominal ultrasound:** Least expensive and least invasive; ultrasound should be the first test done for those with jaundice; it visualizes the bile ducts, echotexture of the liver, gallbladder, and pancreas; normal CBD diameter is 4 mm; when ultrasound is performed with Doppler, direction of portal blood flow and presence of thrombi in the portal system can be determined. $96

→ **CT Abdomen and pelvis:** Noninvasive; good view of the entire abdominal cavity; requires oral and intravenous contrast for best visualization; patient could have allergy to IV dye or have elevated creatinine that would not allow IV dye to be used, thereby hindering the benefits of the study. $334

→ **MRI/MRCP (MRI/magnetic resonance cholangio-pancreatography):** Noninvasive; great look at the soft-tissue structures in the abdomen (liver, pancreas, gallbladder); 85% sensitivity for bile duct stones or debris; can't be done if patients have metal in their bodies or have pacemakers; study can be unfriendly to claustrophobic patients and requires patients to be able to stay still. $446

→ **Endoscopic ultrasound (EUS)–ERCP:** Invasive; best method to look at bile ducts. EUS allows for a close-up look at the pancreas, gallbladder, and liver; biopsy via fine-needle aspiration through the EUS scope can be done to sample the liver, pancreas, adrenal gland, and any unusual nodes seen on imaging. **ERCP** is diagnostic and therapeutic for choledocholithiasis; there is risk of pancreatitis with ERCP. $885, $2044

Clinical Entities	Medical Knowledge

Hepatitis

Pφ Inflammation of the liver with many etiologies including alcohol, herbal drugs, medications, infection (hepatitis A/B/C/E, Epstein-Barr virus [EBV], and cytomegalovirus [CMV]).

TP Patients present with right upper quadrant pain and significant elevations in AST and ALT. The alkaline phosphatase and bilirubin can also be elevated, but usually not as high as the AST and ALT values. Patient will complain of "flulike" symptoms such as malaise, nausea, weakness, decreased appetite, decreased oral intake, fever, night sweats, and chills.

Dx Diagnosis is often made by careful history. Ask about alcohol use, recent travel, new medications, herbal medications, recent sick contacts, acetaminophen usage, and high-risk sexual activity. If a viral etiology is suspected, blood sample should be sent for hepatitis A IgM, hepatitis B surface antigen, hepatitis B core IgM antibody, hepatitis e antigen, hepatitis C RNA, and CMV and EBV serology. Acetaminophen levels are checked if there is suspicion of acetaminophen-induced hepatotoxicity. Abdominal ultrasound will show an enlarged liver, and physical exam may reveal hepatomegaly.

Tx If the source is viral, the treatment is usually supportive care. Most patients recover rather quickly with no remaining sequelae of disease. If hepatitis B or C is the etiology, some of these patients may go on to have chronic liver disease. If acetaminophen toxicity is the etiology, treatment can be initiated with *N*-acetylcysteine. Herbal drugs, alcohol, and inciting medications should all be stopped. If alcohol is thought to be the culprit, be wary of signs of alcohol withdrawal. **See Cecil Essentials 43.**

Cirrhosis

Pφ Long-standing liver disease secondary to either previous or ongoing insults (hepatitis B, hepatitis C, or alcohol) or a primary disease (autoimmune hepatitis, hemochromatosis, Wilson disease, amyloidosis, α_1-antitrypsin deficiency, primary biliary cirrhosis [PBC], primary sclerosing cholangitis [PSC]). Hepatitis B is the most common cause worldwide. Hepatitis C and alcohol are the most common causes of cirrhosis in the western world.

TP Patients with cirrhosis often do not realize they have the disease until they present with sequelae, such as ascites, encephalopathy, hematemesis, or pruritus. These patients are susceptible to infections (pneumonia, bacteremia, and spontaneous bacterial peritonitis) and deep venous thrombosis.

Dx The AST/ALT ratio and total bilirubin can be either normal or elevated. Imaging with abdominal ultrasound, CT, or MRI will demonstrate a nodular liver contour with a coarse echotexture. Because of the prolonged inflammation and resulting fibrosis, the liver is often small and scarred, unlike the picture of acute hepatitis described above. Liver biopsy establishes the definitive diagnosis of cirrhosis.

Tx Treatment depends on the cause of cirrhosis. Clearance of the hepatitis B virus can be attempted with pegylated interferon, lamivudine, adefovir, or entecavir. Clearance of the hepatitis C virus can be attempted with combination therapy of pegylated interferon + ribavirin; the addition of a protease inhibitor (e.g., teleprevir or bocepivir) to standard therapy has been shown to increase response rates and improve outcome. Despite these attempts, clearance of the virus does not reverse the patient's cirrhosis. Stop alcohol intake. Steroids aid in treatment of autoimmune hepatitis. Phlebotomy and deferoxamine have been used for hemochromatosis. Penicillamine has been used for Wilson disease. Ursodiol has been used to slow down the progression of PBC and PSC. Encourage a low-sodium diet. If the patient is retaining fluid in the abdomen or legs, a course of diuretics can be attempted as long as the kidney function is intact. Upper endoscopy is needed in cirrhotics to rule out esophageal and gastric varices. If encephalopathy is present, rifaximin and lactulose have been crucial in improving patients' mental status. Ultimate treatment would be liver transplantation. **See Cecil Essentials 45.**

Choledocholithiasis

Pφ Choledocholithiasis is the presence of gallstones in the bile ducts. The gallstones originate from the gallbladder. Occasionally, stones may form in the bile ducts de novo, but this is difficult to prove unless the gallbladder has been removed for more than 1–2 years. Bile duct stones found less than 2 years from a previous cholecystectomy are referred to as "retained" stones.

TP Patients present with RUQ abdominal pain and jaundice. Intermittent obstruction can occur several times before medical help is sought.

Dx LFTs demonstrate an obstructive pattern. Ultrasound will often show dilated biliary ducts proximal to the obstruction.

Tx The treatment depends on local expertise. Most centers perform a laparoscopic cholecystectomy with a pre- or postoperative ERCP. During the ERCP, stones are extracted with balloon dilatation and sphincterotomy. Another approach is cholecystectomy with bile duct exploration. This can be performed with good results, and it may be preferred by some patients as it requires only a single procedure. **See Cecil Essentials 46.**

Cholangitis

Pφ Cholangitis is usually preceded by choledocholithiasis. Stasis creates a medium for exponential bacterial growth, inflammation of the ducts, and ultimate infection.

TP Patients with cholangitis may appear ill and present acutely with nausea/vomiting, fevers, night sweats, and chills. Decreased oral intake, abdominal pain, weakness, and malaise are common findings. Two eponyms have been associated with cholangitis: ***Charcot triad*** (fever, abdominal pain, and jaundice) and ***Reynold pentad*** (fever, abdominal pain, jaundice, septic shock, and mental status changes).

Dx Bilirubin and alkaline phosphatase are typically more elevated than AST and ALT because of the location of the pathology. Leukocytosis is often present on CBC. Abdominal ultrasound shows dilated biliary ducts and can sometimes localize the area of obstruction. MRCP or EUS can localize the area of obstruction. ERCP is a diagnostic and therapeutic procedure that is the gold standard for biliary obstruction.

Tx Initially, these patients should be kept on a regimen of nothing by mouth, given IV fluids, and treated with IV antibiotics primarily directed toward anaerobes and gram-negative bacilli. ERCP allows removal of the obstructing gallstone and debris, and decompression of the biliary tree. If the biliary obstruction is too high up in the biliary tree or the patient has had previous surgical procedures that make ERCP difficult, percutaneous transhepatic cholangiography (PTC) can be helpful in decompressing the bile ducts. **See Cecil Essentials 46.**

Benign Stricture

Pφ Benign stricture refers to partial obstruction of the biliary tract not due to stones or malignancy. Approach all strictures as if you suspect malignancy. Diseases that can cause strictures include sclerosing cholangitis, previous episodes of pancreatitis, parasites, or previous cholangitis episodes. After cholecystectomy, biliary duct injury (partial transection or cautery burn) can also cause strictures.

TP Patients present with intermittent or progressive jaundice with occasional pain. Alkaline phosphatase is usually elevated.

Dx Abdominal ultrasound is generally the first imaging test, but strictures will be better seen on CT or ERCP/MRCP. The latter two studies will allow for better delineation of the anatomy.

Tx Benign strictures require an exhaustive search for a cause. Via ERCP, the stricture can be stented and biopsy specimens and brushings of the stricture can be obtained. If malignancy can't be excluded, a "blind Whipple" procedure may be necessary. **See Cecil Essentials 46.**

Pancreatic Adenocarcinoma

Pφ Risk factors for pancreatic cancer: age > 60 years, male sex, smoking, diets high in red meat, diets low in vegetables and fruit, obesity, diabetes, family history of pancreatic cancer, *Helicobacter pylori* infection, and chronic pancreatitis.

TP Clinical presentation consists of nonspecific symptoms such as nausea, malaise, decreased appetite, decreased oral intake, and weakness. Weight loss is common. Patients may also note tea-colored urine, pale-colored stools, and diarrhea/steatorrhea. Abdominal pain starts in the epigastric region and radiates to the back, but some patients don't have pain at all and present with "painless jaundice." Development of diabetes may be an early sign of pancreatic cancer. *Trousseau sign*—migratory thrombophlebitis. *Courvoisier sign*—porcelain gallbladder.

Dx AST, ALT, bilirubin, and alkaline phosphatase will all be elevated. Imaging with abdominal ultrasound, CT of abdomen/pelvis, or MRI helps to visualize the mass. As with any cancer, it is crucial to have a tissue diagnosis to confirm disease. EUS gives a very good view of the pancreas, and one can obtain biopsy samples of the pancreatic mass or any surrounding abnormal lymph nodes. An elevated serum CA 19-9 has a 77% sensitivity and an 87% specificity for malignant disease.

Tx If the cancer is localized, a Whipple procedure (pancreaticoduodenectomy) can be done. If the cancer has spread, chemotherapy and radiation are used for treatment. Gemcitabine, oxaliplatin, and erlotinib (Tarceva) are a few of the chemotherapeutic drugs used. Median survival from diagnosis is 3–6 months, and 5-year survival is less than 10%. **See Cecil Essentials 40, 57.**

ZEBRA ZONE

a. **Intraductal papillary mucinous neoplasm (IPMN):** Slow-growing precancerous lesion formed of papillary proliferations of mucin-producing epithelial cells; treat with surgery.

b. **Sarcoidosis:** A collection of abnormal inflammatory cells that congregate to form granulomas; these granulomas can form in the liver, causing eventual obstruction of bile ducts and subsequent jaundice.

c. **Other periampullary tumors:** This refers to four separate tumors with similar surgical treatment: *cholangiocarcinoma, pancreatic adenocarcinoma (see above), ampullary cancer,* and *duodenal cancer.* Cholangiocarcinoma is cancer of the bile ducts, and diagnosis usually occurs at a late stage. When this cancer is present at the porta hepatis, it carries the eponym *Klatskin tumor.* These tumors all grow from their respective locations and, at times, cause obstruction of the biliary ducts and subsequent jaundice. The 5-year survival rates vary greatly: duodenal (60%), ampullary (40%), cholangiocarcinoma (30%), pancreatic cancer (10%).

d. **Sepsis:** Sepsis is more common than these other zebras, but it should be included in the differential diagnosis of jaundice more often; selective defect in the secretion of conjugated bilirubin leads to hyperbilirubinemia and jaundice in these patients. Bilirubin levels normalize with treatment of infection.

e. **Autoimmune pancreatitis:** This is a rare cause of pancreatitis that can eventually cause strictures of bile ducts leading to jaundice. The condition is characterized by an autoimmune pathophysiology involving the IgG_4 antibody. Imaging shows a thick, "sausage-shaped" pancreas; diagnosis made by obtaining tissue by EUS. The disease can be treated successfully with prednisone, but the relapse rate is 40% to 50%.

Practice-Based Learning and Improvement: Evidence-Based Medicine

Title
Transection of the esophagus for bleeding esophageal varices. Prognostic value of Child-Turcotte criteria in medically treated cirrhotics

Authors
Pugh RN, Murray-Lyon IM, Dawson JL, et al.

Reference
Br J Surg 1973;60:646

Problem
Predicting outcome in cirrhotic patients

Outcome/effect

Measure	1 Point	2 Points	3 Points
Total bilirubin, μmol/L (mg/dL)	<2	2–3	>3
Serum albumin (g/dL)	>3.5	2.8–3.5	<2.8
INR	<1.7	1.7–2.2	>2.2
Ascites	None	Mild	Severe
Hepatic encephalopathy	None	Grade I–II (or suppressed with medication)	Grade III–IV (or refractory)

Points	Class	1-Year Survival	2-Year Survival
5–6	A	100%	85%
7–9	B	81%	57%
10–15	C	45%	35%

In 1964, Child and Turcotte proposed a scoring system based on five criteria in an effort to classify the severity of liver disease in cirrhotic patients. Nine years later, Pugh et al. modified the scoring system by replacing nutritional status with PT/INR, thus removing one of the most subjective parts of the score. It was originally created to predict mortality during surgery, but it can also be used to determine necessity for liver transplantation.

Interpersonal and Communication Skills

Give Forethought to the Setting When Delivering Bad News

With a serious medical illness such as unresectable pancreatic cancer, there are times when patients will have little chance for meaningful recovery. In communicating a poor prognosis or bad news in general, it is often helpful to set up a family conference.

Before a family meeting occurs, here are some tips for basic planning:

- Be cognizant of who are the legal decision makers and the influential family members; this may help you anticipate the dynamics of the upcoming conversation.

- Have your facts straight before you begin.
- If possible, invite other members of the health care team, including specialists and nurses, so that information and voices are consistent.
- Choose a setting that is private where everyone can sit down.
- Avoid a seating arrangement that may be seen as confrontational or paternalistic, where the physician is on one side of the table and the family is on the other.
- Be sure that tissues are available.
- Avoid carrying on such conversations at the bedside or in a busy hallway.
- Make arrangements to ensure that you will not be constantly interrupted (e.g., sign out your beeper, silence your cell phone).
- If the family is not primarily English speaking, arrange for an official hospital interpreter to be present or utilize a language line (if available). Avoid having family members translating for other family members, as it is difficult to assess how much they understand and whether the translation is correct.

Professionalism

Maintain Patient Confidentiality

As a physician, your responsibility is to the patient. There will be times when you walk into a patient's room expecting to convey the results of a test, and the room is filled with family and friends. Resist any temptation to deliver the information; it would be essential to ask *privately* if the patient feels comfortable with the others in the room hearing the information. The Health Insurance Portability and Accountability Act (HIPAA) of 1996, effective April 2003, addresses the security and privacy of health data. HIPAA has resulted in health professionals and hospitals being more vigilant in protecting patient data from those not involved in the patient's care. Specific tips for students and resident house staff include:

- Do not discuss cases in public areas (elevators, hallways, cafeterias).
- Do not leave computerized patient lists in areas shared by patients and their families.
- Respond courteously and appropriately to persons asking for information.
- Do not access information on patients that are not under your care (e.g., actors, politicians, sports figures).

Systems-Based Practice

Informed Consent

Procedures may be necessary in cholestatic cases of jaundice. In pancreatic cancer, for example, placement of a biliary stent can help to relieve obstruction in the bile ducts; in cholangitis, an ERCP can remove the stone or debris causing the biliary obstruction. These and all procedures require that an informed consent is obtained before the procedure can be performed. An informed consent signifies that the physician performing the procedure has explained to the patient what the procedure entails, why it is indicated, the potential benefits, the potential risks, and the therapeutic alternatives. The informed consent is a *legal* necessity that gives the physician a formal opportunity to discuss each procedure fully with the patient. When a patient is determined to be incompetent to make his or her own decisions, consent must be obtained from his or her power-of-attorney designee or next of kin.

Suggested Readings

Child III CG, editor. The liver and portal hypertension. Philadelphia: WB Saunders, 1964.

Oullette JR, Schmidt DJ. Surgery: cases in surgical oncology, Section III, 2007.

Section VII
HEMATOLOGIC DISEASES

Section Editor
Marc J. Kahn MD, MBA

Section Contents

33 **Elevated Blood Counts (Case 26)**
Marc J. Kahn MD, MBA

34 **Teaching Visual: The Importance of the Peripheral Blood Smear**
Aarti Shevade MD and Paul Gilman MD

35 **Pancytopenia (Case 27)**
Byron E. Crawford MD

36 **Excessive Bleeding or Clotting (Case 28)**
Rebecca Kruse-Jarres MD, MPH

37 **Lymphadenopathy and Splenomegaly (Case 29)**
Bridgette Collins-Burow PhD, MD

Chapter 33
Elevated Blood Counts (Case 26)

Marc J. Kahn MD, MBA

Case: A 43-year-old healthy woman presents with upper respiratory symptoms characterized by rhinorrhea, a dry cough, and a headache over a period of 3 days. She presented to her primary-care provider, who diagnosed a viral infection; she was told to drink fluids and take acetaminophen as needed, and was given a decongestant. Two days after her visit, she was called by her physician because the complete blood count (CBC) that had been ordered was abnormal, revealing a white blood cell (WBC) count of 14,600/μL, a hemoglobin of 16.7 g/dL, and a platelet count of 1,432,000/μL. The WBC count differential revealed 80% polymorphonuclear cells, 12% lymphocytes, 5% monocytes, 2% eosinophils, and 1% basophils. On further questioning, she reports some menorrhagia but is otherwise completely asymptomatic. She is very worried that she may have leukemia.

Differential Diagnosis

Polycythemia vera (PV)	Essential thrombocytosis (ET)	Chronic myelogenous leukemia (CML)

Speaking Intelligently

Whenever a patient is found to have an abnormal CBC, I always review a peripheral blood smear as the next step. Review of the smear is quick and inexpensive, and can greatly help to narrow a differential diagnosis and to plan further diagnostic tests. It is important to educate the patient that in the absence of immature blood cells, acute leukemia is highly unlikely. Because the patient will be referred to a specialist, it is important that the patient understands your reasoning. This is especially important if the patient is referred to a hematologist/medical oncologist in a cancer center.

PATIENT CARE

Clinical Thinking
- In a patient with elevated blood counts, especially an elevated WBC count, it is important to distinguish a problem with cellular

differentiation, such as acute leukemia, from a problem with cellular proliferation, such as the myeloproliferative disorders (MPDs).

- The peripheral blood smear and WBC differential count are helpful in the case presented, because no immature cells are identified. In this case, acute leukemia is extremely unlikely, and the patient is more likely to have an MPD.
- The MPDs can be roughly divided by the cellular element that is increased: ET (platelets increased), PV (red cells increased), and CML (granulocytes increased).
- Agnogenic myeloid metaplasia (AMM) (fibrous tissue increased in the marrow) is also included as an MPD, but unlike the other three disorders, patients usually present with pancytopenia due to marrow replacement with fibrous tissue.
- Although distinctions by cell type are made, in fact, there is great overlap between the MPDs, and most often an individual patient may present with increases in more than one cellular element.

History
- Typically, patients with MPDs are asymptomatic, and abnormalities in the CBC are detected incidentally on routine blood tests.
- Because splenomegaly can occur in patients with CML and other MPDs, patients may complain of early satiety because the enlarged spleen compresses the stomach.
- Patients with ET may complain of erythromelalgia, which is burning and redness in the palms and soles.
- Patients with ET may additionally have problems with either bleeding or thrombosis.
- Patients with PV may complain of pruritus or headache, and may also present with thrombosis.

Physical Examination
- The physical examination may be normal in patients with MPDs.
- Splenomegaly is found in most patients with CML and is also found occasionally in patients with PV and ET.
- Because the MPDs increase the risk for thrombosis, careful examination of the lower extremities is important to look for evidence of arterial or venous insufficiency.
- Easy bruisability may be a feature of ET or PV.

Tests for Consideration
- **Nucleic acid amplification tests such as polymerase chain reaction (PCR) of peripheral blood for the BCR/ABL transcript**, found in patients with the 9;22 translocation (Philadelphia chromosome), are diagnostic of CML. $315

- **Bone marrow biopsy and aspirate to look at marrow cellular elements:** These can also be used to detect the Philadelphia chromosome [t(9;22)] cytogenetically or by fluorescence in situ hybridization (FISH). $500
- **Assay for the JAK2 V617F mutation**, found in most patients with PV and half of the patients with ET. $375

Clinical Entities	Medical Knowledge

Polycythemia Vera

Pφ PV is a clonal disorder characterized by excessive production of red blood cells. PV is strongly associated with acquired mutations of the gene encoding JAK2, an intracellular signaling molecule. The most common mutation, JAK2 V617F, leads to constitutive activation of JAK2, causing erythropoiesis to become independent of erythropoietin. JAK2 V617F is found in over 90% of patients with PV.

TP Although patients with PV can be asymptomatic, they may complain of headache, pruritus, or fatigue. Shortness of breath, dizziness, and visual changes from increased blood viscosity are also common complaints. Erythromelalgia, burning of the palms and soles, can occur as a result of increased platelets. About 15% of patients may experience arterial or venous thrombosis, manifested as transient ischemic attacks (TIAs), stroke, myocardial infarction (MI), deep venous thrombosis (DVT), and Budd-Chiari syndrome. Epistaxis and gastrointestinal (GI) bleeding can also occur. Patients with PV may be hypertensive, and more than half of patients with PV have splenomegaly.

Dx Patients with PV have low serum erythropoietin concentrations. The CBC is remarkable for an elevated hematocrit. Platelets and WBCs may also be increased. Serum concentrations of vitamin B_{12}, lactate dehydrogenase (LDH), and uric acid are frequently elevated. Over 90% of patients with PV have the JAK2 V617F mutation. Bone marrow evaluation reveals hypercellularity with erythroid hyperplasia. Marrow fibrosis can also be seen.

Tx Phlebotomy is the mainstay of therapy in PV to keep the hematocrit less than 45% in men and less than 42% in women. Low-dose aspirin is also recommended to reduce the incidence of thrombosis. Cytoreductive therapy with hydroxyurea or interferon may be used in patients at high risk for thromboembolic disease, such as those over 60 years of age. **See Cecil Essentials 48.**

Essential Thrombocytosis

Pφ ET is a clonal disorder characterized by increased numbers of megakaryocytes in the bone marrow and platelets in the circulation. ET is the most common of the MPDs. Between 30% and 50% of patients with ET have the JAK2 V617F mutation.

TP At least half of patients with ET are asymptomatic at presentation. Because of the increased platelet numbers, most patients with ET eventually experience vasomotor symptoms such as headache, visual disturbance, acrocyanosis, paresthesias, or erythromelalgia. Only about a quarter of patients with ET have palpable splenomegaly. Patients are at increased risk for both arterial and venous thrombotic complications including first-trimester spontaneous abortions. Because of qualitative platelet defects, patients with ET are also at increased risk of bleeding.

Dx Patients with ET have platelet counts > 600,000/μL without other etiologies for thrombocytosis. Because iron deficiency can cause an elevated platelet count, normal serum ferritin concentrations and stainable iron on marrow biopsy are necessary to make the diagnosis of ET. Detection of either t(9;22) or the BCR/ABL transcript rules out ET in favor of CML. Patients with ET can also have elevations in leukocyte count.

Tx Patients with ET and platelet counts > 1,500,000/μL, those with a history of thromboembolism, and those older than age 60 years are treated with hydroxyurea as a first-line agent to lower the platelet count. Low-dose aspirin is also used unless bleeding or bruising is exacerbated by the addition of aspirin. Anagrelide is a second-line agent to lower the platelet count. Women of childbearing potential can be treated with interferon-α. Platelet apheresis, along with cytoreductive therapy, may be needed in patients with life-threatening symptoms such as stroke, TIA, MI, or GI bleeding. **See Cecil Essentials 48.**

Chronic Myelogenous Leukemia

Pφ CML is characterized by the balanced translocation t(9;22), also called the Philadelphia chromosome. This translocation leads to a fusion gene, BCR/ABL, which functions as a tyrosine kinase. The BCR/ABL protein acts in a number of cellular pathways to promote proliferation of myeloid cells. BCR/ABL is also able to inhibit apoptosis. Over time, the leukemic clone of CML acquires additional abnormalities, which leads to acceleration into a blast phase, characterized clinically as an acute leukemia.

TP Almost all patients with CML present in a chronic phase characterized by an elevated WBC count and elevated platelets. The peripheral WBC count is predominantly myeloid cells without a significant number of blasts. Almost half of patients with CML are asymptomatic at presentation. Most patients with CML have splenomegaly. Thrombotic or hemorrhagic complications are uncommon until blast crises occur; thrombocytopenia leads to purpura and bleeding.

Dx Demonstration of t(9;22) by cytogenetics or BCR/ABL by PCR is required for the diagnosis of CML. Granulocytosis, thrombocytosis, and basophilia may be present on the peripheral smear; in the chronic phase, <10% blasts are seen on the peripheral smear. In the accelerated phase, blast counts are between 10% and 19%. In the blast phase, acute myeloid or, less commonly, acute lymphoblastic leukemia is seen with ≥20% blasts. Serum LDH and uric acid are increased.

Tx Treatment for CML has changed since the introduction of the novel tyrosine kinase inhibitor, imatinib. A complete hematologic remission is seen in >90% of CML patients in chronic phase and >30% of CML patients in accelerated or blast phase who are treated with imatinib. Allogeneic stem cell transplantation is reserved for patients who fail to respond to imatinib. Over time, imatinib resistance can develop. Allogeneic transplantation or use of dasatinib, a second-generation tyrosine kinase inhibitor, can be employed in patients who are no longer responding to imatinib. **See Cecil Essentials 48.**

ZEBRA ZONE

a. **Erythrocytosis** can also be caused by hypoxia (secondary to high altitude, or cardiac or pulmonary disease); high–oxygen affinity hemoglobins, which leads to a shift in the oxygen saturation curve; and erythropoietin-producing tumors (such as pheochromocytoma, hepatic or kidney tumors, or cerebellar hemangiomas); and can occur following renal transplantation or surreptitious use of erythropoietin.

b. **Thrombocytosis** can also be seen in patients with iron deficiency with blood loss, infections, POEMS syndrome (osteosclerotic myeloma characterized by polyneuropathy, organomegaly, endocrinopathy, monoclonal protein, and skin changes), and other inflammatory disorders.

c. **Granulocytosis** can occur in infectious illnesses; the WBC count can be quite high in patients with *Clostridium difficile* infection.

Practice-Based Learning and Improvement: Evidence-Based Medicine

Title
Efficacy and safety of low-dose aspirin in polycythemia vera

Authors
Landolfi R, Marchiolo R, Kutti J, et al.

Institution
Catholic University School of Medicine, Rome, Italy

Reference
N Engl J Med 2004;350:114–124

Problem
Increased arterial and venous thrombosis in patients with PV

Intervention
Low-dose aspirin (100 mg/day) vs. placebo

Quality of evidence
Level I

Outcome/effect
Low-dose aspirin was associated with a reduction in nonfatal MI, nonfatal stroke, pulmonary embolism, major venous thrombosis, and death from cardiovascular disease (relative risk, RR = 0.40, $P = 0.03$) when compared with placebo in patients with PV. There was no significant increased incidence of bleeding in the aspirin group.

Historical significance/comments
Historically, the use of aspirin in asymptomatic patients with PV has been controversial because of the potential risk of increased bleeding complications in treated patients. This is the first randomized, double-blind, placebo-controlled trial to show efficacy of low-dose aspirin in patients with PV.

Interpersonal and Communication Skills

Diffuse the "C" Word

Patients with MPDs are frequently referred to specialists in hematology/oncology because they have a "cancer," a term that causes significant emotional distress for patients and their families. Although MPDs are indeed cancers in that they are clonal, it often helps to let patients know that "all cancers are different" and the patient's prognosis is related to his or her specific disorder. CML, for example, is clearly a cancer and leukemia, but the physician can offer hope to patients and their families by informing them of the high efficacy and low toxicity of the tyrosine kinase inhibitors in the treatment of CML. For patients with PV and ET, it may be emphasized that the natural history of the disease can be quite good. Although honesty with patients and families is essential, the physician should try to find ways to plant seeds of hope in discussions of prognosis and treatment.

Professionalism

Dilemmas in Clinical Trials: Follow Ethical Principles

As more and more tyrosine kinase inhibitors become available for treating diseases such as CML, there will be increased interest in placing suitable patients into clinical trials involving these drugs. As with any clinical trial, specific ethical principles must apply: (1) All clinical trials must be properly registered with, and reviewed by, an appropriate human subject committee and an institutional review board; (2) patients entered into a clinical trial must receive information advising them of the possible risks and benefits of the therapy, and must provide informed consent; (3) patients must be informed that their medical records pertinent to the trial may be made available to outside data-monitoring committees including the US Food and Drug Administration (FDA); and (4) patients must be provided with contact information should they have any questions or concerns about their participation in the clinical trial.

Systems-Based Practice

Be Aware of Community Resources to Help Patients Obtain Medications

Although quite effective for the treatment of CML, imatinib and dasatinib are expensive medications. Additionally, because they are oral medications taken at home, inpatient hospital insurance benefits may not cover the costs associated with their use. As such, for patients with CML and inadequate outpatient prescription coverage, affording proper therapy could be a problem. In this case it is often necessary to pursue programs offered through the pharmaceutical companies so as to get patients the medications they need at reduced or no cost. Additionally, hospital social workers can sometimes assist in finding community resources to help make necessary medications available to patients who cannot otherwise afford them.

Chapter 34
Teaching Visual: The Importance of the Peripheral Blood Smear

Aarti Shevade MD *and Paul Gilman* MD

Objectives

- Describe the value of preparing and examining a peripheral smear.
- List important diagnoses that can be suggested by visual abnormalities of red blood cells (RBCs), WBCs, and platelets on the peripheral smear.

INTRODUCTION

The peripheral blood smear is the often-neglected foundation of the evaluation of a patient with any cytopenia or blood dyscrasia. One would not think of evaluating a patient with chest pain without looking at the electrocardiogram or a patient with cough and fever without looking at the chest radiograph. With hematologic abnormalities there is too often a reliance on numbers and automated results.

This chapter will familiarize the reader with the blood smear in conditions where it is particularly useful. It will provide an understanding of the normal appearance of the different types of WBCs as well as the normal and important abnormal appearances of RBCs. As demonstrated, the ability to perform a quantitative evaluation of platelets on the peripheral smear is an important skill in evaluating the patient with thrombocytopenia.

While detailed and complex analysis of blood smears is the role of the hematologist, a fundamental knowledge of the use of this diagnostic tool will benefit any clinician.

WHITE BLOOD CELLS AND PERIPHERAL SMEAR

Specific to the evaluation of WBCs, a normal peripheral smear should contain a spectrum of mature leukocytes, including lymphocytes, monocytes, neutrophils, eosinophils, and basophils.

Lymphocytes constitute 20% to 25% of the total circulating leukocytes. They are characterized by a clumped acentrically located nucleus and thin rim of blue cytoplasm. Lymphocytes are larger than erythrocytes and are typically 8 to 10 μm in diameter. Atypical lymphocytes are differentiated by a larger cytoplasm. They are often observed in the setting of viral infections (e.g., infectious mononucleosis).

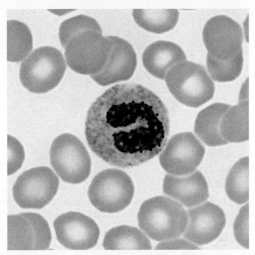

Figure 34-1 Neutrophil band form. (From McPherson RA, Pincus MR: Henry's clinical diagnosis and management by laboratory methods. 22nd ed. Philadelphia: Saunders/Elsevier; 2012. Figure 31-17.)

Neutrophils are the most numerous of the WBCs and are characterized by a three- to four-lobed nucleus and a pink granular cytoplasm. They develop in a systematic fashion from myeloblast, the most immature form, to promyelocyte to myelocyte to metamyelocyte to band form to mature neutrophil. However, only band forms and mature neutrophils are normally present in the peripheral smear. Neutrophils are among the first cells to appear in acute bacterial infections.

Connect the dots outlining the band form in Figure 34-1.

Recognize that this is the immature form of the neutrophil. Its presence in the smear may be a clue to systemic infection, even if the total WBC count is not increased.

Eosinophils constitute less than 5% of all circulating WBCs. They are characterized by orange granules and a bilobed nucleus. Eosinophilia can be seen in allergic states and parasitic infections.

Basophils are the least common of the WBCs. They contain prominent dark-blue to black granules and an S-shaped nucleus. Basophilia can occur in myeloproliferative disorders, hypersensitivity reactions, hypothyroidism, and infection.

Monocytes are the largest of the circulating blood cells and are characterized by a large, acentric, kidney-shaped nucleus that typically has a "moth-eaten" appearance. They remain in circulation for only a few days before migrating into connective tissue, where they differentiate into macrophages.

Myeloblasts are precursors of all three types of **granulocytes**, the eosinophil, basophil, and neutrophil. They are large cells, contain two to

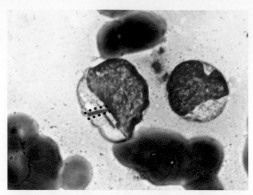

Figure 34-2 Auer rods. (From McPherson RA, Pincus MR: Henry's clinical diagnosis and management by laboratory methods. 22nd ed. Philadelphia: Saunders/Elsevier; 2012. Figure 33-25.)

three nucleoli, and do not contain any granules. Their cytoplasm is characterized by blue clumps in a pale-blue background. Acute myeloblastic leukemia results from uncontrolled mitosis of a transformed stem cell whose progeny do not differentiate into the mature cell but stop at the myeloblast stage. Auer rods are seen within the leukemic blast cells of acute myelogenous leukemia (AML). These rods are clumps of azurophilic granules that are typically needle-shaped or round and are seen within the cytoplasm. Their presence within a blast cell as noted on a peripheral smear is useful in distinguishing between acute lymphocytic leukemia (ALL) and AML. They are virtually pathognomonic for AML.

Connect the dots forming one of the Auer rods in Figure 34-2.

Recognize that Auer rods are elongated bluish red rods composed of fused lysosomal granules. They can be seen in the cytoplasm of myeloblasts, promyelocytes, and monoblasts and in patients with AML.

THROMBOCYTOPENIA

Thrombocytopenia is defined as a platelet count less than 150,000/µL. It can occur as a result of reduced bone marrow production, hemodilution, or splenic sequestration.

The peripheral blood smear may show enlarged platelets when platelet turnover is increased.

Compare the smear with thrombocytopenia in Figure 34-3 vs. the smear with normal platelets in Figure 34-4.

The presence of immature leukocytes in addition to thrombocytopenia may suggest a bone marrow stem cell disorder such as leukemia. The presence of a nucleated erythrocyte with a low platelet count may indicate an invasive bone marrow process.

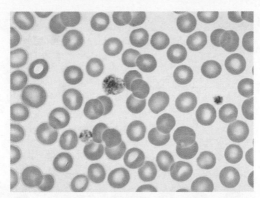

Figure 34-3 Giant platelets. (From McPherson RA, Pincus MR: Henry's clinical diagnosis and management by laboratory methods. 22nd ed. Philadelphia: Saunders/Elsevier; 2012. Figure 30-43.)

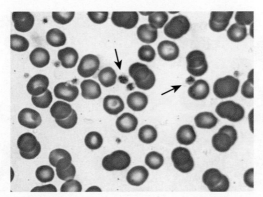

Figure 34-4 Platelets on a peripheral smear. (From McPherson RA, Pincus MR: Henry's clinical diagnosis and management by laboratory methods. 22nd ed. Philadelphia: Saunders/Elsevier; 2012. Figure 30-42.)

Pseudothrombocytopenia, or a falsely low platelet count, is an in vitro phenomenon without clinical relevance. It typically occurs as a result of platelet clumping (Fig. 34-5). If platelet clumping is observed, the platelet count is repeated using a different anticoagulant.

The presence of immature leukocytes in addition to thrombocytopenia may suggest a bone marrow stem cell disorder such as leukemia. The presence of nucleated erythrocytes with a low platelet count may indicate an invasive bone marrow process (Fig. 34-6).

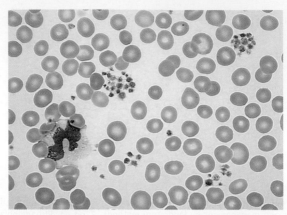

Figure 34-5 Platelet clumping. (From Walsh DT, Caraceni AT, editors. Palliative medicine. Philadelphia: Saunders/Elsevier; 2009. Figure 74-12.)

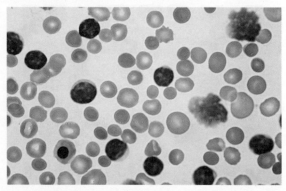

Figure 34-6 Nucleated RBCs. (From Kumar V, Abbas AK, Fausto N, Aster J, et al. Robbins and Cotran pathologic basis of disease. 8th ed. Philadelphia: Saunders/Elsevier; 2010. Figure 13-8.)

ACQUIRED HEMOLYTIC ANEMIA: MICROANGIOPATHIC HEMOLYTIC ANEMIA

Microangiopathic hemolytic anemia is an acquired hemolytic anemia and is characterized by erythrocyte fragmentation that occurs as a result of mechanical destruction. The characteristic finding on peripheral smear is the *schistocyte*. The schistocyte is a fragmented part of an RBC that is formed in the setting of a vascular lesion. These vascular lesions can produce shearing forces causing fragmentation of the RBCs. These

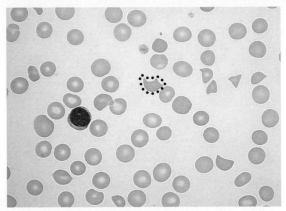

Figure 34-7 Schistocyte. (From Walsh DT, Caraceni AT, editors. Palliative medicine. Philadelphia: Saunders/Elsevier; 2009. Figure 74-2.)

lesions can also cause inflammation of small-vessel walls, in turn generating fibrin strands that sever the circulating RBCs. The resulting RBC, or schistocyte, is irregularly shaped and asymmetrical, and lacks central pallor.

Connect the dots to circle the schistocyte and identify all other schistocytes in Figure 34-7.

Microangiopathic hemolytic anemia is seen in eclampsia, preeclampsia, disseminated intravascular coagulation (DIC), malignancy, aneurysms, and exposure to certain drugs, most notably cyclosporine and ticlopidine. It can also be seen in patients with mechanical heart valves, especially in the setting of a dysfunctional valve. Treatment of this disorder is specific to the underlying cause.

SPHEROCYTES: AUTOIMMUNE HEMOLYTIC ANEMIA, HEREDITARY SPHEROCYTOSIS

Spherocytes are most commonly found in immunologically mediated hemolytic anemias and in hereditary spherocytosis. Spherocytes are characterized by their spherical shape as opposed to the biconcavity of a normal erythrocyte. They typically have a smaller surface area through which oxygen and carbon dioxide can be exchanged. Spherocyte formation involves several different mechanisms. In immune-mediated spherocytosis, antibodies affix themselves to the RBC, marking them for splenic destruction. Splenic macrophages will partially phagocytize the RBC. The remaining membrane of the RBC will re-form, resulting in a smaller, denser, more spherical RBC, or spherocyte.

Autoimmune hemolytic anemia can present related to certain lymphoproliferative disorders, collagen vascular diseases, drugs or

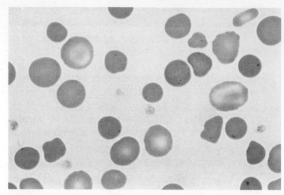

Figure 34-8 Spherocyte. (From Kumar V, Abbas AK, Fausto N, Aster J, et al. Robbins and Cotran pathologic basis of disease. 8th ed. Philadelphia: Saunders/Elsevier; 2010. Figure 14-4.)

medications, malignancy, and viral infections. Not uncommonly, an underlying cause is never identified. This condition occurs when autoantibodies, most often IgG and IgM, bind to erythrocyte antigens.

Hereditary spherocytosis is a congenital hemolytic anemia caused by an abnormality in the erythrocyte membrane protein (Fig. 34-8). In hereditary spherocytosis, a molecular defect in the gene that encodes the RBC membrane protein leads to its abnormal spherical shape. Specifically, hereditary spherocytosis is characterized by spherocytic erythrocytes with increased osmotic fragility. Osmotic fragility refers to the spherocytes' tendency to burst when placed into water. Affected patients may have evidence of splenomegaly, gallstones, and leg ulcers. Folate supplementation is an integral component of therapy, and splenectomy may be required to reduce the amount of hemolysis.

Suggested Readings

Bain BJ. Diagnosis from the blood smear. N Engl J Med 2005;353:498–507.

Burns ER, Lou Y, Pathak A. Morphologic diagnosis of thrombotic thrombocytopenic purpura. Am J Hematol 2004;75:18–21.

Eber S, Lux SE. Hereditary spherocytosis—defects in proteins that connect the membrane skeleton to the lipid bilayer. Semin Hematol 2004;41:118–141.

Poyart C, Wajcman H. Hemolytic anemias due to hemoglobinopathies. Mol Aspects Med 1996;17:129–142.

Westerman DA, Evans D, Metz J. Neutrophil hypersegmentation in iron deficiency anaemia: a case-control study. Br J Haematol 1999;107:512–515.

Chapter 35
Pancytopenia (Case 27)

Byron E. Crawford MD

Case: An unemployed 38-year-old woman presents with recent onset of epistaxis and lethargy. She has previously been diagnosed with gout, for which she takes colchicine, aspirin, and nonsteroidal anti-inflammatory drugs (NSAIDs) during flare-ups. Because of a strong family history of cancer (mother died from breast cancer at any early age, and brother was recently diagnosed with malignant melanoma of his scalp), she is very fearful of having cancer. Physical examination reveals a pulse of 106 beats/minute (bpm), pallor of her nail beds, and several oral cavity and skin petechial hemorrhages. There is no lymphadenopathy or hepatosplenomegaly. Laboratory studies reveal a hemoglobin of 6.5 g/dL, hematocrit of 19%, platelet count of 14,000/μL, WBC count of 1800/μL with an absolute neutrophil count of 1100/μL, and a corrected reticulocyte count of 0.8%. Biochemical studies are normal, including serum LDH and uric acid concentrations.

Differential Diagnosis

Aplastic anemia	AML	Megaloblastic anemia
Myelodysplastic syndromes	Myelofibrosis	

Speaking Intelligently

A very thorough history and physical examination are paramount in patients with pancytopenia, including questions regarding drugs, radiation, chemical and toxin exposure, previous and recent infections, and immunologic disorders. It may require multiple questions to elicit drug, chemical, or toxin history or exposures. Though usually not diagnostic, it is very important to review the peripheral blood smear for additional findings that may help establish a more definitive differential diagnosis. Bone marrow aspirate and biopsy to determine if the marrow is hypocellular or normocellular are also important. Pancytopenia is usually very serious, and discussion with the patient about the differential diagnosis, etiology, utilization of diagnostic tests, and therapy, both definitive and supportive, should occur.

PATIENT CARE

Clinical Thinking

- Determine if the symptoms are due to a process infiltrating the bone marrow (myelophthisic anemia), or due to a primary reduction in the production of blood cells.
- Evaluation of the peripheral smear and bone marrow will usually help provide the etiology of pancytopenia.
- A marrow with an infiltrative process, such as myelofibrosis, will exhibit teardrop-shaped erythrocytes (dacrocytes), nucleated RBCs, and possibly immature myeloid precursors and giant platelets in the peripheral smear.
- The bone marrow biopsy will show increased fibrosis with either hyperplasia of all hematopoietic elements or replacement of the marrow by granulomas, tumor, or fibrosis.
- In patients with aplastic anemia, the marrow will be hypocellular or essentially acellular in regard to hematopoietic tissue, while peripheral values demonstrate pancytopenia.
- Patients with megaloblastic anemia will exhibit a macrocytic anemia with macrocytes, ovalocytes, nucleated red blood cells with nuclear-cytoplasmic asynchrony, and hypersegmented neutrophils on peripheral smear. In these patients the bone marrow will be hypercellular with erythroid hyperplasia and erythroid nuclear-cytoplasmic asynchrony. Nuclear-cytoplasmic asynchrony may also be found in myeloid and megakaryocytic precursors.
- Patients with myelodysplasia exhibit hypogranulated and hyposegmented (pseudo–Pelger-Huët) cells, neutrophils, neutrophils with Döhle bodies, and, possibly, rare blasts. A bone marrow biopsy in these patients will show variable cellularity with ringed sideroblasts, erythroid megaloblastoid dysplastic maturation, megakaryocytic dysplastic maturation, and possibly increased myeloblasts, but less than 20% of the myeloid population of the marrow.
- Patients with acute leukemia with peripheral pancytopenia will have a normocytic, normochromic anemia with hyposegmented and hypogranular neutrophils and possibly rare blasts containing Auer rods in the case of acute myeloblastic leukemia. The bone marrow will be hypercellular with greater than 20% blasts.
- In acute myeloblastic leukemia, the blast will stain or express myeloperoxidase, CD33, and CD15, while in acute lymphoblastic leukemia the blast will stain with periodic acid–Schiff (PAS) or express CD22, CD19, CD10, terminal deoxynucleotidyl transferase (TdT), and Bcl-2.
- Additional laboratory features may be helpful, such as elevated serum LDH and uric acid in megaloblastic anemia, acute leukemia, and myelofibrosis, but the evaluation of the patient's peripheral smear and

bone marrow is paramount in determining the etiology of pancytopenia.

History

- Many patients with pancytopenia will be asymptomatic until the anemia becomes symptomatic with malaise, vertigo, lassitude, palpitations, and weakness.
- With thrombocytopenia, the patient may present with complaints of epistaxis, easy bruising, bleeding gums, or heavy menstruation (in women).
- Other presentations of significance include weight loss (malignancy), early satiety (splenomegaly), numbness of extremities (vitamin B_{12}/folic acid deficiency), and fever (malignancy, infection). Patients with pancytopenia usually do not present with primary infectious processes secondary to leukopenia without signs of significant anemia and thrombocytopenia.
- A medication history might reveal use of pharmacologic agents associated with bone marrow suppression including chloramphenicol, colchicine, NSAIDs, phenothiazines, thiazides, quinine, carbamazepine, phenytoin, phenylbutazone, and sulfonamides.
- Chemotherapy drugs may also result in pancytopenia.
- Chemical or toxin exposure to benzene or arsenic, and previous radiation exposure, may be found.
- Sometimes questions regarding drug, chemical, radiation, and toxin exposure must be asked multiple times in different ways to obtain a positive history.
- Past history of infectious disorders such as tuberculosis, fungal infections, HIV, hepatitis B, hepatitis C, Epstein-Barr virus (EBV), cytomegalovirus (CMV), and rarely hepatitis A may be associated with pancytopenia.
- A previous history of gastrectomy or malabsorption syndrome may be found in patients with vitamin B_{12} or folic acid deficiency leading to pancytopenia.
- A history of Down syndrome or Fanconi anemia may be seen in patients with myelodysplasia.

Physical Examination

- Physical examination is usually limited to features secondary to anemia and thrombocytopenia.
- Physical findings include tachycardia, pallor, possible cardiomegaly, ecchymoses, gingival bleeding, and petechial hemorrhages.
- In patients with leukemia and myelofibrosis, splenomegaly and hepatomegaly may be present.
- In patients with megaloblastic anemia, physical examination may reveal decreased vibratory sensation in the extremities, abnormal reflexes, dementia, and possible features of psychosis.

Tests for Consideration

• CBC with examination of peripheral smear.	$11
• Bone marrow examination.	$500
• Bone marrow cytogenetics.	$485
• Type and screen for packed RBCs.	$8
• Serum LDH, uric acid, B_{12}, and folic acid concentrations.	$8, $6, $21, $20
• Antinuclear antibodies (ANAs), rheumatoid factor, Coombs test.	$16, $8, $8
• Reticulocyte count.	$6

Clinical Entities	Medical Knowledge

Aplastic Anemia

Pφ High-dose radiation and toxins (benzene) result in extrinsic damage to the bone marrow, while effects of moderate doses of drugs cause suppression of the marrow by altered metabolism of the pharmacologic agent. The production of toxic drug intermediates, with genetic inability for drug detoxification, may lead to marrow aplasia. Immune-mediated injury may also have a role, as certain cytokines, such as tumor necrosis factor and interferon, promote apoptosis. Cytotoxic T cells can also promote stem cell destruction.

TP Clinical features of aplasia may have an insidious onset or may present acutely. Signs of anemia include weakness, lassitude, and malaise. The earliest signs of marrow aplasia usually result from bleeding and include epistaxis, petechial hemorrhages, easy bruising, and heavy menstruation (in women). Infections are an unusual initial presentation of aplastic anemia.

Dx The bone marrow will exhibit sparse spicules, and examination will reveal either a very hypocellular marrow or an acellular marrow. Occasional mononuclear cells representing lymphocytes, stromal cells, and predominantly adipose tissue will be found in the marrow. Megakaryocytes, myeloid precursors, and erythroid precursors will be absent or markedly diminished. There will be no evidence of granulomas, infectious etiologies, or marrow infiltrative processes such as tumors. The history is extremely important in determining an etiology. A CT scan of the chest should be performed to look for a thymoma.

Tx Any potential causative agents should be withdrawn. If a thymoma is present, surgical excision can be curative. Bone marrow transplantation is the best therapy if the patient has a fully histocompatible sibling donor. Cyclosporine with anti-lymphocyte globulin or anti-thymocyte globulin is preferred in patients without a suitable donor. Androgens have been shown to be effective in some patients, and splenectomy may occasionally increase blood counts in some patients (relapsed or refractory patients). Human leukocyte antigen (HLA)–matched platelets should be transfused to maintain a platelet count >10,000/µL, and RBC transfusions should be used to treat symptomatic anemia. After repeated RBC transfusions, an iron chelator (deferoxamine or deferasirox) may be added to prevent secondary hemochromatosis. **See Cecil Essentials 47.**

Acute Myelogenous Leukemia

Pφ The pathophysiology of pancytopenia secondary to acute leukemia is unclear but is probably related to a combination of suppression of normal hematopoiesis and replacement of bone marrow by leukemic cells.

TP Patients present with gradual or abrupt onset of signs of leukopenia, anemia, and/or thrombocytopenia including weakness, fatigue, weight loss, and anorexia. Occasionally patients present with fever, easy bruising, lymphadenopathy, or bone pain. Physical examination may reveal sternal tenderness, splenomegaly, hepatomegaly, ecchymoses, poor dentition, and/or petechial hemorrhages. In patients with acute leukemia and pancytopenia, the blood counts and peripheral smear may reveal features of normocytic, normochromic anemia, anisopoikilocytosis, nucleated RBCs, hyposegmented and hypogranular neutrophils, low platelet count (<25,000/µL), and possibly rare immature forms including rare blasts. In aleukemic leukemia, no blasts or immature forms will be present, and bone marrow must be examined. Patients may have elevated serum LDH and uric acid concentrations.

Dx Examination of the bone marrow will reveal a hypercellular marrow with 20% or more blasts (some may contain Auer rods) that stain or express myeloperoxidase, chloroacetate esterase, CD33, and CD15 (AML). Cytogenetics of myeloblasts may exhibit balanced chromosomal translocations including t(8;21), t(15;17), and inv(16). Immunohistochemical stains, flow cytometry, and enzyme cytochemistry are needed to differentiate lymphoblasts; acute lymphoblastic leukemia (B-lymphoblasts are PAS positive, and may express CD22, CD19, CD10, TdT, and Bcl-2).

Tx The most commonly used induction regimen for complete remission in patients with AML is combination chemotherapy such as daunorubicin, etoposide, mitoxantrone, idarubicin, thioguanine, anthracycline, and cytosine arabinoside. If remission is not successful after two courses, an allogeneic stem cell transplant is done if an appropriate donor is available. Post-remission therapy includes high-dose cytosine arabinoside, and allogeneic or autologous stem cell transplantation. Use of granulocyte and granulocyte-macrophage colony-stimulating factors to increase WBC counts is controversial. HLA-matched platelets should be transfused to maintain a platelet count above 10,000–20,000/μL (10,000 if there is no bleeding, fever, or complications), and RBC transfusions should be used to treat symptomatic anemia if the patient has pulmonary or cardiac disease or active bleeding. Blood products should be irradiated to prevent graft-versus-host disease, CMV infection in CMV seronegative patients, and leukocyte depletion by filtration to delay alloimmunization and reduce febrile reactions. Patients who receive stem cell transplants require protective isolation until their WBC counts are >500/μL. Patients with central nervous system (CNS) leukemia require intrathecal chemotherapy. **See Cecil Essentials 48.**

Megaloblastic Anemia

Pφ Megaloblastic anemias are disorders resulting from a deficiency of folic acid and/or vitamin B_{12} (cobalamin), resulting in impaired DNA synthesis. Folic acid is essential for the synthesis of purines, and a deficiency in cobalamin results in impaired ability to convert homocysteine to methionine, thereby inhibiting folic acid metabolism, and purine/DNA synthesis. This results in ineffective hematopoiesis with nuclear-cytoplasmic asynchrony. Etiologies for folic acid deficiency include (1) malabsorption (sprue, phenytoin, barbiturates), (2) impaired metabolism secondary to ethanol and drugs (methotrexate, trimethoprim), and (3) increased requirements (malignancy, pregnancy, hemolytic anemia). Cobalamin deficiencies may be secondary to malabsorption (partial or total gastrectomy, pernicious anemia, sprue, intestinal resection, blind-loop syndrome, and fish tapeworm infections) and inadequate intake.

TP Patients present with signs of anemia and neurologic manifestations. Palpitations, vertigo, weakness, light-headedness, numbness of the extremities, irritability, and forgetfulness may be reported by patients. Physical examination may reveal tachycardia, pallor, and mildly icteric skin with mildly elevated serum total bilirubin concentrations, enlarged heart, rarely purpura if platelets are low, paresthesias of the extremities, diminished or increased reflexes, ataxia, diminished vibratory sense, dementia, and psychosis.

Dx Review of blood cell counts and the peripheral smear will demonstrate a macrocytic anemia with a mean corpuscular volume (MCV) usually >100 fL with reduced platelet and leukocyte counts. RBC morphology reveals macrocytes, ovalocytes, nucleated RBCs with nuclear-cytoplasmic asynchrony, and basophilic stippling. Hypersegmented neutrophils (more than six lobes), when seen, are characteristic of megaloblastic anemia. There may be leukopenia and thrombocytopenia in some patients. Serum LDH concentrations may be markedly elevated with a flipped LDH pattern (LDH$_1$ > LDH$_2$). The anemia may be extremely severe for the clinical symptomatology. A bone marrow examination is indicated in the workup of a patient with suspicion of megaloblastic anemia and will reveal a hypercellular marrow with erythroid hyperplasia. Erythroid and myeloid precursors are large and exhibit immature-appearing nuclei compared to the cytoplasmic maturation (nuclear-cytoplasmic asynchrony). Megakaryocytes also show abnormal morphology. Cobalamin and/or folic acid serum concentrations are reduced (cobalamin <200 pg/mL, folic acid <4 ng/mL). Methylmalonic acid concentrations are elevated in cobalamin-deficient patients. Homocysteine concentrations are increased with both folate and cobalamin deficiency.

Tx In patients with cobalamin deficiency, replacement typically begins with parenteral intramuscular injections of cyanocobalamin. Oral cobalamin can then be given at daily doses of 1000 µg for the rest of the patient's life. In folic acid deficiency, oral replacement with 1 mg/day, and up to 5 mg/day in patients with malabsorption syndromes, is given. Mistakenly treating cobalamin deficiency with folic acid will correct the anemia but not the neurologic symptoms and signs. **See Cecil Essentials 49.**

Myelodysplastic Syndromes

Pφ Myelodysplastic syndromes (MDSs) are abnormal clonal hematopoietic stem cell lesions resulting in impaired cell differentiation and proliferation. They are due to a combination of cytogenetic abnormalities, mitochondrial dysfunction, oncogene activation, and loss of tumor suppressor genes resulting in disordered iron metabolism and ineffective hematopoiesis.

TP About one-half of patients are asymptomatic, with the remainder presenting with fatigue, pallor, weakness, and dyspnea. A history of radiation, chemotherapy, Down syndrome, and Fanconi anemia may be seen in MDS. A family history of sideroblastic anemia and Fanconi anemia may be present. Physical examination may reveal pallor and increased heart rate indicative of anemia. CBC reveals a macrocytic anemia, pancytopenia, or isolated neutropenia or thrombocytopenia. Patients may have a monocytosis.

Dx Evaluation reveals a dimorphic population of RBCs, large platelets that are deficient of granules, hypogranulated neutrophils with hyposegmented (two lobes) pseudo–Pelger-Huët cells, or ringed neutrophils and neutrophils with Döhle bodies. Rare myeloblasts may be found. Examination of the bone marrow may reveal a hypercellular or normocellular marrow; however, in 10% to 20% of cases the marrow is hypocellular. Ringed sideroblasts, erythroid megaloblastoid dysplastic maturation, disordered (dysplastic) maturation of megakaryocytes (micro-megakaryocytes, hypolobation, pawn ball megakaryocytes), and increased myeloblasts, but <20% of non-erythroid cells can be found. Marrow examination may show abnormal localized immature precursors (ALIPs) remote from bone trabeculae. Cytogenetics may show clonal chromosome abnormalities including trisomy 8, monosomy 5 or 7, and deletions of the long arms of chromosomes 20, 5, or 7 (20q-, 5q-, or 7q-).

Tx Only stem cell transplantation offers a cure for the patient, with success related to the patient's International Prognostic Scoring System score. Patients with MDS and trisomy 8 may respond to cyclosporine. Hematopoietic growth factors can improve cell counts in some patients with mild pancytopenia. Erythropoietin with granulocyte colony-stimulating factor has shown increase in hemoglobin levels. Three agents have been approved for treatment of MDS by the U.S. FDA: decitabine, 5-azacytidine, and lenalidomide. The first two have been shown to decrease blood transfusions, and the third (expensive, about $7000 per month) has been approved only for use in patients with 5q-syndrome. HLA-matched platelets should be transfused to maintain a platelet count above 10,000/μL, and RBC transfusions should be used to treat symptomatic anemia if the patient has pulmonary or cardiac disease. After repeated transfusions of RBCs, an iron chelator (deferoxamine or deferasirox) can be added to prevent secondary hemochromatosis. **See Cecil Essentials 47.**

Myelofibrosis

Pφ Myelofibrosis may be primary (agnogenic myeloid metaplasia [AMM]) or secondary to infiltrative diseases such as infections and metastatic malignancies (myelophthisic marrow). Because the marrow is replaced by fibrous tissue and possible infiltrative process of metastatic tumor or infection, there is loss of hematopoietic tissue with increase in extramedullary hematopoiesis (spleen and liver). When primary, there is neoplastic transformation of multipotent stem cells that stimulate (transforming growth factor-β and thrombopoietin) marrow non-neoplastic fibroblasts to produce excess collagen. Marrow failure eventually occurs with resultant pancytopenia.

TP In early stages, patients are usually asymptomatic and are first diagnosed with splenomegaly or from an abnormal CBC. In the later stages, patients develop weight loss, hepatomegaly, malaise, and fever. In primary myelofibrosis, they may present with AML. Rarely, patients develop lymphadenopathy, splenic infarction, or secondary gout. Also, secondary myelofibrosis may be seen in patients exposed to toxins such as benzene and radiation.

Dx Evaluation of the patient's peripheral smear and bone marrow is required to make the diagnosis. Patients may exhibit anemia with or without thrombocytopenia and/or leukopenia. Platelet and leukocyte counts may even be increased. The peripheral smear may reveal nucleated RBCs, teardrop-shaped RBCs, and immature myelogenous cells including myelocytes, promyelocytes, and myeloblasts. Patients may have elevated serum LDH and uric acid concentrations. In patients with myelofibrosis the bone marrow aspirate usually produces a dry tap, requiring a biopsy for evaluation and diagnosis. The bone marrow biopsy will reveal increased marrow fibrous tissue and may exhibit a hypercellular marrow including trilineage hyperplasia. In secondary myelofibrosis, granulomas, osteomyelitis, Hodgkin and non-Hodgkin lymphoma, hairy cell leukemia, or metastatic carcinoma may be found.

Tx   Splenectomy may be indicated in patients with splenomegaly. Androgens and erythropoietin have been used but are not consistently effective. RBC transfusions may be indicated. Allogeneic bone marrow transplantation may be indicated in younger patients. Splenic radiation and chemotherapy have also been used in primary myelofibrosis. In secondary myelofibrosis, appropriate antimicrobial agents are given if fibrosis is due to an infectious agent. In patients with secondary gout, allopurinol is used. **See Cecil Essentials 48.**

ZEBRA ZONE

a. **Visceral leishmaniasis:** Most cases are in patients from India, Bangladesh, Nepal, Sudan, and Brazil. Diagnosis can be made by finding the amastigote form of the organism extracellularly or within histiocytes in the bone marrow, lymph nodes, spleen, or liver.

b. **Paroxysmal noctural hemoglobinuria** should be considered when the patient has pancytopenia with features of intravascular hemolysis, including elevated LDH, hemoglobinuria, hemoglobinemia, and hemosiderinuria. The acidified serum lysis test or Ham test is unreliable; flow cytometry, looking for decreased expression of CD55 and CD59 in peripheral leukocytes, is helpful.

c. **HIV** may be diagnosed serologically and with viral studies. Must first rule out an infectious marrow process in an HIV-infected patient.

d. **Hepatitis A, B, and C:** Pancytopenia secondary to hepatitis B and C is far more common than pancytopenia secondary to hepatitis A. Mortality rate is high in hepatitis-associated pancytopenia.

e. **Gaucher disease:** A prominent infiltrate of lipid-laden histiocytes is present in the bone marrow.

f. **Sarcoidosis:** Though it commonly involves the bone marrow, sarcoidosis only rarely results in pancytopenia. Bone marrow contains non-necrotizing granulomas that are negative for acid-fast bacilli and fungi by stains and cultures.

g. **Systemic lupus erythematosus:** Pancytopenia may occur with anemia secondary to chronic disease state and sometimes hemolysis. Thrombocytopenia is common, and leukopenia is usually secondary to lymphopenia and not neutropenia.

Practice-Based Learning and Improvement: Evidence-Based Medicine

Title
A multicenter randomized study of the threshold for prophylactic platelet transfusions in adults with acute myeloid leukemia

Authors
Rubella P, Finazzi G, Marangoni F, et al.

Institution
Instituto di Ricovero e Cura Carattere Scientifico Osperdal Maggiore, Milan, Italy

Reference
N Engl J Med 1997;337:1870

Problem
Thrombocytopenia in patients with acute myeloblastic leukemia

Intervention
Platelet transfusions

Quality of evidence
Level I

Outcome/effect
The risk of major bleeding during induction chemotherapy in patients with acute myeloblastic leukemia was similar in stable, nonbleeding patients not requiring an invasive procedure and with temperatures less than 38° C, and in patients with platelet transfusion thresholds of 20,000/μL and 10,000/μL. Use of the lower threshold reduced the utilization of platelets by 21.5%.

Historical significance/comments
Platelet transfusions in patients with acute myeloblastic leukemia are routinely given when platelet counts drop below 20,000/μL. There have been observations that in appropriate stable patients the lower thresholds can be used safely as an indication for prophylactic platelet transfusions.

Interpersonal and Communication Skills

Points to Remember When the Discussion Is Complex
Discussions regarding bone marrow disorders can be very complex. The physician must discuss diagnostic tests, the need for a bone marrow evaluation, complex concepts, multiple potential therapies, and potential complications. When having this type of sophisticated

medical discussion with patients, particularly those whose health literacy may be diminished, the following points about good interpersonal and communication skills may prove very valuable:

1. Speak slowly and use language the patient can understand.

2. Maintain eye contact.

3. Whenever possible, draw a picture or a simple diagram.

4. Don't overwhelm the patient with more information than he or she can handle.

5. Check comprehension by having the patient reiterate important points.

6. Avoid making the patient feel ashamed. Remind your patient that many people have difficulty understanding health-care information, especially when the condition is complex.

7. If the patient agrees, have a family member or friend accompany him or her to the office visit.

Adapted from Mann B. Surgery: a competency-based companion. Philadelphia: Elsevier; 2009, p. 183.

Professionalism

Ensure Access to Care: Funding Sources for Expensive Treatments
A stem cell transplant is a complicated technical procedure and can be costly. Health insurance policies generally cover the cost when indicated; however, some patients may require financial assistance. Hospital social services and finance departments can be valuable resources in planning the financial needs of these patients. Local service organizations and federal and state government programs, such as the National Cancer Institute (NCI) and the Cancer Information Service (CIS), may be helpful resources to patients and their families in finding programs for financial assistance. It is our professional responsibility to be aware of both local community and larger national initiatives to ensure access to the care our patients may need.

Systems-Based Practice

Patient Safety: Blood Bank Protocols

Hemolytic transfusion reaction is usually due to ABO incompatibility and results in death in 1 in 600,000 transfusions. The system established to prevent such problems involves a complex, but orderly, interaction among the ordering physician, the nursing staff, the blood bank, and the hospital laboratory. A blood sample is first obtained from the patient to determine blood type and to crossmatch the patient's serum with donated blood to exclude preformed antibodies. It is critically important that the identity of the patient from whom the blood sample was obtained is properly verified before the sample is sent to the blood bank; failure of verification should lead to the sample being discarded and a new sample obtained. The blood product is prepared in the blood bank and carefully labeled for the specific patient. Before the product is administered, two people are required to confirm the identity of the recipient and the designation of the blood product so as to ensure that the correct blood product is given to the correct patient. The patient is carefully monitored during transfusion to identify any signs of a transfusion reaction (e.g., fever, rash, anaphylaxis, and pulmonary edema).

Chapter 36
Excessive Bleeding or Clotting (Case 28)

Rebecca Kruse-Jarres MD, MPH

Case: A 74-year-old woman is in good general health except for hypothyroidism, which is well controlled on thyroid hormone replacement. Over the past month she noticed that she started bruising easily. She had never before had a problem with easy bruising, prolonged bleeding from cuts, or other unusual bleeding. She goes to see her primary-care physician, who orders a bleeding time. She presents to the ED 5 days after the test because she is still bleeding from the test site. She has multiple bruises covering her arms, trunk, and legs.

Differential Diagnosis

Immune thrombocytopenic purpura (ITP)	DIC	Acquired factor VIII deficiency
Drug-induced thrombocytopenia	Vitamin K deficiency	Thrombotic thrombocytopenic purpura (TTP)

Speaking Intelligently

When I encounter a patient with bleeding, the most important approach is to take a detailed history and perform a physical examination. First, I like to establish whether the bleeding disorder is of a chronic nature. Is this a condition the patient had all of his or her life, and do I have to think about congenital causes (such as hemophilia or von Willebrand's disease), or is this of recent onset and more likely an "acquired" condition?

If the problem seems to have been going on for a significant portion of the patient's life, it is crucial to get a good family history of any family member with bleeding tendencies and to draw a pedigree to establish the inheritance pattern.

If the bleeding is of more recent onset, it is critical to elicit any changes in the patient's life that may have been contributory, such as new medications, newly diagnosed other medical conditions, other associated symptoms, and recent travel.

Finally, it is important to separate disorders of primary hemostasis from disorders of secondary hemostasis. Patients with primary hemostatic disorders usually present with superficial bleeding such as easy bruisability, gum bleeding, or menorrhagia; the primary hemostatic system involves platelets, von Willebrand factor, and a vessel wall. Patients with disorders of secondary hemostasis, such as factor deficiencies, usually present with deep bleeding such as cerebral hemorrhage or bleeding into muscles and joints.

PATIENT CARE

Clinical Thinking
- This patient seems to have an acquired problem that started causing symptoms (i.e., bruising) about 1 month before her presentation.
- She also appears to have a disorder of primary hemostasis.
- It is important to investigate any possible triggers for the new symptoms such as recent medication changes or travel.

- The physical exam may point to other possible etiologies, such as a hematologic malignancy, which can cause thrombocytopenia.

History

- In investigating a bleeding disorder, it is essential to differentiate a congenital from an acquired condition.
- Once an acquired condition is suspected, it is crucial to elicit the severity, duration, speed of progression, and associated circumstances. Examples include changes in the patient's health such as new medical diagnoses, newly prescribed medications, and recent surgeries.
- The patient's past medical history is also important; patients with autoimmune disorders, such as thyroid disease or diabetes mellitus, may develop other autoimmune phenomena, such as ITP.
- DIC may accompany disorders such as malignancy or sepsis.
- Medications can also contribute to bleeding problems. For example, if the patient is on warfarin, change in certain other medications or diet could easily increase warfarin concentrations. Changes in diet or recent use of antibiotics can lead to vitamin K deficiency, causing bleeding and bruising.
- Patients with platelet disorders and von Willebrand disease, which are disorders of primary hemostasis, present with mucosal bleeding such as petechiae, mouth bleeding, and heavy menstrual bleeding. Factor deficiencies may lead to soft-tissue bleeding and bleeding from surgical sites.
- Especially in the elderly, a history of bruising has to raise a suspicion for potential physical abuse.

Physical Examination

- Determine the pattern and location of blood loss.
- Look for bruising, petechiae, and bleeding from cuts, surgical sites, and IV access sites.
- Evaluate for possible oropharyngeal, GI, and genitourinary bleeding.
- Remember to assess for the possibility of internal bleeding, such as intracranial hemorrhage, especially if the patient has symptoms or signs of neurologic abnormalities.
- Assess the mouth for signs of "wet" purpura characterized by blood-filled blisters.

Tests for Consideration

- **CBC:** To determine the platelet count and see whether other cell lines (WBCs, RBCs) are normal or abnormal. $11
- **Hemoglobin/hematocrit:** May help in estimating how much bleeding has occurred, if a baseline is available. $7
- **Peripheral smear** is essential in almost every hematologic disorder. $5
    - There could be platelet clumping, ruling out a true thrombocytopenia.
    - Blast cells are worrisome for an acute leukemia.

- Schistocytes could be indicative of the microangiopathic hemolytic anemia of DIC or TTP.
- ITP results in a normal smear except for thrombocytopenia.
- **Prothrombin time (PT):** Assesses the extrinsic and common coagulation pathway (factors II, V, VII, X, and fibrinogen). $6
- **Activated partial thromboplastin time (aPTT):** Assesses the intrinsic and common coagulation pathway (factor II, V, X, VIII, XI, XII, and fibrinogen). $9
- **PT or aPTT mixing study:** Prolongation of either can help to differentiate a factor deficiency from an inhibitor. $6, $9
- **PFA-100 (has now replaced bleeding time in most places):** Screens for a platelet disorder but is not reliable in patients with thrombocytopenia. $5
- **Fibrin degradation products (FDPs) or D-dimer:** Are elevated in DIC. $14
- **Bone marrow aspirate and biopsy:** May be needed to check for platelet production, aplasia, myelodysplasia, or malignancy. $500

IMAGING CONSIDERATIONS

→ **CT or MRI** can be ordered to assess the extent of a hematoma or to evaluate for internal bleeding in a symptomatic patient. $334, $435

Clinical Entities   Medical Knowledge

Immune Thrombocytopenic Purpura

Pφ In ITP, an antibody binds to the platelet surface, causing premature removal of platelets from the circulation by the phagocytic cells of the reticuloendothelial system. The autoantibody causing ITP is most often targeted to platelet glycoprotein (GP) IIb/IIIa or platelet GP Ib/IX; bound antibody leads to platelet removal by binding to Fc receptors on the membrane of macrophages, followed by removal by the spleen. ITP is also characterized by decreased platelet production.

TP There is spontaneous onset of petechiae and/or bruising or other spontaneous bleeding, such as epistaxis. Severe bleeding is rare, despite very low platelet counts.

Dx Usually the platelet count is very low (<5000/μL), PT/PTT are normal, PFA-100 (due to thrombocytopenia) is prolonged, RBC and WBC counts are normal, and a peripheral smear is normal except for thrombocytopenia and large platelets.

This is a diagnosis of exclusion and should be considered if no other cause of thrombocytopenia can be identified. Pseudothrombocytopenia caused by platelet clumping or aggregation around leukocytes when ethylenediamine tetraacetic acid (EDTA) is used in the collection tube should be excluded by repeating the platelet count in a tube containing citrate or heparin as the anticoagulant.

Tx Prednisone 1 mg/kg daily for 2–4 weeks, with a gradual taper, is the initial treatment. If unresponsive to prednisone, most adult patients may require splenectomy or other immunosuppressive therapy (such as cyclophosphamide, azathioprine, or rituximab). Intravenous immune globulin (IVIG) may increase very low platelet counts, but the effect is transient (days to weeks).

Platelet transfusions are **unnecessary**, unless there is severe bleeding. A hematologist should be consulted in patients suspected of having ITP. **See Cecil Essentials 53.**

Disseminated Intravascular Coagulation

Pφ DIC is defined as sustained, disseminated, and excessive coagulation without the ability to neutralize activated products of coagulation. This leads to consumption of coagulation products and platelets, leading to both bleeding and thrombosis. Consumption of platelets causes thrombocytopenia.

TP Consider DIC in a patient with underlying cancer (typically mucin-producing adenocarcinomas), sepsis, trauma, or after obstetric complications. Acute promyelocytic leukemia is also often associated with DIC. Typical patients present with signs of excessive clotting (e.g., deep venous thrombosis) and/or excessive bleeding (e.g., oozing from around IV catheter sites).

Dx Moderately decreased platelet count, prolonged PT and aPTT, elevated D-dimer, decreased fibrinogen, and increased fibrin degradation products.

Peripheral blood smear shows decreased platelets and fragmented RBCs (schistocytes).

Tx Supportive, by treating underlying cause. Patients with bleeding may need fresh-frozen plasma to replace coagulation factors, or platelet transfusion. Heparin is rarely used because of the potential for increasing risk of bleeding, and there is no improvement in outcome. **See Cecil Essentials 53.**

Acquired Factor VIII Deficiency

Pφ Formation of an autoantibody against factor VIII. May occur in older patients and those with autoimmune disease, cancer, lymphoproliferative disorders, and in women during the postpartum period.

TP Spontaneous bleeding occurs, often in soft tissues (such as spontaneous bleeding into joints). Prolonged bleeding from cuts and with surgeries or procedures has also been described.

Dx Prolonged aPTT with a normal PT; no correction with a mixing study. The platelet count is normal. There is decreased factor VIII level (usually <30%), with a detectable factor VIII inhibitor level.

Tx Factor VIII bypassing agents such as activated factor VII or activated prothrombin complex concentrates (which contain factors VII, IX, X, and prothrombin) can be given to stop acute bleeding. Definitive treatment of the inhibitor is difficult and can be achieved through IVIG or immune-suppressive agents such as prednisone, cyclophosphamide, vincristine, or rituximab. **See Cecil Essentials 53.**

Drug-Induced Thrombocytopenia

Pφ Platelets are the first response to epithelial damage. They are activated at the site of injury to form a temporary plug until the coagulation factors can produce a more permanent clot. Certain medications (such as quinine, antibiotics, and heparin) have been associated with development of thrombocytopenia.

TP Patients seldom present with bleeding from thrombocytopenia unless the platelet count is <10,000/μL. At that point, petechiae and mucosal (e.g., GI, epistaxis, gums) bleeding can occur.

Dx Decreased platelet count; normal PT and aPTT.

Tx Stop the offending medication. There is seldom a need for platelet transfusion if the platelet count is >10,000/μL. **See Cecil Essentials 53, 54.**

Vitamin K Deficiency

Pφ Vitamin K is necessary for the synthesis of the extrinsic coagulation factors (factors II, VII, IX, and X). Vitamin K can become deficient during periods of malnutrition or with antibiotic usage that decreases synthesis of vitamin K by bacterial flora.

TP The diagnosis should be considered with bruising or bleeding in a patient with malnutrition, or in a patient on prolonged antibiotic therapy.

Dx Prolonged PT (may also see a prolonged aPTT, if severe); PT mixing study that corrects; low serum albumin in a malnourished patient; and clinical suspicion.

Tx Replace vitamin K by mouth (5–10 mg) or intravenously. Patients with acute bleeding require administration of fresh-frozen plasma to replace the missing clotting factors. **See Cecil Essentials 53.**

Thrombotic Thrombocytopenic Purpura

Pφ TTP is a disorder of the systemic circulation caused by microvascular aggregation of platelets in the brain and other organs. Patients have unusually large multimers of von Willebrand factor (vWF) in their plasma. ADAMTS13, a disintegrin and metalloprotease, cleaves large multimers of vWF; patients with deficiencies or antibodies to ADAMTS13 can develop platelet aggregates in the microvasculature. TTP can also be seen in patients with cancer, transplant recipients, and following administration of chemotherapeutic agents and other drugs.

TP The typical pentad of findings in patients with TTP is thrombocytopenia, microangiopathic hemolytic anemia, fever, renal insufficiency, and neurologic deficits; all five findings do not have to be present to establish the diagnosis.

Dx The diagnosis should always be considered in patients with thrombocytopenia and microangiopathic hemolytic anemia. The main consideration in the differential diagnosis is DIC, which can be excluded in patients with normal PT, aPTT, and D-dimer.

Tx The treatment of choice is urgent plasma exchange transfusion. **See Cecil Essentials 29, 31, 49, 54.**

ZEBRA ZONE

a. **Acquired von Willebrand syndrome:** Described in association with numerous conditions such as myeloproliferative or lymphoproliferative disorders, monoclonal gammopathies, autoimmune disease, acquired or congenital heart disease. Resembles congenital von Willebrand disease with decreased vWF antigen and ristocetin co-factor (functional evaluation of vWF). The aPTT is prolonged.

b. **Platelet aggregation disorders:** For example, Bernard-Soulier syndrome (platelet adhesion disorder due to abnormality in GP Ib/IX/V) or Glanzmann thrombasthenia (platelet aggregation disorder due to abnormality in GP IIb/IIIa).

c. **Afibrinogenemia or dysfibrinogenemia:** Usually results in an abnormal thrombin time.

d. **Other clotting factor inhibitors:** These are rare but should be suspected if mixing studies are prolonged.

e. **Acquired qualitative platelet disorders:** Patients have normal platelet counts but a qualitative defect. Commonly caused by drugs (aspirin, NSAIDs, clopidogrel), and in patients with uremia.

f. **Psychogenic purpura:** This is a rare, not well-understood phenomenon in patients who often have associated psychological disorders. A thorough clinical investigation should be completed before this diagnosis of exclusion is entertained.

Practice-Based Learning and Improvement: Evidence-Based Medicine

Title
Comparison of plasma exchange with plasma infusion in the treatment of thrombotic thrombocytopenic purpura. Canadian Apheresis Study Group.

Authors
Rock GA, Shumak KH, Buskard NA

Institution
Multi-institutional

Reference
N Engl J Med 1991;325:393–397

Problem
The best treatment for TTP is unknown; both plasma infusion and plasma exchange seemed effective.

Intervention
Prospective randomized trial comparing plasma exchange with plasma infusion for the treatment of TTP

Quality of evidence
Level I

Outcome/effect
Plasma exchange is more effective than plasma infusion in the treatment of TTP.

Historical significance/comments
This has established plasmapheresis as the standard of care for the treatment of TTP.

Interpersonal and Communication Skills

Be Prepared for Conversations with Patients
When called to see a patient whose workup is in progress, the consultant may be the first to know that the bone marrow or CT scan ordered by the primary-care team reveals a likely diagnosis of advanced malignancy. In such a situation, a consultant should be very careful when talking with the patient. Consult the primary-care team first to determine who should discuss the diagnosis and in what setting. Before explaining matters to the patient, determine what the patient knows about his or her condition. The patient's answer guides the explanation. Medical students and residents, who are often first to evaluate a requested consultation, should be cognizant of this dilemma and should consult with attending physicians before finding themselves "trapped" in a discussion that they may not be prepared to conduct.

Professionalism

Understand the Patient's Right to Refuse Treatment
A patient of yours with a bleeding disorder has had a large upper GI hemorrhage and presents in the ED with a critically low hemoglobin. While you are obtaining informed consent to begin transfusing packed RBCs, the patient informs you that she is a Jehovah's Witness and cannot accept the transfusion. She is tachycardic and hypotensive. Situations like these can be hard to accept from the treating physician perspective. Learning more about a particular patient's cultural or religious beliefs can be very helpful in understanding the implications of particular recommended therapies on the patient. For Jehovah's Witnesses, accepting blood from a source other than themselves is against the scriptural teachings of their religion. Even in a life-threatening situation, the right answer is always to respect patient autonomy.

Systems-Based Practice

Describe Medication Reconciliation

Patients with bleeding disorders need to be monitored frequently; often they need laboratory work and adjustment of their treatment weekly, if not more frequently. Some of these patients may also have other comorbid conditions that require use of additional medications that may need to be periodically adjusted. Given multiple changes in medication, it is important to adequately reconcile what the patient is taking across the continuum of care. This can be done on an outpatient basis and requires dedicated staff, such as a nurse or nurse practitioner working closely with the patient and their physician. If the patient is hospitalized, a process must be followed for accurate and complete medication reconciliation as follows:

- The home medication list is compared to the current list and reconciled on admission, transfer, and discharge.
- The home medication list should include dose, route, and frequency of administration.
- Any discrepancies must be reconciled and documented.
- The patient must receive an updated list of medications upon discharge.
- The medication list must be provided to the next provider of care upon discharge or transfer to another facility.

Chapter 37
Lymphadenopathy and Splenomegaly (Case 29)

Bridgette Collins-Burow PhD, MD

Case: A 21-year-old healthy woman presents to her gynecologist in March for her yearly Pap smear. Upon further questioning she reports fatigue, persistent upper respiratory symptoms with a nonproductive cough, as well as persistent low-grade fever for several months. She also reports a weight loss of about 10 pounds over the past several months and attributes this to the fact that she was attempting to lose weight. She denies any travel, sick contacts, or high-risk sexual behaviors. Her physical examination is remarkable for two firm, palpable, rubbery, left anterior cervical nodes that measure 2 cm in diameter. She is reassured by her physician and prescribed a 10-day course of oral penicillin.

Four weeks later, these lymph nodes are still present, and she feels that her left neck is "slightly fuller and tender." Clearly upset about the swelling in her neck, she returns to her primary-care physician. In addition to her previous pertinent positive findings, on review of systems, she reports early satiety and night sweats. She has looked on the Internet for alternative explanations for her symptoms, and she is nervous now about the possibility that she may have lymphoma. She has lost an additional 7 pounds and is noted to have a palpable spleen on physical examination, in addition to both cervical and axillary lymphadenopathy. Her CBC and peripheral blood smear are normal.

Differential Diagnosis

Hodgkin lymphoma	Non-Hodgkin lymphoma (NHL)	Mononucleosis/EBV infection
Sarcoidosis	Primary HIV infection	

Speaking Intelligently

When I encounter a patient with lymphadenopathy, I always take a detailed medical history and perform a complete physical examination. Of greatest concern is the possibility of malignancy. While the prevalence of malignancy in the general population presenting with unexplained lymphadenopathy is low, there are both historical and physical clues that can be suggestive of a diagnosis, including the age of the patient, the duration of lymphadenopathy, whether the lymphadenopathy is localized or generalized, the location of the lymphadenopathy, and associated clinical symptoms. Rubbery lymph nodes often suggest the diagnosis of lymphoma, whereas carcinomatous nodes are usually hard. Splenomegaly, in association with lymphadenopathy, focuses the differential on infectious mononucleosis, primary HIV infection, lymphomas, and sarcoidosis. When malignancy is of concern, excisional biopsy of a node is necessary to establish the diagnosis.

PATIENT CARE

Clinical Thinking
- When evaluating a patient with lymphadenopathy, it is first important to obtain a detailed medical history.
- The age of the patient is very important in the evaluation. A majority of healthy young children have palpable cervical, axillary, and inguinal adenopathy; in fact, total lymph node mass reaches a maximum in early adolescence.

- Exposures related to travel, infection, the environment, and occupation are relevant for the evaluation of unexplained lymphadenopathy.
- Physical examination is equally important and must include a complete lymphatic examination with attention to lymphatic drainage patterns, as well as size and character of the lymph nodes.
- Iatrogenic causes of lymphadenopathy, with medications such as phenytoin, can be ruled out by history.
- The presentation of splenomegaly in association with lymphadenopathy in the above case focuses the differential on infectious mononucleosis, primary HIV infection, lymphomas, and sarcoidosis.
- The malignancies of particular concern in our patient's presentation with classical "B" symptoms (i.e., fever, night sweats, and unexplained weight loss) include that of Hodgkin lymphoma and non-Hodgkin lymphoma.

History
- While patients who present with an underlying malignancy may often be asymptomatic, a history of fever, chills, night sweats, and unexplained weight loss should warrant further evaluation and workup.
- A good history should include investigation into infectious etiologies, as well as a detailed exposure history, sexual history, and medication history.

Physical Examination
- A patient who has evidence of an active pharyngitis, otitis media, or other focal infection may require no further evaluation of the lymphadenopathy. Other infectious etiologies of lymphadenopathy, however, may require specific testing, as in the examples of infectious mononucleosis and HIV.
- Important characteristics of lymph nodes on physical examination include the location, whether the lymphadenopathy is localized or generalized, the size and consistency of the node, whether fixed or mobile, and whether the lymph node is tender or nontender.

Tests for Consideration
- **Heterophile antibody test:** This test is sensitive for the diagnosis of EBV infection; however, the test will be negative early after infection and will be negative if the mononucleosis is caused by other infections, such as CMV. If the test is negative, serologic assays for specific agents should be considered. $9
- **HIV RNA testing:** Could be considered in the setting of a high-risk patient with symptoms of acute HIV infection with a negative enzyme-linked immunosorbent assay (ELISA)

and Western blot, which may represent the "window period"
before seroconversion. $120
- **Serum angiotensin-converting enzyme (ACE) concentration:**
  Although some studies report an elevated ACE concentration in
  approximately 75% of patients with sarcoidosis, it is both an
  insensitive and a nonspecific test. $30
- **Excisional lymph node biopsy:** The preservation of the nodal
  architecture is critical in the evaluation of lymphoma. In patients
  with Hodgkin lymphoma, the pathologic interpretation based on
  histology and the putative malignant cell, the Reed-Sternberg
  cell, is necessary for diagnosis. In patients with non-Hodgkin
  lymphoma, histologic, cytologic, and immunologic features as
  well as cytogenetic abnormalities are all instrumental in the
  classification. Fine-needle aspirates are never adequate to
  diagnose lymphoma. $570
- **Bone marrow biopsy and aspirate:** Important in evaluating
  disease involvement outside of the lymphatic system in
  patients with lymphoma. $500

Clinical Entities	Medical Knowledge

Hodgkin Lymphoma

Pφ Hodgkin lymphoma is characterized by the presence of the
Reed-Sternberg cell. The exact mechanism by which these cells
derive and their role in the malignant process remain unclear.
The majority of these cells are monoclonal B cells believed to be
derived from preapoptotic germinal-center cells that have lost the
capacity to express a high-affinity B-cell receptor. Reed-Sternberg
cells are therefore able to subvert the apoptotic process.

TP The typical presentation of Hodgkin lymphoma is a young,
otherwise healthy individual who presents with painless or
slightly tender, rubbery lymphadenopathy in a single group of
lymph nodes. Hodgkin lymphoma has a biphasic incidence with
a peak in young adulthood and in the fifth decade. The most
common nodal areas of involvement in a young patient include
cervical, axillary, and mediastinal nodes. Hodgkin lymphoma can
occur in the presence or absence of B symptoms (i.e., fever,
weight loss, night sweats).

Dx Diagnosis of Hodgkin lymphoma requires an excisional biopsy of
a lymph node with review by a hematopathologist. To make the
diagnosis with certainty, the Reed-Sternberg cell, or a variant,
must be identified. Histologic classification of Hodgkin lymphoma
includes the following: (1) nodular/lymphocyte predominant,
(2) lymphocyte-rich classical, (3) nodular sclerosis, (4) mixed
cellularity, and (5) lymphocyte depleted.

Tx Accurate diagnosis and staging are critical in the treatment of Hodgkin lymphoma. All stages of Hodgkin lymphoma are treated with intent to cure. Hodgkin lymphoma is sensitive to radiation and several chemotherapeutic regimens. ABVD (doxorubicin, bleomycin, vinblastine, dacarbazine) is a commonly used chemotherapeutic regimen. **See Cecil Essentials 51.**

Non-Hodgkin Lymphoma

Pφ NHL is a heterogeneous spectrum of diseases characterized by a malignant clonal expansion of B or T cells that occurs through genetic alterations involving a wide spectrum of proto-oncogenes and/or tumor suppressors.

TP There is a tremendous variation in clinical presentation of this spectrum of diseases. Follicular lymphomas, which constitute approximately one-third of all cases of NHL, are considered a low-grade lymphoma and typically present in mid- to late adulthood, are slow growing, and may evolve over years. The majority of these patients have disseminated disease at diagnosis. On the other hand, diffuse large B-cell lymphoma is an intermediate-grade lymphoma that constitutes approximately 40% of all cases of NHL. These patients typically present with one or more rapidly growing nodal sites, and approximately half have evidence of disseminated disease at presentation.

Dx Diagnosis of NHL requires an excisional lymph node biopsy demonstrating lymphocyte destruction of the normal architecture of the tissue. Histologic, cytologic, and immunologic features, along with cytogenetics, are utilized for further classification.

Tx Treatment of NHL is based on the aggressiveness of each histologic type. The take-home message is that low-grade lymphomas, such as follicular lymphoma, have an indolent course and are characterized by repeated relapses. Generally speaking, it is considered an incurable disease; therefore, the standard of care with regard to treatment in advanced-stage disease in an asymptomatic individual has often entailed an observational approach. The initiation of treatment is dictated by the development of symptomatic disease or development of cytopenias requiring supportive therapy. Many treatment options have been established in the literature, including the use of chemotherapy, monoclonal antibodies, and more recently chemoimmunotherapy with maintenance immunotherapy. In contrast, intermediate- or high-grade lymphomas, such as diffuse large B-cell lymphoma, are considered potentially curable with aggressive therapy. In this setting, chemoimmunotherapy with CHOP-R (cyclophosphamide, doxorubicin, vincristine, prednisone, rituximab) is the standard of care. There are also prognostic indices that can be utilized to define therapy, such as the International Prognostic Index (IPI) and the Follicular Lymphoma International Prognostic Index (FLIPI) scores; these scores are based on pretreatment characteristics found to be independent predictors of death. **See Cecil Essentials 51.**

Mononucleosis/EBV

Pφ It is estimated that approximately 90% of cases of infectious mononucleosis are caused by EBV. B cells become infected upon contact with EBV-infected epithelium of the oropharynx and salivary glands. Enlargement of lymphoid tissue occurs with the expansion of EBV-infected B cells and reactive T cells.

TP While a childhood infection is often subclinical, it is estimated that approximately 30% of adolescents and young adults will present with the classic triad of fever, pharyngitis, and generalized lymphadenopathy. Other reported symptoms and signs include headache, GI symptoms, splenomegaly, hepatomegaly, and rash.

Dx The heterophile antibody test is a diagnostic test for evaluation of infectious mononucleosis due to EBV infection; 90% of cases are heterophile positive. The basis of this test is the Paul-Bunnell antigen, which is present on the surface of EBV-infected cells. In heterophile-negative cases, determination of EBV antibodies may be helpful to establish the diagnosis.

Tx Supportive care. Corticosteroids may be helpful in complicated cases—tonsillar enlargement causing airway compromise, autoimmune hemolytic anemia, severe thrombocytopenia, and aplastic anemia. **See Cecil Essentials 51, 95.**

Sarcoidosis

Pφ Sarcoidosis is a multisystem disorder of unknown cause. Affected organs demonstrate an accumulation of T lymphocytes and mononuclear phagocytes, noncaseating epithelioid granulomas, and distortion of normal tissue architecture.

TP Although sarcoidosis can be discovered as an incidental finding on chest radiograph in an asymptomatic person, many clinical presentations can include constitutional symptoms of fever, fatigue, and weight loss. The typical presentation of sarcoidosis includes cough, dyspnea, chest discomfort, and polyarthritis. Hilar lymphadenopathy has been estimated to occur in 75% to 90% of patients. Splenomegaly has been estimated to occur in 5% to 10% of patients. The eyes and skin may also be involved.

Dx A diagnosis of sarcoidosis is made by clinical presentation, radiographic studies, and the presence on biopsy of noncaseating granulomas, with exclusion of other causes of the abnormalities such as infection.

Tx First-line therapy for sarcoidosis is corticosteroids. The most difficult dilemma is often when and if therapy should be initiated. Spontaneous remission of disease has been reported in up to two thirds of patients. **See Cecil Essentials 18, 95.**

Primary HIV Infection

Pφ The acute HIV syndrome is estimated to occur in approximately 50% to 70% of individuals within 2 to 6 weeks after primary infection. This acute viral syndrome is proposed to be secondary to wide dissemination of the virus and the retrafficking of lymphocytes.

TP The typical presentation is characterized by symptoms consistent with many acute viral syndromes, including such symptoms as fever, pharyngitis, lymphadenopathy, headache, fatigue, weight loss, mucocutaneous lesions, and GI symptoms.

Dx Diagnosis of HIV in the setting of the acute HIV syndrome is particularly difficult because it usually precedes by several weeks the development of HIV-specific antibodies detected by screening measures (ELISA/Western blot analysis). HIV RNA testing could be considered in the setting of a high-risk patient with symptoms of acute HIV infection with a negative ELISA and Western blot, which may represent the "window period" before seroconversion.

Tx There is a lack of randomized clinical data that demonstrate a value in initiating highly active antiretroviral therapy (HAART) during the acute HIV syndrome. **See Cecil Essentials 95, 108.**

ZEBRA ZONE

a. **Other infectious causes of lymphadenopathy and splenomegaly:** include mycobacterial infections such as tuberculosis and disseminated fungal infections such as histoplasmosis. Appropriate stains of excised lymph nodes may confirm the diagnosis.

b. **Autoimmune diseases such as rheumatoid arthritis and systemic lupus erythematosus:** can present with lymphadenopathy and splenomegaly. Specific serologic studies will establish the diagnosis.

c. **Other malignant diseases in which lymphadenopathy and splenomegaly can be observed:** include chronic and acute myeloid and lymphoid leukemia, Waldenström macroglobulinemia, and amyloidosis.

d. In certain **storage diseases**, such as Gaucher disease, as well as in certain endocrinopathies such as hyperthyroidism, lymphadenopathy and splenomegaly may be observed.

Practice-Based Learning and Improvement: Evidence-Based Medicine

Title
Chemotherapy plus involved-field radiation in early-stage Hodgkin's disease

Authors
Ferme C, Eghbali H, Meerwaldt JH, et al.

Institution
EORTC-GELA (Groupe d'Etudes des Lymphomes de l'Adulte) H8 trial results as of January 2006

Reference
N Engl J Med 2007;357:1916–1927

Problem
Radiation therapy with or without combination chemotherapy in treating patients with previously untreated stage I or stage II Hodgkin lymphoma

Intervention

Patients with favorable prognostic features were randomized to subtotal nodal radiation therapy or combination therapy consisting of three cycles of MOPP (mechlorethamine, vincristine, procarbazine, prednisone)-ABV (doxorubicin, bleomycin, vinblastine) plus involved-field radiation therapy. Patients with unfavorable prognostic features were randomized to one of three regimens: six or four cycles of MOPP-ABV plus involved-field radiation therapy or four cycles of MOPP-ABV plus subtotal nodal radiation therapy.

Quality of evidence

Level I

Outcome/effect

In the patients with the favorable prognostic features, the difference in the estimated 5-year event-free survival rate was 24 percentage points (95% confidence interval [CI], 18 to 29; $P < 0.001$), favoring the combination-therapy group consisting of three cycles of MOPP-ABV plus involved-field radiation therapy. There were 19 deaths in the group receiving subtotal nodal radiation therapy and 4 in the combination-therapy group. The 10-year overall survival estimate was significantly higher in the combination-therapy group (97%) than in the group receiving subtotal nodal radiation therapy (92%, $P = 0.001$). In the patients with the unfavorable prognostic features, there were no significant differences in the 5-year event-free survival estimates or estimated overall survival among the three groups.

Historical significance/comments

This study demonstrated that patients with favorable prognostic features can no longer be treated with subtotal nodal radiation therapy alone. The new standard of care should be a combination of chemotherapy and radiation therapy based on an increased event-free survival rate and overall survival. The standard treatment is three courses of doxorubicin-containing regimen followed by involved-field radiation therapy. This study supports the use of four cycles of a doxorubicin-containing regimen and involved-field radiation therapy in patients with unfavorable prognostic features as the standard of care.

Interpersonal and Communication Skills

Avoid Technical Terms and Medical Jargon

When communicating with patients, be mindful to avoid technical terms and medical jargon that you would use with colleagues. This matter is particularly important when discussing oncologic issues. Offer explanations using clear and simple language. Here are a few suggestions to keep in mind when talking to patients.

Instead of saying	Say
Inoperable	Can't be cured by an operation
Malignant	Cancerous
Metastasized	Cancer has spread
Monitor	Keep an eye-on; check
Noninvasive	Without surgery or cutting skin
Oncologist	Cancer doctor
Palliative care	Will provide symptom management
Radiology	X-ray department
Referral	Send to another doctor
Toxic	Poisonous
Ventilator	Breathing machine

From Mann BD. Surgery: a competency-based companion. Philadelphia: Elsevier; 2009, p. 205.

Professionalism

Show Commitment to Professional Excellence and Lifelong Learning

The importance of commitment to lifelong learning in the profession of medicine is clearly illustrated in the fields of hematology and medical oncology. What we know today to be the standard of care will not necessarily remain the standard of care tomorrow. The treatment of Hodgkin lymphoma is a success story in this field. Over the past four decades advances in the field of radiation oncology and the introduction of combination chemotherapy have improved the cure rates of this disease to as high as 80% to 90%. This advancement has been driven by the scientific research that works to gain an understanding of the biology of the disease and in doing so serves as the basis for the establishment of clinical trials.

Systems-Based Practice

Respond to Critical Laboratory Results

In patients with lymphoma who are treated with chemotherapy, certain laboratory parameters may need to be periodically monitored, and critical test results must be addressed in a timely manner (i.e., called to the physician within 60 minutes of the result becoming available) to avoid the possibility of adverse outcome. The following process should be utilized in the hospital setting by the staff informed of the critical value:

- Always use two patient identifiers to ensure the correct patient.
- Listen to the critical result from the diagnostic department.
- Document the critical result in the patient's chart.
- Read back and verify the result and patient identification to the diagnostic department.
- Notify the physician of the result.
- Ask the physician to repeat back the patient identification and result.
- If the physician provides any verbal orders in regard to the critical value, read the order back to the physician.

Section VIII
ONCOLOGIC DISEASES

Section Editor
Mary Denshaw-Burke MD

Section Contents

38 **Breast Mass (Case 30)**
Tamara Donatelli DO, Jennifer Sabol MD, Roxane Weighall DO,
Ari D. Brooks MD, and Mary Denshaw-Burke MD

39 **Prostate Mass (Case 31)**
Amy L. Curran MD and Clifford H. Pemberton MD

40 **Testicular Mass (Case 32)**
Christopher Greenleaf MD, Tamara Donatelli DO,
Jennifer Sherwood MD, and Mary Denshaw-Burke MD

41 **Neck Mass (Case 33)**
Bradley W. Lash MD and Erik L. Zeger MD

42 **Pigmented Skin Lesions (Case 34)**
James G. Bittner IV MD, Joan R. Johnson MD, MMS,
and D. Scott Lind MD

43 **Incidentally Discovered Mass Lesions (Case 35)**
Tami Berry MD and Joseph J. Muscato MD

44 **Oncologic Emergencies (Case 36: A Problem Set of Three**
Common Cases)
Minal Dhamankar MD and Zonera Ali MD

45 **Paraneoplastic Syndromes (Case 37: A Problem Set of Three**
Common Cases)
Nishanth Sukumaran MD and Mary Denshaw-Burke MD

Chapter 38
Breast Mass (Case 30)

Tamara Donatelli DO, Jennifer Sabol MD,
Roxane Weighall DO, Ari D. Brooks MD,
and Mary Denshaw-Burke MD

Case: Breast mass in a 44-year-old female.

Differential Diagnosis

Benign	Malignant
Fibroadenoma	Infiltrating (or invasive) ductal carcinoma
Cyst	Invasive lobular carcinoma
Benign breast nodularity	

Speaking Intelligently

When evaluating a breast mass, we always think about the **triple test** (clinical examination, imaging, pathology). We examine the patient while paying attention to the characteristics of the mass and review the mammogram or ultrasonogram to determine our level of clinical suspicion. If our level of suspicion warrants a tissue diagnosis, we use the least invasive biopsy technique that will yield an accurate diagnosis. In the case of a palpable breast mass, this is most often a fine-needle aspiration biopsy or a core needle biopsy. Although we may occasionally suspect that the mass represents benign breast nodularity, biopsy is still recommended for peace of mind (sometimes ours, often the patient's).

PATIENT CARE

Clinical Thinking
- **Clinical examination**, including a focused history and physical, will determine the first step in the algorithm of diagnosing and treating diseases of the breast. A 44-year-old female who presents with a breast mass will raise my level of suspicion for a malignant mass, as opposed to a 19-year-old female with a palpable mass for whom the likelihood of malignancy is relatively low.

- Any palpable mass should be imaged. In a 44-year-old female, **diagnostic mammography**, including ultrasonography, is indicated for complete evaluation.
- A fine-needle aspiration or core needle biopsy under local anesthesia should be performed on all lesions. If the mass is palpable or seen on ultrasonography, then this can be done in the surgeon's office. Otherwise, the lesion requires visualization by radiography or MRI in a breast center.
- The treatment for a malignant mass requires a multispecialty approach and should involve a team consisting of a surgeon, medical oncologist, and radiation oncologist.

History
- A complete history includes age, race, age at menarche, the number of previous breast biopsies and any diagnosis of atypia, age at first live birth, and the number of first- or second-degree relatives (both maternal and paternal) who have had breast and/or ovarian cancer. In addition, exogenous use of hormones and lactation history should be noted. Many of these risk factors can be applied to the Gail model, which estimates the probability of developing invasive breast cancer over 5 years and a lifetime in a population of women utilizing screening mammography.
- Details regarding the mass should include duration of symptoms, alterations in size, skin changes, relationship to the menstrual cycle and/or pregnancy, associated pain, and nipple discharge.

Physical Examination
- Having a chaperone present is a good idea when performing a breast examination, particularly if you are a male.
- The breast should be palpated systematically in a sweeping motion covering all four quadrants of the breast. You should examine the breasts with the patient upright with arms relaxed and supine with the ipsilateral arm extended over the head. Observe for symmetry, skin changes, dimpling, retraction, and nipple discharge. It is important that palpation extend up the tail of Spence (far upper outer quadrant toward axilla) so as to evaluate all breast tissue.
- The axillary, supraclavicular, and infraclavicular lymph nodes should be palpated, and lymphadenopathy should be documented.
- If a mass is palpable, note its diameter and mobility, and whether it is best described as nodular, smooth, firm, and/or rubbery. Findings are conventionally documented in clock positions with the nipple as the center. For example, "a 2-cm mass at the 10:00 position, 1 cm from the nipple on the right breast."
- In menstruating women with a variable breast mass, it may be appropriate to repeat the exam at different points in the patient's menstrual cycle.
- Be sure to discuss your findings with the patient.

IMAGING CONSIDERATIONS

→ **Bilateral screening mammography:** Used for asymptomatic screening. Screening mammograms have been shown to lower the chance of dying from breast cancer by 35% in women over the age of 50 years, and by 25% to 35% for women between 40 and 50 years. Current recommendations are variable. The US Preventive Services Task Force (USPSTF) recommends imaging beginning at age 50 years for women at average risk of breast cancer. The American Cancer Society recommends yearly mammogram screening beginning at age 40 years for women at average risk of breast cancer. Screening mammography consists of two views of both breasts (craniocaudal and mediolateral oblique). The Breast Imaging Reporting and Data System (BI-RADS) assessment is useful in determining management (see Table 38-1 on the following page for details). $130

→ **Diagnostic mammography:** Indicated for patients with breast complaints, such as a palpable mass or nipple discharge, or abnormality on breast exam or screening mammogram. A radiologist is always actively involved in this examination and relays the outcome to the patient. $157

→ **Ultrasound:** Not used for screening. Useful in determining if a mass is cystic or solid. May be used to guide a needle biopsy. $62

→ **MRI:** Both screening and diagnostic. May be a valuable screening adjunct in genetically high-risk patients (greater than 20% lifetime risk). Also useful to clarify vague mammographic abnormalities. $435

COMMON MAMMOGRAPHIC FINDINGS

Assessment of risk depends on characteristics of findings and time frame of development.

Masses

Benign Mammographic Masses
Well-circumscribed and smooth masses are suggestive of a benign etiology. The typical benign mass is either a cyst or a fibroadenoma. Ultrasonography will differentiate the two.

Table 38-1 Breast Imaging Reporting and Data System (BI-RADS®)	
Category	**Recommendation**
0: Incomplete: Need Additional Imaging Evaluation and/or Prior Mammograms	More information is needed to determine whether a finding is abnormal
1: Negative	Continue routine screening
2: Benign	Continue routine screening
3: Probably Benign	Initial short-interval follow-up suggested (usually 6 months)
4: Suspicious Abnormality	Usually requires biopsy
5: Highly Suggestive of Malignancy	Appropriate actions should be taken (requires biopsy or surgical treatment)
6: Known Biopsy-Proven Malignancy	Appropriate actions should taken

From the American College of Radiology (ACR). ACR BI-RADS®–4th Edition. ACR Breast Imaging Reporting and Data System, Breast Imaging Atlas; BI-RADS. Reston, VA. American College of Radiology; 2003. Reprinted as modified and approved with permission of the American College of Radiology. No other representation of this material is authorized without expressed, written permission from the American College of Radiology.

Malignant Mammographic Masses

See Figure 38-1.

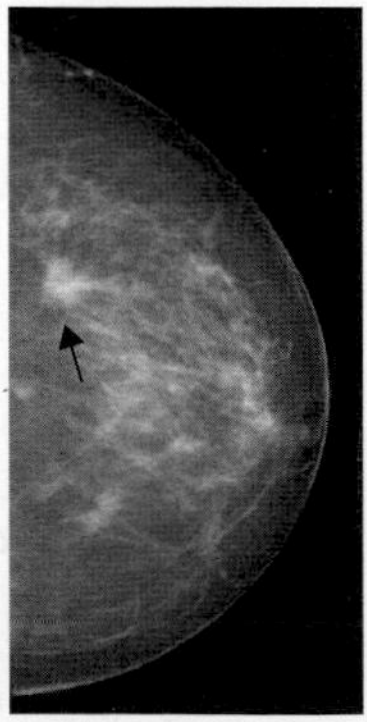

Figure 38-1 Malignant masses. Typically irregular and spiculated, and often contain calcifications. (From Mann B. Surgery: a competency-based companion. Philadelphia: Elsevier; 2009. Figure 20-4.)

Architectural Distortion
See Figure 38-2.

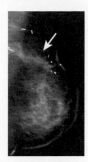

Figure 38-2 Architectural distortion. May be the earliest sign of breast cancer. May also be associated with scars from previous surgery. (From Mann B: Surgery: a competency-based companion. Philadelphia: Elsevier; 2009. Figure 20-5.)

Calcifications
Calcifications are the deposition of calcium in the breast tissue or its elements. Calcifications are divided into three types: benign, indeterminate, and high probability of malignancy (Figs. 38-3 and 38-4).

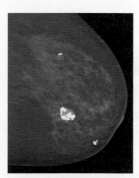

Figure 38-3 Benign calcifications can be coarse, rodlike associated with blood vessels, round, popcorn-shaped, or milk of calcium (concave). (From Mann B: Surgery: a competency-based companion. Philadelphia: Elsevier; 2009. Figure 20-1.)

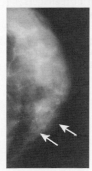

Figure 38-4 Malignant calcifications are more likely to be pleomorphic, heterogeneous, clustered, or branching. (From Mann B: Surgery: a competency-based companion. Philadelphia: Elsevier; 2009. Figure 20-2.)

PATIENT CARE

Biopsy Approaches

- **Fine-needle aspiration biopsy:** Easily done in the office or imaging suite with an 18- to 22-gauge needle under local anesthesia. Interpretation is very dependent on the experience of the pathologist interpreting the slide; cannot distinguish between in situ and invasive cancer. $320
- **Core needle biopsy:** Slightly larger needle but still performed under local anesthesia. Delivers a specimen upon which the tumor's architecture can be determined; hence, the study is able to determine if the lesion is invasive. $320
- **Stereotactic biopsy:** Core needle biopsy utilizing mammography to localize the lesion; requires a specialized table and computer software. Performed as an outpatient procedure under local anesthesia. $570
- **Excisional biopsy:** Should the modalities listed above fail to yield a diagnosis or the biopsy results are discordant with radiologic imaging, surgical excision is indicated. Typically performed as outpatient procedure with IV sedation. $1784

Clinical Entities   Medical Knowledge

Fibroadenoma

Pφ Fibroadenomas are well-circumscribed, solid masses. They contain fibrous and epithelial elements, and are thought to represent benign hyperplastic lobules. The cut surface is white or yellow, and bulging beyond its pseudocapsule.

TP Fibroadenomas can appear at any age. The typical patient is younger than 40 years; fibroadenomas are common in teenagers. Physical exam demonstrates a smooth, well-circumscribed mass that is mobile and rubbery in texture.

Dx Ultrasound shows a mass with smooth margins and benign characteristics. In older women, "popcorn calcifications" may be associated with involuting fibroadenomas. Core needle biopsy can confirm the diagnosis.

Tx Small asymptomatic fibroadenomas do not have to be excised. However, excision is recommended if there is evidence of growth, an inconclusive needle biopsy, size > 2–3 cm, or bothersome tenderness. **See Cecil Essentials 71.**

Cyst

Pφ Cysts are round to oval well-circumscribed masses that can be single or multiple. They are fluid-filled benign sacs located within the fibrous tissue of the breast.

TP Cysts are common in patients undergoing hormonal fluctuations. They are common in premenopausal women and around the onset of menopause. On examination, cysts are smooth and frequently tender.

Dx On mammogram, cysts have a smooth distinct border. An ultrasound will easily confirm the presence of fluid and has a diagnostic accuracy of close to 100%. Cysts may fluctuate in size or presence over serial examinations.

Tx Asymptomatic cysts do not require treatment. Those that are painful or of concern (having septations, intracystic growth, or thick walls) should be aspirated or excised depending on how suspicious they appear. Cyst fluid is typically "straw-colored." Other typical benign fluid colors are white, gray, blue, and green. Bloody aspirate should always be sent for cytology and the patient reevaluated by imaging with the possibility of excisional biopsy in mind. **See Cecil Essentials 71.**

Benign Breast Nodularity

Pφ Normal breast tissue can have a nodular pattern in some women. This is more marked in the upper outer quadrants and is often very tender in response to normal cyclic hormonal variations. This cyclic tenderness is more pronounced as women become perimenopausal, and often one breast is affected more than the other.

TP The typical patient is premenopausal and complains of an intermittently tender mass that seems to fluctuate in size. The pain is characteristically worse in the 7 days before her menstrual period and then begins to abate with the onset of menses.

Dx Mammograms and ultrasonography typically show normal breast tissue. Ultrasonography may show thickened breast tissue approaching the skin in the area of the mass. Women with dense breasts may require a breast MRI scan to rule out carcinoma.

Tx If the palpable mass is believed to be suspicious or if a woman's anxiety level is acute, a biopsy should be performed to exclude malignancy. **See Cecil Essentials 71.**

Malignant Mass

Pφ The common malignant breast masses are invasive ductal carcinoma and invasive lobular carcinoma.

TP **Infiltrating (or invasive) ductal carcinoma:** The typical patient has a firm dominant mobile mass found by self-examination or by a health-care practitioner. The mass may be associated with skin retraction, palpable adenopathy, and/or nipple discharge. In the more advanced stages, the mass may be fixed to surrounding structures and associated with erythema, skin edema, skin ulceration, peau d'orange, and matted axillary nodes. A carcinoma may be nonpalpable and present as an unexpected density on the screening mammogram.

    Invasive lobular carcinoma represents only 5% to 10% of breast cancers and is classically more difficult to identify mammographically as well as on palpation because of its classic single-cell (Indian file) growth histologically. Lobular carcinoma is often perceived as a "thickening" rather than as a discrete mass, and what you feel or see may be only the "tip of the iceberg." The final pathologic size of an invasive lobular cancer is often much greater than anticipated as a result of this growth pattern.

Dx Tissue biopsy is essential to confirm the diagnosis of a malignant mass. If the lesion is palpable, a fine-needle aspiration or percutaneous core needle biopsy can be performed in the office. (Many surgeons prefer to be sure a mammogram is obtained before biopsy because of the risk of hematoma formation.) Ultrasound or stereotactic guidance may be utilized for diagnosis if the lesion is not palpable. Open incisional or excisional biopsies are appropriate when needle biopsy cannot be performed or is inconclusive.

Tx **Management of breast carcinoma:** All patients with newly diagnosed breast cancer should receive a metastatic workup appropriate to clinical stage to rule out distant disease to the most common sites of metastasis, namely bone, lung, and liver. Fewer than 10% of patients will present at stage IV. Once patients appear to have locally resectable disease, the patients are confronted with two main issues: local control and microscopic systemic disease control.

Local control is often the first decision a patient faces and can often be confusing. Try to simplify these choices, and describe the options of mastectomy and breast conservation to the patient.

Mastectomy involves removing all of the breast tissue (simple mastectomy) or breast tissue and surrounding lymph nodes if involved (modified radical mastectomy), while preserving much of the overlying skin. It may or may not include immediate breast reconstruction.

Breast conservation therapy consists of **lumpectomy** to negative margins (for unifocal disease) and **radiation therapy** (either whole or partial breast irradiation).

It is important to note that these two local treatment choices for invasive carcinoma are equivalent in terms of overall survival. Local recurrence after mastectomy is 14%, while it is 5% to 7% following breast conservation.

Some patients may not be considered good candidates for breast conservation therapy if they have multifocal disease, extensive skin involvement such as inflammatory cancer, or inability to complete radiation therapy.

All patients having cancer, with the exception of those with noninvasive cancer, will have evaluation of their lymph nodes at the time of surgery to evaluate the extent of disease. Traditionally, if there is biopsy-proven lymph node involvement, additional surgical therapy has included resection of levels I and II axillary nodes or palpable disease. However, a recent study released by the American College of Surgeons Oncology Group Z-11 Trial has suggested that additional axillary surgery may not be necessary and that the small amount of microscopic disease may be eradicated by chemotherapy. While this is not yet the standard of care, these data may lead to a paradigm shift in the surgical management of breast cancer.

Adjuvant therapy for malignancy: Once the surgery has been performed, physicians now have the information needed to predict the possibility of microscopic systemic disease (i.e., the need for adjuvant systemic therapy). This is a complex decision that is based on many factors and requires a thorough dialogue between the patient and physician. Traditionally, histopathologic features such as tumor size, tumor grade, estrogen receptor (ER) and progesterone receptor (PR) status, *HER2/neu* status, and axillary lymph node involvement have been used to make recommendations about adjuvant chemotherapy. More recently, predictive molecular profiling with either OncotypeDX or MammaPrint assays has been widely used to help with this decision. Patients with low-risk profiles are typically treated with adjuvant anti-estrogen hormonal therapy and can be spared the side effects of chemotherapy.

Adjuvant chemotherapy plays a more significant role in patients who have a tumor that is ER/PR negative, *HER2/neu* positive, or with axillary lymph node involvement. In general, the patients with the greatest risk of disease recurrence obtain the largest absolute benefit from the use of adjuvant chemotherapy. Multiple chemotherapy drug combinations are appropriate in the adjuvant setting, often including anthracyclines and taxanes. For patients with ER- or PR-positive cancers, oral anti-estrogen hormonal therapy for a minimum of 5 years reduces the risk of local and systemic recurrence as well as contralateral breast cancer by 40% to 50%. Premenopausal or perimenopausal women are treated with tamoxifen. Postmenopausal women may be treated with either tamoxifen or aromatase inhibitors; however, aromatase inhibitors are considered the first-line therapy in postmenopausal women. Adjuvant! Online is a wonderful risk assessment tool that can help the clinician assess an individual's risk of dying of comorbid disease versus risk of systemic disease recurrence, and estimates both the impact of anti-estrogen hormonal therapy as well as cytotoxic chemotherapy on overall survival.

Once a patient's systemic risk has been addressed, the final treatment step is radiation therapy if indicated. All patients undergoing breast conservation will require radiation as part of their treatment. Most patients undergoing mastectomy will require radiation only if the tumor size is ≥5 cm, if there are positive margins of resection, if there is extracapsular nodal involvement, or if there is involvement of four or more axillary lymph nodes with metastatic cancer. **See Cecil Essentials 57, 59, 68.**

ZEBRA ZONE

a. **Phyllodes tumors** are stromal tumors that may grow rapidly to large sizes, resembling fibroadenomas microscopically. They may be locally recurrent, and 10% are frankly malignant with the ability to spread hematogenously like sarcomas. Treatment is wide local excision.

b. **Metastatic deposits:** The breast can be a site for metastatic deposits from other malignancies, although this is rare. One of the most common lesions in this category is lymphoma.

c. **Trauma:** A hematoma due to trauma can cause a clinical mass. Later in the course, the mammographic appearance may be similar to that seen in malignancy; "fat necrosis," a frequent consequence of trauma, may leave an irregular mass, often containing calcifications.

d. **Male breast cancer:** Male breast cancer accounts for less than 1% of all breast cancers. Gynecomastia frequently presents as a mass that is smooth, firm, and symmetrically distributed beneath the areola. If a malignant breast mass is suspected in a male, the biopsy approaches are similar to those for women.

Practice-Based Learning and Improvement

The National Surgical Adjuvant Breast and Bowel Project (NSABP) is a multi-institutional and multinational research organization that was founded in 1958 to address controversial issues in breast (and subsequently colon) cancer care. At the time of its establishment, the reigning theory of breast cancer, promulgated in the late 19th century by William Stewart Halstead, was that breast cancer spread in a stepwise local fashion from one point to the next and that this spread had a predictable time line. Based on this principle, the radical mastectomy became the standard of care for all patients with breast cancer, regardless of tumor size. In the 1960s, Bernard and Edwin Fisher recognized circulating tumor cells in the blood of all breast cancer patients and proposed the then radical hypothesis that breast cancer is a "systemic" disease from its inception and that radical surgery may be unnecessary for the majority of patients. The NSABP B-04 trial, initiated in 1971 comparing radical mastectomy and simple mastectomy plus radiation, provided evidence that less radical surgery could provide equal survival, ultimately serving as the foundation principle for breast conservation therapy and thus enhancing quality of life for many women with a diagnosis of breast cancer.

In addition to providing the framework for randomized prospective treatment trials, the NSABP has provided pathologic material for retrospective analyses as new concepts have been advanced in prognostic indicators and response patterns to treatment. The more recent NSABP studies have collected a repository of tumor tissue and blood samples to be used for future research. The National Cancer Institute (NCI) has recognized this database as a "national treasure."

To date, over 500 participating institutions and more than 110,000 patients have participated in clinical trials. For additional information on past, present, and future protocols as well as links to the published data, visit the NSABP website at http://www.nsabp.pitt.edu.

Interpersonal and Communication Skills

Discussing Family History and Its Impact

A major concern for the breast cancer patient is the consideration of how the diagnosis affects other members of her family. For a woman whose mother or sister had breast cancer, there can be up to a three- to fourfold increased risk for developing breast cancer; that risk is further increased if the cancer was bilateral or premenopausal. Therefore, an emphasis should be placed on obtaining a thorough family history as it pertains to breast and ovarian cancers. The USPSTF has recommended that patients be referred for genetic counseling if they have a family history positive for multiple close relatives with breast or ovarian cancer, have a close relative with bilateral or premenopausal breast cancer, have a family history of male breast cancer, or are of Ashkenazi Jewish ancestry. The decision to obtain genetic counseling is often difficult for patients, and they should be counseled on both the indications for testing as well as the management options for individuals who are determined to be carriers of the autosomal-dominant *BRCA1* and *BRCA2* genes. In addition to changes in screening initiation and interval (with mammography and, at times, MRI), many women will consider tamoxifen therapy, and prophylactic mastectomy and oophorectomy, after a positive genetic test. These are often emotionally challenging decisions, and these discussions should always be approached gently with interpersonal sensitivity and specificity.

Professionalism

Commitment to Improving Access to Care
In the realm of health-care reform and at a time when approximately 20 million women in the United States are uninsured, it is the role of the physician to be an advocate for patients by linking them to the numerous philanthropic and government-funded resources that provide free or low-cost mammograms to low-income or uninsured women. For example, the Centers for Disease Control and Prevention (CDC) coordinate the National Breast and Cervical Cancer Early Detection Program, which provides screening services, including clinical breast exams and mammograms, to eligible women throughout the United States and in several US territories. Contact information for local programs is available on the CDC's website at http://apps.nccd.cdc.gov/cancercontacts/nbccedp/contacts.asp or by calling the CDC at 1-800-CDC-INFO (1-800-232-4636). Information about low-cost or free mammography screening programs is also available through the NCI's Cancer Information Service (CIS) at 1-800-4-CANCER (1-800-422-6237).

Systems-Based Practice

Standardizing Clinical Information: The BI-RADS Lexicon
The BI-RADS lexicon is a systems approach to standardize common language and is intended to facilitate communication between radiologists, referring physicians, and patients. Table 38-1 shows a systems-based approach to reporting the results of mammography.

Chapter 39
Prostate Mass (Case 31)

Amy L. Curran MD and Clifford H. Pemberton MD

Editors' Note: The editors felt that the section on oncology should include the issues of (1) recurrent malignant disease, (2) caring for metastatic disease, and (3) care when treatment is no longer efficacious or advised. We chose the chapter on prostate cancer as the chapter in which to integrate these principles.

Case: The patient is a 65-year-old man who presents for an annual examination. He has no complaints, and his only medical condition is well-controlled hypertension. Previously the physician and patient had decided to obtain annual prostate specific antigen (PSA) testing based on the patient's positive family history of prostate cancer. This year the PSA is found to be slightly elevated at 5 ng/mL, compared to a level of 2.1 ng/mL a year ago. On physical exam, his digital rectal exam (DRE) is remarkable for right-sided prostatic induration. The patient undergoes an ultrasound-guided biopsy taken at the suspicious area and sampling throughout the gland. Pathology confirmed adenocarcinoma of the prostate with a Gleason score of 6.

Speaking Intelligently

There are several approaches to treating early-stage prostate cancer, and the optimal treatment must be tailored to the patient. Because a large percentage of patients die *with* prostate cancer, rather than dying *from* prostate cancer, it is important to first determine the patient's life expectancy. Next, one can utilize information about the tumor to assess its recurrence risk. **Low-risk prostate cancer is defined by small tumors (T1 or T2a), Gleason scores ≤ 6, and PSA < 10 ng/mL.**

What Is a Gleason Score?
A Gleason score is assigned to prostate cancer based upon its histopathologic appearance. Gleason grades range from 1 to 5, with 5 having the worst prognosis. A Gleason score of 1 is a well-differentiated cancer that has small, uniform glands, whereas a Gleason grade of 5 represents a poorly differentiated tumor that lacks glands and has sheets of cells. The pathologist assigns a grade to the two most common tumor patterns; the two grades are added together to give a Gleason score (≤6 is well differentiated, 7 is moderately differentiated, and 8–10 is poorly differentiated).

Therapeutic Options for Prostate Cancer

Radical prostatectomy	• For tumors confined to the prostate in patients with a life expectancy >10 years and well enough to undergo major surgery. • Significant risk of incontinence and erectile dysfunction.
External-beam radiation therapy	• Similar progression-free survival to surgery for low-risk patients. • Addition of pelvic lymph node irradiation and/or androgen-deprivation therapy for higher risk groups. • Advantages include avoiding surgical complications, and less incontinence and erectile dysfunction. • Disadvantages include long treatment course, bowel and bladder symptoms during treatment, and late radiation proctitis.
Brachytherapy	• Involves planting radioactive sources into the prostate tissue. • Treatment is completed in 1 day and is effective for low-risk tumors. • Patients with very large or small prostate glands, bladder outlet obstruction, or prior transurethral resection of the prostate (TURP) are not good candidates for brachytherapy. • General anesthesia is required for placement.
Hormonal therapy	• Androgen-deprivation therapy through either administration of a luteinizing hormone-releasing hormone (LHRH) agonist or orchiectomy. • Used routinely with definitive radiation therapy for higher risk disease as well as for metastatic disease. • Adverse effects include osteoporosis with greater incidence of fracture, obesity, insulin resistance, and dyslipidemia.
Active surveillance	• Monitoring course of the disease with the expectation to intervene if the cancer progresses. • Reasonable option for men with low-risk cancers and a short life expectancy.

The patient in this case opted for treatment with external beam radiation and had a complete response with normalization of his PSA. For 9 years he was considered disease free with regard to his prostatic cancer. Unfortunately, 9 years after treatment the patient presented to the ED with severe back pain. The pain began about 4 weeks earlier and had worsened in the past few days, making it difficult for him to sleep. He is taking over-the-counter medications, including acetaminophen and ibuprofen, with little benefit.

Differential Diagnosis

Back Pain in a Patient with a History of Cancer		
Bone pain/spinal cord compression from metastatic disease	Compression fracture	Musculoskeletal low back pain

PATIENT CARE

Clinical Thinking

- Patients with cancer commonly present with pain, especially at original diagnosis or at disease progression. Sometimes the pain can be acute caused by a medical emergency such as spinal cord compression or a bowel obstruction. More frequently, cancer patients have chronic pain and need ongoing care including monitoring of pain medications, referral to pain specialists for procedures, consultation and treatment with radiation oncology, and psychosocial support.
- Although there is a broad differential diagnosis (including disk herniation and spinal stenosis) in patients presenting with back pain, those with a history of cancer should be imaged to rule out metastatic disease to the spine and the possibility of cord compression.
- A dose of corticosteroids should be given before definitive diagnosis, if spinal cord compression is possible.
- Intravenous narcotics are appropriate front-line therapy when a patient presents in severe pain refractory to oral medications. In addition to narcotics, adjuvant medications such as corticosteroids, nonsteroidal anti-inflammatory drugs (NSAIDs), and muscle relaxants can both assist with pain control and allow patients to use lower doses of narcotics.
- Patients with severe chronic pain often require a combination of long-acting narcotics for baseline pain control and short-acting narcotics for breakthrough pain. A common starting point is to prescribe about two thirds of a patient's total daily narcotic dose as long-acting medications and provide about 10% of this dose in short-acting narcotics as needed. One can utilize a "narcotic calculator" to change between IV pain medications and commonly prescribed oral medications.
- A bowel regimen should be started to decrease constipation, which is a common adverse reaction to narcotics.

History

- Develop your own way of taking a pain history. Refer below to the Interpersonal and Communication Skills section, which gives an example of a pain algorithm.

- Whether a patient presents with chest pain from a myocardial infarction, abdominal pain from an acute abdomen, or back pain from metastatic disease, your approach should be similar, modifiable, efficient, and accurate.
- Specifically, for this patient, it is important to elicit the patient's prior history of prostate cancer, the high level of pain that keeps him awake at night, and the fact that his pain is refractory to over-the-counter medications and/or positioning.
- These details should raise your index of suspicion that his back pain might have a serious etiology.

Physical Examination
- **Vital signs and general appearance** are important.
- **Fever** can be a sign of systemic disease (either tumor or infection).
- Perform a thorough **musculoskeletal exam** of the back with attention to tenderness of soft tissue overlying the spinous processes.
- Note limitation in mobility, as well as decreased chest expansion on pulmonary exam.
- A **straight-leg-raising test** should be performed and is positive when the leg cannot be elevated beyond 60 degrees and the test causes sciatic pain.
- A complete **neurologic exam** should be performed, including strength at the ankle and large toe dorsiflexion (L5), plantar flexion strength (S1), and reflexes at both the knee and ankle.
- A **rectal exam** should be performed to ensure normal rectal tone.

Tests for Consideration
- **Metabolic panel** including basic electrolytes, renal function, and calcium. $12
- **PSA**. $26
- **Complete blood count (CBC)**. $11

IMAGING CONSIDERATIONS

→ **MRI of the spine.** Though, in general, low back pain does not mandate early imaging, when you are concerned about metastatic disease, it is important to obtain an MRI scan of the entire spine; it is the test of choice. It is quite common for patients to have multiple foci of disease. $534

Clinical Entities	Medical Knowledge

Bone Metastases/Spinal Cord Compression

Pφ Metastatic disease to the spine typically involves the vertebral body, sparing the disk space.

TP Usually patients are older or have a prior history of cancer when they present with back pain from spine metastases. The pain tends to be severe, is not lessened by lying down, often keeps patients awake at night, and can be refractory to pain medications. Patients presenting with cord compression usually have had back pain for several days or weeks and present with flaccid paraparesis or quadriparesis, early-onset hyporeflexia followed later by hyperreflexia, urinary overflow incontinence and bowel incontinence, and development of a sensory level (change in sensation below a horizontal line across the spine).

Dx Diagnostic tests consist of careful history and physical exam including detailed neurologic exam. If cord compression is considered, an MRI with gadolinium of the entire spine should be performed. If MRI is not available, myelography plus CT is done.

Tx Spinal cord compression is a medical emergency. Corticosteroids should be started in patients immediately, even before definitive testing. The two major treatments are neurosurgical intervention and radiation therapy. Typical patients considered for neurosurgical intervention include those with a single focus of disease who have a reasonable life expectancy. **See Cecil Essentials 58.**

Compression Fracture

Pφ Compression fracture often occurs in elderly patients with a history of osteoporosis. Younger patients with significant trauma can also suffer compression fractures. Sites of lytic lesions from diseases such as multiple myeloma or some metastatic cancer can also present with compression fractures.

TP Localized pain at the site of the compression fracture.

Dx Plain films of the spine will show a compression fracture. In patients with concern of an underlying malignancy, an MRI scan is sometimes indicated to rule out other etiologies.

Tx Pain control is important. Kyphoplasty in select patients can both alleviate pain and support the spine. It is important to treat the patient's underlying disease whether it is from osteoporosis, myeloma, or another malignancy.

Musculoskeletal Low Back Pain

Pφ Musculoskeletal low back pain occurs most frequently as a result of age-related changes in the intervertebral disks and facet joints as well as injury to muscles and ligaments.

TP Back pain is a very common presenting symptom in both the outpatient office and the ED. Low back pain affects both men and women usually between the ages of 30 and 50 years. Increased risks include heavy lifting, twisting, obesity, and poor conditioning.

Dx Patients will often display decreased range of motion of the spine as well as spasm of the paraspinal muscles. The straight leg-raising test should be negative and the patient's neurologic exam normal.

Tx Treatment includes rest from heavy lifting or twisting motions; however, bed rest should be avoided. Patients should maintain activity to keep their muscles and joints from becoming stiff. Additionally, anti-inflammatory medications such as NSAIDs and muscle relaxants can be used. Physical therapy may help some patients, and weight loss should be encouraged for overweight or obese patients. **See Cecil Essentials 119.**

ZEBRA ZONE

a. Osteomyelitis or an **epidural abscess** can also cause severe focal back pain. Infectious processes should be considered in patients who are febrile, bacteremic, have had recent procedures, or have an underlying injection drug use history. Because the usual pathogenesis is from hematogenous dissemination of infection to the back, disease typically involves several vertebral bodies and includes the disk space.

Practice-Based Learning and Improvement: Evidence-Based Medicine

Title
Early palliative care for patients with metastatic non–small cell lung cancer

Authors
Temel JS, Greer JA, Muzikansky A, et al.

Institution
Massachusetts General Hospital (Boston), State University of New York–Buffalo, Columbia University (New York, NY), Yale University (New Haven, CT)

Reference
N Engl J Med 2010;363:733–742

Problem
Metastatic non–small cell lung cancer

Intervention
Early palliative care integrated with standard oncologic care

Comparison/control (quality of evidence)
Randomized controlled study

Outcome/effect
Improved quality of life, fewer depressive symptoms, improved median overall survival in group receiving early palliative care

Historical significance/comments
Medical oncologists have struggled with offering patients concurrent palliative care along with standard oncologic care. There is no surprise that early palliative care improves quality of life and decreases depression; however, the improvement in overall survival was less expected. The current use of palliative care services before hospice is low and tends to be thought of as an alternative to life-sustaining treatment. This trial brings to attention the benefit of early palliative care.

Interpersonal and Communication Skills

Demonstrate Effective and Appropriate Techniques in Eliciting a Pain History

An important skill is to be able to thoroughly and efficiently take a "pain" history from a patient. A similar approach can be utilized whether the patient is presenting with chest pain, abdominal pain, or joint pain. Once you learn a systematic way of eliciting this history, you will get all the pertinent data. Key elements of a pain history include the following:

1. Ask the patient to quantify the level of pain. The standard approach is to have the patient rate his or her pain on a scale of 1 to 10 (Fig. 39-1). There are visual scales using graded faces that are helpful in children, elderly, and disabled patients.

2. Have the patient describe the pain: Quality? Location? Radiation?

3. Ask the patient the timing of the pain. When did it start? Is it constant or intermittent?

4. Determine if anything alleviates or worsens the pain (such as position or medications).

5. Understand how the pain is affecting the patient's quality of life.

6. Is there an underlying psychiatric history, or a history of substance abuse?

7. Determine if the patient has an adequate social support system.

8. Remember that pain must be reassessed frequently.

PAIN RATING SCALE

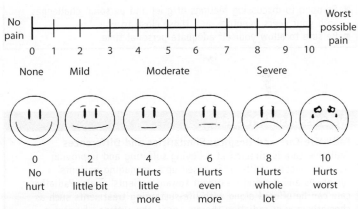

Figure 39-1 Two examples of pain scales. (Adapted from McCaffery M, Pasero C. Pain: clinical manual. St. Louis: Mosby; 1999. Faces pain rating scale modified from Wong DL. Whaley & Wong's essentials of pediatric nursing. 5th ed. St. Louis: Mosby; 1997.)

Professionalism

Self-Regulate Personal Feelings toward Patients That May Impede Effective Communication

In the profession of medicine, you will develop close relationships with your patients. It can be difficult not to allow your personal feelings for a patient or the patient's family to interfere with your professional judgment. All physicians have patients who touch them more deeply than others. When a patient responds well to therapy, it is satisfying for the physician as well as the patient. This can set up a very difficult situation when one of these patients takes a turn for the worse and eventually dies. As caregivers, we cannot grieve for every patient as if they are family members. However, we must acknowledge our grief and learn to confront it or be at risk for burnout or compassion fatigue. We are just as human as our patients and their families. The attributes that make us compassionate doctors also leave us vulnerable in these difficult times. It is often the most compassionate physicians who are most vulnerable to physician burnout, a syndrome that consists of emotional exhaustion, depersonalization, and losing the sense of personal accomplishment. Things you can to do prevent burnout include the following:

- Allow yourself to grieve for the loss of a patient.
- When caring for dying patients, avail yourself of the support of colleagues.
- Be open to discussing feelings of grief and personal challenges with your peers, mentors, and those close to you.
- Be sure to allow yourself adequate personal time.

Systems-Based Practice

Palliative Care and Hospice: Similarities and Differences

Palliative care is directed at relieving suffering and improving patients' quality of life. It is based upon managing patients' symptoms and gearing treatment toward patients' goals. Palliative care can be offered along with life-sustaining treatments such as chemotherapy or radiation therapy, or in the setting of hospice. Palliative care programs are offered in most large US hospitals, but tend to be underutilized. Many physicians erroneously equate **palliative care** with **hospice care** and do not involve a palliative care team (doctors, nurses, social workers, chaplains) early in patient care, but instead wait until a patient is in his or her last weeks of life. Hospice is end-of-life care. Though palliative in nature, once a patient elects **hospice**, life-sustaining treatments are generally stopped. Attention is focused on pain control and symptom management. Hospice care should be directed toward both the patient and the patient's family. Along with supporting the patient and patient's family during the end-of-life period, hospice provides bereavement support for the family.

Suggested Readings

Carragee EJ. Persistent low back pain. N Engl J Med 2005;352: 1891–1898.

Shanafelt T, Adjei A, Meyskens F. When your favorite patient relapses: physician grief and well-being in the practice of oncology. J Clin Oncol 2003;21:2616–2619.

Temel JS, Greer JA, Muzikansky A, et al. Early palliative care for patients with metastatic non–small cell lung cancer. N Engl J Med 2010;363:733–742.

Chapter 40
Testicular Mass (Case 32)

Christopher Greenleaf MD, Tamara Donatelli DO, Jennifer Sherwood MD, and Mary Denshaw-Burke MD

Case: You are consulted by your hospital urologist: "A 19-year-old male presents with a 3.0-cm firm asymptomatic testicular mass of concern. By exam, this does not appear to be a hernia, hydrocele, or varicocele. Please evaluate."

Differential Diagnosis

Benign	Malignant
Inguinal hernia	Seminomas
Hydrocele	Nonseminomatous germ cell tumors
Spermatocele	(NSGCTs)
Varicocele	
Torsion	
Infection: epididymo-orchitis	
Benign tumors: Sertoli-Leydig cell	

Speaking Intelligently

The urologist seeing a patient with an asymptomatic scrotal mass directs the physical examination toward differentiating the benign from the malignant causes. An inguinal hernia can be invaginated at the inguinal ring. A hydrocele will have a cystic consistency. A varicocele will often feel like a "bag of worms." These benign conditions result in relatively soft, compressible masses of the scrotum. A malignant mass, however, palpates as a firm lump with a "woody" or heavy consistency. Almost all scrotal masses should be imaged to further define anatomic features. If the suspicion is high for malignancy, the next step is to obtain an ultrasonogram. A trans-scrotal biopsy should never be performed, because it can disrupt the lymphatic channels and lead to metastases or obscure the anatomy during future inguinal orchiectomy. If a malignant tumor is suspected on exam and imaging, surgical intervention must be instituted quickly (ideally within 48 hours due to the rapid tumor doubling time).

The **medical oncologist** consulted on this patient with a possible testicular cancer suggested by physical exam and ultrasonography should order testing for the *preoperative* tumor markers α-fetoprotein (AFP), lactate dehydrogenase (LDH), and the β subunit of human chorionic gonadotropin (β-hCG). Metastatic workup for a testicular tumor should include a chest radiograph and a CT scan of the abdomen and pelvis, and occasionally a CT scan of the chest.

PATIENT CARE

Clinical Thinking
- All solid/hard scrotal masses are considered malignant until proven otherwise.
- Groin pathology may present as abdominal complaints and vice versa; however, testicular tumors are usually asymptomatic.
- Suspected testicular tumors require urgent surgical removal (radical orchiectomy via an inguinal approach).
- Patients with testicular tumors frequently require additional therapy (such as chemotherapy or radiation therapy), depending on the tumor pathology discovered after resection.
  - After radical orchiectomy, tumor markers (AFP, β-hCG) will have to be monitored until they reach the lowest possible point.

History
- A careful history of the onset and course of a painless mass should be obtained. Particularly helpful are the following questions:

- How long has it been there?
- Does it come and go?
- Has there previously been pain?
- Is there associated erythema or edema?
- If it is persistent, is it staying stable in size or getting bigger or smaller?
- **Review of systems** should focus on the presence of systemic symptoms such as fever and chills, weight loss, and night sweats; back pain; abdominal symptoms such as pain, distension, nausea, and bowel changes; and genitourinary symptoms such as dysuria and urethral discharge.

Physical Examination

The importance of the physical exam is to differentiate benign from malignant processes and to evaluate for possible metastases.

- The physical exam should begin with particular attention to the lymph nodes (especially supraclavicular area). The lungs should be auscultated carefully, particularly with attention to any pulmonary findings that may be problematic for potential future use of bleomycin (a critical chemotherapeutic agent for treatment of testicular cancer).
- The abdominal exam should pay close attention to any scars and/or tenderness in any quadrants. Most importantly, one should carefully feel for any masses (in the setting of testicular cancer, an abdominal mass can indicate massive retroperitoneal lymph node metastases).
- An inguinal exam focuses on signs of lymphadenopathy or inguinal hernias, and potential involvement of the spermatic cord with tumor. The scrotum should be invaginated through the internal ring to inspect for any laxity or bulges within the inguinal canal that may signal an inguinal hernia. The patient should cough and perform a Valsalva maneuver to increase intra-abdominal pressure, which aids in revealing an occult hernia.
- The scrotal exam includes inspection of skin and rugations, and palpation of testicles, epididymides, and spermatic cords. One should evaluate for skin changes (i.e., loss of normal rugation), erythema, edema, induration, and tenderness. The posterolateral portion of the testis is covered by the epididymis, which should be nontender. The spermatic cord runs in the most superior aspect of the scrotum and should be palpated gently between thumb and forefinger. The testes should be examined with the patient in both the recumbent and standing positions. Start at the base of the scrotum and palpate the testes, which should be firm but not hard. It should be noted whether fluid is present around the testicles and whether a mass is palpable (frequently the testicle itself cannot be palpated because of the presence of scrotal fluid or a mass replacing the testicle).

Tests for Consideration
When you have diagnosed a likely testicular cancer by physical exam and ultrasonography:

- Serum markers of **AFP**, **β-hCG**, and **LDH** should be obtained immediately. $24, $21, $9
- Seminomas can be associated with elevated β-hCG (in ~10% of cases), but usually the tumor markers are normal.
- NSGCTs produce AFP and/or β-hCG.
- LDH, a nonspecific marker of tumor burden, may be elevated in patients with either seminomas or NSGCTs.
- These tumor markers should be obtained both before and after orchiectomy, as it is critical to follow their values as a measure of residual disease after initial orchiectomy. Each tumor marker has a specific half-life, and time to normalization of elevated markers is highly predictable. Normalization of tumor markers within the expected time line implies absence of residual disease (in the scrotum/groin and lymph nodes). Persistently elevated tumor markers beyond the date of expected normalization portend a worse prognosis with presence of ongoing cancer (typically lymph node disease).

IMAGING CONSIDERATIONS

→ **Ultrasonography:** For clinically suspicious masses or when unsure of the diagnosis, ultrasonography is the imaging modality of choice for the majority of scrotal masses. It can differentiate solid from cystic masses and testicular from paratesticular masses. $96

→ **MRI:** If the diagnosis is still uncertain, an MRI scan is appropriate and effective. MRI has been reported to have a negative predictive value of 100% and a positive predictive value of 71%. $534

→ **CT scan:** If the mass is found to be malignant, the next step is to obtain a CT scan of the abdomen and pelvis (with IV contrast) and a chest radiograph (posteroanterior and lateral views) to evaluate for metastatic disease. In the event of a positive abdominal CT scan or an abnormal chest radiograph, a chest CT scan would be indicated. **These images will differentiate clinical stages I, II, and III.** $334

- Clinical stage I disease is confined to the testis.
- Clinical stage II disease is characterized by enlarged retroperitoneal lymph nodes.
- Clinical stage III disease involves metastatic disease to any viscera or any disease above the diaphragm.

Clinical Entities*	Medical Knowledge

Seminomas

Pφ A seminoma is derived from spermatogonia/spermatocytes.

TP A tumor may present as a solid, painless mass in the scrotum or along the cord structures within or above the scrotum. With hormone-producing tumors, precocious puberty ensues.

Dx Testicular ultrasonography is indicated if the diagnosis is in question or a solid component is suspected (i.e., bilateral scrotal ultrasonography should be performed in every case of suspected tumor). A chest radiograph, CT of the abdomen and pelvis with IV contrast, and tumor markers (AFP, β-hCG, and LDH) should be obtained preoperatively if tumor is suspected.

Tx Testicular tumors should be treated initially with radical inguinal orchiectomy and may require further medical treatment. Further treatment includes:
- **Clinical stage I seminomas:** Active surveillance (in compliant patients) vs. radiation therapy (XRT) vs. one to two cycles of single-agent carboplatin.
- **Clinical stage II seminomas:** XRT vs. etoposide and cisplatin (EP) for four cycles vs. bleomycin, etoposide, and cisplatin (BEP) for three cycles.
- **Clinical stage III seminomas:** Good risk—EP for four cycles, BEP for three cycles. Intermediate risk—BEP for four cycles.

See Cecil Essentials 72.

*Please note that only malignant diagnoses are presented in the Clinical Entities.

Nonseminomatous Germ Cell Tumors

Pφ NSGCTs can be composed of one or more histologic subtypes that include embryonal carcinoma, yolk sac tumor, choriocarcinoma, and teratoma.

TP A tumor may present as a solid, painless mass in the scrotum or along the cord structures within or above the scrotum. With hormone-producing tumors, precocious puberty ensues.

Dx Testicular ultrasonography is indicated if the diagnosis is in question or a solid component is suspected (i.e., bilateral scrotal ultrasonography should be performed in every case of suspected tumor). A chest radiograph, a CT of the abdomen and pelvis with IV contrast, and tumor markers (AFP, β-hCG, and LDH) should be obtained preoperatively if tumor is suspected.

Tx Testicular tumors should be treated initially by radical inguinal orchiectomy and may require further medical treatment. Further treatment includes:
- **Clinical stage I NSGCT:**
  Stage IA: active surveillance (in a compliant patient) vs. retroperitoneal lymph node dissection (RPLN).
  Stage IB: rarely active surveillance (T2 lesion in a compliant patient) vs. XRT vs. BEP for two cycles.
  Stage IS (persistent elevation of tumor markers): EP for four cycles or BEP for three cycles.
- **Clinical Stage II NSGCT:** EP for four cycles vs. BEP for three cycles.
- **Clinical Stage III NSGCT:** Intermediate risk—BEP for four cycles. Poor risk—BEP for four cycles vs. etoposide, ifosfamide, cisplatin, and mesna (VIP) for four cycles (if patient cannot tolerate bleomycin).

See Cecil Essentials 72.

ZEBRA ZONE

a. Epididymo-orchitis: Although mumps is now rare in the United States because of the widespread use of the MMR vaccine, this viral cause of orchitis should be considered in a young man with scrotal swelling. Orchitis usually develops within 1 week of the onset of parotitis.

b. Hematocele: In addition to physical examination, a history of trauma to the testicles would be suggestive of a hematocele, an accumulation of blood within the scrotal space. Significant testicular trauma may also rupture the tunica, a condition referred to as testicular fracture. Hematoceles may be associated with testicular rupture and occur in as many as 50% of patients with blunt scrotal trauma. The definitive diagnosis of a ruptured testicle is made after surgical exploration. All cases of hematocele require surgical evacuation and exploration to preserve testicular function and fertility.

Practice-Based Learning and Improvement: Evidence-Based Medicine

Title
Improved chemotherapy in disseminated testicular cancer

Authors
Einhorn LH, Donohue JP

Institution
Indiana University Medical Center

Reference
Einhorn LH, Donohue JP. Improved chemotherapy in disseminated testicular cancer. J Urol 117:65–69, 1977

Problem
Patient mortality from testicular cancer was greater than 50% before 1970.

Intervention
Addition of platinum-based drugs to chemotherapy regimens

Comparison/control (quality of evidence)
This study compared the then standard chemotherapy regimen of adriamycin, bleomycin, and vincristine against platinum, vinblastine, and bleomycin.

Outcome/effect
The adriamycin, bleomycin, and vincristine group had an 87.5% overall response rate with a 50% partial remission rate and a 37.5% complete remission rate. The group receiving platinum, vinblastine, and bleomycin (which ultimately became known as the Einhorn regimen) had a 100% overall response rate with a 20% partial remission rate and an 80% complete remission rate.

Historical significance/comments
Testicular cancer has become one of the most curable cancers in the United States. In 1997, there was less than 5% patient mortality.

Interpersonal and Communication Skills

Communicate Effectively about Potential Diagnoses
In the setting of a testicular mass, this patient is already concerned that he may have cancer. During the examination, describe your impression of the testicular exam and explain the implications of this to the patient (who is often accompanied by a parent, given the relatively young age at diagnosis). It is preferable to be direct about the concern for a testicular tumor, if the examination warrants this concern. Communicate to the patient that an ultrasonogram should

be performed to obtain further information. As testicular cancer has a very rapid doubling time and surgery should be performed expeditiously, the patient must be given a clear understanding of the likely diagnosis so that he can cooperate with immediate testing. Throughout this time, support the patient and family by answering any questions and by explaining that should this be diagnosed as a testicular malignancy, it has a very high cure rate.

Professionalism

Maintain Appropriate Patient Relations in Performing a Testicular Exam

In a time when female medical students constitute approximately 50% of medical school classes, many testicular exams will be performed by female physicians. Before approaching the male patient for a genital exam, a female physician should always be accompanied by a chaperone (male or female is acceptable). Privacy and confidentiality should be respected at all times. Great care and professionalism must be conveyed when approaching the patient so as to gain the patient's confidence and establish a level of comfort that will facilitate both a thorough physical exam and a nontraumatic experience for the patient. The female physician might also explain that care of the male patient is what she does on a daily basis and that she is very comfortable in that role. A patient's genitalia should be covered during all parts of the physical exam until the time for the genital exam. Verbalize to your patient what you plan to do and what you are doing throughout the exam. Often this simple "warning" of what is to come will facilitate the exam. If a patient is still uneasy despite your efforts, it is often helpful to emphasize both your role as the physician and the importance of the exam for diagnostic purposes. The most important aspect of this encounter is demeanor; if you convey a sense of serious and confident professionalism, the patient will respond to you appropriately.

Systems-Based Practice

Effective Use of Health Information Resources on Patient Options and Patient Care

In certain clinical circumstances, namely stage IA and IB seminomas and nonseminomas, the patient has the option of aggressive surveillance in lieu of systemic therapy. Surveillance as a management option for early-stage testicular cancer requires a series of regimented studies over several years to monitor disease, so this option is historically reserved only for compliant patients. Reports have indicated that 21% of seminoma patients on surveillance were lost to follow-up after approximately 5 years. One tool that has been instrumental in facilitating compliance with follow-up is the electronic medical record (EMR). EMR has the capacity to organize surveillance schedules and enhance patient compliance with follow-up care. Additionally, it has been suggested that providing effective access to EMR data as a reference source for patients with early-stage testicular cancer contributes to patient reassurance and to enhanced compliance with surveillance.

Chapter 41
Neck Mass (Case 33)

Bradley W. Lash MD *and Erik L. Zeger* MD

Case: A 24-year-old woman presents for evaluation of a painless lump on her right lateral neck. She noticed it first about 3 weeks ago, and since then it has grown slightly in size. She denies any local symptoms such as hoarseness, otalgia, or difficulty swallowing. She has had no recent infections or high fevers. She denies drenching night sweats or weight loss.

Differential Diagnosis

Infectious or inflammatory lymphadenopathy	Lymphoma (Hodgkin and non-Hodgkin lymphoma)	Squamous cell carcinoma of the head and neck
Thyroid cancer	Benign neoplasms and congenital anomalies	

Speaking Intelligently

A new neck mass is a relatively common problem in primary-care medicine. The differential diagnosis is broad, and the workup can be challenging. Often the only history is a new "lump" that is found incidentally. Infectious or inflammatory causes are the most common etiologies in children and young adults. The incidence of malignancy increases with age, particularly in patients over the age of 40 years. The type of malignancy varies with age as well, with lymphomas being more prevalent in patients under the age of 40 and carcinomas being more common in patients over age 40 years. A logical and disciplined evaluation is necessary to ensure that nothing is overlooked and that the workup is cost-effective. Even though lymphoma is of concern in the patient presented above, it is appropriate to start with a fine-needle aspiration (FNA) and reserve excisional biopsy for when results are inconclusive.

PATIENT CARE

Clinical Thinking
- The most common causes of neck masses in young adults are infectious/inflammatory, lymphomas, and congenital lesions.
- The incidence of malignancy increases with age and with risk factors such as tobacco or alcohol use.

History
- The lesion's onset and growth pattern should be noted. Stable lesions present for a long time are likely to be congenital or benign neoplasms. Conversely, rapidly appearing painful lesions are likely to be infectious/inflammatory or a manifestation of lymphoma.
- Human papillomavirus (HPV) infection increases the risk of head and neck cancer even in those without traditional risk factors such as tobacco or alcohol use.
- Prior radiation exposure (i.e., in the treatment of Hodgkin lymphoma) increases the risk of thyroid cancer.
- Local symptoms such as hoarseness, otalgia, recurrent infections, and dysphagia should be noted.
- Assess for "B" symptoms: fevers, drenching night sweats, and greater than 10% weight loss.
- The lymphadenopathy associated with malignancy (both solid and hematologic tumors) is usually painless; one notable exception is pain associated with alcohol consumption in cases of Hodgkin lymphoma.
- Recent skin infections, dental infections, and sick contacts should be noted.
- A new neck mass in a patient over 40 years old should be considered malignant until proven otherwise.

Physical Examination

- A **complete general examination** is necessary to search for any source of infection, to look for hepatosplenomegaly, and to evaluate all other nodal areas.
- The **location of the enlarged node** is helpful. The neck is generally divided into three regions: the anterior triangle, posterior triangle, and central neck. Nodes in each of these areas suggest potential etiologies.
- Examine the mouth, the entire neck including vascular structures, the thyroid, and skin.
- **Note the characteristics of the mass:** a mass that is rock-hard and fixed to adjacent structures is much more likely to be malignant. A tender, rubbery lesion is more likely to be infectious. A pulsatile lesion suggests a vascular aneurysm.
- **Direct laryngoscopy** is part of the evaluation in most patients, especially those with risk factors for carcinoma.

Tests for Consideration

- **FNA** is the first test. It can be performed with local anesthesia and under ultrasound guidance. Using a fine (21-gauge) needle, several passes through the mass are performed, with samples sent for cytologic evaluation. Studies have suggested both a high sensitivity and a high specificity of this test, even for lymphoma. $320
- **Open biopsy** is performed with complete excision of the mass and allows for the most accurate diagnosis. In cases of lymphoma, tissue examination is critical, as it defines nodal architecture. In cases of Hodgkin lymphoma, the malignant cell represents a small fraction of cells in the lymph node and, therefore, FNA may not establish a conclusive diagnosis. $570
- **Bone marrow aspirate and biopsy:** If a lymphoma is found, a bone marrow aspirate and biopsy are needed for staging purposes. $500
- **Routine laboratory studies** rarely lead to a diagnosis but are often helpful. Studies to consider include:
  - **CBC**, **comprehensive metabolic panel**, **erythrocyte sedimentation rate**, **LDH**, and **testing for various infectious causes** $11, $12, $4
    such as **Epstein-Barr virus (EBV)** and **HIV**. $9, $19, $13
  - While there are other serologic tests available, they rarely add meaningful information. The one exception might be a test to assess for tuberculous infection such as an **interferon-γ release assay** in patients at risk. $88

IMAGING CONSIDERATIONS

→ Various imaging studies can be done at the time of initial evaluation or as part of the workup once a diagnosis is established. In cases of lymphoma (both Hodgkin lymphoma and non-Hodgkin lymphoma), the following are helpful:

- **CT scan of the chest, abdomen, and pelvis with IV contrast:** This allows for complete staging and provides detailed anatomic locations of pathologic involvement. $334
- **PET scanning:** Not only does this allow for determining the exact extent of disease, but it can help in determining response to treatment. $1037

Clinical Entities	Medical Knowledge

Infectious or Inflammatory Lymphadenopathy

Pφ Cervical adenitis is the most common cause of a neck mass in children and young adults. Often a clear source of infection is found (i.e., a recent viral syndrome, cellulitis, or dental infection).

TP Infectious causes of cervical adenitis often present as acute, painful swelling of one or more nodes. Inflammatory disorders such as sarcoidosis, connective tissue diseases, or salivary gland stones can present with rapidly developing painful lymphadenopathy much like infectious etiologies. History and physical might suggest the diagnosis, but often biopsy (in cases of sarcoidosis), imaging (in cases of stones), or laboratory testing (in cases of autoimmune diseases) are needed.

Infectious causes can be divided into bacterial, viral, fungal, and protozoal causes:

- Bacterial causal agents are often staphylococcal or streptococcal species; however, less common agents such as typical and atypical mycobacteria should be considered in appropriate contexts.
- Viruses are the most common causal agents of infectious lymphadenopathy. Infectious mononucleosis from EBV or atypical mononucleosis from cytomegalovirus (CMV) should be considered. Of note, acute retroviral syndrome in HIV can mimic these disorders.
- Fungal infections are uncommon causes, but histoplasmosis and other pathogens should be considered if appropriate.
- Protozoal causes are unusual, but toxoplasmosis should be considered in the right clinical setting.

Dx The diagnosis is usually made by history and physical examination, but serologic testing may be necessary. If there is concern for EBV, a monospot test can be ordered. HIV testing should be strongly considered in those with risk factors. Routine cultures are often not necessary.

Tx Most cases of inflammatory or infectious adenitis resolve without intervention. If a bacterial infection is considered, a single course of appropriate antibiotics should be given. If the patient's node does not resolve with antibiotics, biopsy should be undertaken. **See Cecil Essentials 51, 95.**

Squamous Cell Carcinoma of the Head and Neck

Pφ If a cervical biopsy reveals squamous cell carcinoma, it signifies locally advanced disease. While metastatic disease from other primary sites can present with cervical lymphadenopathy, the most common primary site is in the head and neck.

TP Head and neck cancer often presents in patients over the age of 40 years who have risk factors (tobacco and alcohol abuse) and is often a painless, enlarging mass. Of note, recent data have shown an increase in this disease in younger patients; in these cases, HPV infection seems to be a possible etiology. Often a primary site is found by history or examination, but occult primaries do occur. Localizing symptoms such as otalgia, hoarseness, or dysphagia might point to a primary site.

Dx The diagnosis is established by complete head and neck examination including panendoscopy (which includes direct laryngoscopy, esophagoscopy, bronchoscopy, and endoscopic evaluation of the nasopharynx). This is most often performed by a surgeon. Imaging studies help to stage the disease and plan surgical resection.

Tx The treatment depends on the site of origin. As general rule, surgery is the mainstay of treatment. Complete radical resection with lymph node dissection is the most common procedure. In cases where the primary is not known or in cases where the surgery would be too morbid, chemotherapy and radiation therapy are used. **See Cecil Essentials 57.**

Lymphoma (Hodgkin and Non-Hodgkin)

Pφ Lymphomas are common causes of lymphadenopathy in all age groups. It may be localized or disseminated at diagnosis. Non-Hodgkin lymphoma is more common than Hodgkin lymphoma; however, in some series, up to 80% of patients with Hodgkin lymphoma had cervical node involvement as part of their presentation.

TP Lymphoma often presents as a painless, slowly enlarging mass. Since in most cases it is a systemic disease at diagnosis, associated symptoms known as "B" symptoms (fever, night sweats, >10% weight loss) may be present.

Dx The diagnosis is made by biopsy. FNA is able to diagnose lymphoma fairly well. If the FNA is positive for lymphoma or suspicious for lymphoma, a lymph node excision is needed to subtype the lymphoma. Additional diagnostic testing includes CT scan, PET scan, and bone marrow aspiration and biopsy.

Tx There are numerous classification systems for the various lymphomas. One way of thinking about non-Hodgkin lymphomas is to classify them based on their aggressiveness:
- *Indolent lymphomas:* Chronic lymphocytic leukemia (CLL), lymphoplasmacytic lymphoma, hairy cell leukemia, follicular lymphoma, nodal and extranodal marginal-zone lymphoma, T-cell large granular lymphocyte leukemia, mycosis fungoides.
- *Aggressive lymphomas:* Diffuse large B-cell lymphoma, mantle cell lymphoma, peripheral T-cell lymphoma, anaplastic large cell lymphoma.
- *Highly aggressive lymphomas:* Burkitt lymphoma, acute lymphoblastic lymphoma/leukemia.

The treatment is based on the type of lymphoma found and the stage at diagnosis. Surgery has no role except in the initial diagnosis. The mainstays of therapy are chemotherapy and radiation therapy. **See Cecil Essentials 51.**

Benign Neoplasms and Congenital Anomalies

Pφ Benign neoplasms (lipomas, fibromas, neuromas, and hemangiomas) and congenital anomalies (brachial cleft cysts and thyroglossal duct cysts) occur within the neck. While congenital lesions are more common in children, they can be found in adults.

TP In the case of benign neoplasms, the typical presentation is that of a slowly enlarging mass, which is generally painless. They are typically present for many years and are problematic only if they cause problems with surrounding structures or are cosmetically bothersome.

For congenital anomalies, presentation depends on the type. Classically brachial cysts will be present in the lateral neck, and patients may have a history of recurrent infection or drainage. Thyroglossal duct cysts are found in the midline and move with protrusion of the tongue.

Dx Often history and physical examination are sufficient to make the diagnosis, although radiographic imaging may be needed. For certain lesions, malignancy can only truly be ruled out at the time of biopsy.

Tx Treatment is either observation or surgical correction. The choice depends on histology, the location of the lesion, and patient preference.

Thyroid Cancer

Pφ Cancer of the thyroid is an uncommon cancer in adults, but the incidence is increasing. It is about four times more common in women than in men. The only consistent risk factor is prior radiation exposure. Thyroid cancer can be divided into three broad histologic categories: differentiated (including papillary, follicular, Hürthle cell), medullary, and anaplastic.

TP The typical patient presentation is somewhat dependent on histologic type:

- *Differentiated:* Most commonly found either incidentally on imaging or as a mass in the thyroid. Local symptoms such as hoarseness can rarely occur.
- *Medullary:* Often found in patients with a positive family history (multiple endocrine neoplasia (MEN) syndromes, *RET* oncogene mutations). Usually is an asymptomatic mass but can present as paraneoplastic hypercalcemia from calcitonin secretion.
- *Anaplastic:* Rare, but extremely aggressive. It is locally destructive, often causing airway compromise. It is by definition incurable and stage IV at diagnosis, even if it has not spread beyond the thyroid.

While the incidence is increasing, mortality has not changed for the differentiated types of thyroid cancer. This is probably a manifestation of a lead time bias secondary to incidental diagnosis on imaging.

Dx After physical examination and/or imaging finds a nodule, the next step is to determine the thyroid status. If a patient has hyperthyroidism, no further workup is needed, as the nodule is unlikely to be cancer. If a nodule is found in a euthyroid or hypothyroid patient, FNA of the lesion should be done.

Tx Treatment is initially surgical. There are controversies over which surgery should be done and whether lymph node dissection should be performed. Postoperatively, a radioactive iodine scan can be done to look for metastatic disease. **See Cecil Essentials 66.**

Practice-Based Learning and Improvement: Evidence-Based Medicine

Title
The accuracy of fine-needle aspiration biopsy in the diagnosis of head and neck masses

Authors
Carroll CM, Nazeer U, and Timon CI

Institution
St. James Hospital, Dublin, Ireland

Reference
Ir J Med Sci 1998;167:149–151

Problem
To assess the diagnostic accuracy of FNA biopsy in diagnosis of masses in the head and neck

Intervention
Retrospective comparison of the results of FNA biopsies performed at a single center over a 2-year period

Comparison/control
The comparison was excisional biopsies from the same patient. The investigators compared the results of the initial FNA with the final pathology.

Quality of evidence
Level II by Oxford Criteria

Outcome/effect

Of the 130 patients who underwent FNA biopsy, 78 eventually had an excisional biopsy performed. Results demonstrate an 87% concordance between the two techniques if the lesion was malignant, and 95% if the lesion was benign. Of note, there were no complications from the procedure.

Historical significance/comments

This study is one of several studies that established FNA biopsy as the standard of care for initial sampling of lymph nodes or masses in the head and neck. The technique is highly sensitive and involves little morbidity. It will help direct the workup and management for a majority of patients who present with a neck mass.

Interpersonal and Communication Skills

Obtaining Informed Consent Should Be a Structured Dialogue

In the practice of medicine, patient autonomy is paramount. This is demonstrated in the process of obtaining informed consent for a procedure or for medication administration. Informed consent should not be viewed as "just getting a signature on the consent form." Informed consent should be a **structured dialogue** between the physician and patient regarding the risks, benefits, and alternatives to treatment. Obtaining consent is a matter of ethics (i.e., demonstrating the core value of patient autonomy), but there are important legal reasons as well. There has been an increase in the number of malpractice cases that allege improper consent. Informed consent serves to verify that the patient has been appropriately apprised of potential complications and informed of the possibility of an adverse outcome. Even the most skilled physician occasionally has a bad outcome that could not have been prevented. Be sure to sit down with the patient and carefully review the consent form patiently and in detail. Ensure that the patient has had a chance to ask questions regarding the risks. Strongly consider procedure-specific consent forms that can provide the patient with more detailed information.

Professionalism

Remain Current with Practice Guidelines

One major focus of the recent health-care debate is cost control. The challenge facing clinicians is which tests to order and when. In oncology there are well-established guidelines on how to evaluate and treat patients with many specific cancers. These guidelines are updated yearly by the National Comprehensive Cancer Network (NCCN) and are evidence-based and written by experts from oncology, radiation therapy, radiology, pathology, and surgery so as to provide uniform recommendations on evaluation and treatment. Guidelines such as these serve as an excellent reference for practicing clinicians to stay current on the best evidence available for treatment of their patients.

Systems-Based Practice

Reimbursement: Medicaid

The finding of a neck mass, and the need for additional diagnostic procedures and therapeutic interventions, will have substantial financial consequences for the patient. Insured patients will probably have coverage for the costs of biopsy and therapy. For those patients without health insurance and for those who fall below certain income levels, **Medicaid** will cover a portion of the costs of treatment. Medicaid is the federal insurance program designed to cover health care for individuals and families with low incomes and resources. Established in 1965, the program is run and funded as a joint federal-state program, with states electing to participate. Statistics from the Centers for Medicare & Medicaid Services show that Medicaid spending increased from $187 billion in 2000 to $346 billion in 2009. The federal government provides certain guidelines that states must follow, but the individual states establish their own programs, each with a state-specific name and its own set of eligibility requirements and coverage. The federal government then funds half or more of the total cost of the program, depending on the poverty level of the state. *Given the current financial challenges and budget shortfalls in many states, significant cuts to Medicaid funding may occur, leading to decreased access to care for vulnerable populations.* Medicaid is contrasted with the federal insurance program designed to care for the elderly and disabled, known as Medicare. There are many similarities between Medicaid and Medicare, but a few key differences are worth noting: Medicaid is administered at the state level, generally covers a broader range of health-care needs, and generally provides long-term care benefits; therefore, a significant number of the elderly living in nursing homes eventually go on Medicaid, since Medicare does not cover long-term care. (See Systems-Based Practice: Reimbursement: Medicare, Chapter 46.)

Chapter 42
Pigmented Skin Lesions (Case 34)

James G. Bittner IV MD, Joan R. Johnson MD, MMS, and D. Scott Lind MD

Case: A 68-year-old woman presents with a pigmented skin lesion on her right thigh.

Differential Diagnosis

Basal cell carcinoma (BCC)	Atypical nevus
Squamous cell carcinoma (SCC)	Actinic keratosis
Malignant melanoma	Benign nevus

Speaking Intelligently

When asked to see a patient who presents with a pigmented skin lesion, we start by asking the patient what she thinks the lesion may be and reassuring her that as a team we will "find out" the answer. This allows us to quickly assess the patient's level of concern regarding the pigmented skin lesion. Next, we find out when she first noticed the lesion; if it has changed in shape, size, or color; whether or not it is painful; and whether the patient noticed any similar lesions recently or in the past. We also ask whether the lesion has been itching or bleeding and whether she has had any prior biopsies, laboratory tests, or imaging studies ordered by other physicians. It is important to ask about a prior personal or family history of skin cancer.

PATIENT CARE

Clinical Thinking

- Most patients think cancer first (perhaps rightfully so), and they want an answer—yesterday. That said, it is up to you, the physician, to reassure the patient that the ideal scenario is a correct diagnosis based on clinical, radiographic, and pathologic evidence. A timely but inaccurate answer may result in lost credibility, increased patient anxiety, and a strain on the physician-patient relationship. Most of all, you don't want to miss a skin cancer. Therefore, if a lesion is suspicious, you should perform a biopsy. If a biopsy is required, be

sure to check the patient's history for coagulopathy or medications that might cause bleeding such as clopidogrel, aspirin, and warfarin.
- Different pigmented skin lesions present differently. It is very important to understand the natural history and clinical presentation of malignant melanoma. In other words, when the history and physical exam are equivocal, consider melanoma and evaluate accordingly.
- Any patient who presents with a skin lesion should be offered education about the sources and hazards of ultraviolet radiation as well as the importance of sun-safe behaviors.

History
It is crucial to obtain a thorough history, including past medical history, family history (especially including skin cancers), surgical history, and medications; of particular interest are the following skin cancer risk factors:
- **Age and gender:** Forty-five percent of men with melanoma have trunk or back lesions, while 42% of women have lower extremity lesions. In addition, women with melanoma have an improved survival rate compared to men (82% 10-year survival compared to 61% 10-year survival in stage I disease).
- **Skin and hair color:** Fair-skinned people, especially with blond or red hair, are more likely to develop melanoma.
- **Skin history:** Is there a history of severe sunburns (especially as a child), tanning bed exposure, or previous melanomas? Bullous skin disease and decubitus ulcers or other nonhealing wounds or ulcers all have an increased risk of becoming malignant. When these lesions become cancerous, they are referred to as Marjolin ulcers.
- **Anatomic location:** Melanoma limb lesions have a better prognosis than head/neck or trunk lesions (82% compared to 68% overall survival rate).
- **Occupation:** Patients with prolonged ultraviolet exposure are at increased risk.
- **Location:** Persons who spend a significant amount of time in areas of the world that receive more sunlight are at increased risk.
- **Chemical carcinogens:** Exposures to tar, arsenic, nitrogen mustard, and soot are significant risk factors.
- **Radiation:** History of industrial, therapeutic, and occupational exposure constitutes high risk.
- **Medications:** Topical acne medications may predispose to skin sloughing, and anticoagulants may affect surgical planning.
- **Immunosuppression:** Patients with HIV, AIDS, and patients on chronic immunosuppression, such as solid-organ transplant patients, are at increased risk of developing malignant skin lesions.

Physical Examination
- Most patients with a skin lesion present with **normal vital signs**.
- **A complete skin examination** in a well-lighted room includes inspection from the scalp to the toes, paying careful attention to those areas most notable for harboring cutaneous malignancies such

as the face, neck, upper back, upper and lower extremities, and dorsal and ventral aspects of the hands and feet.

- Document the anatomic location, size, shape, color (pigmentation), presence or absence of ulceration, blanching, bleeding, or evidence of inflammation. A photograph of the lesion can also be helpful. Benign pigmented lesions such as freckles should be followed for increased melanoma risk.
- When evaluating a patient with a pigmented skin lesion, the findings of *A*symmetry (one half of the lesion is different from the other half), *B*order irregularity, variegated *C*olors (multiple colors such as black and blue), larger *D*iameter (>5 mm), and *E*volution (change in size, color, or erythema, onset of pruritus, and ulceration) raise the suspicion for malignancy (ABCDE of melanoma). You need only one of these findings for the lesion to be concerning.
- A rigorous search for palpable lymph nodes is a must. Pay close attention to the path of lymphatic drainage particular to the skin involved.

Tests for Consideration

- **CBC:** Useful to evaluate for preoperative thrombocytopenia or anemia if surgery is considered. $11
- **PT/INR and PTT:** Help with procedural planning in patients taking anticoagulants or those with potential coagulopathy. $15
- **Punch biopsy:** A 6-mm punch biopsy is appropriate for small (<5 mm) benign-appearing lesions that will be entirely removed or for larger lesions (2 cm or more) that will require wide local excision. Do not perform a shave or partial-thickness biopsy, because depth of invasion is the most important prognostic feature. $105
- **Excisional biopsy:** This type is preferred for all malignant-appearing lesions at least 5 mm in diameter where complete excision is possible. A full-thickness biopsy is obtained to determine depth of invasion. Care must be taken to orient the incision in a fashion compatible with future wide local excision. $310
- **Wide local excision:** Every primary malignant melanoma requires wide local excision to decrease the risk of loco-regional recurrence. Current recommendations for excision margins are: $580
  - Lesion ≤ 1 mm in depth, excise 1-cm tumor-free margin.
  - Lesion 1.01–2 mm in depth, excise 1- to 2-cm tumor-free margin.
  - Lesion 2.01–4 mm in depth, excise 2-cm margin.
  - Lesion > 4 mm in depth, excise 2- to 3-cm margin.
- **Sentinel lymph node biopsy:** This is an accurate, minimally invasive method for staging patients with malignant melanoma. The sentinel node(s) is the first or principal site of lymphatic tumor spread to the nearest basin draining the affected skin. $570

IMAGING CONSIDERATIONS

→ **Chest radiograph:** Performed for preoperative evaluation and to evaluate for pulmonary metastases if melanoma is diagnosed. $45

→ **CT scan:** When melanoma depth of invasion is >4 mm or ulcerated >2 mm, palpable lymph nodes are present, and/or symptoms suggest metastatic disease, a CT scan of the chest, abdomen, and pelvis should be performed. $334

→ **PET scan** to evaluate for metastases. It can be combined with regular CT scan to more precisely localize metastatic lesions if clinically indicated. $1037

→ **CT/PET** of chest, abdomen, and pelvis if melanoma depth is >2 mm with ulceration or >4 mm without ulceration. $1037

Clinical Entities	Medical Knowledge

Basal Cell Carcinoma

Pφ BCC is the most common skin cancer worldwide. It is a slow-growing tumor that arises from abnormal epidermal keratinocyte growth and is divided into three types: nodular (70%–80%), superficial, and morpheaform. The histology is unique for aggregations of basophils at the tumor periphery called "peripheral palisading."

TP Nodular BCC usually presents as a waxy, raised, pearl- or cream-colored lesion with heaped borders and often exhibits central ulceration. Superficial BCC presents as an erythematous, scaling lesion usually on the trunk. BCC may also contain pigment and appear tan or black. These lesions must be differentiated from melanoma by biopsy.

Dx Most lesions can be diagnosed based on clinical presentation, but biopsy of any pigmented BCC is required to exclude melanoma.

Tx The gold standard treatment for BCC is complete surgical excision with negative margins. However, newer therapies include curettage/electrodesiccation, Mohs micrographic surgery, cryosurgery, radiation, and topical chemotherapy or immunomodulator therapy. Mohs surgery can be offered to patients with BCC size >2 cm, contiguous lesions in high-risk locations (eyelids, ears, nose), recurrent tumors, and tumors with little metastatic potential. **See Cecil Essentials 57.**

Squamous Cell Carcinoma

Pφ SCC is the second most common skin cancer worldwide. It arises from abnormal epidermal keratinocyte growth and is divided into two types—in situ (Bowen disease or erythroplasia of Queyrat) and invasive. The histology demonstrates atypical squamous cells of the epidermis with possible extension into the reticular dermis.

TP SCC most often presents as a hyperkeratotic, raised, flesh-colored lesion with associated ulceration and erythema commonly located on the face, ear, trunk, or regions of skin pathology. Predisposing skin lesions for SCC include Marjolin ulcers, decubitus ulcers, bullous disease, and areas of chronic osteomyelitis.

Dx Most lesions can be diagnosed based on clinical presentation, but biopsy of any SCC is required to exclude amelanotic melanoma.

Tx The gold standard treatment for SCC is complete surgical excision with negative margins with or without lymph node biopsy. However, newer therapies include curettage/electrodesiccation (if epidermis involvement only), Mohs micrographic surgery, cryosurgery, and topical chemotherapy or immunomodulator therapy for multiple lesions. Mohs surgery can be offered to patients with SCC diameter > 2 cm, contiguous lesions in high-risk locations (eyelids, ears, nose, lips), recurrent tumors, and tumors with little metastatic potential. Radiation can be used alone for moderate-risk locations (with lesions < 20 mm diameter) and high-risk locations (<15 mm diameter), or in combination with cisplatin-based chemotherapy regimens. Postoperative chemotherapy and radiation are used for high-risk lesions, nodal involvement, and incompletely resected margins. **See Cecil Essentials 57.**

Malignant Melanoma

Pφ Malignant melanoma is now the fifth most common cancer in men and seventh in women, with approximately 68,000 new cases of invasive melanoma diagnosed and 8400 deaths reported annually in the United States. At the time of diagnosis, about 84% present with localized disease, 8% have regional disease, and 4% have distant metastases. Melanoma arises from mutated melanocytes, and four common types are classified: superficial spreading (70%), nodular (15%–30%), lentigo maligna (4%–15%), and acral lentiginous (5%).

TP **Superficial spreading melanoma** presents as a flat, pigmented lesion with variegated pigmentation, irregular borders, and areas of tumor regression anywhere on the body except the hands and feet. **Nodular melanoma** typically contains more pigmentation and appears raised without evidence of radial spread. The **lentigo maligna** type occurs on the face, neck, and hands of elderly patients. **Acral lentiginous** type occurs on the palms and soles as well as the subungual region of predominantly dark-skinned people (African Americans, Asians, and Hispanics).

Dx Most lesions can be grossly diagnosed based on clinical presentation, but biopsy of every melanoma is required for type-specific identification. Breslow depth of invasion determines the T classification using the TNM system: T1 lesion < 1 mm in depth, T2 lesion 1–2 mm in depth, T3 lesion 2–4 mm in depth, and T4 lesion > 4 mm in depth. Current pathologic T staging differentiates between (a) nonulcerated and (b) ulcerated. Also, pathologic N staging differentiates between (a) micrometastasis, (b) macrometastasis, and (c) in-transit metastasis.
- Stage IA   (T1a, N0, M0)   (90%–98% 5-year survival)
- Stage IB   (T1b-2a, N0, M0)
- Stage IIA   (T2b-3a, N0, M0)   (60%–70% 5-year survival)
- Stage IIB   (T3b-4a, N0, M0)
- Stage IIC   (T4b, N0, M0)
- Stage IIIA   (T1-4a, N1a/N2a, M0)
- Stage IIIB   (T1-4a, N1b/N2b/N2c, M0; or T1-4b, N1a/N2a, M0)
- Stage IIIC   (T1-4b, N1b/N2b/N2c, M0; or Any T, N3, M0)
- Stage IV   (any T, any N, M1)   (5%–15% 5-year survival)

Tx The gold standard treatment for malignant melanoma is wide local excision with tumor-free margins. For patients with melanoma of stage IB or higher, consider sentinel lymph node biopsy. Systemic treatment options for advanced or metastatic melanoma include a clinical trial, interferon-α, ipilimunab, vemurafenib, dacarbazine, temozolomide, high-dose interleukin-2, paclitaxel, cisplatin, or carboplatin. Genetic testing is available and should be offered to patients who meet any of the following criteria:
- Patients with strong personal or family history of melanoma
- Patients diagnosed with melanoma + family history of melanoma
- Patients diagnosed with multiple primary melanomas
- Patients diagnosed with multiple dysplastic nevi + family history
- Patients with relatives who tested positive for p16 mutation
  See Cecil Essentials 57.

Atypical Nevus

Pφ Atypical nevi are either inherited or sporadic precursors to cutaneous malignant melanoma with a prevalence of 2% to 5% in light-skinned people in the United States. The greater the number of atypical nevi present, the higher the risk of developing melanoma; however, the greatest risk is a strong family history of atypical nevi and melanoma.

TP Atypical nevi present as large, variably pigmented lesions with ill-defined borders most commonly in sun-exposed areas similar to melanoma. Ultraviolet light exposure is an independent risk factor for the development of sporadic atypical nevi.

Dx Most lesions can be grossly diagnosed based on clinical presentation, but biopsy of a melanoma precursor is required for identification. Only the most concerning lesion should be excised with narrow margins for histologic identification.

Tx The gold standard treatment for atypical nevi is excision.

Actinic Keratosis

Pφ Actinic keratosis is the most common sun-related premalignant skin lesion worldwide, with prevalence directly related to ultraviolet light exposure and light skin color. Histologically, epidermal changes include acanthosis and cellular atypia of keratinocytes.

TP Actinic keratosis presents as a discrete, verrucous, hyperkeratotic lesion usually on a sun-exposed area of the face, ears, forearms, and hands. More advanced lesions form keratotic horns. Ultraviolet light exposure is an independent risk factor for the development of actinic keratosis.

Dx Most lesions can be grossly diagnosed based on clinical presentation, but biopsy of a melanoma precursor is required for identification.

Tx The gold standard treatment for advanced actinic keratosis is surgical excision. However, early small lesions may be treated initially with topical 5-fluorouracil for approximately 1 month. If the lesion continues to improve with medical management, a repeat course of 5-fluorouracil is indicated before excision. For smaller lesions that fail repeated attempts at medical management, cryotherapy with liquid nitrogen is an effective means of removing the cutaneous lesion.

Benign Nevus

Pφ Benign melanocytic nevi represent nests of neural crest–derived melanocytes with no evidence of cytogenetic flaws or contact inhibition, which are present in most dysplastic nevi. In light-skinned individuals, benign nevi are so prevalent that they may not even be considered pathologic.

TP Benign melanocytic nevi present as small (<1 cm), well-circumscribed, uniformly pigmented, flat lesions usually on sun-exposed areas. Ultraviolet light exposure is an independent risk factor for the development of benign melanocytic nevi.

Dx Most lesions can be grossly diagnosed based on clinical presentation, but biopsy of a benign melanocytic nevus is required for identification.

Tx The gold standard treatment for benign melanocytic nevus is to rule out malignancy. Since these lesions may be difficult to distinguish from melanoma clinically, an appropriate biopsy should be performed. Medical management is usually ineffective and generates no pathologic specimen for lesion identification.

ZEBRA ZONE

a. **Nevi of Ota and Ito:** Nevus of Ota is a hamartoma of dermal melanocytes that usually appears on the face, and nevus of Ito is a dermal melanocytic condition of the shoulder.

b. **Metastatic carcinoma of the skin:** The breast (most common), stomach, lungs, uterus, and colon are potential primary sources of cutaneous metastatic carcinoma.

c. **Keratoacanthoma:** Low-grade malignancy that resembles SCC.

d. **Spitz nevus:** Childhood benign pigmented lesion with a rapid growth phase followed by a quiescent phase during which color changes, pruritus, and bleeding may occur. This lesion is often confused with childhood melanoma.

e. **Giant hairy nevus:** A pigmented skin lesion with large, dark, hairy patches and an increased risk of melanoma.

Practice-Based Learning and Improvement: Evidence-Based Medicine

Title
Excision margins in high-risk malignant melanoma

Authors
Thomas JM, Newton-Bishop J, A'Hern R, et al.

Institution
United Kingdom Melanoma Study Group

Reference
N Engl J Med 2004;350:757–766

Problem
Controversy exists regarding the appropriate margin of resection for cutaneous melanoma of 2 mm or greater in depth. This multicenter, prospective, clinical trial investigated the significance of excision margins on loco-regional recurrence and disease-free survival in high-risk melanoma patients. Loco-regional recurrence was defined as recurrence within 2 cm of the excision site, in-transit recurrence, and regional node metastases.

Intervention
Using the intention-to-treat principle, eligible adults with cutaneous melanoma greater than or equal to 2 mm in depth on the trunk/limbs and no prior history of cancer or immunotherapy were randomized to resection with 1-cm or 3-cm margins. No sentinel lymph node biopsies or lymphadenectomies were performed. Patients did not receive adjuvant interferon.

Quality of evidence
Like the Swedish Melanoma Study Group, which supports 2-cm margins of excision for melanomas 0.8–2 mm in depth, and the Intergroup Melanoma Surgical Trial, which recommends 2-cm margins for tumors 1–4 mm in depth, the quality of evidence for this study is high.

Outcome/effect
In adults with cutaneous malignant melanoma of the trunk or limbs at least 2 mm in depth, a 1-cm margin of excision increases risk of loco-regional recurrence but does not alter disease-free survival compared to 3-cm margins. Overall survival decreased in those patients who did experience recurrence after excision with 3-cm margins.

Historical significance/comments
This article supports the use of wide local excision with margins greater than 1 cm for all cutaneous melanomas of the trunk and limbs at least 2 mm in depth. It stands to reason that patients who develop melanoma greater than 4 mm in depth may benefit from wider margins (3 cm) than those with tumor of 4 mm or less in depth. This is because deeper tumors (>4 mm) have a significantly higher rate of loco-regional recurrence and decreased overall survival.

Interpersonal and Communication Skills

Preoperative and Postoperative Discussions Are Essential to the Patient-Physician Relationship
Preoperatively, patients with pigmented skin lesions are usually concerned with the overall risk of the procedure, the aesthetic results, and the likelihood of cure. A realistic, positive discussion addressing the risks and benefits, as well as the scar and aesthetics, is the best approach. Postoperatively, a candid and compassionate disclosure of the pathologic results, the disease stage if completely determined, the natural history of the disease process, and appropriate future management facilitates patient satisfaction and promotes an ongoing physician-patient relationship.

Professionalism

Cell Phone Etiquette: A Skill to Develop
You are in the process of discussing a new diagnosis and prognosis with a patient, and your cell phone rings. Do you answer it? What if you see on the face of your phone that it is a medical student? What if it is the chief resident? The attending physician? What do you do if it's a text message, "Call me ASAP about Mr. Jones."? These are difficult questions to answer definitively. Although, of course, patients are aware that a physician's beeper or cell phone might ring—after all, this is how they reach the doctor in an emergency—certain conversations will not lend themselves to interruption. In the case of an emergency, simply explaining that fact and excusing yourself momentarily may be the best option. As a medical community, it will become important to cultivate behavioral guidelines for our use of technology so that our technologic achievements in communication do not interfere with physician-patient interactions.

Systems-Based Practice

Community Education Benefits Community Health
Individual and community-based education programs specifically outlining the independent risk factors of cutaneous malignancy significantly impact the overall prevention of skin neoplasms. School-aged children and adolescents should be taught about the use of ultraviolet protection in sun-exposed areas, minimizing unprotected time in the sun during the midday, and performing early skin self-examination. Adults should receive similar education, with particular attention to close observation of existing pigmented skin lesions. Finally, community-based programs designed to screen individuals at risk are available and aid in early diagnosis and possibly improved mortality associated with malignant skin neoplasms.

Chapter 43
Incidentally Discovered Mass Lesions (Case 35)

Tami Berry MD and Joseph J. Muscato MD

Case: A 42-year-old woman presented to her family physician with right lower quadrant discomfort of 2 days' duration and was sent for a CT scan of the abdomen and pelvis to "rule out appendicitis." The CT scan revealed a normal appendix and no acute abnormality. The patient's acute problem was self-limited, and she felt better the following day. However, the radiologist noted an "incidental finding," and the family physician was promptly notified.

Differential Diagnosis

Adrenal masses	Ovarian mass	Renal mass	Hepatic mass	Pulmonary nodule
• Cortisol-secreting				
• Aldosterone-secreting				
• Pheochromocytoma				
• Primary adrenocortical adenocarcinoma				

Speaking Intelligently

An incidentally discovered mass, or "incidentaloma," will be experienced by every physician, both during training and during practice. The unsuspected mass that appears on imaging done for some other purpose can present a great conundrum for clinicians. As our population ages and both the frequency and resolution of radiologic imagery increase, there will consequently be more incidental mass findings. Clinicians must be prepared to manage these safely and effectively. The focus of evaluation is a balance of minimizing untoward stress or risk to the patient without missing something important that requires additional diagnostic evaluation.

PATIENT CARE

Clinical Thinking
- Incidental lesions force the clinician to "work backwards," by re-examining the patient's history and clinical picture to determine whether the finding validates a concern, warrants a more extensive evaluation, or requires surveillance.

History and Physical Examination
- Specific points of history, possible findings on examination, and specific tests for diagnosis are covered separately under Clinical Entities below.

Clinical Entities   Medical Knowledge

Adrenal Mass

Pφ An adrenal "incidentaloma" is an adrenal mass > 1 cm in size that is discovered on radiologic imaging performed for reasons unrelated to the adrenal glands.

TP Prevalence of an incidental adrenal mass found on abdominal CT imaging is 4% and in those aged ≥ 70 years is ~7%. A compelling theory is that as people age there is increased likelihood of undergoing imaging and that the effects of local ischemia and atrophy lead to the development of cortical nodules or lesions.

Dx Three questions should be investigated when evaluating an incidental adrenal mass: (1) Is the tumor active or functional? (2) Does the radiologic phenotype suggest malignancy? (3) Is there a history of a previous malignant lesion?

Radiologic phenotypic features that aid our characterization of the mass include size, shape, symmetry, and heterogeneity or homogeneity of tissue density measured in Hounsfield units (HU). Adenomas tend toward smooth edges, symmetry, and homogeneous density.

FNA of the mass is recommended only in patients with suspicious radiologic phenotypic malignant features in the background of a prior oncologic process. FNA is also reasonable in patients refusing the recommendation for surgery, if the findings would alter management. FNA should proceed only after a pheochromocytoma has been ruled out, as hypertensive crisis and physiologic collapse may occur.

Tx If any of the above diagnostic questions can be answered affirmatively, then a multidisciplinary approach is prudent, inclusive of an endocrinologist, surgeon, and medical oncologist. Refer to the following Clinical Entities on specific workup for hypercortisolism, hyperaldosteronism, pheochromocytoma, and primary adrenocortical adenocarcinoma. Excess production of androgen or sex hormones is rarely asymptomatic and is not included in our discussion on incidental adrenal masses.

Incidental adrenal lesions that are inactive and measuring over 4–6 cm warrant both radiologic and biochemical follow-up. Radiologic follow-up is fashioned to elicit whether the lesion is either dormant or rapidly proliferating; radiologic evaluations are recommended at 6-, 12-, and 24-month intervals. Annual biochemical assays, over a 5-year duration, are warranted for any nonfunctional adrenal mass measuring over 4–6 cm because there is a positive relationship between adrenal mass size and hormonal functionality. **See Cecil Essentials 67.**

Cortisol-Secreting Adrenal Mass

Pφ These lesions display autonomous glucocorticoid production and can be termed subclinical hypercortisolism (SCS) when the patient is asymptomatic or lacks the signs and symptoms of the Cushing syndrome.

TP SCS is the most common biochemical abnormality detected in patients with an adrenal incidentaloma (~9%) and can be accompanied by arterial hypertension, obesity, dyslipidemia, glucose intolerance, and osteoporosis.

Dx An overnight 1-mg dexamethasone suppression test is done to screen for elevated cortisol levels in patients with suspected Cushing syndrome or SCS; a serum cortisol > 5 μg/dL after a 1-mg (low-dose) dexamethasone suppression test is considered positive (specificity 91%). If the screening test is positive, then confirmatory testing is warranted. This can be done with measurement of a 24-hour urinary free cortisol (UFC), midnight salivary cortisol, or a 48-hour 2-mg (high-dose) dexamethasone suppression test.

Tx Medical therapy remains the mainstay of treatment. Surgical adrenalectomy is reserved for patients who are young (<40 years) and those with recent onset or worsening hypertension, glucose intolerance, dyslipidemia, obesity, or osteoporosis. **See Cecil Essentials 67.**

Aldosterone-Secreting Adrenal Mass

Pφ Almost 1% of incidental adrenal masses are aldosterone-secreting adenomas, warranting biochemical evaluation in those with hypertension or other signs or symptoms consistent with autonomous aldosterone production.

TP Patients with hypertension should undergo evaluation for hyperaldosteronism. In those with hypokalemia and mild hypernatremia, you may elicit a history of nocturia, polyuria, muscle cramping, and palpitations.

Dx Measure the ambulatory morning plasma aldosterone concentration (PAC) to plasma renin activity (PRA) ratio while the patient is upright. A PAC/PRA ratio > 20 is consistent with hyperaldosteronism (note: spironolactone and mineralocorticoid antagonists can result in false positive results). A positive screen is followed with confirmatory measurement of mineralocorticoid secretory autonomy with oral sodium loading, IV saline infusion, or a fludrocortisone suppression test.

Tx Any lesion autonomously producing aldosterone should be referred for surgical removal. **See Cecil Essentials 13, 67.**

Pheochromocytoma

Pφ Pheochromocytoma is associated with high rates of morbidity and mortality.

TP History may include episodic (paroxysmal) rapid heart rate, tremor, headache, or diaphoresis. These episodes may be precipitated by anxiety, extreme postural changes, or medications (metoclopramide and anesthetic agents).

Dx Initial evaluation should include measurement of plasma free metanephrines (sensitivity 98% and specificity 92%), and/or 24-hour total urinary metanephrines and fractionated catecholamines. A total plasma catecholamine of at least 2000 pg/mL is diagnostic of a pheochromocytoma. Generally a positive plasma fractionated metanephrine test deserves confirmation with either urinary fractionated metanephrines or a clonidine suppression test. When plasma free metanephrines, 24-hour urinary metanephrines, and fractionated catecholamines are elevated, the sensitivity is 100% and specificity 96.7%, with a negative predictive value of 100%. False positive results can occur in patients with congestive heart failure, cerebrovascular accident, acute alcohol or clonidine withdrawal, cocaine use, or use of medications such as tricyclic antidepressants, phenoxybenzamine, bromocriptine, labetalol, and α_1-adrenergic receptor blockers.

Tx The mainstay of treatment for pheochromocytoma is surgical resection after several weeks of α-adrenergic blockade. **See Cecil Essentials 13, 67.**

Primary Adrenocortical Adenocarcinoma

Pφ Primary adrenocortical adenocarcinoma is found in 4.7% of patients and is metastatic in 2.5%. The prognosis is very poor, with mean survival at the time of diagnosis of only 18 months.

TP There may be a history of some degree of discomfort secondary to mass effect or other vague symptoms related to secretion of any the adrenals' hormonally active substances. Patients may have signs of osteopenia, osteoporosis, hypertension, glucose intolerance, diabetes mellitus, hyperlipidemia, and leukocytosis or lymphopenia. Only 50% to 60% of adrenocortical adenocarcinomas are hormonally active. Furthermore, patients with hormonally inactive adrenocortical adenocarcinomas rarely present with weight loss, fever, or anorexia, or other symptoms of back or abdominal pain.

Dx The mass size and radiologic appearance are the two major predictors of malignant disease. A diameter > 4 cm is consistent with an adrenocortical carcinoma with a sensitivity of 90% (specificity only 24%). Risk of malignancy rises with increasing size of adrenal masses: those <4 cm confer 2% risk for malignant potential, 4–6 cm 6% risk for malignant potential, and >6 cm a 25% risk for malignant potential. Based on size alone, surgical removal is advocated for adrenal masses > 4–6 cm. Once adrenocortical carcinoma is suspected, size matters even more, because the smaller the lesion at the time of diagnosis, the lower will be the tumor stage, which correlates with a better overall prognosis.

Tx Referral to both medical and surgical oncologists is appropriate. **See Cecil Essentials 67.**

Ovarian Mass

Pφ Any adnexal mass identified by a primary-care physician or gynecologist should be considered potentially malignant in patients in any age group.

TP In terms of gynecologic cancer, ovarian cancer is the leading cause of death. In 2007 an estimated 22,500 women were newly diagnosed and there were more than 15,000 deaths. Mortality rises with advanced stage; the 5-year survival in those with stage I cancer approaches 90%, while the 5-year survival in those with stage III or IV is between 30% and 55%.

Dx Most incidentally discovered adnexal masses are benign, especially those that are unilocular cystic masses in premenopausal or perimenopausal women. Cystic lesions measuring >5–6 cm should be followed up radiologically in the premenopausal age group, as they are at risk of torsion. Referral to a gynecologic oncologist is recommended when complex cysts of any size are found in postmenopausal women (risk of malignancy 3%). Tumor volume doubling time for ovarian cancer is <3 months; thus, repeat imaging (ultrasound or MRI) should occur in 6 weeks on any lesions with solid components or any lesion in postmenopausal women.

Society of Gynecologic Oncologists and American College of Obstetrics and Gynecology guidelines for referral in women with a newly detected adnexal mass (2002)

Premenopausal woman	Postmenopausal woman
CA-125 > 200 U/mL	CA-125 > 35 U/mL
Ascites	Ascites
Evidence of abdominal or distant metastasis	Evidence of abdominal or distant metastasis
Family history of breast or ovarian cancer (in a first-degree relative)	Family history of breast or ovarian cancer (in a first-degree relative)
	Nodular or fixed pelvic mass

Reprinted from Journal of the American College of Radiology, 4/10, Miller JC, et al., Evaluating adnexal lesions: Which need follow-up?, pages 725–729, 2007, with permission from American College of Radiology. http://www.sciencedirect.com/science/journal/15461440.

Tx Operative indications and referral are warranted in patients who are symptomatic and those who display increasing size of the lesion over time. **See Cecil Essentials 57.**

Renal Mass

Pφ Incidental renal tumors have emerged as a new clinical entity with modern imaging. Small renal masses measure <4 cm and enhance on imaging. Renal masses are covered in greater detail in Chapter 25.

TP The frequency of small renal masses has risen quite steeply. A recent review by the US National Cancer Data Base (NCDB) shows that the proportion of tumors measuring <4 cm increased by >10% between 1993 and 2004.

Dx There are no concrete guidelines on evaluation, management, and surveillance of small renal masses. The consensus is that elderly or infirm patients, with an expected short life expectancy, can undergo surveillance with imaging every 6–12 months. Several studies have supported a positive correlation between renal cell tumor growth and increasing malignancy and higher tumor grade. Percutaneous biopsy (PCB) has been utilized to distinguish benign from malignant lesions, but this falls short on accuracy (20% remain indeterminate) and thus should be used only if the result will change management.

Tx Pathologic grading is traditionally done at the time of surgical removal. Surgical excision has been the mainstay of treatment for renal masses especially in those under the age of 70 years with a significant life expectancy. Young, healthy individuals with lesions that are >1 cm generally are referred for surgical removal. Treatment options include radiofrequency ablation and cryoablation, although long-term data on efficacy are not yet available. Nephron-sparing surgery (NSS) is appropriate for many patients. **See Cecil Essentials 30, 57.**

Hepatic Mass

Pφ Liver lesions can be quite common. Most of them will be benign and appear as a simple cyst, hemangioma, focal fat, or focal nodular hyperplasia (FNH). Incidental liver masses are challenging in patients with cirrhosis, fibrosis, and hemochromatosis, as there is a slightly higher propensity for malignant potential.

TP These lesions are discovered at the time of right upper quadrant ultrasound or upon CT performed for reasons other than those related to liver abnormalities.

Dx Workup of incidental liver lesions follows an algorithm based on the clinical and radiologic pictures correlating positively with malignant potential. Classic benign lesions contain fat or serous contents (simple cyst, hemangioma, FNH). Patients with a previous history or risk factors for hepatic malignancy warrant MRI with contrast, or helical CT with contrast, including delayed portal venous phases. Patients with lesions that correlate both clinically and radiologically with malignancy should be evaluated with serum tumor markers and/or percutaneous core biopsy.

Tx Malignant confirmation warrants referral to both surgical and medical oncologists for directed treatment and management.

Solitary Pulmonary Nodule

Pφ A solitary pulmonary nodule is an approximately round lesion that is between 1 and 3 cm in diameter and completely surrounded by pulmonary parenchyma. When warranted, workup is critical because of the high mortality rate (85%) in those with lung cancer. Pulmonary nodule is covered in greater detail in Chapter 17.

TP Concern for malignant potential should be raised in those with a social history of smoking (total pack-years is directly proportional to incidence of cancer). Other risk factors include prior malignancy (testicular, melanoma, sarcoma, or colon), pulmonary fibrosis, and HIV infection.

Dx Stable radiologic findings over a 2-year period support a benign etiology. Reviewing old images is prudent and may negate further workup. Lesions with spiculated margins and calcifications that are stippled, eccentric, diffuse, or amorphous warrant further workup with either FNA or core biopsy (if lymphoma is suspected). CT with IV contrast that demonstrates nodule enhancement <15 HU is strongly indicative of a benign etiology (positive predictive value, ~99%). An excellent prediction model is available at http://www.chestx-ray.com.

Tx If malignant features are present, staging must be performed to determine the appropriate treatment. **See Cecil Essentials 24.**

Practice-Based Learning and Improvement: Evidence-Based Medicine

Title
Adrenal lesion frequency: a prospective, cross-sectional CT study in a defined region, including systematic re-evaluation

Authors
Hammarstedt L, Muth A, Wangberg B, et al.; on behalf of the Adrenal Study Group of Western Sweden

Institution
Sahlgrenska Academy at the University of Gothenburg, Southern Alvsborg Hospital, Kungalv Hospital, Northern Alvsborg Hospital

Reference
Acta Radiol 2010;10:1149–1156

Problem
The investigative goal was to prospectively estimate and validate the prevalence of detected adrenal incidentalomas in patients undergoing abdominal CT evaluations in the clinical setting.

Intervention
During their 18-month collection period, 30,000 CT scans were performed in western Sweden (population 1.6 million). Initial reported frequency was compared to the frequency of detection on systematic re-evaluation by blinded interobserver assessments performed by experienced radiologists.

Comparison/control (quality of evidence)

Approximately 30,000 CT scans were performed in western Sweden during the 18-month collection period. The initial reportable frequency of adrenal lesions was 0.9% (range 0%–2.4% among hospitals). The systematic re-evaluation of 3801 randomly selected cases showed a mean frequency of 4.5% (range 1.8%–7.1% among hospitals). On the systematic re-evaluation, 177 cases of incidental adrenal lesions were found; 47% of these had not been reported by the radiology department.

Outcome/effect

This study concludes that adrenal lesions are under-reported in clinical practice.

Historical significance/comments

The results of this study imply that the medical community has largely under-recognized the incidence of adrenal lesions that are found on CT imaging. Consequently, we also underappreciate the prevalence of adrenal masses. This may have broader implications on the clinical management approach when we acknowledge that much of the natural history of incidental adrenal masses may be largely unknown.

Interpersonal and Communication Skills

Physician-Patient Joint Decision Making Follows the Model of Patient-Centered Care

A discussion about an unexpected finding is a challenge. The finding of a potentially serious, but asymptomatic, lesion requires a straightforward and gentle delivery. Your words should reassure the patient that many of these findings are not serious, but you should outline whatever further evaluation may be necessary. Choosing the right language can be difficult. Remember that the process of shared, informed decision making is the essence of patient-centered care and guides physicians and patients under conditions of uncertainty and risk. Under this model, the physician provides information of clinical probability (based on thorough history, physical examination, and review of pertinent studies), weighing the risks and benefits of different management strategies. Ultimately the physician and patient identify the management option that best aligns with the patient's values and elicits the most appropriate course of action.

Professionalism

Uphold the Primacy of Patient Welfare
Primum non nocere. Above all do no harm. The finding of an incidental mass on a radiologic study engenders concern in the patient. It is often necessary to be clear with patients about the need for careful radiologic follow-up evaluation, as some of these findings, when properly monitored, will lead to better outcomes. However, these potential benefits must be balanced with the risks of radiation exposure. Overly frequent imaging carries the risks of cumulative radiation exposure, which has potential for long-term negative consequences. In these circumstances, physicians should adhere to evidence-based recommendations to ensure the greatest benefit, while minimizing risk to the patient.

Systems-Based Practice

Be Mindful of the Benefits and Risks of Testing
The frequency of incidentally detected adrenal lesions will grow as the population ages and more refined investigative tools are utilized for assessment. Adrenal lesions are now probably underreported in all clinical settings. Managing an adrenal lesion should be approached by characterizing the lesion to determine whether it is probably malignant and by assessing possible hormonal production. Most adrenal lesions are benign and hormonally inactive, but reliable identification and reporting in the primary radiologic investigation is a prerequisite for further characterization and management. Given the widely publicized concerns about excessive radiation exposure related to CT scans and other imaging modalities, compliance with guidelines to minimize radiation exposure is important in the follow-up of these lesions.

Suggested Readings

Berland LL, Silverman SG, Gore RM, et al. Managing incidental findings on abdominal CT: white paper of the ACR Incidental Findings Committee. J Am Coll Radiol 2010;7:754–773.

Hammarstedt L, Muth A, Wangberg B, et al., on behalf of the Adrenal Study Group of Western Sweden. Adrenal lesion frequency: a prospective, cross-sectional CT study in a defined region, including systematic re-evaluation. Acta Radiol 2010;10:1149–1156.

MacMahon H, Austin JHM, Herold CJ, et al. Guidelines for management of small pulmonary nodules detected on CT scans: a statement from the Fleischner Society. Radiology 2005;237:395–400.

Mues AC, Landman J. Small renal masses: current concepts regarding the natural history and reflections on the American Urological Association guidelines. Curr Opin Urol 2010;20:105–110.

Patard JJ. Incidental renal tumours. Curr Opin Urol 2009;19:454–458.

Tien L, Giede C. Initial evaluation and referral guidelines for management of pelvic/ovarian masses. Joint SOGC/GOC/SCC Clinical Practice Guideline No. 230, July 2009.

Winer-Muram HT. The solitary pulmonary nodule. Radiology 2006; 239:34–49.

Zieger MA, Thompson GB, Quan-Yang D, et al. American Association of Clinical Endocrinologists and American Association of Endocrine Surgeons (AACE/AAES) medical guidelines for the management of adrenal incidentalomas. Endocrine Pract 2009;15(Suppl 1):1–20.

Chapter 44
Oncologic Emergencies (Case 36: A Problem Set of Three Common Cases)

Minal Dhamankar MD and Zonera Ali MD

Case 1: A 77-year-old man with history of CLL presents with severe fatigue, nausea, and mild abdominal discomfort. He is found to have an elevated white count, splenomegaly, and bulky lymphadenopathy. He is admitted and started on chemotherapy. His basic metabolic panel is as follows: potassium 6.8 mEq/L, calcium 8.1 mg/dL, phosphate 7.0 mg/dL, LDH 28,900 U/L, uric acid 14.3 mg/dL, and creatinine 2.6 mg/dL (baseline creatinine before treatment was 1.0 mg/dL).

Differential Diagnosis

Renal Failure in Cancer Patients		
Tumor lysis syndrome (TLS)	Infiltration of kidneys by the underlying neoplastic process	Renal failure secondary to nephrotoxic chemotherapeutic agents
Prerenal azotemia from volume depletion	Ureteral obstruction due to adenopathy	

Case 2: A 56-year-old man with history of osteoarthritis presents with a 1-month history of back pain that radiates down his legs. Pain wakes him at night and is more severe with recumbency. On physical exam, there is point tenderness at the level of the first lumbar vertebra, but range of motion is normal. The straight leg–raising test on the right side is positive. A radiograph of his lumbar spine reveals age-related degenerative changes. He receives a presumptive diagnosis of lumbosacral strain and is advised to take NSAIDs. A month later, he wakes up with leg weakness. Clinical exam reveals bilateral leg weakness, an enlarged, nodular prostate, and a PSA of 45 ng/mL.

Differential Diagnosis

Low Back Pain and Leg Weakness in a Cancer Patient	
Brain metastasis	Asthenia
Lambert-Eaton myasthenic syndrome	Spinal cord compression (SCC)

Case 3: A 55-year-old man with a history of acute myelogenous leukemia (AML) presents for a scheduled routine red blood cell (RBC) transfusion and reports fatigue. He is also receiving outpatient chemotherapy via a peripherally inserted central venous catheter (PICC). His temperature is 101°F, and blood pressure is 82/58 mm Hg with orthostatic changes. He is given 1 L of IV fluids and has routine laboratory samples drawn as he is transferred to the hospital. Upon admission, he is having rigors. His lab work shows a white blood cell count of 200 cells/μL and an absolute neutrophil count of 60 cells/μL.

Differential Diagnosis

Fever in a Cancer Patient		
Tumor fever	Neutropenic fever	Transfusion reaction
Catheter-related sepsis	Drug fever	

Speaking Intelligently

Patients with cancer are subject to developing a unique set of complications that require emergent evaluation and treatment. These oncologic emergencies can be broadly classified as those resulting from the disease itself and those resulting from therapy directed against the cancer; however, they can also be classified according to organ systems to facilitate recognition and management as follows (selected emergencies are discussed in more detail in the Clinical Entities section).

Metabolic Emergencies	Neurologic Emergencies	Cardiovascular Emergencies	Hematologic Emergencies	Infectious Complications
Hypercalcemia	Malignant SCC	Malignant pericardial effusion	Hyperviscosity syndrome (monoclonal gammopathy)	Neutropenic fever
TLS	Increased intracranial pressure due to brain metastasis	Superior vena cava syndrome (SVCS)	Hyperleukocytosis and leukostasis	Catheter-related sepsis

PATIENT CARE

Clinical Thinking

- Oncologic emergencies may manifest over hours, causing devastating outcomes such as paralysis and death, while some are insidious and may take months to develop.
- Various clinical symptoms often are evident before an emergency occurs; therefore, a patient-focused approach that includes education and cancer-specific monitoring is needed.
- Ability to recognize these conditions, a focused initial evaluation, and institution of appropriate therapy can be lifesaving and may spare patients considerable morbidity.
- The approach to definitive therapy is commonly multidisciplinary, involving surgeons, radiation oncologists, medical oncologists, and other medical specialists.

History

- In patients with **TLS**, symptoms largely reflect the underlying metabolic derangements, including nausea, vomiting, diarrhea, anorexia, lethargy, and fatigue. Urine output may decrease, and the patient may manifest symptoms of uremia or volume overload. Hypocalcemic tetany and seizures can occur. Muscular symptoms may include muscle weakness, cramps, and parasthesias. Life-threatening arrhythmias in the form of ventricular tachycardia or fibrillation can lead to syncope and sudden death.
- New back pain that is not responding to routine pain medication, worsens when the patient lies down, or is associated with the

development of leg weakness, urinary incontinence, and loss of
sensory function warrants consideration of **epidural SCC**.
- Fever can be the only symptom in patients with **neutropenic fever**.
A focused history to identify any localizing symptoms should be
obtained. Presence of rigors is usually indicative of bacteremia.
Diarrhea is usually associated with a gastrointestinal source, and
persistent headaches might prompt a workup to rule out meningitis.
It is important to know when the patient received his last
chemotherapy, as the neutrophil nadir typically occurs 5 to 10 days
after the last dose. Usually, white blood cell recovery occurs within 5
days of this nadir.

Physical Examination
- In **TLS**, physical exam may reveal signs of renal failure and acidosis.
In cases of severe renal failure, there may be signs of fluid overload
secondary to aggressive hydration in the setting of oliguria/anuria.
- In patients presenting with epidural **SCC**, symmetrical motor weakness
is typical. If the lesion is at or above the conus medullaris, extensors
of the upper extremities are affected. Lesions above the thoracic
spine cause weakness from corticospinal dysfunction and affect flexors
in the lower extremities. Patients may be hyperreflexic below the
lesion and have extensor plantar responses. There may be absent
sensation below the level of spinal cord involvement.
- In patients with **neutropenic fever**, the oral cavity should be
examined carefully, looking for erythema and mucosal ulcers. All sites
of IV catheters and tunneled catheters should be inspected, looking
for erythema, tenderness, and purulent exudates. The perianal area
should be inspected and palpated gently.

Tests for Consideration
Laboratory studies include:
- **CBC with differential count:** Neutropenia is usually
defined as an absolute neutrophil count (ANC) of less than
500 cells/μL or less than 1000 cells/μL with a predicted
nadir of less than 500 cells/μL. $11
- **Basic metabolic profile:** Tumor lysis syndrome leads to a
large number of metabolic derangements. $12
- **Serum uric acid levels:** Large amounts of uric acid are
released when tumor cells lyse and should be closely
monitored whenever there is a high suspicion of TLS. $6
- **Microbiologic evaluation:** Blood cultures should be obtained
as soon as possible. Urine should be collected for culture,
and sputum should be sent for cultures if there is a
productive cough. Stool and cerebrospinal fluid should
be collected and cultured, if there is clinical suspicion
of infections of these sites. $45

IMAGING CONSIDERATIONS

→ **Plain radiographs:** Chest radiographs should be obtained but are commonly normal or show nonspecific findings in patients with neutropenic fever. In patients with back pain where there is a concern for epidural SCC, radiographs of the spine are simple and inexpensive but have high false negative rates. $45

→ **CT scan:** High-resolution CT may be helpful in febrile neutropenic patients with suspected lung infection and a normal chest radiograph. The role of CT scan in diagnosing epidural SCC is limited, as focused CT imaging can miss clinically inapparent lesions; CT myelography is useful but involves a lumbar puncture and hence is contraindicated in patients with brain metastases, thrombocytopenia, or coagulopathy. $334

→ **MRI:** MRI of spine is the standard of care in the diagnosis of spinal cord compression. It is noninvasive, allowing imaging of the entire spine and the thecal sac. $534

Clinical Entities	Medical Knowledge

Tumor Lysis Syndrome

Pφ Initiation of cytotoxic chemotherapy in malignancies with high proliferative rate, large tumor burden, and/or a high sensitivity to treatment can result in the rapid lysis of tumor cells. This releases massive quantities of intracellular contents into the systemic circulation, leading to hyperkalemia, hyperphosphatemia, secondary hypocalcemia, hyperuricemia, and acute renal failure.

Hyperuricemia is a consequence of the catabolism of purine nucleic acids to hypoxanthine and xanthine, and then to uric acid via the enzyme xanthine oxidase. Overproduction and overexcretion of uric acid in TLS lead to crystal precipitation and deposition in the renal tubules, with resultant acute renal failure.

Rapid tumor breakdown can lead to **hyperphosphatemia**, as phosphorus concentration in malignant cells is higher than in normal cells, which can cause secondary **hypocalcemia**. Allopurinol blocks the catabolism of xanthine; this can result in xanthine stone formation and resultant acute renal failure despite adequate hydration.

TP Patients generally have a history of recently started chemotherapy. The tumors most frequently associated with TLS are high-grade non-Hodgkin lymphomas and acute lymphoblastic leukemia (ALL). Underlying hypovolemia or renal failure predisposes to TLS. The symptoms largely reflect the associated metabolic abnormalities. These include nausea, vomiting, diarrhea, anorexia, lethargy, hematuria, heart failure, cardiac dysrhythmias, seizures, muscle cramps, tetany, syncope, and possible sudden death.

Dx The Cairo-Bishop definition, proposed in 2004, provides specific laboratory criteria for the diagnosis of TLS both at presentation and within 7 days of treatment.
   Laboratory TLS is defined as any two or more serum values revealing the following abnormalities:
- Serum uric acid ≥ 8 mg/dL or 25% increase from baseline
- Serum potassium ≥ 6.0 mmol/L or 25% increase from baseline
- Serum phosphate ≥ 6.5 mg/dL in children, ≥ 4.5 mg/dL in adults, or a 25% increase from baseline in either age group
- Serum calcium ≤ 7 mg/dL (1.75 mmol/L) or 25% decrease from baseline

These abnormalities must be present within 3 days before and 7 days after instituting chemotherapy in the setting of adequate hydration (with or without alkalinization) and use of a hypouricemic agent. Clinical TLS is defined as laboratory TLS plus one or more of the following that was not directly attributable to a therapeutic agent: increased serum creatinine concentration (≥ 1.5 times the upper limit of normal [ULN]), cardiac arrhythmia/ sudden death, or a seizure.

Tx The risk of TLS can be reduced by maintaining adequate hydration status and administering allopurinol for 2 to 3 days before planned chemotherapy. Patients at high risk, such as those with tumors of high proliferative rate, high baseline uric acid, large tumor burden, and chemosensitive disease, may benefit from IV recombinant urate oxidase (rasburicase).
   Patients with established TLS need hospital admission and may need cardiac monitoring. IV fluids should be given to maintain urine output of ≥ 100 mL/m^2 per hour.
   Aggressive treatment of **hyperkalemia** is indicated. Calcium gluconate and sodium bicarbonate should be used in addition to insulin, dextrose, and sodium polystyrene sulfonate (Kayexalate), as severe hyperkalemia is associated with cardiac conduction disturbance.

Alkalinization of the urine has been recommended in the past, but its usefulness remains controversial. Uric acid is more soluble in alkaline urine, but the solubility of xanthine and hypoxanthine decreases with alkalinization. Urine alkalinization could possibly lead to formation of urinary xanthine crystals, resulting in obstruction of renal tubules if allopurinol is used concurrently. Rasburicase, a urate oxidase, degrades uric acid to allantoin, which is a much more water-soluble compound. It causes rapid reduction in the uric acid levels and lowers both new and previously produced uric acid. This is in contrast to the effect of allopurinol, which decreases uric acid formation and does not acutely reduce the serum uric acid concentration. Rasburicase is considered superior to allopurinol in preventing and treating TLS. Cautious use of diuretics in the euvolemic patient can help to increase urine output.

Hyperphosphatemia can be treated by restricting phosphate intake and with phosphate binders such as aluminum hydroxide.

Dialysis is indicated in severe cases, including patients with oliguric renal failure, congestive heart failure, or severe hyperkalemia, or in patients who do not respond to medical therapy.

Hypocalcemia should not be treated unless symptomatic.
See Cecil Essentials 32, 48, 51, 74, 87.

Spinal Cord Compression

Pφ SCC develops when tumors metastasize to the vertebral bodies and subsequently erode into and encroach on the spinal cord. The thoracic spine is the most common location. Some lung cancers, lymphomas, and sarcomas, which may not cause bony destruction, can lead to spinal cord damage; these tumors occupy the paraspinous space and may enter the spinal canal through the intervertebral foramen, leading to cord compression. The mechanism of injury to the spinal cord from an epidural tumor is due to direct compression of the neural elements interrupting axonal flow or via a vascular mechanism. Venous plexus obstruction can cause marked cord edema, whereas tumor occlusion of the arterial blood supply to the spinal cord creates an acute infarction, leading to abrupt and irreversible cord ischemia. Multiple inflammatory mediators and cytokines can increase the edema and the ischemia, resulting in irreversible neuronal injury.

TP The most common presenting symptom is back pain. Pain is often worse with recumbency, secondary to distension of the epidural venous plexus. Other symptoms include radicular pain, motor weakness that is usually symmetrical, gait disturbance, and dysfunction of bladder and bowel function. Sensory involvement is less common. Because neurologic deficits may not improve with treatment, it is imperative to consider the possibility of SCC before neurologic dysfunction develops.

Dx The diagnosis depends upon the demonstration of a neoplastic mass that extrinsically compresses the thecal sac. MRI of the entire spine is the preferred modality for the initial evaluation of a patient with a suspected SCC. It can provide an accurate evaluation of the extent of disease within the thecal sac and of involvement of adjacent soft tissues and bone. CT myelography can be used if MRI is contraindicated or not available.

Tx Therapy should be initiated as soon as possible. Glucocorticoids should be given immediately if there is a delay in performing the imaging studies. Dexamethasone is typically given as an initial IV dose of 10 to 16 mg followed by 4 mg every 6 hours. Higher doses (up to 100 mg) may be associated with slightly better outcome but have a higher incidence of adverse effects. Patients without motor deficits or massive invasion of the spine on imaging studies may do well without corticosteroids. Radiation therapy has been the mainstay of the treatment, but recent studies have challenged that belief. Surgery is generally considered for patients with a good performance status and the ability to withstand an extensive operation, gross instability of the spine, rapidly progressive symptoms, progressive symptoms during radiation therapy, or when tissue for diagnosis is needed. **See Cecil Essentials 58.**

Neutropenic Fever

Pφ Most episodes of febrile neutropenia occur in patients receiving chemotherapy. Less commonly, patients with acute leukemias, myelodysplastic syndromes, or other diseases that create leukopenias may present de novo with febrile neutropenia. The risk of developing febrile neutropenia depends on both the depth and the duration of the neutrophil nadir, as well as comorbid conditions or complications such as mucositis. The neutrophil nadir typically occurs 5–10 days after the last dose. Usually, white blood cell recovery occurs within 5 days of this nadir.

Multiple gram-positive and gram-negative bacteria can cause infections in neutropenic patients; however, an infectious source is identified in only 30% of cases. Enteric gram-negative bacilli have historically been the bacteria most commonly recovered from the bloodstream of febrile neutropenic patients, but gram-positive bacteria are assuming more importance due to use of long-term indwelling lines and empirical and prophylactic antimicrobials that are primarily active against gram-negative pathogens. Viral infections, especially human herpesviruses, and fungal pathogens are also common in this patient population.

TP Fever is commonly the only symptom, but patients may also have localizing symptoms and physical findings. Common infections may present atypically as a result of the lack of neutrophils. Skin infections may manifest as a subtle rash or erythema. Patients with meningitis may not have the typical physical findings such as nuchal rigidity; furthermore, urinary tract infections may be asymptomatic, and there may be no pyuria. Moreover, because of profound neutropenia, patients can have lung infections without pulmonary infiltrates.

Dx A complete workup to identify the source of infection should be undertaken as noted previously.

Tx Once febrile neutropenia is diagnosed, antibiotics should be administered immediately once the necessary cultures have been obtained. Initial antibiotic selection should be guided by the patient's history, allergies, symptoms, signs, recent antibiotic use, culture results, and institutional nosocomial infection patterns. Ideally, antibiotics should be bactericidal. There is no clear optimal choice for empirical antibiotic therapy; combination therapy and monotherapy have led to similar outcomes.

Monotherapy: Cefepime or ceftazidime, or a carbapenem (meropenem or imipenem).

Dual therapy: Aminoglycoside plus anti-pseudomonal β-lactam (piperacillin or piperacillin/tazobactam), cephalosporin (cefepime or ceftazidime), or a carbapenem (meropenem or imipenem).

Antibiotic therapy should be altered if there is evidence of progressive disease or a new complication. Routine use of gram-positive antibiotic coverage (e.g., vancomycin or linezolid) is not recommended except in the following circumstances: presence of hypotension, mucositis, skin or catheter site infection; history of methicillin-resistant *Staphylococcus aureus* (MRSA) colonization; recent quinolone prophylaxis; or overall clinical deterioration. Antifungal or antiviral drugs are usually not needed as a part of initial therapy. The echinocandins (e.g., caspofungin) are used as a first-line antifungal therapy in neutropenic patients with no obvious source of infection who are persistently febrile for 5 days despite broad-spectrum antibacterial therapy. Routine use of prophylactic antibiotics or colony-stimulating factors is not recommended. The latter have not been shown to decrease mortality and beneficial effects are quite modest, but they may be used in critically ill patients such as those with pneumonia, hypotension, or organ dysfunction, and in patients whose bone marrow recovery is expected to be especially prolonged. **See Cecil Essentials 58, 95, 109.**

ZEBRA ZONE

a. **Hypercalcemia:** This is discussed in Chapter 45, Paraneoplastic Syndromes.

b. **Increased intracranial pressure due to brain metastases:** Commonly caused by lung cancer, breast cancer, and melanoma. Occurrence of brain metastases portends a poor prognosis, and symptom control is achieved with IV dexamethasone and anticonvulsants if there are seizures.

c. **SVCS:** Obstruction of the SVC as can be caused by external compression (masses in the lung and mediastinum) or by thrombus, or by a combination of both processes. It is not a true emergency unless there is central airway obstruction or severe laryngeal edema causing respiratory compromise. Chemosensitive tumors may respond rapidly to chemotherapy alone. Other tumors may require radiation therapy.

d. **Hyperviscosity:** This can occur secondary to high levels of IgM paraproteins in patients with monoclonal gammopathies. It can cause mental status and visual changes secondary to impaired perfusion of the brain and the eyes. Plasmapheresis is used to decrease plasma viscosity. Treatment of the underlying disease with corticosteroids and chemotherapy can prevent recurrent symptoms.

e. **Hyperleukocytosis and leukostasis:** In acute leukemias, plasma viscosity can be increased due to leukocytosis; leukapheresis followed by initiation of chemotherapy is the mainstay of treatment.

Practice-Based Learning and Improvement: Evidence-Based Medicine

Title
Direct decompressive surgical resection in the treatment of spinal cord compression caused by metastatic cancer: a randomized trial

Authors
Patchell RA, Tibbs PA, Regine WF, et al.

Institution
Department of Surgery (Neurosurgery), University of Kentucky Medical Center, Lexington, Kentucky

Reference
Lancet 2005; 366:643–648

Problem
Radiation therapy has been the mainstay of the treatment, but recent studies have challenged that belief. This study showed that direct decompressive surgery followed by radiation therapy is superior to radiation therapy alone.

Intervention
In this randomized, multi-institutional, nonblinded trial, patients with SCC caused by metastatic cancer were randomly assigned to either surgery followed by radiation therapy ($n = 50$) or radiation therapy alone ($n = 51$). Radiation therapy for both treatment groups was given in 10 fractions of 3 Gy each. The primary end point was the ability to walk. Secondary end points were urinary continence, muscle strength and functional status, the need for corticosteroids and opioid analgesics, and survival time.

Comparison/control (quality of evidence)
The group receiving surgery followed by radiation therapy was compared to the group receiving radiation therapy alone.

Outcome/effect
Significantly more patients in the surgery group (42/50, 84%) than in the radiation therapy group (29/51, 57%) were able to walk after treatment (odds ratio 6.2; 95% confidence interval 2.0–19.8; $P = 0.001$). Patients treated with surgery also retained the ability to walk significantly longer than did those with radiation therapy alone (median 122 days vs. 13 days, $P = 0.003$). Thirty-two patients entered the study unable to walk; significantly more patients in the surgery group regained the ability to walk than patients in the radiation group: 10/16 (62%) vs. 3/16 (19%); $P = 0.01$. The need for corticosteroids and opioid analgesics was significantly reduced in the surgical group.

Historical significance/comments
Direct decompressive surgery plus postoperative radiation therapy is superior to treatment with radiation therapy alone for patients with SCC caused by metastatic cancer.

Interpersonal and Communication Skills

Alert Patients to Potential Complications of Treatment
Educating patients proactively about potential oncologic emergencies in a language that they understand will encourage them to seek timely help and prevent catastrophes. For example, educating patients about neutropenia related to chemotherapy and instructing them to notify the health-care provider of any fever while being treated can lead to earlier intervention, reducing the likelihood of an adverse outcome. A reminder to patients about adequate hydration before and during chemotherapy is also helpful in preventing metabolic derangements.

Professionalism

Inform Patients and Families When Requesting Consultation
In cases of oncologic emergencies, the approach to definitive therapy is multidisciplinary, involving surgeons, radiation oncologists, medical oncologists, and other specialists. Appropriate guidance should be sought from consultants in a timely manner and often on an emergent basis. It is important to inform the patient and family about whom you have consulted for help and why. When things happen quickly in the care of a patient, this matter is often overlooked. Families and patients become anxious quickly when multiple new physicians are suddenly involved. Keep everyone informed and up to date with your plan of management.

Systems-Based Practice

Consider Patient Compliance in Outpatient Treatment
Selected patients with fever and neutropenia can be treated in the outpatient setting. Close follow-up and unrestricted access to health-care personnel are essential when patients are receiving outpatient therapy. Situations such as a history of noncompliance, inability to care for oneself, lack of caregivers, no telephone, or lack of reliable transportation are contraindications for outpatient treatment. The best-studied oral regimen used in outpatient

treatment for fever/neutropenia is a combination of ciprofloxacin (500 mg every 8 hours) and amoxicillin/clavulanate (500 mg every 8 hours). When using such a regimen, patients should be assessed daily for the first 3 days to assess compliance, response to therapy, and development of any adverse effects. All patients should be given clear instructions as to when and how to seek medical attention.

Suggested Readings

Bosly A, Sonet A, Pinkerton CR, et al. Rasburicase (recombinant urate oxidase) for the management of hyperuricemia in patients with cancer. Cancer 2003;98:1048–1054.

Cairo MS, Bishop M. Tumor lysis syndrome: new therapeutic strategies and classification. Br J Haematol 2004;127:3–11.

Coiffier B, Mounier N, Bologna S, et al. Efficacy and safety of rasburicase (recombinant urate oxidase) for the prevention and treatment of hyperuricemia during induction chemotherapy of aggressive non-Hodgkin's lymphoma: results of the GRAAL1 (Groupe d'Etude des Lymphomes de l'Adulte Trial on Rasburicase Activity in Adult Lymphoma) study. J Clin Oncol 2003;21:4402–4406.

Freifeld AG, Bow EJ, Sepkowitz KA, et al. Clinical practice guideline for the use of antimicrobial agents in neutropenic patients with cancer: 2010 update by the Infectious Diseases Society of America. Clin Infect Dis 2011;52:e56–e93.

Halfdanarson TR, Hogan WJ, Moynihan TJ. Oncologic emergencies: diagnosis and treatment (abstract). Mayo Clin Proc 2006;81: 835–848.

Loblaw DA, Perry J, Chambers A, Laperriere NJ. Systematic review of the diagnosis and management of malignant extradural spinal cord compression: the Cancer Care Ontario Practice Guidelines Initiative's Neuro-Oncology Disease Site Group. J Clin Oncol 2005;23:2028–2037.

Patchell RA, Tibbs PA, Regine WF, et al. Direct decompressive surgical resection in the treatment of spinal cord compression caused by metastatic cancer: a randomised trial. Lancet 2005;366:643–648.

Schiff D, O'Neill BP, Wang CH, O'Fallon JR. Neuroimaging and treatment implications of patients with multiple epidural spinal metastases. Cancer 1998;83:1593–1601.

Chapter 45
Paraneoplastic Syndromes (Case 37: A Problem Set of Three Common Cases)

Nishanth Sukumaran MD and Mary Denshaw-Burke MD

Case 1: A 70-year-old man presents to the ED with confusion and dehydration. Family members report a weight loss of 30 pounds over the last 6 months and increased forgetfulness over the last several weeks. He has a 50-pack-year smoking history. He has dry mucous membranes on examination. Laboratory values reveal a blood urea nitrogen (BUN) of 50 mg/dL, serum creatinine of 2.5 mg/dL, and serum calcium of 17 mg/dL. Chest radiograph shows a 5 cm × 4 cm mass in the right upper lobe.

Differential Diagnosis

Hypercalcemia and Abnormal Chest Radiograph	
Tumor secretion of parathyroid hormone–related peptide (PTHrP)	Bone metastasis
Tumor secretion of calcitriol	Ectopic secretion of parathyroid hormone (PTH)

Case 2: A 65-year-old woman presents to the ED with progressive confusion. Laboratory values reveal serum sodium of 120 mEq/L, serum osmolality of 245 mOsm/kg water, urine osmolality of 600 mOsm/kg water, and urine sodium of 65 mmol/L. A CT scan of the chest shows a mass in the right middle lobe.

Differential Diagnosis

Hyponatremia in Malignancy		
Poor dietary intake	Increased gastrointestinal losses from tumor or treatment	Syndrome of inappropriate secretion of antidiuretic hormone (SIADH)
Renal failure or congestive heart failure secondary to chemotherapy	Adrenocortical insufficiency from tumor metastasis to adrenal glands	

Case 3: A 68-year-old man presents to his family doctor with a 2-month history of dry cough. He also reports a 1-year history of difficulty in getting up from a chair and climbing stairs. He describes muscle aches and cramping, especially after long walks. Chest radiograph shows a left upper lobe mass.

Differential Diagnosis

Weakness in Malignancy	
Asthenia	Brain metastasis
Lambert-Eaton myasthenic syndrome (LEMS)	Spinal metastasis with cord compression

Speaking Intelligently

Paraneoplastic syndromes are diseases or symptoms that are the consequence of the presence of cancer in the body, but they are not directly due to the local presence of cancer cells. These phenomena are mediated by humoral factors (hormones and cytokines) secreted by the tumor cells or an immune response directed against the tumor. Paraneoplastic syndromes may parallel the underlying malignancy, and successful treatment of the malignancy may lead to disappearance of the syndrome. However, many paraneoplastic syndromes, especially of immunologic or neurologic etiology, may not respond predictably to treatment of the underlying malignancy. Selected paraneoplastic syndromes are discussed in more detail in the Clinical Entities section.

PATIENT CARE

Clinical Thinking
- Paraneoplastic syndromes may be the presenting symptom in someone who has not yet been diagnosed with cancer or may develop during the course of treatment for cancer.
- The incidental finding of a possible paraneoplastic syndrome should lead to a prompt workup to rule out an underlying malignancy.
- The identification and treatment of the underlying malignancy not only improves symptoms from the paraneoplastic syndrome but also may improve survival if the malignancy is diagnosed at an earlier stage.

- In some patients with a known malignancy, the discovery of a paraneoplastic syndrome may indicate a worse outcome.

History
- Patients with paraneoplastic syndromes may be either acutely symptomatic needing emergent care or asymptomatic.
- Some patients present with mental status changes such as confusion and coma. The history can be obtained from the patient's spouse or other family members in the event that the patient is too obtunded to provide any history.
- History of clinically significant weight loss, anorexia, and smoking should draw attention to malignancy as an underlying cause.
- Once a malignancy is suspected, it is imperative to elicit a focused history related to identifying the underlying malignancy.
- A history of drenching night sweats and pruritus could indicate a lymphoproliferative disorder.
- Symptoms such as hemoptysis, persistent cough, hoarseness, and shortness of breath could be indicative of a lung malignancy.
- History should always include questions regarding age-appropriate screening.
- A comprehensive social history including smoking, alcohol use, and occupational exposure to various chemicals should be obtained.
- Family history of malignancies, especially at a younger age, may indicate a genetic link.

Physical Examination
- Patients with hypercalcemia of malignancy have a very high serum calcium level and generally present with signs of volume depletion, such as hypotension, tachycardia, confusion, and dry mucous membranes.
- Patients with SIADH are euvolemic and may present with confusion.
- Patients with LEMS present with proximal muscle weakness.
- The presence of confluent macular erythema (heliotrope rash) and discrete erythematous papules overlying the metacarpophalangeal and interphalangeal joints (Gottron papules) suggests a diagnosis of dermatomyositis, which may be associated with an underlying malignancy.
- Brown to black velvety hyperpigmentation of skin, usually found in body folds, is termed acanthosis nigricans. When seen in individuals over 40 years of age, it is suggestive of an internal malignancy, especially of the gastrointestinal tract.

- Explosive onset of multiple seborrheic keratoses (sign of Leser-Trélat) is a sign of possible internal malignancy of the gastrointestinal tract, breast, or lung.
- Physical exam findings suggesting malignancy also include clubbing, lymphadenopathy, palpable breast mass, and hepatosplenomegaly.

Tests for Consideration

- **Comprehensive metabolic profile:** Used to diagnose hyponatremia, hypercalcemia, and renal failure either secondary to hypercalcemia or from volume depletion. It may also provide a clue to diagnosis of underlying pancreatic and hepatobiliary malignancies.　　　　　　$12
- **CBC with differential count:** Eosinophilia is commonly associated with Hodgkin lymphoma and mycosis fungoides. Basophilia is associated with chronic myelogenous leukemia and other myeloproliferative disorders.　　　　　　$11

IMAGING CONSIDERATIONS

→ **Chest radiograph**, **CT scanning**, and **MRI** can help identify the tumor. They are most often used along with **bone scans** or **PET** to stage tumors.　　　$45, $334, $534, $247, $1037

Clinical Entities　　　　　　　　　　Medical Knowledge

Hypercalcemia of Malignancy

Pφ There are four subtypes of malignancy-associated hypercalcemia: (1) local osteolytic hypercalcemia due to bone metastases from solid tumors or marrow invasion by primary hematologic malignancies, typically in patients with lymphoma, myeloma, and breast cancer; (2) hypercalcemia due to production of calcitriol $(1,25(OH)_2D)$ by lymphomas; (3) ectopic secretion of authentic PTH by rare malignancies (ectopic hyperparathyroidism); and (4) humoral hypercalcemia of malignancy (HHM).

Paraneoplastic syndrome–related hypercalcemia includes all of the above except local osteolytic hypercalcemia. HHM is caused by systemic secretion of PTHrP by malignant tumors; it is commonly associated with squamous cell carcinoma of the lung. Some tumors also cause hypercalcemia by secretion of cytokines such as transforming growth factor-β, tumor necrosis factor-α, and interleukin-1.

TP Patients with mild hypercalcemia (<12 mg/dL) may be asymptomatic or present with nonspecific symptoms such as fatigue, depression, and constipation. However, patients with hypercalcemia associated with malignancy present with much higher calcium levels and are frequently obtunded. They usually present with confusion and even coma. Although these patients usually have a known malignancy, hypercalcemia may be the presenting finding leading to diagnosis.

Dx The following is the diagnostic approach to hypercalcemia:
- Serum calcium is bound to albumin, and the measured total calcium levels may be underestimated or overestimated depending on decreases or increases in albumin. A rough estimation of corrected calcium is determined by adding 0.8 mg/dL to total calcium for every 1 mg/dL of serum albumin below 3.5 mg/dL.
- Serum ionized calcium measurement should be considered when there is doubt about the validity of the total calcium measurement.
- Intact PTH should be routinely measured in all cases of hypercalcemia. Levels are elevated in primary hyperparathyroidism and some cases of HHM, where the tumor produces PTH. However, in most cases of HHM, the serum PTH is normal.
- Although most patients with HHM have elevated levels of PTHrP, the diagnosis is usually obvious on clinical grounds. Therefore, PTHrP measurement should be undertaken only in the few cases where the diagnosis is uncertain.
- Plasma 1,25(OH)$_2$D should be measured when sarcoidosis, other granulomatous disorders, or the 1,25(OH)$_2$D lymphoma syndrome is considered in the differential diagnosis

Tx The following is the approach to management of hypercalcemia of malignancy:
- General measures include discontinuation of calcium from parenteral feeding solutions, discontinuation of medications that cause hypercalcemia (e.g., calcium and vitamin D supplements, thiazide diuretics, and lithium), increased weight bearing by the patient if possible, and discontinuation of sedative medications.
- Normal saline, at a rate of 200–500 mL/hr, should be administered depending on the degree of hypercalcemia, baseline level of volume depletion, renal impairment, and cardiovascular status.
- Loop diuretics are administered only after full hydration is achieved. Loop diuretics such as furosemide block the reabsorption of calcium in the loop of Henle, aiding in the excretion of calcium.
- Bisphosphonates work by blocking osteoclastic bone resorption. As oral bisphosphonates are poorly absorbed, only IV preparations are used for hypercalcemia. In the United States, the two drugs approved for use by the Food and Drug Administration (FDA) in mild to severe hypercalcemia are pamidronate and zoledronic acid.
- Serum phosphate and creatinine should be closely monitored to keep phosphate levels between 2.5 and 3.0 mg/dL, serum creatinine in the normal range, and the calcium × phosphate product in the range of 30–40.
- Agents such as glucocorticoids, calcitonin, and mithramycin are either infrequently used or are used when the use of bisphosphonates is ineffective or contraindicated.
- In selected patients who are likely to respond to treatment but have acute or chronic renal failure, and aggressive fluid infusion is not possible, dialysis may be a reasonable option.
See Cecil Essentials 24, 58, 74.

Syndrome of Inappropriate Secretion of Antidiuretic Hormone

Pφ ADH is secreted from the posterior pituitary gland to prevent water loss in the kidneys. When water is ingested, the resulting dilution of plasma and decrease in plasma osmolality is sensed by the osmoreceptors in the hypothalamus, and ADH secretion is switched off. In SIADH, the release of ADH is not inhibited by decreased plasma osmolality. The principal malignancy associated with SIADH is small cell lung cancer, accounting for

75% of the cases. Other less frequently associated malignancies include those of the duodenum, pancreas, and head and neck. The tumors cause ectopic secretion of ADH leading to symptoms and signs of SIADH.

TP Most patients are asymptomatic or experience minimal symptoms, and hyponatremia is discovered incidentally on routine laboratory evaluation. When symptoms develop, they generally reflect central nervous system toxicity. In early stages patients complain of fatigue, headaches, anorexia, and mild altered mental status. As the syndrome progresses, patients may experience continued delirium, confusion, and seizures. Ultimately, patients may suffer refractory seizures or coma, and, in rare cases, death.

Dx Patients with SIADH present with hyponatremia and are found to have a low serum osmolality and elevated urine osmolality. The urine sodium concentration is usually >40 mEq/L. The serum BUN and uric acid concentrations are low, with normal acid-base and potassium balance. Patients have normal renal, adrenal, and thyroid function.

Tx Asymptomatic hyponatremia is treated with fluid restriction of 500 to 1000 mL/day. Severe, symptomatic, or resistant hyponatremia requires administration of 3% hypertonic saline, the effects of which can be enhanced if given with a loop diuretic. The rate of correction should not exceed 8–10 mEq/L on any day of treatment to prevent the development of central pontine myelinolysis. Demeclocycline can be used in resistant cases. Conivaptan, a vasopressin receptor antagonist, was approved by the FDA for treatment of hypervolemic hyponatremia. Treatment of small cell carcinoma of the lung with chemotherapy is generally associated with improvement of SIADH. **See Cecil Essentials 28, 58.**

Lambert-Eaton Myasthenic Syndrome

Pφ LEMS is an autoimmune disorder associated with antibodies directed against the presynaptic voltage-gated calcium channels (VGCCs) of the neuromuscular junction. Blockade of calcium channels leads to inhibition of acetylcholine release from the presynaptic vesicles, thus affecting muscle contraction. Approximately 50% of LEMS cases are associated with small cell carcinoma of lung.

TP Patients present with slowly progressive proximal muscle weakness. The typical presentation is that of alteration in gait, as well as difficulty rising from a chair or climbing stairs. Muscle aches and cramping are common. Autonomic dysfunction is often present and could be a clue to diagnosis. Dry mouth is the most common autonomic symptom, and erectile dysfunction is common in men. In contrast to myasthenia gravis, the symptoms of LEMS are worse in the morning and improve as the day progresses.

Dx Maximal isometric contraction of the relevant muscles for 10–15 seconds can lead to temporary improvement of muscle weakness, a phenomenon known as post-exercise or post-activation facilitation. Radioimmunoassay is utilized to detect antibodies against the VGCCs. An incremental response to repetitive nerve stimulation on electrophysiologic studies is also observed.

Tx Treatment of underlying malignancy is essential in the treatment of paraneoplastic LEMS. Often, this may be the only treatment needed. For mild symptomatic disease, pyridostigmine, either alone or in combination with 3,4-diaminopyridine or guanidine, can be used. Immunosuppressive agents such as corticosteroids and azathioprine have been used with limited success. More significant or refractory weakness may require treatment with IV immunoglobulin or plasmapheresis. **See Cecil Essentials 24, 58, 132.**

ZEBRA ZONE

a. **Cowden disease:** Autosomal-dominant syndrome with numerous tumors of the hair follicles called trichilemmomas located on the face. These patients have a high risk of breast and thyroid carcinomas.

b. **Gardner syndrome:** Autosomal-dominant familial adenomatous polyposis, a colorectal cancer syndrome characterized by hundreds of colorectal polyps, which lead to colon cancer by the age of 40 years.

c. **Sweet syndrome:** Consists of acute onset of fever, neutrophilia, and appearance of painful red cutaneous papules on the face, neck, and upper extremities. Association with malignancy, including acute myelogenous leukemia, occurs in 20% of cases.

Practice-Based Learning and Improvement: Evidence-Based Medicine

Title
Zoledronic acid is superior to pamidronate in the treatment of hypercalcemia of malignancy: a pooled analysis of two randomized, controlled clinical trials

Authors
Major P, Lortholary A

Institution
Hamilton Regional Cancer Centre, Hamilton, Ontario, Canada

Reference
J Clin Oncol 2001;19:558–567

Problem
Is zoledronic acid superior to pamidronate in the treatment of hypercalcemia of malignancy?

Intervention
Patients were randomized to treatment with either a single dose of zoledronic acid (4 or 8 mg) via a 5-minute IV infusion or pamidronate (90 mg) via a 2-hour IV infusion.

Comparison/control
Two identical, concurrent, parallel, multicenter, randomized, double-blind trials were conducted at centers in the United States/Canada and Europe/Australia. A total of 287 patients were randomized in the two trials.

Quality of evidence
Level I

Outcome/effect
Zoledronic acid was found to be superior to pamidronate. Zoledronic acid at a dose of 4 mg is the dose recommended for initial treatment of hypercalcemia of malignancy and 8 mg for relapsed or refractory hypercalcemia. The safety profile of zoledronic acid was similar to that of pamidronate. However, renal adverse events were reported somewhat more frequently in the zoledronic acid groups compared to the pamidronate groups.

Historical significance/comments
Before this study, pamidronate was the standard of care for hypercalcemia of malignancy. This study proved that zoledronic acid provides a more effective and more convenient treatment for hypercalcemia of malignancy.

Interpersonal and Communication Skills

Deliver News of Worsening Prognosis in a Sensitive Manner
The diagnosis of a paraneoplastic syndrome may lead to discovery of a new cancer or may suggest a poorer prognosis in a patient known to have a malignancy. Breaking news about an underlying cancer is the most critical conversation you will have with your patient. Be prepared that patients will respond in various ways including denial, anger, intellectualization, and feelings of guilt. It is important to recognize these various responses, and it is vital to approach the subject as sensitively and empathetically as possible. When possible, and at the discretion of the patient, family members and other supportive persons should be present during these conversations, which may help to comfort the patient when first hearing about the diagnosis of cancer. When concluding initial discussions, it is important to assure both the patient and family that you will be available to answer follow-up questions as they arise.

Professionalism

Telephone Challenges: Maintain Patient Confidentiality
When you give a diagnosis of cancer to a patient, it is necessary to state the facts honestly and sensitively, and the patient's confidentiality must be respected at all times. You must ask the patient specifically with which family members and/or friends you may discuss medical issues. *Especially when a patient is in the intensive care unit*, it is not uncommon that the physician will end up fielding phone calls from those inquiring about the patient's condition. While it may seem difficult or unfair, unless you have specific permission to discuss the matter with the caller, the correct answer is to state that you are unable to discuss the patient's medical issues with anyone without the patient's permission.

Systems-Based Practice

Consider Costs and Benefits When Prescribing Medications
In the United States there are two drugs that are approved for use in hypercalcemia of malignancy and considered agents of choice in mild to severe hypercalcemia: pamidronate (Aredia) and zoledronic acid (Zometa). Although a relative superiority of zoledronic acid over pamidronate has been demonstrated, these differences may be of minor clinical significance for the individual patient. The choice of one agent over the other is currently based on convenience and cost. The standard dose of zoledronic acid is 4 mg given over a 15-minute

period, whereas pamidronate is given at a dose of 60–90 mg over a 2-hour period. Pamidronate is currently less expensive; however, zoledronic acid is more convenient to use. Both agents have been associated with impairment of renal function, and monitoring of renal function should be a routine practice.

Suggested Readings

AAEM Quality Assurance Committee. American Association of Electrodiagnostic Medicine. Literature review of the usefulness of repetitive nerve stimulation and single fiber EMG in the electrodiagnostic evaluation of patients with suspected myasthenia gravis or Lambert-Eaton myasthenic syndrome. Muscle Nerve 2001;24:1239–1247.

Burtis WJ, Wu TL, Insogna KL, Stewart AF. Humoral hypercalcemia of malignancy. Ann Intern Med 1988;108:454–457.

Dau PC, Denys EH. Plasmapheresis and immunosuppressive drug therapy in the Eaton-Lambert syndrome. Ann Neurol 1982;11:570–575.

Ellison DH, Berl T. Clinical practice. The syndrome of inappropriate antidiuresis. N Engl J Med 2007;356:2064–2072.

Fleisch H. Bisphosphonates: mechanisms of action (review). Endocr Rev 1998;19:80–100.

Johnson BE, Chute JP, Rushin J, et al. A prospective study of patients with lung cancer and hyponatremia of malignancy. Am J Respir Crit Care Med 1997;156:1669–1678.

Lang B, Newsom-Davis J, Wray D, et al. Autoimmune etiology for myasthenic (Eaton-Lambert) syndrome. Lancet 1981;2:224–226.

Major P, Lortholary A. Zoledronic acid is superior to pamidronate in the treatment of hypercalcemia of malignancy: a pooled analysis of two randomized, controlled clinical trials. J Clin Oncol 2001;19:558–567.

Motomura M, Johnston I, Lang B, et al. An improved diagnostic assay for Lambert-Eaton myasthenic syndrome. Neurol Neurosurg Psychiatr 1995;58:85–87.

Ralston SH, Gallagher SJ, Patel U, et al. Cancer-associated hypercalcemia: morbidity and mortality: clinical experience in 126 treated patients. Ann Intern Med 1990;112:499–504.

Ratcliffe WA, Hutchesson AC, Bundred NJ, Ratcliffe JG. Role of assays for parathyroid-hormone-related protein in investigation of hypercalcaemia. Lancet 1992;339:164–167.

Robertson GL. Regulation of arginine vasopressin in the syndrome of inappropriate antidiuresis. Am J Med 2006;119(7 Suppl 1):S36–S42.

Sterns RH, Nigwekar SU, Hix JK. The treatment of hyponatremia. Semin Nephrol 2009;29:282–299.

Stewart AF. Hypercalcemia associated with cancer. N Engl J Med 2005;352:373–379.

Section IX
ENDOCRINE DISEASES

Section Editor
Mansur Shomali MD

Section Contents

46 **Polyuria and Polydipsia (Case 38)**
   Kavita Iyengar MD

47 **Hypoglycemia (Case 39)**
   Shadi Barakat MD

48 **Weight Gain and Obesity (Case 40)**
   Elizabeth Briggs MD

49 **Weight Loss (Case 41)**
   Pamela R. Schroeder MD, PhD

50 **Amenorrhea (Case 42)**
   Amy Rogstad MD

51 **Fragility Fracture (Case 43)**
   Paul Sack MD

Chapter 46
Polyuria and Polydipsia (Case 38)

Kavita Iyengar MD

Case: The patient is a 68-year-old woman with a medical history of hypertension, hyperlipidemia, and obesity. She presents to the outpatient office because for the last few weeks she has been more tired than usual and feels that she has been drinking more water. She has also been going to the bathroom more frequently, particularly at night. In addition, she has blurry vision and headaches. Her husband is also your patient. He has trouble maintaining control over his blood sugar and is also obese. Both the patient and her husband often miss scheduled follow-up appointments.

The patient's medications are hydrochlorothiazide, atorvastatin, and an aspirin. Her father had hypertension and coronary artery disease, and her mother was recently diagnosed with type 2 diabetes mellitus. The patient works as an administrative assistant. She smokes half a pack of cigarettes a day and drinks a glass of wine occasionally.

On examination she is pleasant and conversant and appears comfortable. She states that she thinks she may have "a little sugar" like her husband. Her vital signs are within normal limits, but her body mass index (BMI) is 37. Her lungs are clear to auscultation, and heart sounds are normal. Her abdomen is obese. Her neurologic exam is normal except for a decreased monofilament sensation in her feet.

Differential Diagnosis

Diabetes mellitus, type 1	Diabetes mellitus, type 2	Diabetes insipidus (DI)
Hypercalcemia	Gestational diabetes	

Speaking Intelligently

Polyuria is most often caused when the kidneys are subjected to an increased osmotic load, such as that from glucose or calcium. Alternatively, it may be due to endocrine disorders of fluid regulation such as vasopressin (antidiuretic hormone, ADH) deficiency. Conditions that cause bladder irritability or obstruction such as cystitis or prostatic enlargement can cause increased urinary frequency, but usually not polyuria. When most clinicians are assessing an obese patient with polyuria and polydipsia, type 2 diabetes mellitus, which affects over 20 million persons in the United States, is the first diagnosis that comes to mind. A point-of-care capillary glucose by finger-stick or a urinalysis can quickly make the diagnosis of uncontrolled diabetes, so that this patient can quickly get the appropriate care.

PATIENT CARE

Clinical Thinking

- Diabetes mellitus is diagnosed with two fasting blood glucose measurements greater than 125 mg/dL or a random value greater than 200 mg/dL in a patient with symptoms. At this point, you have to determine how sick the patient is and whether the patient needs inpatient management to treat symptomatic hyperglycemia or has life-threatening complications such as diabetic ketoacidosis (DKA) or a nonketotic hyperosmolar state.
- Patients with type 1 diabetes may present to the emergency department in DKA, with an elevated blood glucose, or an anion gap metabolic acidosis with positive serum ketones and electrolyte imbalances.
- Patients with type 2 diabetes may present in a hyperosmolar state with severe volume depletion, hypernatremia, and very high blood glucose levels.
- If the glucose and calcium are normal, other conditions such as DI or primary polydipsia should be considered.

History

- Hyperglycemia can present as a spectrum from one in which the patient is completely asymptomatic to one in which the patient has DKA or a hyperosmolar state.
- In an asymptomatic patient, hyperglycemia may be an incidental finding on laboratory work done for other reasons, or it could be seen in a patient admitted to the hospital in acute stress (e.g., from a myocardial infarction or severe infection). At times, medications such as corticosteroids can be the cause.
- If a patient's blood glucose has been consistently high for some time, symptoms such as polydipsia, polyuria, and nocturia can be seen, since excess glucose delivered to the kidneys causes an osmotic diuresis. Hyperglycemia can also manifest as blurry vision from the effects of glucose on the lens, or tingling and numbness in the toes from peripheral neuropathy. Other symptoms that should be sought are weight loss and fatigue.
- A patient who presents in DKA or a hyperosmolar state may be too sick to give a history but may have an obvious inciting insult such as

infection or a myocardial infarction. Nausea, vomiting, and abdominal pain are common symptoms in patients with DKA.
- A family history of diabetes can be found, which is more common in patients with type 2 diabetes.
- Patients with DI may have pituitary tumors; they should be questioned about headaches and visual changes, and other endocrinopathies. Patients with primary polydipsia may be drinking excessive amounts of water because of a psychiatric or central nervous system (CNS) disorder.

Physical Examination
- Look for signs of complications of long-standing hyperglycemia.
- Patients with type 2 diabetes are typically overweight, while those with type 1 diabetes are often not.
- An exam of the skin may reveal signs of insulin resistance such as acanthosis nigricans and skin tags.
- Patients with type 1 diabetes may have other signs of autoimmune disorders such as vitiligo and goiter.
- Screening for chronic complications of diabetes should include a monofilament exam looking for sensory neuropathy, a foot exam assessing for peripheral vascular disease, and a dilated funduscopic exam screening for retinopathy.
- In a patient admitted to the hospital with DKA, Kussmaul respirations and ketotic breath may be noted; very sick patients may present with mental status changes and signs of volume depletion such as hypotension and tachycardia.

Tests for Consideration
- **Fasting plasma glucose:** Obtained to diagnose diabetes. A value of 100 to 125 mg/dL indicates pre-diabetes, while a value above 125 mg/dL obtained twice indicates diabetes. $7
- **Random plasma glucose:** Can also be used to diagnose diabetes. A value of 140 to 200 mg/dL indicates pre-diabetes or glucose intolerance, while a value above 200 mg/dL, in the presence of symptoms, is diagnostic of diabetes. $7
- **Fingerstick blood glucose:** Checked by the patient at home, using a glucometer. This should typically be checked once daily in patients on oral hypoglycemic agents and three to four times a day in patients on insulin. This could also be checked in an emergency, while awaiting serum blood glucose values from the lab. $5
- **Hemoglobin A$_{1c}$ (HbA$_{1c}$ or glycosylated hemoglobin):** Gives an idea of the average blood glucose over the 3- to 4-month period before the blood sample is drawn. The average blood sugar of a normal person should be less than 120 mg/dL, which corresponds to an HbA$_{1c}$ of 6%. For every point increase in HbA$_{1c}$, a 30-point increase in the average blood glucose can be expected. For example, an HbA$_{1c}$ of 8% would suggest the

patient's blood glucose averaged 180 mg/dL over the previous 3 months. An HbA$_{1c}$ of less than 7% suggests good blood sugar control. $14

- **Urine microalbumin-to-creatinine ratio:** Elevated in early diabetic nephropathy. $14
- **Serum creatinine:** Elevated in later stages of diabetic nephropathy. $6
- **Arterial blood gas and serum ketones:** Used to assess patients with DKA in which an anion gap metabolic acidosis (pH < 7.30) and positive serum ketones are seen. $27, $12
- **Sodium:** The osmotic effect of hyperglycemia can shift water from the extravascular to the intravascular space, which is measured as hyponatremia. This is particularly evident in the hyperosmolar state. As a general rule, for each 100 mg/dL of glucose over 100 mg/dL, the serum sodium concentration is lowered by approximately 1.6 mEq/L. Conversely, when glucose levels fall, the serum sodium level rises by a corresponding amount. $6
- **Urine and serum osmolality:** Patients who have lost excessive free water because of hyperglycemia or hypercalcemia will have high serum osmolality. Patients with DI usually have high serum osmolality and low urine osmolality. Patients with primary polydipsia will have normal or even low serum osmolality and appropriately dilute urine. $18
- **Potassium:** Hyperkalemia may be seen in patients with DKA. Hypokalemia can be expected on treating an acutely ill patient with insulin. An electrocardiogram (ECG) may be used to evaluate the cardiac effects of extremes in serum potassium. $6
- **Bicarbonate:** Used in conjunction with the anion gap to assess the degree of acidosis. $6
- **Phosphorus:** Should be checked and repleted while treating DKA.
- **Blood urea nitrogen (BUN):** Elevated in patients with volume depletion. $6
- **Serum osmolality:** Measured as 2(Na$^+$) (mEq/L) + glucose (mg/dL)/18 + BUN (mg/dL)/2.8. Values above 330 mOsm/kg H$_2$O are typically seen in hyperosmolar patients. $9
- **Complete blood count (CBC):** An elevated white blood cell (WBC) count may indicate infection as a precipitating cause of hyperglycemia. $11
- **Urinalysis:** To look for glycosuria and ketonuria. $4
- **Amylase and lipase:** Elevated in pancreatitis. $19
- **Calcium and albumin, ionized calcium:** Total calcium is elevated in patients with hypercalcemia. If the albumin is low, total calcium can be mathematically corrected for albumin, or ionized calcium may be measured. $14
- **Parathyroid hormone (PTH):** Elevated in patients with hyperparathyroidism; low in patients with hypercalcemia of malignancy or vitamin D intoxication. $59

- **C-peptide level and glutamic acid decarboxylase (GAD) antibodies:** Used to diagnose type 1 diabetes. In these patients C-peptide may be low, since no insulin is being secreted in vivo, and GAD antibodies are positive, suggesting autoimmune destruction of the insulin-producing cells of the pancreas. $60
- **Lipids:** Should be in the normal range; low-density lipoprotein (LDL) cholesterol, in particular, should be as close to 70 mg/dL as possible to lower the risk of cardiovascular disease. $19
- **Ankle-brachial index:** Should be assessed in patients with poor lower extremity pulses to evaluate for peripheral arterial disease. $65

Clinical Entities	Medical Knowledge

Diabetes Mellitus Type 1

Pφ Destruction of the β-cells of the pancreas from autoimmune, environmental (virus, toxin, stress), or other causes. This results in insulin deficiency; patients are symptomatic when the majority of the β-cells are destroyed.

Previously called IDDM (insulin-dependent diabetes mellitus) or juvenile-onset diabetes mellitus.

TP Patients are younger at diagnosis, sometimes just 10–14 years of age. Signs and symptoms of hyperglycemia include the following: increased thirst and hunger, frequent urination especially at night, weight loss, and fatigue. Often, a DKA picture at diagnosis.

Dx High blood and urine glucose, elevated HbA$_{1c}$, positive GAD antibodies, and nondetectable C-peptide level. In patients with DKA, anion gap metabolic acidosis, low serum bicarbonate, high serum and urine ketones.

Tx Insulin, subcutaneously with frequent fingersticks to monitor blood glucose. This can be given as multiple daily injections or via an insulin pump. Patients should receive basal insulin (e.g., glargine or detemir) once or twice daily, and prandial (mealtime) insulin (e.g., lispro, aspart, or glulisine) with each meal. Insulin pumps contain short-acting insulin, set for basal doses to be running continuously and bolus doses to cover meals. In addition, diet, exercise, and diabetes and nutrition education are critical.

Patients presenting with DKA require IV fluid hydration and IV insulin infusion, with close monitoring of blood glucose and serum electrolytes; particular attention must be given to potassium and phosphorus repletion. **See Cecil Essentials 69.**

Diabetes Mellitus Type 2

Pφ Usually a combination of insulin resistance at the periphery, decreased insulin production from the pancreas, and excess glucose production by the liver. Previously called NIDDM (non–insulin-dependent diabetes mellitus) or adult-onset diabetes mellitus.

TP Patients are typically obese, with a sedentary lifestyle and a strong positive family history in first-degree relatives. They are usually over 30 years of age at diagnosis, but this is now frequently seen at younger ages as well. There is a higher incidence in African Americans, Hispanics, and Native Americans. Patients usually have hyperglycemia for several months before diagnosis. They may have symptoms of hyperglycemia as in type 1 patients and frequently also have blurred vision, tingling/numbness in the feet, and poor wound healing. Other features associated with insulin resistance/metabolic syndrome, such as acanthosis nigricans, hyperlipidemia, and hypertension, may be seen. Sometimes, with uncontrolled hyperglycemia, patients may present in a hyperosmolar state, with severe dehydration and high serum osmolality; serum ketones are usually absent.

Dx High blood and urine glucose, elevated HbA_{1c}. Diagnosis is made with at least two fasting blood glucose measurements > 125 mg/dL or random blood glucose > 200 mg/dL with symptoms of hyperglycemia.

Tx Diet and exercise play an important role in management, and all patients should receive diabetes and nutrition education. Oral hypoglycemic agents should be started, with a goal HbA_{1c} of <6.5% or 7.0%. Typically, metformin is the first agent of choice. Patients could also use one of the secretagogues, sulfonylureas, and meglitinides, which stimulate the pancreatic β-cells to secrete insulin. Other agents used are thiazolidinediones and α-glucosidase inhibitors. More recently, the dipeptidyl peptidase IV inhibitor sitagliptin and the incretin mimetic exenatide, which have been proven to have other beneficial effects in addition to blood glucose control, are gaining popularity.

For a patient presenting in a hyperosmolar state, IV hydration and IV insulin should be started, although it is important to volume-resuscitate the patient adequately before insulin is administered, because intracellular fluid shifts following reduction in serum glucose may worsen systemic tissue perfusion. Electrolyte imbalances are common, so close monitoring and repletion with correct use of IV fluids are crucial.

During outpatient follow-up, patients should have annual eye and foot exams to detect retinopathy and neuropathy/vascular disease, respectively. In addition, patients should be advised to take a low-dose aspirin daily to prevent cardiovascular complications. Urine microalbumin-to-creatinine ratio should be checked routinely and the patient started on an angiotensin-converting enzyme (ACE) inhibitor or angiotensin receptor blocker (ARB) if early nephropathy is found. Blood pressure control and cholesterol lowering are crucial for the reduction of cardiovascular risk. **See Cecil Essentials 69.**

Gestational Diabetes Mellitus

Pφ Insulin resistance during pregnancy.

TP Abnormal fasting or oral glucose tolerance on routine blood tests performed at prenatal visits. Patients are usually asymptomatic or may have symptoms of hyperglycemia.

Dx Fasting blood glucose > 95 mg/dL, or 100 mg oral glucose tolerance test with the following results: >180 mg/dL at 1 hour, >155 mg/dL at 2 hours, and >140 mg/dL at 3 hours.

Tx Diet and exercise through diabetes and nutrition education. Insulin is the mainstay of therapy during pregnancy; metformin could be used in the first trimester. Postnatal follow-up, with at least an annual fasting blood glucose measurement, should be performed, keeping in mind that these patients are at a high risk of developing type 2 diabetes in the future. **See Cecil Essentials 69, 71.**

Diabetes Insipidus

Pφ Deficiency of ADH (also known as vasopressin) from either a hypothalamic-pituitary disorder (central DI) or renal resistance to the action of ADH (nephrogenic DI). ADH is synthesized in the hypothalamus and secreted by the posterior pituitary, so damage to these areas (from trauma, tumor, infection, infiltration, or vascular lesion) results in ADH deficiency and central DI. On the other hand, impaired renal tubule response to ADH can result in nephrogenic DI, which may be inherited or acquired. A common acquired cause is from a side effect of the drug lithium.

TP Insidious onset of polydipsia and polyuria at any age. Alternatively, with an insult to the hypothalamus or pituitary, the onset of symptoms may be acute, resulting in volume depletion and hypernatremia.

Dx ADH levels (not routinely measured) are low in central DI and high in nephrogenic DI. Diagnostic tests should include measurement of serum electrolytes and osmolality as well as urine specific gravity and osmolality. The water deprivation test reveals the inability to concentrate urine; injecting vasopressin improves symptoms and increases urine osmolality in central DI but not in nephrogenic DI.

Tx Desmopressin (a synthetic analogue of ADH) treats central DI effectively. Diuretics (i.e., thiazides), which may reduce distal sodium delivery in the renal tubules, may improve nephrogenic DI. Intake of free water, a low-salt, low-protein diet, and correcting the underlying cause, if possible, may be helpful in management. **See Cecil Essentials 27, 28, 65.**

Hypercalcemia

Pφ Hypercalcemia may be PTH-mediated (hyperparathyroidism with increased intestinal calcium absorption) or non–PTH-mediated (localized bone destruction or via PTH-related peptide activity from malignancies, granulomatous disorders, and medications such as thiazides or lithium). Other causes are prolonged immobilization, milk-alkali syndrome, ingestion of calcium supplements, vitamin A or D excess, multiple myeloma, Paget disease, familial hypocalciuric hypercalcemia, and hyperthyroidism.

TP Patients with mild hypercalcemia may have no symptoms. In more severe cases the patient may have nausea, vomiting, abdominal pain, constipation, altered mental status, headache, muscle/joint aches, and polyuria. These symptoms are more common in the elderly. On exam, hyperreflexia, tongue fasciculations, altered mental status, abdominal tenderness, proximal muscle weakness, and volume depletion may be seen.

Dx High serum calcium, after correcting for albumin. Ionized calcium levels may also be measured. Other helpful lab tests, including PTH, phosphorus, vitamin D levels, creatinine, and 24-hour urine calcium, should be done to evaluate for the potential cause. If suspected, malignancy should be ruled out.

Tx Adequate hydration followed by loop diuretics (furosemide), bisphosphonates, steroids, calcitonin, and calcimimetics may be used. Treatment of the underlying cause is also important for management. **See Cecil Essentials 74.**

ZEBRA ZONE

a. **Psychogenic polydipsia (primary polydipsia):** Patients with psychiatric illnesses (e.g., schizophrenia) may drink large volumes of water in the absence of a physiologic stimulus, with resulting low ADH levels and polyuria. They may excrete over 6 L of urine daily, without nocturia, and with resulting hyponatremia. If necessary, these patients should be admitted and severe hyponatremia managed appropriately.

Practice-Based Learning and Improvement: Evidence-Based Medicine

Title
Executive summary: standards of medical care in diabetes—2012

Authors
Numerous. Expert opinion reviewed and approved by the Professional Practice Committee and the Executive Committee of the Board of Directors

Institution
American Diabetes Association

Reference
Diabetes Care 2012;35:S4–10.

Problem
Controversies in the diagnosis and treatment of diabetes mellitus, including the most cost-effective approach, prevention of its complications, and the role of nutrition

Intervention
Meta-analysis of best evidence

Quality of evidence
Level III (see below)

Outcome/effect
The listed guidelines are itemized, and each is graded according to the quality of evidence available.

Historical significance/comments
This is a comprehensive set of diabetes guidelines revised and published annually, based on available clinical evidence. Physicians and health-care professionals use these guidelines in the management of patients for optimal control of blood glucose and prevention of complications.

Interpersonal and Communication Skills

Involve Families in the Patient Care Plan

When dealing with diabetic patients and their families, try to keep the following points of communication in mind:

- Close relatives and/or household members should understand the goals of care and how to reach those goals.
- The patient requires family support and encouragement in matters of adhering to regimens of diet and exercise.
- Significant others can be supportive by doing activities together with the patient: attending nutrition classes, encouraging weight loss, and exercising.
- Careful consideration of the family environment may be required in selecting the type of medication used for treatment. Older patients who depend on insulin, for example, may have trouble with self-injections because of visual impairment, arthritis, or inability to use syringes; help from a family member may be required.
- The same principle of family engagement applies to young patients with type 1 diabetes. Parental knowledge of insulin dosing and hypoglycemia is crucial.

Professionalism

Empower Your Patients to Manage Their Disease

Because of modifications in diet, daily injections, and blood glucose testing, diabetes involves the lifelong commitment of the patient. Undoubtedly, the patient may at times be discouraged or indifferent, and may refuse to make the lifestyle modifications required. Occasionally this calls for compromise, which may be difficult for physicians to accept. The physician should understand and respect the patient's need to feel in control.

Systems-Based Practice

Reimbursement: Medicare

Medicare, enacted in 1965, is the federal insurance program that provides care for the elderly and disabled; in 2006 the program cost $400 billion. Administered by the Centers for Medicare & Medicaid Services (CMS), the program consists of four parts, as follows:

- Part A covers hospitalizations and is centered on a system of diagnosis-related groups (DRGs), which are codes that represent the diagnosis of a patient; the hospital is reimbursed a certain amount for each admission depending upon the patient's DRG.

- Part B pays for physician office visits, outpatient care, and durable medical equipment; physicians are paid based on current procedure technology (CPT) codes, among which is a subset of evaluation and management (E&M) codes that provides for different levels of patient visits.
- Part C, or Medicare Advantage, allows Medicare recipients to choose to have their Medicare coverage provided by a private payer; these plans are typically HMO-type plans that are able to save money by limiting their coverage to networks of providers with savings used to offer greater coverage of preventive care and drug benefits. To qualify, persons must be enrolled in both Medicare parts A and B.
- Part D is the prescription drug benefit of Medicare and is being administered by private insurance plans that are reimbursed by CMS. Recipients must elect to participate unless they are dual-eligible (i.e., eligible for Medicare and Medicaid), in which case they are automatically enrolled. Of note is that the legislation prevents the government from negotiating discounts on drugs that might otherwise be available to entities that make mass purchases; there is also a gap in coverage for costs between $2250 and $5100.

Chapter 47
Hypoglycemia (Case 39)

Shadi Barakat MD

Case: The patient is a 35-year-old athletic woman who works as nurse. She has been healthy except for mild depression and anxiety that have not required treatment. She presents for evaluation of recurrent episodes of fatigue, palpitations, tremor, and sweating, without loss of consciousness, that started 4 weeks ago. Each episode lasted for a few minutes and subsided quickly after she ate a snack. Usually these episodes occurred at work shortly before lunchtime. During one of the episodes, she appeared confused and her co-workers tried to obtain a fingerstick glucose, but she refused, claiming that she would be fine. She blamed the episodes on her bad eating habits. She exercises every morning for 1 hour before coming to work, and she does not eat breakfast. For lunch she eats some steamed vegetables with a diet drink. Her coworkers were concerned about her and urged her to make an appointment for evaluation.

Upon further questioning, she mentioned that her boyfriend broke up with her 2 months ago, and that has been a difficult time for her. She recently started to take a couple of drinks of alcohol before she goes to bed. She doesn't smoke, and she denies illicit drug use.

On exam, she is pleasant and in no apparent distress. Her height is 65 in. and her weight is 115 lb. (Her BMI is 19.) Her vital signs and the rest of her exam are negative for any abnormalities.

Differential Diagnosis

Medications (diabetic patients)	Alcoholic hypoglycemia	Non–insulin-secreting tumors
Medications (nondiabetic patients)	Insulin-secreting tumors	
Factitious administration of hypoglycemic agents	Counter-regulatory hormones deficiency	

Speaking Intelligently

Symptoms of hypoglycemia can be grouped as (1) adrenergic symptoms such as palpitations, tremor, and anxiety; (2) cholinergic symptoms such as sweating, hunger, and parasthesias; and (3) neuroglycopenic symptoms including behavioral changes, confusion, fatigue, seizure, and loss of consciousness. When asked to evaluate a patient like this, it is essential to document a measurement of the patient's blood glucose while symptomatic. However, maintaining a broad differential diagnosis is important since other disorders may trigger autonomic and psychiatric symptoms when the blood glucose is normal.

PATIENT CARE

Clinical Thinking

- In a patient presenting with adrenergic, cholinergic, and neuroglycopenic symptoms that resolve with eating, hypoglycemia should be highly suspected but must be documented.
- Hypoglycemia can best be approached by subdividing it into fasting (post-absorptive) hypoglycemia, reactive (post-parandial) hypoglycemia, and factitious hypoglycemia (which can happen any time).
- Reactive hypoglycemia is most commonly seen after abdominal surgeries including gastrectomy and roux-en-Y gastric bypass; in

addition, it is often seen in thin, young healthy individuals and in patients with early diabetes or pre-diabetes who have insulin-secretory dysfunction.

- Factitious hypoglycemia should be suspected in health care workers and relatives of patients with diabetes. It is caused by the accidental or intentional administration of insulin or an insulin secretagogue.
- The causes of fasting hypoglycemia may be due to (1) endogenous hyperinsulinism, as in patients on diabetes medications or with insulin-secreting tumors; (2) exogenous hyperinsulinism; (3) decreased insulin clearance, such as in patients with renal or liver failure; (4) increased utilization of glucose, as in sepsis; or (5) decreased production of glucose either due to organ failure or to counter-regulatory hormone deficiencies (i.e., cortisol, glucagon, or growth hormone deficiency).

History
- Considering the wide differential diagnosis for a patient who is presenting primarily with adrenergic symptoms, it is important to take a detailed history with a focus on the circumstances in which the symptoms occur and how they progress.
- A social and psychiatric history.
- Episodic symptoms of palpitations, tremors, and headache in a patient with hypertension should raise the consideration of pheochromocytoma.
- Symptoms that occur always in public and under stressful condition may indicate panic attacks.
- The fact that the patient is a health care worker means that she has access, skills, and knowledge of how to induce hypoglycemia, and how to treat it; factitious hypoglycemia should be suspected.
- Occurrence of symptoms always during fasting should trigger a workup for post-absorptive hypoglycemia.
- Hypoglycemia in diabetic patients should be approached carefully since it is the direct result of trying to tightly control blood glucose, and patients tend to develop non-adherence to medication if they encounter hypoglycemic episodes.
- Any recent changes in the dosage, timing of administration of the medication, or patient activity.
- A history of heart, kidney, or liver failure can be contributing to hypoglycemia in some patients. Excessive alcohol intake is important to note.

Physical Examination
- Common signs of hypoglycemia include diaphoresis, tremor, and pallor.
- Heart rate and blood pressure are usually elevated.
- Transient focal neurological deficits occasionally occur.
- If hypoglycemia is severe and has persisted for a long time, patients may develop altered consciousness and coma.
- However, the physical exam is otherwise unremarkable between episodes.

Tests for Consideration

- The first step in evaluating a patient with hypoglycemia is to **confirm that hypoglycemia is the cause of the patient's symptoms**; the diagnosis can be best established by **Whipple Triad:** (1) symptoms consistent with hypoglycemia; (2) a low serum glucose level (<55 mg/dL); and (3) relief of symptoms after ingestion/administration of glucose and serum glucose level is raised.

- Hypoglycemia in patients with diabetes mellitus treated with either insulin or a secretagogue warrants dose adjustment and does not require workup in most cases.

- In a non-diabetic patient, if a hypoglycemic episode is observed, the **appropriate blood samples should be drawn while the blood glucose level is still low**, if possible. The management here should be directed toward correcting the hypoglycemia, by administering oral or parenteral glucose, and treating the underlying disease.

- In an apparently healthy patient who presents with a history of symptoms suggestive of hypoglycemia, a **supervised prolonged fasting** of up to 72 hours, which requires hospital admission, should be done. The fast should be stopped when blood glucose drops below 55 mg/dL. Once symptoms of hypoglycemia are observed, blood samples should be collected immediately and sent to the lab to check for simultaneous blood glucose, C-peptide, and insulin levels.

- An **elevated insulin level when the blood glucose is low** is essential to establish hyperinsulinism as the cause of hypoglycemia. However, it does not establish the etiology of the increased insulin level, which can be either endogenous (e.g., an insulinoma or sulfonylureas ingestion) or exogenous (e.g., surreptitious use of insulin). The patient's **blood should be screened for oral hypoglycemic agents**. A positive serum test can establish the diagnosis of factitious ingestion of diabetes medications, while a negative serum test should trigger the evaluation for the presence of an insulinoma. $18

- **Transabdominal ultrasonography**, **endoscopic ultrasonography**, **spiral CT**, and **arteriography** can be used to locate an insulinoma. $96, $154, $334, $2086

Clinical Entities	Medical Knowledge

Medications (Diabetic Patients)

Pφ Medications are the most common cause of fasting hypoglycemia. Insulin causes hypoglycemia through its action of inducing glucose utilization. Sulfonylureas and meglitinides are secretagogues; they act by increasing insulin secretion from the pancreas. Some of them have active metabolites and long durations of action.

TP Insulin-treated diabetic patients usually encounter hypoglycemia when the insulin dose exceeds their needs and is mostly seen when the dose is adjusted to better control high blood glucose. The insulin dose can also exceed the requirement in several other scenarios, such as when patients change their physical activity without adjusting the insulin dose, or when they fail to have a meal or a full meal after they administer a mealtime insulin dose. Also, it is not uncommon for hypoglycemia to occur as a result of the administration of a higher insulin dose by mistake, especially if the patient has a vision problem.

Diabetic patients using sulfonylureas can encounter hypoglycemia in similar circumstances. Both insulin and sulfonylurea doses become higher than the requirement when the patient's kidney function worsens.

Dx Most diabetic patients can recognize and report their hypoglycemic symptoms. However, the physician should always check fingerstick blood glucose when possible before taking any action when hypoglycemic symptoms occur. Demonstration of Whipple triad is easy and confirms the diagnosis.

Tx Diabetic patients are almost always instructed to carry sugar tablets at all times and are educated to recognize and manage hypoglycemia. Most hypoglycemic episodes can be reversed by ingesting 15 g of sugar. Insulin-treated patients who present to the emergency department with hypoglycemia can be treated with IV dextrose and observation for the duration of action of the insulin they are using after other confounding factors such as sepsis and worsening kidney function, which will require inpatient management, have been ruled out. Insulin dose should be adjusted to prevent future events. Special attention should be paid to patients who are using a secretagogue. Sulfonylurea-induced hypoglycemia can be best described as severe, prolonged, and relapsing, and often requires stopping all hypoglycemic agents and instituting inpatient observation for 1 day or more. Keep in mind that one of the main reasons for nonadherence to medication in patients with diabetes is frequent episodes of hypoglycemia. **See Cecil Essentials 70.**

Medications (Nondiabetic Patients)

Pφ Although insulin and secretagogues cause hypoglycemia in diabetic patients through the action of insulin on glucose metabolism, other non-antihyperglycemic medications can cause hypoglycemia by different mechanisms. Large doses of salicylates can cause hypoglycemia by inhibiting glucose production.

Sulfonamides and quinine can stimulate insulin production. Pentamidine causes dysglycemia and is considered toxic to β-cells. Patients can develop hypoglycemia, diabetes mellitus, or hypoglycemia initially and diabetes later. Disopyramide, cibenzoline, and fluoroquinolones (particularly gatifloxacin) have all been reported to cause hypoglycemia.

TP Patients are usually being treated for diseases such as malaria, *Pneumocystis jirovecii* pneumonia, other infections, or arrhythmias. Patients are usually symptomatic, or the hypoglycemia is documented during fingerstick blood glucose determination. Patients being treated with quinine may present with severe hypoglycemic coma.

Dx Diagnosis can be established by the Whipple triad in patients who are being treated with one of the medications that is known to cause hypoglycemia.

Tx Rapid correction of blood glucose with IV dextrose is very important in the acute setting. Glucagon can also be used. Patients should be monitored closely for up to 3 days for recurrence of hypoglycemia. They should be educated about recognizing the symptoms of hypoglycemia and should keep sugar tablets with them at all times. Pentamidine-treated patients should be monitored for the development of diabetes. Diazoxide can be used as an outpatient regimen in patients whose medical condition necessitates continuing the offending agent. **See Cecil Essentials 70.**

Alcoholic Hypoglycemia

Pφ Ethanol blocks gluconeogenesis and causes hypoglycemia.

TP Individuals with ethanol-induced hypoglycemia manifest a variety of neurologic signs. Coma, seizures, and hemiparesis have been described. They may also manifest adrenergic signs and symptoms, such as tachycardia and tremor. However, the repeated exposure to ethanol may deplete the catecholamine stores, resulting in absence of the adrenergic response to hypoglycemia. Most of these patients are chronic alcoholics who present a few days after binge drinking with little food intake. Ethanol-induced hypoglycemia is not related to the degree of ethanol-induced liver damage.

Dx Hypoglycemia should be suspected in any comatose and/or alcoholic patient. Fingerstick and analysis for blood glucose should be routinely done. A low blood glucose level establishes the diagnosis. A urine dipstick is usually positive for ketones.

Tx Patients usually respond immediately to IV glucose infusion and do not require prolonged periods of infusion or observation so long as they can maintain modest carbohydrate intake. In alcoholic patients, physicians should always remember to replace thiamine, along with the infusion of glucose, to avoid the serious side effect of further depleting thiamine stores. **See Cecil Essentials 70.**

Insulin-Secreting Tumors (Insulinoma)

Pφ Though β-cell tumors (insulinomas) are the most common of the pancreatic endocrine neoplasms, they are very rare. The incidence was estimated as low as 4 per 1 million per year. They occur in both genders and have been described in persons from 8 to 82 years of age. They are most often found within the pancreas as a single small (<2 cm) encapsulated tumor. Rarely, they arise from ectopic pancreatic tissues. It is estimated that 10% of insulinomas are malignant.

TP Insulinoma should be suspected in patients who present with Whipple triad who are not being treated with insulin and/or hypoglycemic agents. A typical patient will be a middle-aged and otherwise healthy individual who presents with episodes of hypoglycemia symptoms.

Dx Considering how rare insulinomas are, it is important to keep in mind the wide differential diagnosis, especially the factitious use of insulin or secretagogues. Patients should be observed during fasting for symptoms of hypoglycemia. Sometimes it is necessary to admit the patient to the hospital for a prolonged period of fasting for 48–72 hours. Once symptoms are observed, blood should be drawn and sent for blood glucose, insulin, and C-peptide levels. A high insulin-to-glucose ratio, in the presence of a negative assay for the presence of secretagogues, makes the diagnosis more likely. The next step is localization of the tumor using transabdominal ultrasonography or spiral CT. Endoscopic ultrasonography, arteriography, and arterial stimulation with hepatic venous sampling can be used to localize the tumor if the first two modalities are unsuccessful. The preoperative studies, along with intraoperative ultrasonography and palpation, can identify 98% of all tumors.

Tx Management is surgical by excision of the tumor or tumors. Resection is also indicated for isolated metastatic tumors. In patients who fail surgery, diazoxide can be used. Somatostatin analogues can be effective in diazoxide-refractory symptomatic patients. **See Cecil Essentials 70.**

Non–Insulin-Secreting Tumors

Pφ Several case reports have described patients with non–islet cell tumors with severe hypoglycemia and without hyperinsulinism. The proposed mechanisms of hypoglycemia include the following: inhibition of gluconeogenesis, replacement of the liver and the adrenal tissue with tumors, and excessive utilization of glucose in the skeletal muscles or by the tumors that was linked in most cases to increased secretion of incompletely processed insulin-like growth factor II (IGF-II).

TP Non–islet cell tumor-induced hypoglycemia has been described in patients with a wide variety of tumors and was reported in association with carcinomas of the breast, colon, esophagus, lung, ovary, pancreas, and prostate, as well as other tumors such as carcinoid, hepatoma, lymphoma, multiple myeloma, meningioma, and mesothelioma. These tumors are usually large in size, with an average weight of 2–4 kg.

Dx It is usually easy to establish the diagnosis of hypoglycemia in patients with a known history of a tumor that is known to cause hypoglycemia. Further workup to determine the mechanism is not necessary.

Tx Treatment should be directed to the underlying malignancy, along with correction of hypoglycemia in the acute setting. Patients who respond well to glucagon and who continue to experience hypoglycemia can be treated with a continuous glucagon infusion. **See Cecil Essentials 70.**

Counter-Regulatory Hormones Deficiency

Pφ The first self-defense mechanism against hypoglycemia is to decrease insulin secretion. This is usually followed by increased secretion of hormones that counteract the action of insulin on glucose, attempting to return the serum glucose levels to normal. These counter-regulatory hormones are glucagon, epinephrine, cortisol, and growth hormone.

TP Most of the patients are diabetics on treatment, and they present with other illnesses depending on the organ system involved. Diabetic patients with cirrhosis are a good example and are frequently encountered in acute care facilities. Hypoglycemia due to anterior pituitary insufficiency is seen in neonates and infants more than adults. Patients with adrenal insufficiency present with signs and symptoms of Addison disease. They are extremely sensitive to fasting of any period of time; patients with Addison disease may lack the adrenergic signs and symptoms when they develop hypoglycemia.

Dx Clues to the diagnosis can be obtained by taking a good history and by performing a thorough physical exam. Addison disease patients present with hypotension and hyperpigmentation of the skin and the mucous membranes, along with specific electrolyte imbalances (specifically hyperkalemia). A patient with a history of chronic hepatitis or chronic ingestion of alcohol who presents with ascites should be monitored for hypoglycemia, especially if he or she is a diabetic on treatment. When counter-regulatory hormones deficiency is suspected, appropriate hormonal studies should be ordered. The cosyntropin stimulation test with measurements of cortisol is a very good method for evaluating patients with suspected adrenal insufficiency.

Tx Hypoglycemia secondary to endocrine deficiencies is a medical emergency. In the acute setting, rapid correction of plasma glucose using 50 mL of 50% dextrose should be done as soon as the diagnosis is suspected. Patients should be monitored closely for recurrence. The preferred IV fluids are 5% dextrose in normal saline. Glucagon can also be used to correct hypoglycemia. Parenteral hydrocortisone should be administered immediately if Addisonian crisis or hypopituitarism is suspected. Treatment should be directed to the underlying disease. Doses of hypoglycemic agents should be adjusted as needed. **See Cecil Essentials 70.**

Factitious Administration of Hypoglycemic Agents

Pφ Although this is an induced hypoglycemia, it represents a psychological pathology that warrants treatment. Patients with factitious disorder deliberately induce or falsify illness for the sole reason of playing the sick role. There is no secondary gain from faking the disease in factitious disorder. Stress, personality disorder, and psychodynamic factors have been described as factors in the pathogenesis of factitious disorder.

TP The typical patient with factitious disorder who uses hypoglycemic agents is a female in the third or fourth decade, nondiabetic, health-care worker, or the family member of a diabetic patient. It has also been described in diabetic patients on treatment. Some patients present with a confabulated history describing symptoms of hypoglycemia, while others actually administer a hypoglycemic agent and develop signs and symptoms of hypoglycemia.

Dx The diagnosis should be suspected in all patients undergoing workup for hypoglycemia, especially when the episodes happen randomly in relation to meals. An elevated insulin level with a low level of C-peptide confirms the administration of an exogenous source of insulin. Elevated insulin and C-peptide levels, with positive serum assay for sulfonylureas and/or meglitinides, confirm the use of secretagogue to induce hypoglycemia. However, the diagnosis is more difficult to establish if the patient is a diabetic on treatment. Insulin concentrations > 100 μU/mL suggest factitious use of hypoglycemic agents, since insulin levels are rarely >100 μU/mL in patients with insulinomas.

Tx No specific therapy for factitious disorder has been established. Management should be directed to correcting the hypoglycemia and protecting the patient from self-harm or harmful procedures. **See Cecil Essentials 70.**

ZEBRA ZONE

a. There are two rare etiologies for endogenous hyperinsulinism not caused by insulinomas. One is a **cervical cancer** that was proved to be secreting insulin. Also, in rare cases, hyperinsulinism can be caused by autoantibodies to insulin or insulin receptors.

b. Pheochromocytoma: A tumor most commonly arising from catecholamine-producing chromaffin cells of the adrenal medulla and classically presenting with headache, diaphoresis and palpitations in the setting of paroxysmal hypertension. Symptoms are usually episodic and tend to progress as the tumor grows. The majority of these tumors are benign. Approximately 90% arise in the adrenal gland. The remainder of pheochromocytomas are extra-adrenal in origin and usually arise in the abdomen.

Practice-Based Learning and Improvement: Evidence-Based Medicine

Title
Hypoglycemia and clinical outcomes in patients with diabetes hospitalized in the general ward

Authors
Turchin A, Matheny ME, Shubina M, et al.

Institution
Brigham and Women's Hospital, Boston, Massachusetts; Clinical Informatics Research and Development, Partners HealthCare System, Boston, Massachusetts; Harvard Medical School, Boston, Massachusetts; Vanderbilt Medical Center, Nashville, Tennessee; Tennessee Valley Healthcare System, Veteran's Administration, Nashville, Tennessee; Massachusetts College of Pharmacy and Health Sciences, Worcester, Massachusetts; Medco Health Solutions, Inc., Franklin Lakes, New Jersey.

Reference
Diabetes Care 2009;32(7):1153-1157

Problem
Hypoglycemia may be harmful to hospitalized patients. This has been demonstrated in patients with critical illness and acute myocardial infarction.

Intervention
This study was a retrospective cohort study of 4,368 hospital admissions of patients with diabetes.

Quality of evidence
Level II-2

Outcome/effect
Hypoglycemia is common in diabetic patients hospitalized in the general ward. Patients with hypoglycemia have increased length of stay and higher mortality both during and after admission.

Historical significance/comments
Measures should be undertaken to decrease the frequency of hypoglycemia in high-risk patients with diabetes who are admitted to the hospital.

Interpersonal and Communication Skills

Communicate Proactively Regarding Possible Episodes of Hypoglycemia

Hypoglycemic episodes may occur at any time and during different situations of daily life. Acknowledge proactively the potential consequences of hypoglycemia. If episodes occur during sleep, patients may have nightmares that are both frightening and disruptive to their sleep cycle. Patients will be very concerned about experiencing a hypoglycemic episode while they are driving. They may become overwhelmed by the sudden development of adrenergic and cholinergic symptoms. Some patients will express the fear of "dying during the next episode" if they have experienced palpitations, tremors, and sweating. Physicians should address fears and explain to patients how to abort such episodes. The approach to education also depends on the patient and the situation. Be aware that young patients with type 1 diabetes are at risk of developing hypoglycemia because of their usually active life-style; to avoid hypoglycemia they tend to cut down on their insulin doses or even stop it completely, putting themselves at risk for diabetic ketoacidosis. Should patients with type 2 diabetes who are on secretagogues develop recurrent episodes of hypoglycemia, they should be encouraged to seek medical attention, as their episodes might be severe and require hospitalization. In such situations, medications that regulate glucose but do not cause hypoglycemia should be considered. All diabetic patients on treatment with a secretagogue or insulin, as well as all patients who are experiencing hypoglycemia, should be instructed to have sugar tablets with them at all times.

Professionalism

Maintain Patient Confidentiality

Patients disclose vital information about their lives to their physicians, and it is very important that we do all that we can to protect our patients' right to confidentiality. Suppose your patient works at a hospital with which you are affiliated. Her illness is complicated. You run into her supervisor or a co-worker who is concerned, curious, or just inquiring about the seriousness of the patient's medical condition. Under the patient's right to confidentiality, you may not discuss your findings with anyone without the patient's permission. In fact, even acknowledging her as your patient in public might be considered a disclosure of her *protected health information* (PHI) under the Health Insurance Portability and Accountability Act (HIPAA). If the patient's supervisor requests a summary of your evaluation "to make sure that the patient does not have any medical condition that might limit her ability to perform her duties," you should require the supervisor to follow the appropriate procedures recommended by your institution to obtain such a report.

Systems-Based Practice

Reduce Medication Errors
The Joint Commission has introduced standards to reduce medication prescriber errors that are related to use of unapproved abbreviations. These include abbreviations such as QD for once daily, QOD for once every other day, use of a trailing zero after a decimal point, or use of a decimal point without a leading zero. A significant prescriber error results from the use of "U" for units, which is one of the most frequently cited reasons for the incorrect administration of insulin. The "U" may be mistaken for a "zero," which has the potential to lead to administration of 10 times the ordered dose. Therefore, the word "units" should always be written. There is significant hope that the likelihood of a medication prescriber error will be obviated following widespread utilization of an electronic medical record.

Chapter 48
Weight Gain and Obesity (Case 40)

Elizabeth Briggs MD

Case: The patient is a 38-year-old woman who is referred to you for evaluation of a 40-pound weight gain over 2 years. She tells you that she had weighed about 110 pounds from age 18 until age 24 years, when she gained 25 pounds over the course of a successful pregnancy. By 6 months after this pregnancy, she had lost 15 lb and had been stable at about 120 lb until the past 2 years. She says that she has tried to decrease her intake of calories and increase her exercise, but these measures haven't been effective in slowing her weight gain. In addition, she has been noticing facial hair, as well as hair on her chest and abdomen, which is new for her. She is clearly distressed over the changes she sees physically. Her menstrual cycle, usually regular since menarche, has been less so, with eight to nine menses per year and occasional months with 5 to 8 days of menstrual bleeding, which is longer than what she was used to until 3 years ago. On further questioning, she complains of easy bruising, acne, emotional lability, and difficulty walking up stairs due to leg weakness.

On physical examination, her blood pressure is 150/102 mm Hg, weight 164 pounds, height 62 in., and BMI 30. She has an obese trunk with relatively thin extremities. She has a rounded face with ruddy cheeks and excess supraclavicular and dorsocervical fat. She has hair on her chin, upper lip, chest, abdomen, back, and upper thighs, as well as acneiform lesions on her face, chest, and upper back. She has purple-red striae, 1 cm in diameter, on her abdomen, proximal thighs, and axillae, and ecchymoses on her upper and lower extremities. She has proximal weakness in her upper and lower extremities.

Differential Diagnosis

Exogenous obesity	Cushing syndrome
Hypothyroidism	Polycystic ovarian syndrome (PCOS)

Speaking Intelligently

Weight gain is a common problem encountered in clinical practice. When I evaluate a patient for weight gain I consider what could be its cause, as well as the potential consequences of the weight gain. Weight gain and obesity are very common; about one third of American adults are classified as overweight and about one third as obese. Obesity increases the risk for several disorders, including type 2 diabetes, hypertension, obstructive sleep apnea, dyslipidemia, atherosclerosis, osteoarthritis, and several cancers. Patients are often distressed by weight gain because of societal pressures to attain thinness. Interventions for weight loss include dietary modification, exercise, medications, and weight loss surgery. As clinicians, our responsibility is to identify factors contributing to weight gain and remove them if possible, attenuate risks associated with obesity, and facilitate safe and sustainable weight loss.

PATIENT CARE

Clinical Thinking

- When I evaluate a patient for weight gain, I first consider what has been the change in body composition. In most cases, patients have an increase in fat mass, but they should be examined for other causes, such as fluid retention, as might be seen with congestive heart failure.

- Weight gain caused by increase in fat mass, simplistically, reflects relatively more energy intake than expenditure.
- Most patients who gain weight have increased caloric intake, decreased energy expenditure, or both, perhaps in the context of a genetic predisposition to obesity.
- Occasionally, weight gain may be a sign of another underlying disorder.
- Patients should be evaluated with history and examination for possible causes of weight gain, and clues to possible diagnoses should be followed up with appropriate testing.

History

- In evaluation of weight gain, history should include lifetime weight history and time line and quantity of weight gain, such as was obtained for our patient.
- The pace and amount of weight gain vary with different etiologies and should be considered in the context of life and health events, such as pregnancy, change in environment, and new life stressors.
- Ask about symptoms of possible contributing disorders, such as glucocorticoid excess, psychiatric disease, androgen deficiency in males, growth hormone deficiency, and hypothyroidism.
- Additionally important is medication history, as multiple medications, including antihyperglycemic agents, glucocorticoids, and antipsychotic medications, are known to be associated with weight gain.
- In reviewing the dietary history, ask patients to recall intake and, if possible, to keep a food diary. These tools often will reveal that a patient is taking in more calories than he or she recognizes and will identify components in the diet that can be eliminated or substituted.
- Ask the patient to describe exercise history, including frequency, type, intensity, duration, and limiting injuries.

Physical Examination

- Physical exam should focus on the degree of obesity, signs of potential causative disorders, and signs of conditions caused or exacerbated by excess weight.
- Calculate the BMI for the patient (body weight in kilograms/(height in meters)^2) to classify underweight (<18.5), normal weight (18.5–24.9), overweight (25–29.9), and obesity (>30).
- Track the pace of weight gain, if possible, with an objective record.
- Assess the patient's body habitus. Truncal obesity (apple-shaped) might reflect glucocorticoid excess, and this pattern of obesity is

more commonly associated with metabolic syndrome than is gluteal-femoral obesity (pear-shaped).

- Look for potential signs of glucocorticoid excess (truncal obesity, rounded face, increase in supraclavicular and dorsocervical fat, hirsutism, red-purple wide striae, ecchymoses), hypothyroidism (puffy face; yellowish hue; delayed relaxation phase of reflexes; dry, cool skin; rough elbows), and male hypogonadism (fine wrinkles at corners of eyes, gynecomastia, soft or small testes).
- Examine for edema, which could reflect another cause for weight gain than increase in fat mass (congestive heart failure, cirrhosis, nephrotic syndrome).
- With respect to conditions exacerbated by obesity, look for signs of insulin resistance (acanthosis nigricans, skin tags), hypertension, PCOS (hirsutism), and type 2 diabetes (signs of insulin resistance, complications of diabetes–peripheral neuropathy, infections, carpal tunnel syndrome).

Tests for Consideration

- Testing should generally be guided by clinical suspicion generated by clues on history and physical examination.
- Obesity is common, and Cushing syndrome is rare. Screening for Cushing syndrome is thus associated with false positive and false negative test results. Specific features of Cushing syndrome, as noted in our patient case, should be identified in order to proceed with screening, which consists of three potential tests:
  - **Midnight salivary cortisol:** In normal subjects, midnight cortisol is very low as a consequence of diurnal variation, which is lost in syndromes of endogenous hypercortisolism. $23
  - **24-hour urine free cortisol** $24
  - **1 mg overnight dexamethasone suppression test** $23
  - When clinical suspicion is high, two of the three above tests should be requested to increase diagnostic accuracy.
- **Thyroid-stimulating hormone (TSH):** Elevated in primary hypothyroidism. $24
- Consider screening for associated metabolic disorders with **fasting glucose** and a **fasting lipid panel**. $7, $19
- A **sleep study** should be requested in most obese patients if they have fatigue or hypersomnolence, since obstructive sleep apnea is often undiagnosed. $795
- **Specific genetic testing** for genes that predispose patients to obesity is not widely available and has unproven clinical utility; future research may some day demonstrate that gene testing coupled with early clinical interventions is helpful for patients.

| **Clinical Entities** | **Medical Knowledge** |

Exogenous Obesity

Pφ Results from relatively more energy intake than expenditure; more likely in patients with a genetic predisposition to obesity (usually polygenic).

TP Patients have usually been overweight through adulthood, often from childhood, though weight gain can present in a previously normal-weight person who has increased caloric intake, decreased exercise, or both. Weight gain tends to be more gradual. Patients can have either truncal or gluteal-femoral obesity.

Dx Diagnosis is made by taking a dietary and exercise history and ruling out other causes for weight gain.

Tx • **Hypocaloric diets:** All compositions of diet are modestly effective; the most important factor is adherence to the diet, and weight tends to be regained after patients stop the diet.
  • **Increased physical activity:** Improves fitness and helps patients maintain weight loss.
  • **Weight loss medications:** Currently approved medications include:
    ○ Sibutramine: Serotonin uptake inhibitor that suppresses appetite; approved for long-term use and is moderately effective, but patients tend to regain weight after stopping the medication.
    ○ Orlistat: Reduces fat absorption by blocking pancreatic lipase activity in the gut. Available by prescription and in a reduced-dose over-the-counter (OTC) preparation. Moderately effective; main side effect is oily stool, and fecal urgency and leakage.
  • **Bariatric surgery:** Most effective intervention for obesity (effectiveness varies with surgical procedure), 0.1% to 1% operative mortality, frequent remission of type 2 diabetes, reduced long-term mortality. **See Cecil Essentials 60.**

Cushing Syndrome

Pφ Excess of glucocorticoid. Most common etiology is treatment with systemic glucocorticoids. Endogenous hypercortisolism is most commonly Cushing disease, which is caused by an adrenocorticotropic hormone (ACTH)–secreting pituitary tumor. Other causes are cortisol-producing adrenal adenoma, nodular adrenal hyperplasia, and ectopic ACTH secretion.

TP Presentation can range from subclinical to overt and rapidly progressive. The symptoms of hypercortisolism seen with any etiology are weight gain, hyperglycemia, muscle weakness, easy bruising, violaceous striae, moon facies, increased dorsocervical and supraclavicular fat pads, and facial plethora. Patients with ectopic ACTH secretion can have weight loss (due to underlying malignancy), hyperpigmentation, and hypokalemic metabolic alkalosis.

Dx Screening tests for endogenous hypercortisolism:
- **Midnight salivary cortisol**
- **24-hour urine free cortisol**
- **1-mg overnight dexamethasone suppression test**

If positive, measure ACTH. Should be low with exogenous glucocorticoids and cortisol-producing adrenal neoplasm.

If ACTH is high, request pituitary MRI to evaluate for pituitary adenoma. Invasive sampling procedures can be done in specialized centers if the diagnosis is unclear. If ectopic ACTH secretion is suspected, pursue imaging for the primary tumor.

Tx
- **Exogenous glucocorticoids:** Limit dose as much as possible; taper off if possible.
- **Pituitary Cushing:** Trans-sphenoidal resection of pituitary adenoma.
- **Cortisol-producing adrenal adenoma:** Unilateral adrenalectomy.
- **Micronodular adrenal hyperplasia:** Bilateral adrenalectomy.
- **Ectopic ACTH:** Resection of primary tumor if possible. If not possible, drugs to block steroid synthesis (ketoconazole, metyrapone). If necessary, bilateral adrenalectomy. **See Cecil Essentials 65, 67.**

Hypothyroidism

Pφ Most commonly due to autoimmune (Hashimoto) thyroiditis. Other causes of primary hypothyroidism include prior radioactive iodine treatment for hyperthyroidism, thyroidectomy, and drugs (lithium, amiodarone, interferon). Central hypothyroidism is caused by a pituitary disorder (adenoma, infiltrative disease, pituitary surgery) or hypothalamic disorder (rare).

TP Hypothyroidism can cause modest weight gain (generally less than 10–20 pounds). Patients may have fatigue, constipation, cold intolerance, and menorrhagia. On exam, hypothyroid patients may have coarse hair; cool, dry skin; puffy face; delayed relaxation phase on reflex testing; bradycardia; and a yellowish hue due to accumulation of carotene. Patients with subclinical hypothyroidism (normal free thyroxine with elevated TSH) should not have weight gain attributable to thyroid disease.

Dx • **TSH:** The most reliable test for primary hypothyroidism.
• **Free thyroxine and free triiodothyronine (T_3):** These tests are primarily used to evaluate for hypothyroidism due to pituitary or hypothalamic disease (in which case TSH is unreliable).

Tx Replacement with synthetic levothyroxine to target thyroid function in the normal range. Supraphysiologic doses of levothyroxine or T_3 to induce weight loss are not indicated. Lean mass is lost preferentially to fat mass in the hyperthyroid state, and side effects include risk for arrhythmia and loss of bone mass. **See Cecil Essentials 66.**

Polycystic Ovarian Syndrome

Pφ PCOS does not cause weight gain but is exacerbated by obesity and should be considered as a differential diagnosis in our patient. It is characterized by chronic anovulation and increased ovarian androgen production. Patients with PCOS have high rates of insulin resistance and have improvement in ovulation with weight loss and treatment with insulin sensitizers. They have increased risk of cardiovascular disease and diabetes.

TP Women with PCOS generally have had irregular periods since menarche. They may have acne and hirsutism, reflecting hyperandrogenism.

Dx Diagnostic criteria for PCOS include the following: chronic anovulation, clinical or biochemical hyperandrogenism, and polycystic ovaries (need two of these criteria), *and* exclusion of other causes for these symptoms including Cushing syndrome, congenital adrenal hyperplasia (CAH), and an androgen-secreting tumor.

Tx Diet and exercise interventions should be undertaken to improve metabolic risk. If fertility is desired, an insulin sensitizer, such as metformin, can be tried to allow ovulation. Ovulation induction with clomiphene is also effective. If pregnancy is not desired, oral contraceptives regulate menses, reduce endometrial cancer risk, and improve acne and hirsutism. Spironolactone can also be used to treat acne and hirsutism, and patients may seek cosmetic hair removal. **See Cecil Essentials 71.**

ZEBRA ZONE

a. **Monogenic obesity (leptin deficiency, melanocortin 4 receptor mutations):** Tend to present with severe obesity in childhood.

b. **Growth hormone deficiency:** Fairly common in patients with other pituitary disorders; isolated growth hormone deficiency is less common. Growth hormone deficiency results predominantly in truncal weight gain.

Practice-Based Learning and Improvement: Evidence-Based Medicine

Title
A descriptive study of individuals successful at long-term maintenance of substantial weight loss

Authors
Klem ML, Wing RR, McGuire MT, Seagle HM, Hill JO

Institution
University of Pittsburgh School of Medicine

Reference
Am J Clin Nutr 1997;66:239–246

Problem
What are the diet and exercise habits of people who have been successful at maintaining weight loss?

Intervention
This study describes the demographics, diet, and exercise habits of 784 patients (80% women) in the National Weight Control Registry (a registry of people who have maintained a greater than 30-lb weight loss for longer than 1 year).

Quality of evidence
Level II-3

Outcome/effect
These patients, who have been successful with weight control, consumed an average of 1380 kcal daily and reported 2825 kcal of exercise per week.

Historical significance/comments
Many types of interventions allow short-term weight loss, but maintaining weight loss is more difficult. This study suggests that to maintain weight loss, continued moderate caloric restriction and regular exercise are important.

Interpersonal and Communication Skills

Successful Intervention for Weight Gain Requires Getting to Know Your Patient

To establish a successful plan of care for patients with weight gain, you must take a careful history and get to know your patient's habits. First, entertain medical disorders that could cause weight gain. Consider the psychological context of and your patient's feelings about weight gain. Identify psychiatric and behavioral disorders, such as depression and eating disorders, that may hinder weight loss efforts. These must be addressed if interventions are to succeed. In establishing a plan for diet and exercise modification, be sure you have your patient's input and agreement. Remember, it is the *patient* who will have to implement the changes. Patients should be given behavioral goals (e.g., engaging in physical activity for more than 30 minutes 5 days a week and increasing intake of fruits and vegetables). Be sure the goals are realistic and then check in regularly with your patient to provide positive reinforcement and to troubleshoot problems.

Professionalism

Be Nonjudgmental with Patients

Weight gain and obesity are exceedingly common. Obesity is an emotionally charged subject in American culture. Most patients will be distressed by significant weight gain, though often patients may not want to address it as a problem. It is important that we as physicians are honest with patients about the health risks associated with being overweight, but it's important not to be judgmental about an individual's inability to control his or her weight. We should target interventions that we know to improve these risks and target *health* rather than *slenderness*. A strategy of addressing obesity as a chronic disease rather than blaming the patient is most effective.

Systems-Based Practice

EMTALA: Ensuring Access to Emergency Services

Serious complications can unexpectedly occur in patients with obesity who undergo bariatric surgery, necessitating urgent care at emergency rooms of hospitals where they do not receive their usual care. If the patient lacks insurance coverage, there may be the desire to transfer the patient to his or her usual facility for provision of care. There are

Speaking Intelligently

Upon initially encountering a patient who reports weight loss, I first quantify the amount of weight lost over a specified time frame and determine whether this was intentional or unintentional weight loss. Clinically significant weight loss is defined as over 10 pounds or greater than 5% of body weight in 6 to 12 months. I like to know what kind of appetite the patient has. Causes of unintentional weight loss with an increased appetite usually involve either an underlying medical cause or a significant increase in rigorous exercise, leading to calorie loss despite increased appetite. Examples in this category include malabsorption, uncontrolled diabetes mellitus, and hyperthyroidism. I also like to find out if there is any history of cancer, if patients are up to date on their general medical screenings (e.g., Papanicolaou test, or PAP smear; mammogram; colonoscopy), and if there are gastrointestinal symptoms, fever, psychiatric symptoms, substance abuse or heavy smoking, rigorous exercise, medications, and chronic illnesses. As there is a broad differential diagnosis, the key is to narrow down the possible causes with a thorough history and physical exam.

PATIENT CARE

Clinical Thinking
- If the weight loss is intentional—as, for example in an obese patient (BMI > 30) who is now exercising and modifying the diet—then this patient should be encouraged and the weight loss is not concerning.
- If the patient is overly concerned about the weight loss and exhibits a distorted self-image, excessive exercise, decreased food consumption, laxative abuse, or induced vomiting, one should be concerned about psychiatric conditions such as anorexia nervosa or bulimia.
- Always ask about occupation; for example, a ballet dancer or gymnast may be more likely to exhibit these behaviors.
- A complete medication history, including OTC medications and herbal supplements, is essential, as a number of drugs can cause weight loss.
- I then want to know if appetite is increased or decreased. Since the majority of causes of weight loss are associated with decreased appetite, if the patient's appetite is increased, this can help narrow down the potential underlying pathologies.

History
- Quantify the amount of weight loss and the onset with time frame (over what period of time the weight was lost; how rapidly the weight was lost).

- Determine if symptoms are intentional or unintentional.
- Determine if appetite is increased or decreased.
- Ask about any known chronic medical conditions or history of cancer.
- Ask if up to date on general medical screening (e.g., colonoscopy, mammogram).
- Ask about occupation and hobbies (e.g., excessive exercise, wrestler, gymnast, ballet dancer).
- Ask about medications, including OTC (e.g., laxative abuse).

Physical Examination

- Note the patient's appearance, including cachexia, and clues to mood and affect (e.g., disheveled appearance, flat affect).
- For exam of the head, ears, eyes, nose, and throat, pay attention to any signs suggestive of an underlying disorder like lipodystrophy in HIV and ophthalmopathy in Graves disease.
- For the neck exam, feel for lymphadenopathy, thyroid size, and nodules.
- In women, examine the breasts for any lumps, discharge, or peau d'orange skin suggestive of breast cancer.
- In the pulmonary exam, look for signs of COPD, like "pink puffers" from emphysema with cachexia, pink skin, and use of accessory muscles of respiration.
- During the cardiovascular exam, pay attention to any signs of chronic heart failure, such as jugular venous distension, crackles, S_3 gallop, murmurs, and peripheral edema.
- When performing the abdominal exam, look for jaundice, ascites, hepatomegaly, or any abdominal pain or masses on palpation, as some of these findings can be seen in patients with hepatitis, colon cancer, or inflammatory bowel disease.
- In the genitourinary exam be sure to check the rectum for masses, prostate enlargement, or blood in the stool, which could be suggestive of colon or prostate cancer.
- Be sure to check reflexes for hyperreflexia and note any tremors, both of which could suggest thyrotoxicosis.
- Include a mini mental status exam with the neurologic exam because elderly patients with dementia often present with weight loss.
- Examine the extremities for clubbing, which can be seen in COPD or lung cancer, and edema, which is seen in congestive heart failure (CHF).
- During your examination of the skin, note any ecchymoses, jaundice, rashes, erythema, dryness, and diaphoresis.

Tests for Consideration

- Use clinical judgment when ordering tests based on degree of clinical suspicion for the disease.

Thyrotoxicosis

Pφ Thyrotoxicosis is the clinical syndrome associated with excess thyroid hormone, from either endogenous or exogenous sources. Hyperthyroidism is the endogenous production of too much thyroid hormone, such as occurs in Graves disease or with a toxic adenoma. Graves disease is caused by thyroid-stimulating immunoglobulins binding to and stimulating the thyroid to produce thyroid hormone. Toxic adenomas are often due to mutations in the Gs α-subunit or the TSH receptor, causing activation of the pathway leading to thyroid hormone production.

TP Typically patients present with unintentional weight loss and increased appetite with other symptoms and signs of thyrotoxicosis, including heat intolerance, diaphoresis, tremors, palpitations, hyperdefecation, and difficulty concentrating.

Dx The diagnosis is made clinically based on symptoms and signs and confirmed with thyroid function tests. Physical exam can be helpful. For example, if a diffuse goiter and exophthalmos are seen, this suggests Graves disease. A palpable nodule supports toxic adenoma. TSH should be suppressed with a high free T_4 and/or total T_3. Thyroid uptake and scan is helpful to determine the degree of overactivity from the uptake; the pattern from the scan confirms the etiology. There is a diffuse pattern in Graves disease and multiple hot nodules in toxic multinodular goiter.

Tx Treatment of hyperthyroidism is with antithyroid medications, such as methimazole or propylthiouracil, or radioactive iodine; most experts prefer radioactive iodine. Most patients are also given β-adrenergic-blocking agents, unless contraindicated. Surgery is rarely indicated and is performed in cases refractory to medical therapy. **See Cecil Essentials 66.**

Anorexia Nervosa

Pφ The underlying pathogenesis of anorexia nervosa is unclear, although psychological, genetic, and environmental factors are all thought to contribute to its development.

TP Typically, patients present with disturbed body image, where they fear weight gain, are in denial about the illness, refuse to maintain a normal weight (for height and age), and have amenorrhea or oligomenorrhea in females after menarche.

Dx The diagnosis is made with the clinical history meeting the *Diagnostic and Statistical Manual IV of Mental Disorders* (DSM-IV) criteria and a thorough physical exam looking for findings (e.g., on gastrointestinal or neurologic exam) to rule out other causes of chronic weight loss and vomiting (e.g., brain tumor, inflammatory bowel disease, new-onset diabetes mellitus). Basic laboratory values, as above, are also checked (e.g., BUN, creatinine, electrolytes, glucose, β-human chorionic gonadotropin [HCG]) to look for dehydration and rule out other causes.

Tx Treatment includes weight gain, calcium supplements, daily multivitamins, and possible estrogen/progesterone replacement. Markedly underweight persons may require a hospital-based program to achieve weight restoration; if patients refuse to eat, nasogastric feeding may be used. Psychotherapy is the mainstay for treatment when adequate nutrition is restored. **See Cecil Essentials 61.**

ZEBRA ZONE

a. **Adrenal insufficiency** occurs when the adrenal gland is not functioning (primary) or if the pituitary gland is not sending the signal (i.e., ACTH; secondary) to the adrenal gland to make cortisol. In primary adrenal insufficiency, patients are also deficient in the other hormones synthesized in the adrenal glands such as aldosterone. In addition to weight loss, patients may present with weakness, malaise, fatigue, myalgias, arthralgias, nausea, vomiting, abdominal pain, dizziness, and hypotension. In primary adrenal insufficiency, patients can also have hyperpigmentation. Laboratory findings can include hyponatremia, hyperkalemia, hypoglycemia, eosinophilia, lymphocytosis, and neutropenia. Although adrenal insufficiency is uncommon, clinical suspicion must be high, because administering corticosteroids may be lifesaving in acute adrenal insufficiency and will improve the symptoms of chronic adrenal insufficiency.

> ## Systems-Based Practice
>
> ### Radiation Safety for Patients and Families
> Though radioactive iodine has been used to treat patients with hyperthyroidism since the 1940s, there are a number of patient safety concerns regarding its use. Properly following safety instructions at the time of treatment should minimize radiation exposure to individuals other than the patient, such as family members and visitors. Patients who have been treated should be informed to avoid young children and pregnant women. Mothers with young children will often need to make special arrangements for child care following therapy. Patients may remain detectably radioactive for several days and even weeks and should carry a doctor's note in case sensitive radiation detectors at airports or government buildings are triggered. As a precaution, pregnant or nursing women should not receive radiation, and women who are treated should not become pregnant for 6 to 12 months following treatment.

Chapter 50
Amenorrhea (Case 42)

Amy Rogstad MD

Case: A 28-year-old woman presents with amenorrhea after discontinuing her oral contraceptive pills (OCPs). She desires pregnancy but has not conceived after 9 months of unprotected intercourse with her husband. Further questioning reveals a history of menarche at 13 years of age and normal development of secondary sexual characteristics. She believes breast development began around age 11 years. The patient's menses were initially irregular; during the first year following menarche, she had fluctuations in cycle length and intermittently light and heavy menses. By the age of 15 years, however, her menses had become regular, occurring every 28 to 30 days and lasting about 5 days. She started OCPs when she was 20 years old both for contraception and to help with premenstrual cramping and mood swings. She continued on combination estrogen-progestin OCPs until the age of 27 years. Since stopping her OCPs, she has not had any regular menstrual cycles, with only two occasions of light bleeding lasting about 2 days each.

The patient has been feeling anxious about her inability to conceive and about her absent menses. Her husband has been evaluated and has been found to have a normal semen analysis. The patient reports that she has a history of headaches that began while she was in college but have worsened in the past 2 years. Currently she has headaches almost daily that are retro-orbital, dull, and aching. She denies any recent vision problems but has noticed occasional discharge from her breasts, which sometimes has a white, milky appearance. She has maintained a stable weight and is eating a balanced diet. She has not been sleeping well for the past 3 months, which she attributes to stress, and often feels fatigued during her workday as a high school teacher. She becomes tearful during the interview, and her husband, who accompanied her to the visit, holds her hand throughout the evaluation.

Differential Diagnosis

Hypothalamic amenorrhea (HA)	Prolactinoma	Pituitary adenoma
Primary ovarian insufficiency (POI)	PCOS	
Hyperthyroidism	Hypothyroidism	

Speaking Intelligently

Amenorrhea refers to the absence or abnormal cessation of the menstrual cycle. Evaluation for primary amenorrhea, the absence of menarche, should be initiated when there is failure to menstruate by 15 years of age in the presence of normal secondary sexual characteristics or within 5 years after breast development if that occurs before 10 years of age.

Secondary amenorrhea, cessation of menses after menarche that lasts 3 months or more, should be evaluated, but sometimes it should be evaluated after 1 to 2 weeks in patients with regular cycles to exclude pregnancy. Oligomenorrhea, less than nine menstrual cycles per year, also requires investigation. Pregnancy, lactation, and menopause account for about 96% to 97% of secondary amenorrhea. Of the remaining 3% to 4%, most will have one of several common causes for amenorrhea including hypothalamic-pituitary-ovarian (HPO) axis disorders, structural abnormalities, and disorders of androgen excess.

PATIENT CARE

Clinical Thinking
- When evaluating a patient for amenorrhea, determine whether the problem is genetic, structural, or hormonal.

IMAGING CONSIDERATIONS

→ **Pelvic and/or transvaginal ultrasound:** To evaluate the uterus and ovaries if internal genital exam is not possible or is inconclusive. $96

→ **MRI of the brain and/or pituitary:** To evaluate for mass lesions or other abnormalities. $534

→ **CT scan of the abdomen and pelvis:** To evaluate the adrenal glands and ovaries if there is a concern for adrenal Cushing syndrome, nonclassical CAH, or an androgen-secreting tumor in the adrenal gland or ovary. $334

Clinical Entities	Medical Knowledge

Hypothalamic Amenorrhea

Pφ Amenorrhea caused by hypothalamic dysfunction probably represents a spectrum of related disorders including functional hypothalamic amenorrhea (FHA), amenorrhea in the female athlete, and amenorrhea associated with eating disorders. The precise mechanism of these disorders is not known, but all share a reduction in hypothalamic gonadotropin-releasing hormone (GnRH) production. FHA accounts for about 15% to 35% of cases of amenorrhea, making it one of the most common causes. The blunted GnRH release pattern leads to decreased FSH and LH but an increased FSH/LH ratio similar to that seen before puberty. Estradiol levels are also decreased, and patients are usually anovulatory. Leptin, an adipocyte hormone that acts as a satiety factor and a cofactor in the maturation of the reproductive system, has been implicated in the development of HA. Leptin can stimulate GnRH pulsatility and gonadotropin secretion and is decreased in patients across the spectrum of HA.

TP Amenorrhea in the female athlete is part of the "female athlete triad," which also includes disordered eating and osteoporosis. Elite athletes in sports such as gymnastics, diving, and marathon running, as well as ballet dancers, are particularly vulnerable to this triad. In these patients, body fat often is below the 10th percentile.

Patients with anorexia nervosa also have severely reduced body fat, and often their body weight is <85% of normal for age and height. These patients have a distorted body image, fear weight gain, and exist in a self-imposed starvation state. In addition to low body weight and wasting, they may also have bradycardia, hypothermia, constipation, and dry skin. Patients with bulimia may have normal weight and physical exam findings but can still have neuroendocrine abnormalities leading to irregular menses.

Dx FHA can be related to strenuous exercise or poor nutrition without falling into either of the previous two categories but can also result from psychological stress. Often, these patients are high achievers with an impaired ability to cope with the stress of daily life and/or acutely stressful situations.

GnRH pulsatility cannot be measured, so LH pulsatility is used as a surrogate, and in clinical practice the FSH/LH ratio is used to assess problems with hypothalamic function. In HA, the FSH/LH ratio is >1 in the setting of hypoestrogenemia, although the absolute concentrations of both gonadotropins are decreased. In patients with FHA who have mild perturbations in the HPO axis, these lab data may be normal. In that case HA can be diagnosed when other causes of anovulation are ruled out and the history of amenorrhea coincides with increased physical or psychological stress.

Tx Treatment of the underlying problem with counseling, behavior modification, stress management strategies, or inpatient care in the case of eating disorders should be tailored to the patient's individual needs. With elite athletes with amenorrhea, the underlying problem will probably not be corrected until they retire from competition. All patients with HA should be treated with cyclic estrogen-progestin therapy to protect against bone loss caused by estrogen deficiency. Patients desiring pregnancy should target optimal weight and nutrition, but may need ovulation induction with clomiphene citrate to stimulate endogenous gonadotropins or treatment with exogenous gonadotropins or pulsatile GnRH. **See Cecil Essentials 61, 71.**

Prolactinoma

Pφ Hyperprolactinemia accounts for 15% to 30% of amenorrhea. About 50% of patients with elevated prolactin levels have evidence of a pituitary mass on MRI, and about 40% to 50% of these masses are prolactinomas. Under normal circumstances, prolactin release is under tonic inhibition by dopamine, but these

Tx Treatment for pituitary adenomas depends on the size and location of the mass, as well as any associated symptoms. Non–prolactin-secreting tumors do not respond well to medical therapy. Trans-sphenoidal resection is the treatment of choice for macroadenomas and is usually performed urgently if the patient has evidence of optic chiasm compression and visual field defects. Microadenomas do not require urgent surgery and sometimes can be observed with serial pituitary MRI scans to assess for growth. If the adenoma is producing another type of hormone, resection is recommended in most cases. Additional therapy may be needed after resection for further management of hormone excess caused by any tumor that is left behind.
See Cecil Essentials 65, 71.

Hypothyroidism

Pφ Primary hypothyroidism is caused by decreased production of thyroid hormone by the thyroid gland, most often secondary to autoimmune destruction of the thyroid cells. Low circulating thyroid hormone levels lead to increased thyrotropin-releasing hormone (TRH) production by the hypothalamus and increased TSH release by the pituitary, but also act on lactotrophs to increase prolactin secretion. If the primary hypothyroidism persists, prolactin levels can rise significantly enough to cause menstrual irregularities.

TP Patients may present with galactorrhea, as well as menstrual irregularities, if the prolactin level is high enough. Symptoms typical of hypothyroidism including weight gain, fatigue, constipation, cold intolerance, brittle nails, coarse and dry hair, and dry skin may also be experienced.

Dx Because thyroid dysfunction is common in women, TSH is part of the routine testing done at initial screening for causes of amenorrhea. Patients with an elevated prolactin level should be tested for TSH level, if not already done, to determine whether hypothyroidism could be the cause for the prolactin elevation. The TSH will be elevated in hypothyroidism, with a low thyroid hormone (free T_4) level.

Tx Treatment of the hypothyroidism with levothyroxine will reverse the thyroid dysfunction and correct the menstrual irregularities.
See Cecil Essentials 66, 71.

Hyperthyroidism

Pφ Primary hyperthyroidism results from overproduction of thyroid hormone by the thyroid gland. Most commonly this is due to Graves disease, an autoimmune process mediated by antibodies that bind to the TSH receptor and stimulate thyroid hormone release. The mechanism(s) causing irregular menses in hyperthyroid patients is not known.

TP Patients with hyperthyroidism can present with weight loss, fatigue, irritability, impaired concentration, tachycardia, palpitations, diarrhea, heat intolerance, diaphoresis, hair loss, and warm, moist skin, and addition to amenorrhea.

Dx As is the case with hypothyroidism, TSH level should be used as a screening tool for all women presenting with amenorrhea. Primary hyperthyroidism is diagnosed with an elevated free T_4 and a low or undetectable TSH.

Tx Treatment is aimed at reversing the hyperthyroid state. This can be accomplished with medication, radioactive iodine ablation of the overactive thyroid, and, rarely, surgery. Once the thyroid abnormality is corrected, the menstrual irregularities will resolve. **See Cecil Essentials 66, 71.**

Polycystic Ovarian Syndrome

Pφ Androgen excess accounts for over 30% of amenorrhea and up to 75% of anovulation and is most often caused by PCOS. In 1990 the National Institutes of Health (NIH) developed criteria for the diagnosis of PCOS that included chronic anovulation and clinical and/or biochemical signs of hyperandrogenism with exclusion of other etiologies. In 2003 the Rotterdam consensus conference amended the criteria to require two out of three of the following: oligo-ovulation or anovulation, clinical and/or biochemical signs of hyperandrogenism, and polycystic ovaries with exclusion of other etiologies (i.e., CAH, androgen-secreting tumors, Cushing syndrome). Hyperinsulinemia does seem to play a major role in the pathogenesis of PCOS, with a prevalence of 50% to 60% in this population, compared with 10% to 25% in the general population. Also, increasing evidence points to a strong genetic component to disease development.

ZEBRA ZONE

a. **Asherman syndrome:** Patients have intrauterine adhesions that obliterate the uterine cavity and result from damage to the endometrial basal layer, most commonly after a surgical procedure that disrupts the uterine lining. Patients can have a range of menstrual disturbances, infertility, and spontaneous abortions. Treatment involves lysis of adhesions and hormonal therapy.

b. **Nonclassical CAH:** The clinical features of this disease are similar to those observed in PCOS, including menstrual irregularities, hyperandrogenism, and polycystic ovaries. CAH is an autosomal-recessive disorder that is most often caused by mutations in the gene encoding 21-hydroxylase, an enzyme in the steroidogenesis pathway. Most patients with nonclassical CAH do not have cortisol deficiency or ACTH excess. The diagnosis can be made by measuring early-morning 17-hydroxyprogesterone levels. This is the substrate for 21-hydroxylase and will be elevated, usually over 800 ng/dL, in CAH. Treatment for nonclassical CAH is similar to that for PCOS.

c. **Androgen-secreting tumors:** These can be present in the adrenal gland or ovary, and should be suspected with rapid onset of androgenic symptoms and with associated symptoms like weight loss, anorexia, and bloating. Elevated testosterone > 200 ng/dL and DHEAS > 700 ng/mL raise suspicion for a tumor and should be followed by abdominal and pelvic CT. Pelvic ultrasonography can also help make the diagnosis of an ovarian tumor. Treatment involves surgical resection, mitotane (an adrenal cortex suppressor), and steroid synthesis inhibitors.

d. **Kallmann syndrome:** This syndrome occurs most often in an X-linked recessive inheritance pattern. It involves a mutation of the *KAL1* gene, which codes for anosmin, an adhesion molecule involved in migration of GnRH and olfactory neurons to the hypothalamus. The specific mutation has not been identified in females, but it results in GnRH deficiency and amenorrhea. Patients are treated with hormone replacement therapy to stimulate secondary sexual characteristics and to increase bone mineral density. If pregnancy is desired, patients will be treated with exogenous pulsatile GnRH or exogenous gonadotropins.

Practice-Based Learning and Improvement: Evidence-Based Medicine

Title
Revised 2003 consensus on diagnostic criteria and long-term health risks related to polycystic ovary syndrome

Authors
The Rotterdam ESHRE/ASRM-Sponsored PCOS Consensus Workshop Group

Institution
Various

Reference
Fertil Steril 2004;81:19–25

Problem
Need for a broader definition of PCOS

Intervention
Revision of 1990 NIH diagnostic criteria

Quality of evidence
Level III

Outcome/effect
Increased number of patients meeting criteria for PCOS diagnosis

Historical significance/comments
This is the consensus statement that guides current diagnosis of PCOS, one of the most common causes of amenorrhea.

Interpersonal and Communication Skills

Tailor the Encounter to the Individual
Menstrual irregularities and matters concerning fertility may cause significant psychological distress. In these instances, tailor the interview to the needs of the patient, as follows:

- For those with fertility issues, try to decipher their specific issues, be a good listener, and offer as much reassurance as is legitimated by the medical circumstance.
- For those presenting for the evaluation of amenorrhea, schedule follow-up appointments to review results of screening tests. If further testing is necessary, be careful to convey results in person rather than over the phone, because the patient may have many questions about the implications of her test results and ultimate diagnosis.

PATIENT CARE

Clinical Thinking

- Peak bone mass usually occurs in the third decade of life, and then bone mass diminishes with age.
- Estrogen deficiency accelerates this process, which is why women are more likely to have osteoporosis and osteoporotic fractures.
- Other conditions that can lead to accelerated bone loss or fragility fractures are hyperthyroidism, hyperparathyroidism, steroid excess (either exogenous or endogenous), vitamin D deficiency, and testosterone deficiency (in men).
- Other processes that can result in fragility fractures that are not necessarily due to osteoporosis include metastatic cancer, multiple myeloma, and Paget disease. Therefore, when a patient presents with a fragility fracture, it is important to rule out these other causes.
- Once the diagnosis of osteoporosis has been established and secondary causes have been either excluded or treated, the main goal of therapy is to decrease the risk of a future fracture.

History

- Osteoporosis is frequently a silent disease until a fracture occurs. As a result, many patients will not have any specific complaints. The history should therefore focus on identifying risk factors as well as potential secondary causes of osteoporosis.
- In a woman, estrogen deficiency is the main cause of osteoporosis. Late menarche, amenorrhea, and early menopause are important risks. If a woman is postmenopausal, determining the age of menopause and how much time (if any) the patient was on estrogen replacement therapy is important.
- In a man with osteoporosis, identifying causes, such as testosterone deficiency, are common. Therefore, specific questions regarding sexual drive (libido), erectile function, shaving habits, muscle strength, and overall energy are essential.
- Ascertain the patient's intake of calcium and vitamin D; this includes intake of dairy products as well as OTC calcium and vitamins. Sunlight exposure should also be assessed, as lack of sunlight is a major risk factor for vitamin D deficiency. Vitamin D deficiency is also more common in patients with celiac disease, so it is important to note any symptoms of malabsorption.
- Certain medications may cause bone loss. The main offenders are glucocorticoids such as prednisone. Doses of prednisone over 10 mg/day for more than a few months will lead to worsening bone density. Phenytoin (Dilantin) diverts vitamin D to inactive forms, resulting in vitamin D deficiency and decreased calcium absorption. Androgen deprivation therapy medications used for treating prostate cancer will decrease testosterone production.

- Endocrinopathies that cause osteoporosis must be considered. To rule out hyperthyroidism, question patients about tremor, palpitations, heat intolerance, weight loss, and hair loss. Primary hyperparathyroidism is another silent disease, but the patient with hyperparathyroidism may have a history of kidney stones and hypercalcemia. Excessive weight gain, easy bruising, wide abdominal stretch marks, proximal muscle weakness with difficult-to-control diabetes or hypertension suggest Cushing syndrome (excess endogenous steroid production).
- Both smoking and excessive alcohol use, defined as more than three drinks a day, are risks for osteoporosis. A detailed family history for osteoporosis is important. While the family member may not have been officially diagnosed with osteoporosis, he or she may have had a hip fracture or severe kyphosis.
- The patient's own history of fragility fractures is important. A hip fracture during a car accident is not considered an osteoporotic fracture, but a hip fracture after slipping on ice is. If there has been a vertebral compression fracture, patients will complain of localized, midline, sharp pains that may be disabling. Patients may also have height loss, scoliosis, or kyphosis as the vertebrae compress and change the contour of the spine. Pain is generally not associated with osteoporosis unless a fracture has already occurred.

Physical Examination
- The height measurement is essential when assessing the osteoporotic patient. An attempt should be made to determine if there has been height loss.
- Examine the spine for point tenderness, thoracic kyphosis, and an exaggerated cervical lordosis (dowager's hump).
- The remainder of the physical exam should be focused on including or excluding the secondary causes of osteoporosis. Signs of hyperthyroidism include proptosis, an enlarged thyroid, tremor, tachycardia, warm and moist skin, and proximal muscle weakness. Cushing syndrome presents with central obesity, thin arms and legs, supraclavicular fat pads, a dorsocervical fat pad, widened purplish abdominal stretch marks, proximal muscle weakness, and hypertension.

Tests for Consideration
- **25-OH Vitamin D:** This is the inactive or storage form of vitamin D. The vitamin D level should be at least above 32 ng/mL, and some experts are arguing for even higher levels. It is not recommended to check the active form ($1,25$-dihydroxyvitamin D_3) in patients with normal kidney function. In patients with vitamin D deficiency as indicated by a low 25-OH vitamin D level, the active vitamin D can sometimes still be in the low normal range. $55
- **Intact PTH:** In the setting of a normal or low calcium level, an elevated PTH level may indicate vitamin D deficiency.

→ **Nuclear bone scan:** This study is indicated to find areas of active Paget disease or if metastatic cancer to the bone is suspected. $247

→ **MRI:** This may be used if the suspected fracture is not seen on plain radiographs. In addition, it is used to assess the spine in patients with multiple myeloma. $534

Clinical Entities   Medical Knowledge

Primary Osteoporosis

Pφ Primary osteoporosis is defined by a significantly low bone density without identification of any secondary causes. Bone loss starts to occur after the third decade of life but accelerates with the loss of estrogen or testosterone. Therefore, women are much more likely to have osteoporosis after menopause as a result of their advancing age and low estrogen. Genetic factors, calcium intake, and age are important determinants of one's bone density as well.

TP Osteoporosis is typically a silent disease and is usually found on routine screening with a DXA scan. The first symptom is usually a fracture. Therefore, patients who have a suspicious, low- or no-trauma fracture should be screened for osteoporosis.

Dx A T-score of −2.5 or less defines osteoporosis. In addition, a clinical diagnosis of osteoporosis can be made if the patient has a fragility fracture in the absence of other causes of that fracture. One can calculate the patient's future fracture risk by using a calculation tool called FRAX (Fracture Risk Assessment Tool, found at http://www.shef.ac.uk/FRAX). This gives a 10-year estimated risk for a hip fracture or any osteoporotic fracture. This calculation uses the bone mineral density at the femoral neck as well as clinical information about the patient, including age, sex, weight, tobacco use, alcohol intake, family history of hip fracture, prior personal history of fracture, rheumatoid arthritis, secondary causes of osteoporosis, and steroid use. Treatment should be considered when the 10-year risk is above 3% for a hip fracture and 20% for any fracture.

Tx All patients with primary osteoporosis should receive an adequate amount of calcium and vitamin D. This generally means 1500 mg of calcium a day and at least 800–1000 IU/day of vitamin D. Bisphosphonates are the first-line prescription medication for osteoporosis. These medications decrease bone resorption (breakdown by osteoclasts) while allowing bone formation to continue. This results in a net increase in bone density. Examples of oral bisphosphonates are alendronate, risedronate, and ibandronate. Zolendronate and ibandronate can be given as IV medications for those who cannot tolerate the gastrointestinal side effects of the oral bisphosphonates. Teriparatide is an anabolic agent, given as a daily subcutaneous injection, that increases bone formation and is indicated for those patients with extremely poor bone density who are at very high risk for fracture. Another antiresorptive medication, denosumab, was approved for treatment of osteoporosis in 2010. Denosumab is a RANK ligand inhibitor that is given as an IM injection twice a year. **See Cecil Essentials 76.**

Osteoporosis Secondary to Medical Conditions

Pφ Hyperthyroidism, primary hyperparathyroidism, and glucocorticoid excess states (either endogeneous from Cushing syndrome or exogenous from prolonged use of high-dose steroids) all can cause increased bone turnover. Because bone formation takes much longer than bone resorption, the net effect in all of these conditions is decreasing bone density. Both estrogen and testosterone deficiencies can also lead to increased bone turnover and bone loss.

TP Hyperthyroidism presents with tachycardia, weight loss, tremor, palpitations, anxiety, and heat intolerance. Primary hyperparathyroidism is usually silent and is diagnosed only with an elevated calcium and intact PTH level. Cushing syndrome presents with central weight gain, uncontrolled hypertension and diabetes, excessive fat pads above the clavicle and in the posterior neck, central large and purplish stretch marks, and proximal muscle weakness. Cushing syndrome may also be asymptomatic and must be considered in unusual cases of unexplained low bone density. Estrogen deficiency is obviously an issue in an older woman, but a younger woman with anovulation and hot flashes should be evaluated with lab work for estrogen deficiency.

Dx An elevated alkaline phosphatase level is the blood test result that suggests Paget's disease. However, an elevated alkaline phosphatase level can also be seen in severe osteomalacia, liver disease, and metastatic cancers to the bone. A GGT (γ-glutamyl transpeptidase) level should be checked if the alkaline phosphatase level is elevated. An elevated GGT indicates a hepatic origin of the alkaline phosphatase elevation, while a normal GGT points toward a skeletal etiology. A nuclear bone scan can then identify hypermetabolic areas of the skeleton. This should be followed with radiographs of the affected areas to make sure there is no evidence of cancer at these sites.

Tx The active bone turnover of Paget disease can be halted with bisphosphonates. Oral daily alendronate for 6 months, or daily risedronate for 2 months, is approved for this disease; a one-time zolendronate IV infusion is the most effective. The arthritis and bony deformities will not improve with treatment. These must be individually treated based on symptoms. **See Cecil Essentials 77.**

Multiple Myeloma

Pφ Multiple myeloma is a plasma cell neoplasm. The bone lesions of multiple myeloma are caused by activation of the osteoclasts and increased bone resorption.

TP The presentation can be varied. Multiple myeloma usually presents with bone pain but can also present with anemia, hypercalcemia, pathologic fractures, renal failure, and/or spinal cord compression.

Dx The diagnosis may be suspected from other laboratory studies but SPEP and UPEP are the best tests for confirming the diagnosis. A skeletal series, including the skull, is necessary to determine the extent of the disease affecting the bones. An MRI may be useful to evaluate the spine and spinal cord.

Tx Although multiple myeloma is not curable, it can be treated with chemotherapy and bone marrow transplantation. Bisphosphonates have been found to be helpful in fracture prevention. **See Cecil Essentials 51.**

ZEBRA ZONE

a. **Osteogenesis imperfecta:** This is a genetic disorder that is characterized by an abnormality of type 1 collagen that results in bone fragility. It is usually diagnosed in childhood.

b. **Metastatic cancer to the bone:** Most cancers have the potential to metastasize to the bone, but common cancers include lung, breast, and prostate. The areas of metastasis can lead to fractures at that site.

Practice-Based Learning and Improvement: Evidence-Based Medicine

Title
Fracture risk reduction with alendronate in women with osteoporosis: The Fracture Intervention Trial

Authors
Black DM, Thompson DE, Bauer DC, et al., for the Fit Research Group

Institution
Multiple sites

Reference
J Clin Endocrinol Metab 2000;85:4118–4124

Problem
What is the reduction in fracture risk in women with established osteoporosis while on alendronate?

Intervention
Women with an existing vertebral fracture and women with a T-score less than −2.5 were randomly assigned placebo or alendronate at 5 mg/day for the first 2 years and then 10 mg/day for another 2–3 years. Bone mineral density by DXA scan and new fractures were evaluated yearly.

Quality of evidence
Level I

Outcome/effect
There was a significant reduction of clinical fractures in patients receiving alendronate for both women with an existing vertebral fracture and women without a vertebral fracture who had osteoporosis on DXA scan. Vertebral fractures were reduced by 45%, hip fractures by 53%, and wrist fractures by 30%.

Historical significance/comments
This study showed that pharmaceutical treatment of high-risk patients, even those who have already had significant fractures, can greatly benefit patients by reducing their risk for future fractures.

Interpersonal and Communication Skills

Educate Patients about the Implications of a Fragility Fracture
Fragility fractures can result in significant morbidity. The initial goal is to address the acute fracture, but at some point early in the process the underlying cause of the fracture must be determined. Having just undergone major surgery to repair a fracture, some patients will not understand why it is necessary to have additional blood work, a bone density scan, and other radiographic studies. It is important to explain that the initial goal was to fix the fracture, and now it is essential to identify the underlying cause so as to prevent future fractures. **Osteoporosis** is the most common disease causing the fracture, and while it is not as concerning as **metastatic cancer** or **multiple myeloma**, the physician must ensure that the patient understands the importance of treating this silent disease. Without this understanding, most patients will not follow through with the basic treatments of calcium and vitamin D.

Professionalism

Show Commitment to Professional Excellence
It is the physician's role to promptly identify patients at risk for osteoporosis and initiate treatment for their low bone density. The National Osteoporosis Foundation (NOF) and the American Association of Clinical Endocrinologists (AACE) recommend DXA scans for all women over the age of 65 years, because the risk of fracture begins to increase dramatically in this age group. In addition, a DXA scan should be done in any postmenopausal woman with other risk factors such as family history, vitamin D deficiency, or previous fracture. Those patients on chronic steroids, who have primary hyperparathyroidism, and who have had a suspicious fracture or significant height loss, should also be screened. However, many DXA scans are ordered on patients who do not meet these criteria. While men have significantly less risk for an osteoporotic fracture, there are still millions of men with osteoporosis who are at risk for fracture, but there are no guidelines (and therefore poor insurance coverage)

for screening DXA scans. There are elderly men, especially those with risks such as testosterone deficiency, who should have DXA scans. Well-meaning physicians are ordering these tests in premenopausal women who have no major risks or symptoms. Even when decreases in bone density are found in these women, it is unclear what treatment is most beneficial when they are still young. Therefore, it is imperative for physicians to understand the DXA scan and to be educated as to the limitations and the usefulness of this test in certain patients.

Systems-Based Practice

Accountable Care Organizations Should Enhance Quality and Reduce Costs

Management of fragility fractures requires that all members of the patient's health-care team are working together to enhance quality in a cost-effective manner. Introduced as part of the new health-care reform legislation in March 2010, Accountable Care Organizations (ACOs) are being created to provide better care for individuals, better health for populations, and slower increases in costs through improvements in care.[1] In an ACO, a set of health-care providers will share responsibility for the quality and cost delivered to a defined population of patients; these providers can include a hospital, a group of primary-care providers, specialists, and possibly other health-care professionals. Together these providers will manage the continuum of care across different institutional settings, including outpatient, inpatient, and possibly post-acute care. ACOs are meant to control the growth of costs while maintaining or improving the quality of care of a population of patients by using evidence-based medicine. The incentives of an ACO are different from the current fee-for-service reimbursement system: the focus of the ACO will be to streamline its processes of care while exceeding the norm on quality and outcomes. If the ACO spends less than projected, all members share in bonus payments.

Reference

1. Berwick DM. Making good on ACO's promise—the final rule for the Medicare Shared Savings Program. N Engl J Med 2011;365: 1753–1756.

Section X
RHEUMATOLOGIC DISEASES

Section Editor
Allan R. Tunkel MD, PhD, MACP

Section Contents

52 **Acute Joint Pain (Case 44)**
   Robin Dibner MD, *Joel Mathew* MD, *and Jessica L. Israel* MD

53 **Chronic Joint Pain (Case 45)**
   Robin Dibner MD, *Joel Mathew* MD, *and Jessica L. Israel* MD

Chapter 52
Acute Joint Pain (Case 44)

Robin Dibner MD, Joel Mathew MD,
and Jessica L. Israel MD

Case: A 45-year-old man presents to the emergency department
complaining of pain, swelling, and redness in his right knee and
inability to walk for 1 day. The symptoms appeared acutely yesterday
without any history of trauma. No other joints were painful. He also felt
feverish but did not take his temperature; he had no relief with
acetaminophen. Past medical history is significant for hypertension
controlled with hydrochlorothiazide and a kidney stone 5 years ago. He
was recently divorced but has been sexually active, and he has had no
recent travel or insect bites. He drinks two to three glasses of wine
nightly. There is no family history of arthritis or gout. The review of
systems is negative for rash, sore throat, history of heart murmur, recent
dental work, inflammatory bowel disease, urethral discharge, or any
recent infection. Physical examination shows a temperature of 101°F
and a tender, warm, erythematous, swollen right knee.

Differential Diagnosis

Nongonococcal septic arthritis	Gonococcal arthritis	Gout
Pseudogout/calcium pyrophosphate dihydrate (CPPD) deposition	Viral arthritis	

Speaking Intelligently

When seeing a patient with acute arthritis, it is necessary to think
first of the potential emergencies: undiagnosed trauma and septic
joint. The former diagnosis, which is handled by orthopedic surgeons,
is usually easily eliminated by the physical exam, negative
radiographs, and non-bloody joint fluid. Septic joints, which require
laboratory confirmation, are an emergency because antibiotics must
be initiated quickly and the fluid drained from the joint to reduce
the risk of damage from inflammatory mediators and collagenases.
Untreated septic joints can show radiographic changes in as little as
a week, and there may be irreversible joint damage if drainage is
inadequate; the general approach is to treat presumptively while
awaiting confirmation by Gram stain and culture.

PATIENT CARE

Clinical Thinking

- When evaluating a patient with a new monoarthropathy, the most important focus is to obtain joint fluid for an accurate diagnosis.
- If the patient has a septic joint and appropriate therapy is not initiated as soon as possible, there is a risk of permanent joint destruction and disability.
- In cases in which aspiration of the affected joint is not possible (perhaps because of available resources or experience), treating for the possibility of septic arthritis until a definitive diagnosis can be made is extremely important.

History

- A prior history of an acute episode of arthritis suggests a crystal-induced process. Fifty percent of gout patients have a first episode in the first metatarsophalangeal (large toe) joint; historically, that classic presentation is called podagra. Middle age (older for women), obesity, alcoholism, thiazide or cyclosporine use, and a family history of gout are all risk factors.
- Pseudogout (CPPD deposition disease) is associated with hypothyroidism, hyperparathyroidism, hemochromatosis, and osteoarthritis.
- Obtaining a history of a prior diagnosis or current symptoms of a sexually transmitted disease (STD) is critical, as disseminated gonococcal infection is a common cause of septic arthritis.
- Any history of underlying joint abnormality, such as prior arthritis or prosthetic joint replacement, puts the patient at higher risk of septic arthritis.

Physical Examination

- The pattern of joint involvement is important in suggesting a diagnosis.
- Fifty percent of first attacks of gout occur in a first metatarsophalangeal joint, the classic presentation called podagra. The knee and ankle are the next most common; upper extremity involvement is rarely seen unless the disease is long-standing.
- Tophi, deposits of uric acid seen in some patients with long-standing untreated gout, are palpable subcutaneous deposits of uric acid usually felt in the olecranon bursa or along the proximal ulnar surface.
- Pseudogout generally affects the knees and wrists.
- As the vast majority of septic arthritis is caused by hematogenous spread, any joint can be involved. The knee is the most common.

- Infection of an axial skeletal joint, such as the sternoclavicular joint, is characteristic of the high-grade bacteremia that can be seen in patients with *Staphylococcus aureus* endocarditis.
- Clinical findings in gonococcal arthritis depend on the stage of the disease. Classically the earlier infection is characterized by a migratory joint pattern where one joint is inflamed but resolves before another is involved. Extensor tenosynovitis of the wrist or ankle is common. There is often a rash in this phase with a very small number of individual pustules, each on an erythematous base. A monoarticular septic joint is considered a later manifestation but often is present at the time of diagnosis.

Tests for Consideration

- **Synovial fluid analysis** is most important and is characterized primarily based on the types of cells found: normal, inflammatory, infectious, hemorrhagic. $7
- **Gram stain** of joint fluid, other stains if indicated; culture. $6
- **Polarized microscopy** examination of joint fluid for crystals. $10
- **Blood cultures** if septic joint is suspected or patient is febrile. $15
- **Panculture/DNA probe** for gonorrhea. $50
- If gonorrhea is suspected or diagnosed, tests for other STDs, including **HIV**, should be performed. $13
- **Serum uric acid level** is usually not helpful during an acute gout attack. $6

Clinical Entities	Medical Knowledge

Nongonococcal Septic Arthritis

Pφ   The overwhelming majority of these cases are caused by staphylococci and streptococci as a result of hematogenous dissemination. Acute joint infection can also be the result of trauma to the joint or may have spread from other localized areas where there may be an infection, such as bursitis, overlying cellulitis, or a nearby abscess or osteomyelitis. Rarely, a patient can develop a septic joint as a complication of a diagnostic or therapeutic arthrocentesis via direct inoculation or following use of contaminated tissue allografts. Risk factors for the development of a nongonococcal septic arthritis include rheumatoid arthritis (RA), immunodeficient states, immunosuppressive therapy, diabetes, preexisting joint damage, age, injection drug use, prosthetic joints, indwelling catheters, tissue allograft surgery, and malignancy.

Tx Gout attacks usually last about a week and are often self-limited. Treatments for an acute exacerbation include nonsteroidal anti-inflammatory drugs (NSAIDs), corticosteroids, and colchicine. It becomes important to treat underlying hyperuricemia in patients who have had multiple attacks of gout, kidney stones, or the development of tophi. The goal is to lower the uric acid level below 6.0 mg/dL. Allopurinol or febuxostat are the agents of choice to lower uric acid levels in most patients. It is also important to modify risk factors for the disease. This includes limiting alcohol use, restricting dietary purine intake, losing weight, and occasionally discontinuing certain prescription medications (e.g., thiazide diuretics or salicylates). **See Cecil Essentials 87.**

Pseudogout/CPPD Deposition

Pφ CPPD crystals form in patients with alterations of inorganic pyrophosphate metabolism and abnormalities in calcium metabolism. CPPD crystals precipitate in cartilage and provoke an inflammatory response. Other conditions commonly associated with CPPD arthritis include hypophosphatemia, hypomagnesemia, hypothyroidism, hemochromatosis, and hyperparathyroidism.

TP Many patients are asymptomatic, but when the disease presents as an inflammatory arthropathy it mimics the presentation of gout—thus the nickname pseudogout. These attacks are often seen in postsurgical patients or following an illness. Knees and wrists are the most common joints involved.

Dx Diagnosis depends on the presence of weakly positive birefringent CPPD crystals in a joint aspirate. Inflammatory synovial fluid is characteristic of pseudogout. Patients may also have chondrocalcinosis on radiography.

Tx The treatment for CPPD deposition disease is essentially the same as the treatment for acute gout, with NSAIDs as the mainstay of treatment and maintenance therapy with colchicine for some patients. Evaluation for possible associated conditions will be appropriate in some cases. **See Cecil Essentials 73.**

Viral Arthritis
Pφ The most common viral joint pathogens are parvovirus B19, rubella, and hepatitis B and C viruses.
TP Viral arthritis typically presents as a mild to moderate polyarthritis. Parvovirus B19 usually involves the small joints of the hands and feet and the knees, and may mimic the pattern of RA. It is usually self-limited and sometimes associated with a rash. Acute rubella has a concomitant rash, fever, and lymphadenopathy. Patients can develop a polyarthritis after a rubella vaccination, usually about 2 weeks after immunization.
Dx Parvovirus B19 is diagnosed by the presence of specific serum IgM antibodies. These patients may also develop autoantibodies such as rheumatoid factor and antinuclear antibodies that can persist for years.
Tx Viral arthritis is self-limited and care is supportive, although symptoms can persist for some time. The arthritis is nonerosive in nature. **See Cecil Essentials 79, 104.**

ZEBRA ZONE

a. Rarer forms of septic arthritis from tuberculosis and fungi can be seen in immunocompromised patients. These entities, though sometimes accompanied by fever, develop more gradually and inflammation is less intense than with the usual bacterial organisms or crystal-induced arthritides.

b. Patients with chronic renal failure may develop symptoms of acute arthritis from oxalate crystal deposition. Knees or hands are the most characteristic sites for inflammation. In contrast to gout and pseudogout, synovial fluid WBC counts are generally <2000 cells/mm^3.

Practice-Based Learning and Improvement: Evidence-Based Medicine

Title
Does this adult patient have septic arthritis?

Authors
Margaretten ME, Kohlwes J, Moore D, Bent S

Institution
University of California–San Francisco, California

Chapter 53
Chronic Joint Pain (Case 45)

Robin Dibner MD, Joel Mathew MD,
and Jessica L. Israel MD

Case: A 32-year-old generally healthy woman complains to her primary-care physician of pain and swelling in her hands. She has noticed for 3 months that her fingers feel stiff in the morning, and she has to place them under warm water to loosen them up. She has difficulty with small buttons when dressing, but by the time she gets to work she feels better and can work on the computer. She has tried over-the-counter ibuprofen with some benefit but feels it is causing dyspepsia. She has not had fevers, rashes, travel, tick bites, or any other new symptoms. She is quite worried, because she has an aunt with arthritis who has "twisted fingers" and a lot of pain. "I think I am too young to have arthritis, right?" she asks.

Differential Diagnosis

Osteoarthritis	Systemic lupus erythematosus (SLE)	Fibromyalgia
RA	Systemic sclerosis	Seronegative spondyloarthropathies

Speaking Intelligently

In taking a history from a patient whose arthritis is subacute or chronic, it is important to determine whether the symptoms have been present for longer than 6 weeks. For briefer durations of disease, self-limited entities such as viral arthritides, viral illnesses (e.g., from hepatitis B), and other serum sickness–like reactions from immune complex deposition must also be considered. Infective endocarditis, with an indolent organism such as a viridans streptococcus, is an example of the latter.

PATIENT CARE

Clinical Thinking
- It is important to consider the pattern of joint involvement in a patient who appears to have developed a chronic

process—symmetrical or asymmetric? Large or small joints? Upper or lower extremity? The spine?

- A very complete review of systems is critical, looking for the other findings that can be seen in diseases that manifest with chronic arthritis.
- A difficult part of understanding the different disease entities has to do with the amount of overlap between the diseases, particularly the inflammatory arthritides of an autoimmune etiology, which go by the misnomers collagen vascular diseases and connective tissue diseases.
- Because of the heterogeneous nature of the rheumatic diseases, the American College of Rheumatology has developed criteria for several of the major diagnoses that are highly sensitive and specific. However, there is a great deal of overlap, and early in the course of these diseases there may not be many manifestations.
- Rheumatologists often tell such patients who do not fulfill the criteria for any of the conditions that they have undifferentiated connective tissue disease if they have inflammatory arthritis and a positive antinuclear antibody (ANA) test but insufficient other criteria to fulfill the diagnosis of SLE.
- There are many other rheumatologic signs and symptoms such as alopecia and Raynaud phenomenon that are seen in a variety of conditions and are therefore too nonspecific to be included in any criteria.

History

- Patient characteristics are important: women of childbearing age have SLE 10 times more commonly than men.
- Women are also affected by RA more often than men.
- Osteoarthritis frequency increases with age.
- The chief complaint defines the specific joints and the pattern of involvement.
- The history of the present illness must clarify the onset of the symptoms, which is important in deciding when criteria for RA have been met.
- More than an hour's duration of morning stiffness is pathognomonic of active inflammatory arthritis.
- Past medical history can give clues to other systemic diseases that can cause chronic arthritis such as psoriasis and sarcoidosis.
- Medication history may suggest drug-induced lupus, a specific entity caused by an immunologic reaction to numerous medications.
- Response to prior treatments is also revealing.
- Family history will frequently reveal others with autoimmune disease, though not necessarily the same as the patient's.
- The review of systems is tailored to the likely diagnosis and may include further probing for autoimmune disease such as evidence of Raynaud symptoms, hypothyroidism, or hyperthyroidism.
- A functional history can help guide treatment goals.

Physical Examination
- Involved joints should be examined for swelling, tenderness, range of motion, and deformity.
- Symmetrical joint involvement is characteristic of RA, lupus, and some other inflammatory conditions.
- Inflamed joints often have palpable synovial thickening, which feels doughy.
- The most characteristic joint involvement in RA is involvement of the metacarpophalangeal joints.
- Osteoarthritis is never purely symmetrical; however, it may appear so if many joints are involved. The joints may appear swollen, but the enlargement is bony and represents proliferation of osteophytes.
- Effusions are more common in inflamed joints but can be present in noninflamed joints.
- The skin exam may show characteristic findings, such as the classic erythematous butterfly rash of lupus over the cheeks and bridge of the nose, psoriatic plaques and nail pits, or subcutaneous rheumatoid nodules on the proximal ulnar aspect of the forearm.
- There may be other extra-articular manifestations such as the bluish fingertip discoloration of Raynaud syndrome, crackles of interstitial lung disease, the rub of pericarditis, edema in patients with nephrotic syndrome, or red eyes in episcleritis or scleritis seen in some RA patients.

Tests for Consideration
- **Complete blood count (CBC):** Will usually show a normochromic, normocytic anemia secondary to chronic inflammation. $11
- **Chemistry panel:** Important to determine whether there is renal involvement in lupus. $12
- **Liver function** abnormalities are a potential contraindication to certain medications. $12
- **Urinalysis:** To evaluate for renal lupus. $4
- **Rheumatoid factor (RF):** Seventy-five percent of patients have RF positivity at some point in the disease; high titers of RF are associated with extra-articular manifestations and poor outcome. It may be negative in early disease and is negative in the spondyloarthropathies such as reactive arthritis, psoriatic arthritis, and ankylosing spondylitis. $8
- **Anti-CCP (antibodies to cyclic citrullinated peptide):** Positive in about 65% of patients with RA, is more specific than RF, and may be positive before the RF. In such cases it has been shown to be a predictor of rapid progression to erosions and poor prognosis. $18
- **ANA:** Positive in more than 95% of patients with lupus. $14
- **ESR or CRP** $4, $7
- **Creatine phosphokinase (CPK)** $9
- **Thyroid-stimulating hormone (TSH)** $24
- Consider **serologies** for *Borrelia burgdorferi*, $24, $32, **hepatitis B**, **hepatitis C**, and **HIV**. $22, $13

IMAGING CONSIDERATIONS

→ It generally takes at least 6 months for erosions to be visible on plain radiographs in patients with RA, so early radiographs are not helpful in establishing a diagnosis. Erosions can be seen much earlier on MRI, but this is rarely necessary except in drug studies where the timing of the development of erosions needs to be assessed. In a patient with established disease, plain radiographs may be helpful in distinguishing among RA, psoriatic arthritis, and lupus, among others. Osteoarthritis has characteristic radiographic findings distinct from those of inflammatory diseases.

Clinical Entities	Medical Knowledge

Osteoarthritis

Pφ Osteoarthritis occurs as the structural integrity and the chemical composition of joint cartilage wear down and change over time. As this process occurs, there is less protection from friction created as bones rub against other bony structures in the joint. Age, obesity, and chronic repetitive motion on particular joints are all considered risk factors.

TP Osteoarthritis typically affects the large weight-bearing joints, distal and proximal interphalangeal joints, and the first carpometacarpal joint of the hand. Patients usually complain of pain with activity that is relieved with rest. Pain at rest, or pain specifically worsening at night, is related to more serious advanced disease. Some patients also present with morning stiffness, but this stiffness generally lasts <30 minutes. Joint swelling is not usually a major feature, but some patients can develop bony outgrowths on the distal (Heberden nodes) and proximal (Bouchard nodes) interphalangeal joints. These can be painful and limit motion. In osteoarthritis of the knee, the examiner may feel crepitus when passively flexing the joint.

Dx Osteoarthritis is a clinical diagnosis. The physical findings are surprisingly minimal, especially in early disease. Osteoarthritis of the knees can be reliably diagnosed if the patient is over 50 years of age, has stiffness lasting <30 minutes, crepitus, bony tenderness or enlargement of the joint, and no palpable warmth (American College of Rheumatology clinical criteria). Radiographs of the affected joints may show joint space narrowing, but the findings do not correlate well with disease symptoms.

Tx Nonpharmacologic treatments include weight loss and changes in activity if repetitive actions are an issue. Physical therapy benefits hip and knee osteoarthritis. Assistive devices (such as jar openers and special kitchen utensils) may also be helpful. Pharmacologically, acetaminophen and NSAIDs are frequently used as a first line, with tramadol and opioids as a second-line therapy. More intensive treatments include corticosteroids and hyaluronan joint injections. Joint replacement therapy is considered when medical therapy is no longer helpful or when the arthritis-related debility has a serious and limiting impact on the patient's quality of life. **See Cecil Essentials 88.**

Rheumatoid Arthritis

Pφ RA is a complex disease, the cause of which is not completely understood, although much is known about the pathologic process in the joints. The pathology occurs most likely in response to an antigenic trigger. Synovial membranes become thickened and inflamed in the process, and multiple inflammatory mediators are involved. Involved cell types include B lymphocytes, macrophages, and T lymphocytes in the joint space. Cytokines, such as TNF-α and interleukins, also play a major role. Some patients have a clear genetic risk for the disease.

TP The disease course and symptoms at presentation can be highly variable. Most patients with persistent synovitis will develop erosive disease in the joints that leads to significant functional limitations. Work disability occurs in a variety of patients within 5 years of diagnosis. The peak age of onset is in the mid-50s, and women are affected more than men. RA usually involves the small joints of the hands and feet symmetrically (wrists, metacarpophalangeal, and proximal interphalangeal joints). Knees are also commonly involved. The joints become painful, swollen, and tender. Sometimes affected joints are warm on examination. Morning stiffness lasting more than 1 hour is also a characteristic feature of active disease. Systemic symptoms can also occur, such as malaise and fatigue. Subcutaneous nodules on extensor surfaces can be palpated in some patients. Extra-articular manifestations of RA include scleritis and episcleritis, pleuritis, pericarditis, secondary Sjögren syndrome, and vasculitis of small and medium vessels. Patients with RA may also have cervical instability at the atlantoaxial articulation, which can be diagnosed with extension and flexion radiographs of the neck.

Dx A new diagnosis of RA is made based on the history of symptoms for longer than 6 weeks, characteristic patterns of joint swelling and tenderness, and supporting serologic abnormalities including RF positivity and/or anti-CCP positivity. Elevation of the acute-phase reactants ESR or CRP is supportive evidence but neither sensitive nor specific. The American College of Rheumatology and the European Union League Against Rheumatism developed new ACR-EULAR classification criteria for RA in 2010, in part to aid in earlier diagnosis and treatment. Radiographic bone erosion is no longer mentioned in the new criteria, as it is often not evident in early disease. Arthrocentesis is not needed for diagnosis but can be useful to rule out other etiologies of arthritis.

Tx Early and aggressive treatment is essential to slow the progression of the illness and prevent long-term complications. Damage to joints is irreversible, even in the face of disease-modifying agents. Early symptoms may be treated with NSAIDs and corticosteroids. However, early initiation of disease-modifying antirheumatic drugs (DMARD therapy) has been shown to reduce long-term disability and is now the standard of care. Examples of DMARD therapy include hydroxychloroquine, sulfasalazine, and methotrexate, alone or in combination, as well as biologic agents. Biologic agents used in RA include TNF-α inhibitors (etanercept, infliximab, and adalimumab). Patients who do not respond to TNF-α inhibitors may be candidates for abatacept (a T-cell co-stimulation inhibitor) or rituximab (an anti-CD20 monoclonal antibody). Other new biologic agents for RA continue to become available. Patients should be evaluated for latent tuberculosis before starting treatment with a biologic agent and carefully monitored for development of infections. Surgical intervention, including synovectomy or joint replacement, is helpful in patients with advanced or severely destructive joint disease. **See Cecil Essentials 79.**

Systemic Lupus Erythematosus

Pφ SLE is an autoimmune disease characterized by a complex dysregulation of the immune system and loss of self-tolerance. Polyclonal B-cell activation, abnormal apoptosis, clearing of cellular debris and immune complexes, and unbalanced production of numerous cytokines are a few of the recognized pathologic mechanisms. This manifests with the presence of autoantibodies, and humoral and cellular inflammation affecting many target organs (kidneys, skin, joints, blood cells, nervous system, and serosal surfaces).

keratitis), lungs (apical pulmonary fibrosis), vascular system (aortitis), gastrointestinal (GI) tract (inflammatory bowel disease), and genitourinary tract.

Ankylosing spondylitis occurs more commonly in men usually in the teenage years and the 20s. Concurrent arthritis of the hips is very common with this condition.

Reactive arthritis presents within a few weeks after an episode of bacterial gastroenteritis, urethritis, or cervicitis. The classic triad at presentation of this illness is arthritis, conjunctivitis, and urethritis. The onset of symptoms is acute and is usually an asymmetric arthritis of the lower extremities with or without back pain. Heel pain and swelling from Achilles tendinitis is also common.

Enteropathic arthritis accompanies Crohn disease and ulcerative colitis. The arthritis may even develop before the GI component of the disease. The presentation may be an asymmetric large-joint arthritis, usually of the lower extremities, or the spine may be predominantly involved resembling ankylosing spondylitis. The peripheral arthritis activity usually follows the course of the bowel disease, but spine involvement may progress despite remission of the GI symptoms. Extra-articular manifestations are common, especially in the eyes and skin, particularly erythema nodosum.

Psoriatic arthritis occurs in 20%–40% of patients with psoriasis, with extensive skin involvement being a marker for risk. The psoriasis predates the development of arthritis by many years in most patients, but it is possible to see the arthritic changes before skin involvement. The typical presentation is a symmetrical polyarthritis that can look very similar to RA. In psoriatic arthritis, however, the distal interphalangeal joints are often involved. Patients often have characteristic pitting and onycholysis in the fingernails. RF is negative in these conditions.

Dx Spinal changes can be seen in radiographic studies. Vertebral bodies appear squared, and ossified ligaments lead to the appearance of a "bamboo spine." MRI of the spine is the best test to detect early spinal inflammation. Peripheral joints may show erosions and destruction, especially in psoriatic arthritis, after chronic involvement.

Tx TNF-α inhibitors are the first-line therapy for ankylosing spondylitis, as they can be helpful in both the spinal disease and the peripheral joint and extra-articular components. Traditional immunosuppressants (such as methotrexate and sulfasalazine) help with peripheral and extra-articular disease but not the spinal arthritis. NSAIDs and exercise are also indicated for symptomatic relief and functional improvement.

Reactive arthritis is usually treated with NSAIDs and corticosteroids. Antibiotics are used to treat any residual infection but generally do not help the arthritis itself. Methotrexate and sulfasalazine can be helpful in cases that are recurrent or chronic.

Enteropathic arthritis therapy is now often linked to the treatment of the underlying bowel disease, as the immunosuppressive agents are the same. Corticosteroids, sulfasalazine, azathioprine, and methotrexate may be used for the bowel disease and peripheral arthritis, but treatment of severe bowel disease and spinal involvement often necessitates use of biologic agents such as the TNF-α inhibitors.

Psoriatic arthritis treatment is similar to the immuno-suppressive treatments used for RA, including methotrexate, sulfasalazine, and TNF-α inhibitors. Corticosteroids are generally not used in this setting, because tapering has been associated with significant flares in skin disease. NSAIDs may help symptom-atically but do not alter the disease course or prevent disease progression. **See Cecil Essentials 80.**

Fibromyalgia

Pφ The cause of fibromyalgia is not understood but is possibly related to dysregulation of neurotransmitters or central pain sensitization in the central nervous system. Fibromyalgia is associated with low socioeconomic status, poor functional status, and disability. Often there is a preceding history of trauma or an accident before the onset of symptoms. Chronically disturbed, nonrestorative sleep and physical deconditioning may be predisposing factors. "Secondary fibromyalgia" is used to describe symptoms in patients with another defined autoimmune disease who also experience characteristic fibromyalgia symptoms.

TP Fibromyalgia presents as chronic widespread musculoskeletal pain for at least 3 months without another diagnosis and symptoms of fatigue, waking unrefreshed, and sometimes cognitive symptoms and a variety of somatic symptoms (e.g., headache, irritable bowel, numbness, and tingling). It is most commonly seen in women, particularly between the ages of 20 and 50 years, although it does also occur in men. The patient's physical examination is usually normal, except for tenderness to pressure. Previously tenderness at defined "tender points" was used to diagnose the condition, but more recently the combination of chronic pain and other severe subjective symptoms in the absence of another diagnosis is adequate to fulfill criteria for diagnosis.

GI symptoms may be alleviated with prokinetic agents and gastric acid suppression. Oral cyclophosphamide improves pulmonary symptoms in patients with systemic sclerosis and interstitial lung disease. Pulmonary artery hypertension is treated with anticoagulation, vasodilatation with sildenafil and endothelin antagonists (bosentan and ambrisentan) or prostacyclin analogues (epoprostenol, iloprost, and treprostinil), and oxygen. The cornerstone of treatment for scleroderma renal crisis is early and aggressive blood pressure control with angiotensin-converting enzyme inhibitors. **See Cecil Essentials 83.**

ZEBRA ZONE

a. Sarcoidosis is a systemic inflammatory disease. The hallmark is the presence of noncaseating granulomas. Acute sarcoidosis may present as the classic Lofgren triad: erythema nodosum, acute arthritis (often ankles), and bilateral hilar adenopathy. Fever and uveitis may be present. This presentation has an excellent prognosis and usually resolves with minimal treatment. Chronic sarcoid arthritis is seen in less than 1% of cases but can be deforming.

b. Adult-onset Still disease is similar to the systemic onset of RA seen in children. Usually first presenting with high fevers with an evening temperature spike, the systemic manifestations may precede the joint pain, making the diagnosis difficult. Weight loss, adenopathy, serositis, organomegaly, a faint rash, marked leukocytosis and thrombocytosis, and an elevated ESR are all characteristic, leading in most cases to an extensive workup for infection or even malignancy. If the arthralgias are prominent, or frank arthritis (most commonly knees and wrists) develops, the diagnosis becomes evident. RF and ANA are negative. Extremely high serum ferritin levels (>3000 ng/mL) are characteristic of this condition and support the diagnosis in suspected cases when infection has been excluded. The course is variable, ranging from complete remission to the development of progressive joint destruction.

Practice-Based Learning Improvement: Evidence-Based Medicine

Title
Cardiovascular morbidity and mortality in women diagnosed with rheumatoid arthritis

Authors
Solomon DH, Karlson EW, Rimm ED, et al.

Institution
Brigham and Women's Hospital, Harvard Medical School, Boston, Massachusetts

Reference
Circulation 2003;107:1303–1307

Problem
Do patients with RA have a higher incidence of coronary artery disease (CAD) and stroke?

Intervention
Prospective Cohort Study (The Nurses' Health Study, 2.4 million person-years of follow-up)

Quality of evidence
Level II-2

Outcome/effect
Women with RA had a significantly increased risk of myocardial infarction but not stroke compared to women without RA.

Historical significance/comments
This very large study showing RA as a potent risk factor for CAD has had significant clinical implications. It and other confirmatory studies have been used to justify aggressive CAD risk factor management in RA and to support the hypothesis that aggressive control of inflammation could reduce CAD risk in these patients.

Interpersonal and Communication Skills

Take a Functional History
It is essential to encourage patients with a diagnosis of arthritis to remain active and maintain a healthy lifestyle. Take a "functional history" at every visit. We always ask, "What are the things you have difficulty doing that you would like to be able to do better?" Try to suggest practical solutions to help your patient maintain functionality. If necessary, have the patient evaluated for use of an assistive device. Understand that some patients will refuse to use canes, tripods, and walkers due to personal vanity. Encourage patients to become educated, active partners in the options available for treatment.

Section XI
INFECTIOUS DISEASES

Section Editor
Patricia D. Brown, MD

Section Contents

54 Infections Presenting with Rash (Case 46)
  Patricia D. Brown, MD

55 Skin and Soft-Tissue Infections (Case 47)
  Patricia D. Brown, MD

56 Upper Respiratory Tract Infections (Case 48)
  Patricia D. Brown, MD

57 Genital Ulcers (Case 49)
  Patricia D. Brown, MD

58 Vaginitis and Urethritis (Case 50)
  Patricia D. Brown, MD

59 Fever in the Hospitalized Patient (Case 51)
  Patricia D. Brown, MD

Professionalism

Be Aware of Legal Provisions for the Treatment of the Disabled

Disabilities Act provides many protections for people with disabilities. In the employment setting, for example, companies of a certain size must make "reasonable" accommodations for an employee who is or becomes disabled. If the worker is able, with accommodation, to perform the essential functions of the job, the law states that specific accommodations must be made in order for the employee to continue to do his or her clinical job properly and avoid undue strain on the arthritic wrist. It is important for physicians to be familiar with these provisions and to be certain that their patients are receiving such consideration. Another important provision of the law is the Family Medical Leave Act, which allows patients to take time off without pay for medical reasons for as long as 3 months and still be able to return to employment with their original position. Among other provisions, this Act allows patients to take the time in small increments; hence, a patient requiring physical therapy two afternoons a week, for example, might take time off from work and not lose her job.

Patient Identification and Patient Safety

Patients with chronic joint pain may be diagnosed with conditions that will require joint replacement for optimal therapy. Misidentification of patients, though rare, can be a major source of catastrophic error in those undergoing surgical procedures. Accurate patient identification should be accomplished by matching two identifiers of the patient to two identifiers linked to the procedure. One identifier can be the patient's name, if the patient can articulate it. Do not address a patient by name and look for confirmation; "Are you Johnny Jones?" Rather, ask a patient, "What is your name?" For the patient who is unable to answer or is otherwise unable to provide safe information, other identifiers can be used. The second identifier can be a birth date, address, telephone number, identification number (such as a medical record number), or labeled photograph, depending on what is available in the record. The procedure-linked identifiers should match both patient identifiers. For those patients undergoing joint replacement, often the patient is asked to make a mark and the orthopedic surgeon should also *sign his or her name on the skin over the joint area to be replaced* to ensure that the operation is performed on the correct side.

Chapter 54
Infections Presenting with Rash (Case 46)

Patricia D. Brown MD

Case: A 68-year-old man presents in late August with a complaint of skin rash. Two days earlier, the patient first noticed several red, raised lesions on the left chest wall; the morning of presentation he awoke with a burning pain in that area and noticed multiple lesions, some of which appeared to be filled with fluid. He denies fever or any other specific complaints. His past medical history is remarkable only for hypertension, for which he has taken lisinopril for the past 3 years. He is retired and has no pets. The patient is a resident of Boston who travels frequently to his vacation home on Cape Cod; his last visit there was 6 weeks ago. Three days ago he returned from a family reunion in a rural area of Arkansas. He golfed and fished, spending large amounts of time outdoors, but recalls no insect bites. He is widowed and has not been sexually active for many years. He has no sick contacts. He received the 23-valent pneumococcal polysaccharide vaccine at age 65 years and receives the influenza vaccine yearly; his last tetanus shot was 8 years ago, and he has received no other vaccinations. On physical exam the patient has normal vital signs but appears in mild discomfort secondary to pain. The only abnormal finding is a rash that extends from the midchest to the midback, appearing to follow the T6 dermatome. The rash consists of papular and vesicular lesions on an erythematous base; some lesions are filled with clear fluid, and others appear pustular.

Differential Diagnosis

Viral infections including varicella zoster (shingles)	Rocky Mountain spotted fever (RMSF)
Lyme borreliosis	Disseminated gonococcal infection (DGI) in patients who are sexually active

Speaking Intelligently

The differential diagnosis of a rash is extraordinarily broad, including both infectious and noninfectious etiologies. Numerous viral and bacterial infections can manifest as skin lesions; patients presenting with skin lesions may rarely have a disseminated fungal infection.

Dx The diagnosis of herpes zoster can usually be made based on the history and the typical clinical appearance of the rash. If the diagnosis is uncertain, a viral culture can be obtained; direct fluorescent antibody testing is also available for VZV. Older age may be the only factor that predisposes a patient to reactivation; however, the history and physical exam should be thorough to determine if there is any suggestion of underlying immunodeficiency that would require further evaluation.

Tx Several antiviral agents can be used for the treatment of VZV infection (acyclovir, valacyclovir, and famciclovir). Valacyclovir and famciclovir are often preferred because of less frequent dosing than acyclovir (three times vs. five times daily). Treatment is considered optional in individuals <50 years of age with mild symptoms; those >50 years of age should receive antiviral therapy if it can be initiated within 72 hours of the onset of the rash. All patients with ophthalmic involvement require treatment. The use of corticosteroids in conjunction with antiviral therapy remains controversial; corticosteroids may shorten the duration of acute neuralgia. A live attenuated vaccine is now available for the prevention of zoster and is recommended for individuals who are ≥60 years of age, even if they have a previous history of herpes zoster. **See Cecil Essentials 101.**

Lyme Borreliosis

Pφ Lyme disease is caused by *Borrelia burgdorferi*, a spirochete. Infection is maintained in nature through the horizontal transmission of the organism from infected nymphal ticks to the white-footed mouse, and then from the mouse to the larval ticks. The nymphs are primarily responsible for the transmission of infection to humans. In the United States, Lyme disease is endemic in the northeast (Massachusetts to Maryland), upper Midwest (Wisconsin, Minnesota), and Pacific Northwest (northern California, southern Oregon). Lyme disease is transmitted to humans via the bite of the *Ixodes* tick. The organism multiplies at the site of inoculation, eliciting a local host inflammatory response. The organism may then disseminate via the bloodstream; involvement of the myocardium and the central nervous system (CNS) may occur during early disseminated disease, and involvement of the joints is characteristic of late disseminated disease.

TP The skin lesion of early localized Lyme disease is referred to as erythema migrans (EM). The lesion begins as an erythematous macule or papule that expands to form a large annular lesion, often with a more intensely erythematous border and central clearing. EM lesions are generally not painful. Secondary skin lesions may develop in patients with early disseminated infection, who may present with neurologic (aseptic meningitis, peripheral seventh-nerve palsy) or cardiac (conduction abnormalities) involvement. Because the *Ixodes* tick is small, patients may not recall a history of tick bite.

Dx The diagnosis of Lyme disease should be made based on clinical grounds with an appropriate epidemiologic history (outdoor exposure in an endemic area) and compatible clinical findings. Serologic tests are available, but they are neither sensitive nor specific in early infection and should be used only in selected cases.

Tx Treatment depends on the stage of infection. Early localized disease may be treated with doxycycline or amoxicillin (either is preferred) or cefuroxime axetil (alternative) for 14–21 days. **See Cecil Essentials 95.**

Rocky Mountain Spotted Fever

Pφ RMSF is caused by *Rickettsia rickettsii*, an obligate intracellular pathogen. The disease is endemic in the south Atlantic and east south central regions of the United States, but cases have been reported from almost every state. The organism is transmitted by a tick bite (several tick species are reservoirs for infection). After introduction into the skin, the pathogen disseminates hematogenously and infects vascular endothelial cells, inducing vascular injury that can affect almost any organ.

TP The incubation period for RMSF is 2–14 days. The illness begins with nonspecific symptoms including fever, headache, and generalized malaise. Three to five days later the characteristic rash appears: an erythematous, petechial rash that begins in the periphery of the bite and then spreads centrally. Involvement of the palms and soles is characteristic, but may appear only later in the course of illness. Up to 10% to 15% of patients may not have a rash (so-called spotless RMSF); absence of rash is associated with delay in diagnosis, so it is important to consider this entity in the patient with febrile illness in the correct epidemiologic setting.

commonly in the groin, axilla, or perineum. The lesion begins as an erythematous macule that becomes indurated and then forms a hemorrhagic bullous lesion. The lesion ulcerates, forming a black eschar with surrounding erythema.

c. **Fungal pathogens:** Disseminated fungal infections may be associated with skin lesions that provide an important clue to the diagnosis as well as readily accessible material for histopathologic examination and culture. *Cryptococcus neoformans* infection can present with small papular lesions with central umbilication. Disseminated histoplasmosis is associated with papular and pustular lesions, and oral ulcers. Disseminated coccidioidomycosis commonly manifests with skin lesions, including papules and ulcerative lesions. Skin lesions are the most common extrapulmonary site of blastomycosis. Verrucous, crusted lesions with abscess formation and ulcerative lesions are described.

Practice-Based Learning and Improvement: Evidence-Based Medicine

Title
A vaccine to prevent herpes zoster and postherpetic neuralgia in older adults

Authors
Oxman MN, Levin MJ, Johnson GR, et al.

Institution
Veterans Administration San Diego Healthcare System

Reference
N Engl J Med 2005;352:2271–2284

Problem
Both the incidence and the severity of herpes zoster and PHN increase with age.

Intervention
Adults 60 years of age and older were randomized to receive a live attenuated varicella zoster vaccine or a placebo injection. The primary end point was the burden of illness due to herpes zoster; the secondary end point was the incidence of PHN.

Quality of evidence
Level I

Outcome/effect
The burden of illness due to herpes zoster was significantly reduced in study subjects who received the vaccine. This reduction resulted from both a reduction in the incidence of herpes zoster and a significant reduction in the incidence of PHN in those who developed zoster despite vaccination. The vaccine was safe and well tolerated.

Historical significance/comments
Varicella zoster (shingles) causes significant morbidity in the elderly, and older patients are at a higher risk of developing PHN. The pain of PHN can be extraordinarily difficult to manage and may have a major impact on quality of life. The vaccine was most effective at preventing zoster in those 60 to 69 years of age and most effective at preventing PHN in those over 70 years of age.

Interpersonal and Communication Skills

Document Medical Information Accurately
The differential diagnosis for a patient with illness presenting as a rash can be very broad. Arriving at the correct diagnosis, therefore, requires careful history taking and meticulous attention to detail. Often the patient will make a temporal association between a particular event or exposure and the onset of the rash. It is important to ensure that a thorough chronology of the illness is explored before arriving at a diagnosis. This information, including both pertinent positive and pertinent negative results, must be carefully documented in the patient's medical record.

Professionalism

Provide Accurate Documentation
When it has been determined that a rash was caused by a medication, the physician must ensure that the patient understands the need to report an allergy to that medication in the future. Document the allergy (including the reaction) carefully in the medical record; give the patient written documentation that includes the name of the medication, the date prescribed, and a description of the reaction to keep for his or her own personal health records. When taking a history, the physician should strive to document the reaction for each medication allergy that the patient reports. Often the "allergy" is actually an intolerance (e.g., gastrointestinal upset) that would not preclude the use of that agent or related medications in the future. It is our responsibility to the patient and to the next physician who may care for that patient to accurately and clearly document medical problems to ensure the safest and most informed care.

bite, or any preexisting skin lesion such as venous stasis ulcers or ulcers due to arterial insufficiency.

- A common and often overlooked portal of entry in patients with cellulitis of the lower extremity is tinea pedis, leading to small cracks in the skin between the toes.
- Patients with chronic lower extremity edema, those who have undergone saphenous vein harvest for coronary artery bypass grafting, and those who have lymphedema secondary to pelvic surgery or radiation therapy are also predisposed to SSTI.
- A previous episode of severe cellulitis may lead to scarring of the lymphatics and predispose the patient to recurrent episodes of cellulitis.
- Recurrent cellulitis of the upper extremity in women who have undergone mastectomy with extensive lymph node dissection is seen less frequently now that breast-conserving surgery and limited lymph node dissection are more commonly performed.
- Any history of environmental exposures that may suggest uncommon pathogens should be noted; a patient with SSTI presenting as multiple skin abscesses, suggestive of CA-MRSA, should be questioned about exposure to others with SSTI.
- SSTIs that occur following bite wounds have a microbiology that includes pathogens that are part of the normal oral flora of the animal (or person) that bit the patient.
- Symptoms that would suggest a more severe infection such as necrotizing fasciitis include severe pain that is out of proportion to the clinical findings and a history of a rapidly spreading infection.
- SSTI due to either *S. aureus* or *S. pyogenes* may also predispose the patient to toxic shock syndrome.

Physical Examination
- Review the vital signs; although fever is not unexpected, hypotension is suggestive of sepsis and/or necrotizing fasciitis.
- Perform a careful inspection of the involved area, noting the presence of ulcers, abscesses, blisters, or bullae, and looking for the presence of lymphangitis, which causes linear erythematous streaks along the course of the lymphatic drainage.
- Note the presence of regional lymphadenopathy. Carefully palpate the area of cellulitis; crepitance (palpable gas in the tissues) suggests necrotizing fasciitis, as does diminished sensation or the presence of large bullae, ecchymosis, or skin necrosis. Areas of fluctuance suggest an underlying abscess.
- Note the presence of tinea pedis in patients with lower extremity cellulitis, as treatment may prevent recurrent infections.
- Examine the other extremity, and note the presence of chronic edema or evidence of venous or arterial insufficiency.
- Many clinicians will use a pen to mark the extent of erythema to help discern if the infection is rapidly spreading. Careful documentation of

the extent of erythema is particularly important in settings where the patient will be referred to another physician, who will then need to determine the response to therapy. However, it is not uncommon for the extent of cellulitis to worsen within the first 24 hours of appropriate treatment.

Tests for Consideration

- A microbiologic diagnosis is usually not confirmed in a patient with cellulitis.
- If purulent drainage is noted from a wound or abscesses are present, one should submit material for **Gram stain** and culture to confirm a specific microbiologic diagnosis and guide antibiotic therapy. $6
- When cellulitis occurs in the setting of a chronic ulcer, clinicians may be tempted to send swabs from the ulcer for culture; however, organisms present in a chronic ulcer may be colonizers and not reflective of the pathogen causing the surrounding SSTI. $15
- Patients with severity of illness sufficient to warrant hospital admission should have **blood cultures**; a recent study found that up to one third of patients hospitalized with cellulitis who had an underlying comorbidity such as diabetes mellitus, peripheral vascular disease, or congestive heart failure had concomitant bacteremia. $15

IMAGING CONSIDERATIONS

→ If the history is suggestive, obtain a **plain radiograph** to exclude the possibility of a foreign body. Obtain plain films with diabetics or other patients with sensory neuropathy who have cellulitis of the foot to exclude the possibility of a foreign body. $45

→ Plain radiographs can also reveal evidence of underlying osteomyelitis in patients with a chronic ulcer complicated by infection. $45

→ **CT or MRI scan:** May be needed if there is a concern that cellulitis has been complicated by formation of a deeper abscess. $334, $534

→ While imaging with CT or MRI may reveal findings supportive of the diagnosis of necrotizing fasciitis, it must be emphasized that the possibility of necrotizing fasciitis is an emergency that requires urgent surgical evaluation; this evaluation should not be delayed while sending the patient for imaging studies.

TP A soft-tissue abscess may form in an area of cellulitis. An abscess should be suspected if there is an area of more intense edema or fluctuance, or if the cellulitis is failing to respond to appropriate antibiotic therapy. Frequently development of an abscess is apparent on examination; occasionally CT scan or MRI is required to evaluate for an abscess in the deeper soft tissues that may not be readily apparent clinically. CA-MRSA SSTIs most commonly present as multiple abscesses, although a single abscess may occur. Patients will frequently report that they have "spider bites" or give a history of a household member with "spider bites." Outbreaks of CA-MRSA skin infection have been described among prisoners, men who have sex with men, and athletes (wrestlers, football players); however, many patients do not have a specific risk factor for CA-MRSA infection, so the diagnosis must be suspected based on the clinical presentation.

Dx As discussed above, a skin and soft-tissue abscess can frequently be diagnosed based on the clinical examination. In situations where abscess is suspected clinically but is not clearly present on exam, CT or MRI can confirm the presence of a collection of pus. Abscess drainage should always be cultured to confirm the microbiologic diagnosis and direct appropriate antibiotic therapy. A Gram stain can provide rapid initial information regarding the microbiology of the infection.

Tx Surgical drainage is as important as antimicrobial therapy in the management of skin and soft-tissue abscess. Sometimes surgical drainage may be all that is required for abscesses that are small (<5 cm in diameter) and not associated with a significant area of surrounding cellulitis. When an abscess occurs in the setting of typical cellulitis, initial antibiotic coverage directed toward *S. aureus* and streptococci should be sufficient pending further information from cultures. Trimethoprim-sulfamethoxazole (TMP-SMX) has emerged as the treatment of choice for CA-MRSA infections; clindamycin and doxycycline are alternatives. Abscesses in injection drug users and those that complicate diabetic foot infections (discussed below) will require broader spectrum coverage to include treatment for gram-negative organisms and anaerobes. **See Cecil Essentials 101.**

Necrotizing Fasciitis

Pφ Necrotizing fasciitis is an SSTI that has spread beyond the dermis to the deeper subcutaneous tissues and fascia. Necrotizing fasciitis type I is a polymicrobial infection that can include gram-positive, gram-negative, and anaerobic organisms; type II is caused by *S. pyogenes*. The elaboration of toxins (e.g., streptococcal pyrogenic exotoxin) is important in the pathogenesis of this rapidly progressive and fulminant infection.

TP Necrotizing fasciitis must be suspected when a patient with cellulitis has a rapidly spreading infection, especially when associated with signs of severe systemic toxicity or severe pain that seems out of proportion to the clinical findings. Rapidly forming bullae, ecchymosis, cutaneous anesthesia, and evidence of skin necrosis may occur; palpable crepitance is strongly suggestive of necrotizing fasciitis. Occasionally, patients may present just with severe pain in the involved area and signs of systemic toxicity.

Dx The possibility of necrotizing fasciitis is a medical and surgical emergency, and surgical consultation should be obtained promptly. The diagnosis can be suggested by findings on imaging with CT or MRI, but surgical evaluation should not be delayed to obtain these studies; the diagnosis can only be confirmed with certainty at the time of surgery. Blood cultures should always be obtained in patients with suspected necrotizing fasciitis.

Tx Patients with suspected necrotizing fasciitis must be managed initially with broad-spectrum antibiotics to ensure coverage of gram-positive bacteria (including MRSA), gram-negative bacteria, and anaerobes (e.g., vancomycin or daptomycin, with either piperacillin-tazobactam or a carbapenem). Clindamycin should also be used in the regimen for patients with group A streptococcal necrotizing fasciitis, as it will inhibit the production of toxin, which is important in the pathogenesis of this infection. Many experts recommend the use of IV immunoglobulin to treat the accompanying streptococcal toxic shock–like syndrome. Extensive surgical debridement is frequently required; antibiotic therapy can then be adjusted based on the results of tissue cultures obtained at the time of surgery. **See Cecil Essentials 101.**

Practice-Based Learning and Improvement: Evidence-Based Medicine

Title
Emergence of community-acquired methicillin-resistant
***Staphylococcus aureus* USA 300 clone as the predominant cause of skin and soft tissue infections**

Authors
King MD, Humphrey BJ, Wang YF, et al.

Institution
Emory University School of Medicine, Atlanta, Georgia

Reference
Ann Intern Med 2006;144:309–317

Problem
The incidence of SSTIs due to CA-MRSA has increased dramatically in the past several years, although specific risk groups for CA-MRSA SSTI have been described.

Intervention
This large, epidemiologic study documents the emergence of CA-MRSA as a major cause of SSTI due to *S. aureus*.

Quality of evidence
Level II

Outcome/effect
The majority of community-onset *S. aureus* SSTIs were found to be due to the USA 300 clone of CA-MRSA. A significant proportion of these patients received initial empirical antibiotic therapy that was inadequate for this pathogen.

Historical significance/comments
This study documents the emergence of CA-MRSA as a major cause of SSTIs. The emergence of this pathogen has had a major impact on the approach to the empirical therapy of these infections and underscored the essential importance of obtaining specimens for culture and susceptibility testing in patients with SSTIs associated with abscess formation.

Interpersonal and Communication Skills

The Team Approach of Medicine Requires Interpersonal Skills
In patients with diabetic foot infections, successful treatment requires a multidisciplinary team approach, often including a vascular surgeon, podiatrist, infectious disease specialist, endocrinologist, and, of course, the primary-care physician who should provide the "medical home" for the patient. Here are a few simple tips that are

useful for encouraging better communication among health-care teams:

- Listen.
- Respect the opinions of others.
- Try to understand another's perspective.
- Don't take things personally.
- Cooperate and assume your colleague is acting in good faith.
- Don't be judgmental.
- Learn to compromise.
- Seek a diplomatic approach to conflict resolution.
- Learn to admit when you are wrong.

From Mann BD: Surgery: a competency-based companion. Philadelphia: Elsevier; 2009, pp 467–468.

Professionalism

Show Commitment to Professional Excellence

Patients with infections caused by MRSA should be kept in contact isolation while hospitalized, so that the resistant organism is not spread to other hospitalized patients who may be vulnerable to developing invasive infection; some institutions utilize contact precautions for patients infected with multidrug-resistant pathogens. Unfortunately, health-care workers do not always observe appropriate infection control practices by donning gowns and gloves when caring for isolated patients. It is incumbent upon other care providers to point out lapses in infection control practices and provide feedback to ensure the proper approach to infection control. This may decrease the risk of development of serious infections in hospitalized patients.

Systems-Based Practice

Complications of Disease Impact the System as Well as the Patient

Diabetic foot infections have a substantial impact on the health-care system. Besides causing substantial morbidity and even mortality for patients, these infections are responsible for the largest proportion of hospital days in patients with diabetes. **The importance of prevention cannot be overemphasized.** The best prevention is optimization of glycemic control before the development of neuropathy and vascular insufficiency. Diabetics must be carefully screened for evidence of neuropathy, and once it is detected, they must be provided with education regarding appropriate footwear, foot care, and daily careful self-examination of the feet.

- In patients with acute coughing illness, the presence of pleuritic chest pain should prompt further investigation to exclude pneumonia.
- Influenza virus can cause VRS and acute pharyngitis.

Physical Examination

- Evaluate the temperature, respiratory rate, and pulse.
- Examine the upper respiratory tract, including palpation over the maxillary and frontal sinuses, and carefully examine the posterior pharynx for the presence of tonsillar enlargement, erythema, and exudates.
- Note conjunctival injection.
- Examine the tympanic membranes in adults whose complaints include ear pain or fullness, and palpate the neck for the presence of adenopathy.
- Perform careful auscultation and percussion of the lungs to exclude the presence of focal findings that would suggest pneumonia.
- In patients with severe symptoms suggestive of sinusitis, the presence of periorbital swelling, conjunctival injection, proptosis, or deficits of the extraocular movements suggests extension of infection beyond the sinuses and requires emergent evaluation.
- In a patient with severe symptoms of pharyngitis, diffuse swelling on one side of the neck or asymmetric tonsillar enlargement with medial displacement suggests a suppurative complication such as a peritonsillar abscess.

Tests for Consideration

- In most patients with acute cough, the absence of any abnormality of vital signs (no fever, tachycardia, or tachypnea) or any focal auscultatory finding on lung examination (focal crackles, bronchial sounds) is sufficient to exclude a diagnosis of pneumonia on clinical grounds. Patients with an abnormality of one of the vital signs listed above or focal findings on auscultation should have a **chest radiograph** to exclude the possibility of pneumonia. $45
- In patients with symptoms suggestive of acute sinusitis, radiographs are not recommended routinely, as they will not assist in the differentiation of viral from bacterial infection. **CT of the sinuses** is reserved for selected situations, such as when extension of infection beyond the sinuses is suspected. $334
- A **rapid antigen detection test (RADT) or culture** should be performed to confirm the diagnosis of streptococcal pharyngitis; in adults, a negative result on the RADT is sufficient to exclude the diagnosis of streptococcal pharyngitis. $15
- Rapid tests are also available for the diagnosis of influenza; however, when influenza is known to be circulating in the community, clinical diagnosis is quite accurate. $15

Clinical Entities	Medical Knowledge

Viral Rhinosinusitis or Common Cold

Pφ Viruses responsible for the majority of common colds include rhinoviruses (most common), coronavirus, influenza virus, respiratory syncytial virus, parainfluenza virus, and adenovirus. These viruses are thought to be spread mainly by direct contact with secretions on skin and environmental surfaces; dissemination by infectious secretions in the form of droplet nuclei or larger particles can also occur. The pathogenesis of the common cold is actually poorly understood. Biopsy samples of nasal mucosa from individuals with experimentally induced rhinovirus colds do not reveal evidence of viral cytopathic effect. It is believed that cytokines (interleukins 1, 6, and 8) and other inflammatory mediators play an important role in pathogenesis.

TP The incubation period of the common cold is short (<3 days). Patients present with sneezing, nasal discharge, and symptoms of nasal obstruction, along with sore or scratchy throat. Mild systemic symptoms, such as low-grade fever, myalgias, and malaise, may be present. Cough may develop during the first few days of illness. Influenza is characterized by the abrupt onset of fever, chills, headache, and myalgia, with the systemic symptoms predominating over the respiratory symptoms.

Dx A diagnosis of the common cold (often referred to as nonspecific URI) is made on clinical grounds. Influenza may be confirmed by RADTs, but (as discussed above) when influenza is known to be circulating in the community, clinical diagnosis is both sensitive and specific. Weekly reports of influenza activity in the United States can be found at http://www.cdc.gov/flu/weekly/index.htm. Many state health departments also post weekly reports of regional influenza activity on their websites.

Tx Treatment of the common cold is symptomatic. Nonsteroidal anti-inflammatory drugs (NSAIDs) can relieve systemic symptoms and sore throat, and may reduce cough. A recent Cochrane review concluded that zinc lozenges reduce the duration and severity of the common cold, but there is currently insufficient data to make recommendations regarding the formulation, dose, and duration of therapy. Two agents available for the treatment of influenza are oseltamivir and zanamivir; both work through inhibition of viral neuraminidase. If used within the first 48 hours of symptoms, these drugs may shorten the duration of illness by 1 to 1.5 days. A greater benefit may be seen in older individuals and those with risk factors for complicated infection. Amantadine and rimantidine are no longer recommended for the treatment of influenza because of a high prevalence of resistance. **See Cecil Essentials 98.**

Acute Community-Acquired Bacterial Sinusitis

Pφ The nasopharynx of healthy individuals may be colonized with bacteria that cause ACABS (e.g., *S. pneumoniae*); besides *S. pneumoniae*, *Haemophilus influenzae* (mainly untypable) and *Moraxella catarrhalis* are most commonly implicated. Obstruction of the sinus ostia, which may occur as a result of an antecedent VRS, plays an important role in the pathogenesis of ACABS. It is believed that blowing the nose creates a sudden increase in intranasal pressure that forces fluid that may contain these bacteria from the nasal cavity into the sinuses.

TP Patients present with nasal congestion, purulent nasal discharge, and facial pain/pressure, which may be worsened by leaning forward. There may be maxillary tooth pain in maxillary sinusitis and retro-orbital headache in ethmoid and sphenoid sinusitis; unilateral symptoms are especially suggestive of bacterial sinusitis. Patients may have fever. There is often a history of antecedent symptoms suggestive of VRS, which either fail to improve or begin to improve and then worsen again after 7–10 days of illness.

Dx The diagnosis of ACABS is mainly clinical. Patients with severe symptoms of sinusitis may need antibiotic therapy early in the course of disease; those with mild to moderate symptoms who are not improving by the second week of illness should also be assumed to have a bacterial infection and receive antibiotics. Studies utilizing sinus puncture have been performed to define the microbiology of ACABS; in clinical practice this invasive procedure can be utilized in severely ill patients (especially those with nosocomially acquired sinusitis), but it is not routinely performed. Antibiotics are chosen empirically based on knowledge of the microbiology of bacterial infection of the sinuses. Culture of purulent nasal secretions is not recommended. As discussed above, sinus radiographs cannot distinguish bacterial from viral infections and are not routinely recommended.

Tx Analgesics and decongestants can provide symptomatic relief. Although a number of newer broad-spectrum antimicrobials have shown efficacy in the treatment of ACABS, older agents such as amoxicillin, doxycycline, and TMP-SMX are sufficient for the majority of patients who need antibiotic therapy. **See Cecil Essentials 98.**

Acute Bronchitis

Pφ Infection of the tracheobronchial epithelium leads to acute inflammation and the release of cytokines. The same viruses implicated in the common cold can cause acute bronchitis. The one bacterial pathogen that may be considered in certain patients is *Bordetella pertussis* (discussed in the Zebra Zone section). Inflammation of the tracheobronchial epithelium leads to airway hyperresponsiveness that manifests as persistent cough and wheezing. The production of purulent sputum reflects inflammation and does not indicate a bacterial infection.

TP Patients present with cough and may have mild systemic symptoms and wheezing; an antecedent history of symptoms suggestive of the common cold may be present. Auscultation of the chest may reveal diffuse coarse rhonchi and wheezing.

Dx The diagnosis of acute bronchitis is made clinically; some patients with acute cough may require a chest radiograph to exclude the diagnosis of pneumonia, as discussed above under Tests for Consideration.

Tx Inhaled β_2-agonists can be beneficial for the treatment of persistent cough and wheezing. The benefit of cough suppressants is questionable. Nine randomized placebo-controlled trials have failed to show a benefit of antibiotic therapy in the treatment of acute bronchitis. **See Cecil Essentials 17.**

Pharyngitis

Pφ The pathogenesis of viral pharyngitis is similar to that of the common cold. The inflammatory mediator bradykinin is thought to play a key role in the pathogenesis of sore throat. The pathogenesis of streptococcal pharyngitis is not well understood. The organism is often found colonizing the pharynx in asymptomatic individuals. The factors that lead from colonization to infection are not well elucidated, although a number of extracellular factors produced by *S. pyogenes*, including hemolysins, hyaluronidase, and pyrogenic exotoxins, are probably important in the pathogenesis of disease. The common cold viruses are also implicated as causes of pharyngitis; in addition, patients with Epstein-Barr virus (EBV), cytomegalovirus (CMV), and acute HIV infection can present with pharyngitis accompanied by a mononucleosis-like syndrome. Bacteria are responsible for only 5% to 10% of cases of pharyngitis in adults; the most common is *S. pyogenes* (group A β-hemolytic streptococcus [GABHS]).

TP Patients with viral pharyngitis may present with complaints of sore throat along with other symptoms suggestive of URI. In patients with pharyngitis due to GABHS, sore throat and pain in the throat when swallowing are the presenting complaints. Patients may have quite impressive systemic complaints (including fever and chills, abdominal pain, and headache) or may be only mildly ill. On examination, the posterior pharynx will be markedly erythematous with patches of yellow exudates on the tonsils. There may be redness of the tongue with prominence of the papillae (strawberry tongue) and tender enlargement of the cervical lymph nodes.

Dx The presence of the Centor criteria (fever, exudates, tender cervical adenopathy, and absence of cough) can increase the pre-test probability of GABHS pharyngitis; however, the diagnosis should be confirmed by a RADT or a throat culture. Because the prevalence of GABHS infection in adults is lower than in the pediatric population, the diagnosis can be excluded based on a negative RADT.

Tx Analgesics to relieve throat discomfort can be beneficial in viral pharyngitis. For cases confirmed to be secondary to GABHS, penicillin or amoxicillin remain the first-line therapy; a macrolide can be utilized in patients with penicillin allergy. **See Cecil Essentials 98.**

Otitis Media

Pφ The middle ear communicates with the eustachian tube and mastoid air cells, the nasopharynx, and the nares. Any process that interferes with eustachian tube function, such as edema of the mucosa from a viral infection, can predispose to fluid accumulation in the middle ear, and if this fluid contains bacteria (e.g., *S. pneumoniae*) that can normally be found colonizing the nasopharynx, infection of the middle ear (OM) can ensue. Viruses associated with the common cold may also cause OM; bacterial infections are most frequently caused by *S. pneumoniae*, followed by *H. influenzae* and *M. catarrhalis*.

TP Adults with OM typically present with pain in the ear, which may be accompanied by decreased hearing, drainage from the ear, and fever. Tinnitus and vertigo may also occur. There may be an antecedent history of URI symptoms.

Dx The tympanic membrane (TM) can be erythematous in any infection of the upper respiratory tract, and this finding alone is insufficient to make a diagnosis of OM. In acute OM, the TM is opaque and may be bulging or retracted. Decreased mobility of the TM with pneumatic otoscopy is consistent with fluid in the middle ear.

Tx A wide variety of antimicrobials could be utilized to treat the bacterial pathogens that commonly cause acute OM; however, amoxicillin remains the first-line choice; amoxicillin-clavulanate and cefuroxime axetil are alternatives. **See Cecil Essentials 98.**

ZEBRA ZONE

a. Rarely, ACABS may be complicated by extension of the infection to the orbit and cause **cavernous sinus thrombosis**. Patients present with ptosis, proptosis, and chemosis; there may be deficits of cranial nerves III, IV, and VI. This is a medical emergency and requires emergent imaging by MRI scan and evaluation by otolaryngology and ophthalmology specialists.

b. In recent years it has been recognized that immunity to **pertussis** may wane in adulthood, and *B. pertussis* has been increasingly recognized as a cause of persistent cough in adults. The illness begins with typical URI symptoms, followed by the onset of cough, which occurs in paroxysms that may be associated with sweating, flushing, and post-tussive emesis. Culture or polymerase chain reaction (PCR) of a nasopharyngeal swab can confirm the diagnosis.

c. Though an extremely rare cause of pharyngitis in the United States, **diphtheria** can occur in individuals who did not receive appropriate immunization. A characteristic grayish membrane is present over the pharyngeal mucosa and the tonsils.

Practice-Based Learning and Improvement: Evidence-Based Medicine

Title
Empirical validation of guidelines for the management of pharyngitis in children and adults

Authors
McIsaac WJ, Kellner JD, Aufricht P, et al.

Institution
Mt. Sinai Hospital, Toronto, Ontario, Canada

painful. He has been sexually active with several female partners over the past year (vaginal sex and receptive oral sex), and he admits that he has been inconsistent with the use of condoms. He has no knowledge of any sexually transmitted disease (STD) diagnosis in his previous or current sexual partners. On further questioning, he recalls that he may have experienced several similar episodes of burning and tingling in the same region in the past but never noticed any similar lesions. He is otherwise healthy and denies any prior history of STDs. He believes that he was tested for HIV infection 3 years ago during a visit to his primary-care physician for a routine physical examination. His physical examination is remarkable only for the genital exam, which reveals a cluster of five small, shallow ulcers, each on an erythematous base; there is shotty nontender inguinal adenopathy. The patient is very concerned about the possibility of an STD and also requests testing for HIV.

Differential Diagnosis

Herpes simplex virus (HSV) infection	Chancroid	Syphilis

Speaking Intelligently

The differential diagnosis of genital ulcers includes both infectious and noninfectious etiologies. Ulcers may occur as part of a systemic disease. Among the infectious etiologies, STDs are most common, although infections that are not transmitted sexually can rarely cause genital ulcers. The differential diagnosis can be generated based on the history and clinical characteristics of the lesion and then narrowed on the basis of selected diagnostic testing. It is important to emphasize that a patient diagnosed with an STD is at increased risk for other STDs, including HIV, and to offer screening for these diseases.

PATIENT CARE

Clinical Thinking

- When evaluating a patient with genital ulcers, prioritize the differential diagnosis based on the patient's history, including a careful review of the sexual history and any travel history, the presence of any systemic symptoms, and the symptoms associated specifically with the genital lesions, including the temporal progression of symptoms and the evolution of the lesions.

- Perform a thorough general physical examination, including inspection of the oral mucosa, skin, and anus, and evaluate for adenopathy. Carefully describe the location and appearance of the ulcer(s).
- Although a presumptive diagnosis can usually be made on clinical grounds, selected diagnostic testing is usually necessary to confirm the diagnosis, although treatment may have to be initiated on the basis of the clinical diagnosis.
- Advise the patient about partner notification, provide counseling regarding future risk reduction, and inform the patient regarding the need for disease reporting.

History
- A prior history of recurrent genital ulcers is suggestive of HSV infection.
- The sexual history should include type of sexual activity, since trauma (including sexual assault) can be the etiology of genital ulceration.
- Note any associated systemic symptoms such as fever, arthralgias, oral lesions, or skin lesions.
- Obtain a travel history as well as information regarding symptoms in sexual partners.
- Ulcers secondary to HSV are typically painful; a prodrome of itching, burning, or tingling often occurs, and some patients may complain only of these symptoms despite the presence of ulcers. Ulcers secondary to chancroid are also painful.
- The ulcer associated with primary syphilis (chancre) and lymphogranuloma venereum (LGV) is usually painless.
- Noninfectious causes of genital ulcers include ulcers associated with autoimmune diseases such as Behçet syndrome and inflammatory bowel disease, and aphthous ulcers related to HIV infection; these ulcers are typically painful.

Physical Examination
- Carefully examine the oral mucosa, the skin, and all lymph node groups.
- Carefully note the appearance of the genital ulcer, as the ulcer appearance will provide important clues regarding the etiology of the lesion.
- Note if there is a single ulcer or multiple ulcers.
- In a female, even if lesions are present on the external genitalia, perform a pelvic examination to look for additional lesions.

Tests for Consideration
Although a preliminary diagnosis can be made based on history and physical examination, it is important to utilize diagnostic testing to confirm the etiology of genital ulcers.
- Patients should have **serologic testing for syphilis** (important to screen for a concomitant STD even if an alternative etiology of the ulcer is confirmed). $6

- **Culture or antigen-detection** testing should be done to rule out **HSV**. $17
- In some settings, such as STD clinics, **dark field examination for *Treponema pallidum*** is available. $16
- Testing for *Haemophilus ducreyi* (chancroid) and LGV should be limited to certain epidemiologic settings (discussed in the Chancroid Clinical Entity). $17
- Although type-specific serologic tests for HSV subtypes 1 and 2 are available, serologic testing is not of value in the diagnosis of genital ulcer disease during the acute presentation.

Clinical Entities	Medical Knowledge

Herpes Simplex Virus

Pφ HSV is a dsDNA virus; there are two different HSV subtypes, HSV-1 and HSV-2. Although HSV-1 has typically been associated with herpes labialis (cold sores) and HSV-2 with genital ulcers, an increasing proportion of cases of genital HSV have been documented to be due to HSV-1. HSV viral replication occurs first in epidermal and dermal cells at mucosal surfaces or abraded skin. Virus then enters nerve endings and is transported intra-axonally to nerve cell bodies, most commonly in the sacral root ganglia. Viral replication occurs in the ganglia and surrounding tissues, followed by centrifugal spread back to mucosal surfaces via the peripheral sensory nerves. After the primary infection has resolved, HSV DNA can be found in a small proportion of ganglion cells. When reactivation occurs, peripheral sensory nerves transport virus back to the mucosal surface, and recurrent genital lesions appear. Many individuals with evidence of HSV-2 infection, based on positive serology, may never have clinically recognizable genital ulcer disease, yet these individuals may still intermittently shed virus and transmit the infection to their partners. It is important to emphasize to patients that viral shedding (and therefore transmission to partners) occurs even in the absence of visible lesions.

TP Patients with symptomatic primary genital infection present with multiple bilateral genital lesions characteristically in various stages of evolution from vesicles to pustules to shallow ulcerations; lesions have an erythematous base. The cervix and the urethra may be involved, and patients may complain of dysuria and vaginal discharge. Tender inguinal lymphadenopathy is common, and patients may have significant systemic symptoms including fever, headache, myalgias, and generalized malaise. Recurrent disease is much milder, with fewer lesions that are usually unilateral without systemic symptoms. Recurrence occurs in 90% of those with symptomatic primary infection.

Dx A presumptive diagnosis of genital HSV can be made based on history and physical examination; however, the clinician should attempt to confirm the diagnosis with a viral culture or antigen detection test. It is currently believed that up to 50% of primary genital HSV infections are due to HSV-1; in HSV-1 genital infection, recurrences and subclinical viral shedding are much less common than with HSV-2 infections. This information is important when counseling patients regarding risk of recurrent disease and transmission. The type-specific serologic tests (those that reliably distinguish between HSV-1 and HSV-2) may be useful in some clinical settings, including patients who have recurrent ulcers with a negative culture or those with a past clinical diagnosis of genital HSV that was never virologically confirmed.

Tx Antiviral medication can reduce the symptoms of both primary and recurrent infections and reduce the frequency of recurrence when given as chronic suppressive therapy; chronic therapy can also reduce the risk of transmission to sexual partners. Primary infections may be treated with acyclovir, valacyclovir (a formulation of acyclovir with improved bioavailability), or famciclovir; 7–10 days of therapy are recommended. Episodic therapy for recurrent episodes can be utilized; a 5-day course is recommended. It is important that therapy be started within a day of the appearance of lesions, or during the period of prodromal symptoms before the appearance of lesions. Patients who have frequent recurrences (six or more per year) can be offered daily suppressive therapy, which is effective at reducing the frequency of recurrences. It is important that patients understand that antiviral therapy is not curative in any of these circumstances. Physicians should counsel patients with a diagnosis of genital HSV regarding the natural history of the disease, emphasizing the potential for asymptomatic viral shedding in the absence of lesions, which may result in transmission to sexual partners. Both women and men require education regarding the risk of neonatal HSV infection. **See Cecil Essentials 107.**

Syphilis

Pφ *T. pallidum*, a spirochete, is the causative organism of syphilis and can penetrate intact mucosal surfaces or gain entry into the tissues through abraded skin. The organism disseminates via the lymphatics and the bloodstream; virtually every organ can be affected. Disease is classified into the following stages: incubating syphilis, primary, secondary, latent, and tertiary. An ulcer at the site of inoculation (chancre) is the major manifestation of primary disease. On histopathology, chancres demonstrate infiltration by plasma cells with proliferation of endothelial cells and fibroblasts of small blood vessels, leading to the classic histopathologic finding of obliterative endarteritis.

TP Chancres are usually single ulcers, but several lesions may occur; the lesion is typically painless and therefore may not be noticed by the patient. Chancres are round lesions with raised regular borders that have firm induration on palpation. The ulcer base does not have an exudate. Nontender inguinal adenopathy is frequently found. Genital lesions may also occur in secondary syphilis, where the generalized rash appears as raised, moist papular lesions.

Dx A definitive diagnosis of syphilis may be established by dark field examination or direct fluorescent antibody testing of exudate from the ulcer base. This testing is not available in many settings; therefore, serologic testing can allow a presumptive diagnosis in a patient with a compatible clinical presentation. A two-step serologic testing strategy is as follows: Nontreponemal (nonspecific) tests are the Venereal Disease Research Laboratory (VDRL) and rapid plasma reagin (RPR) tests; these tests are reported qualitatively as a titer. If this test is positive, it is confirmed with a treponemal (specific) test such as the fluorescent treponemal antibody absorbed (FTA-ABS) or the *T. pallidum* particle agglutination (TP-PA) test.

Tx A single intramuscular (IM) dose of benzathine penicillin (2.4 million units) is the recommended treatment for primary and secondary syphilis. Doxycycline, tetracycline, and azithromycin are potential alternative therapies for individuals with penicillin allergy. Follow-up consists of following the titer of the nontreponemal serologic test; a fourfold drop in the titer (i.e., a drop of two dilutions) is considered clinically significant and indicates an appropriate therapeutic response. Ideally, the nontreponemal test should become negative; treponemal antibody tests will generally remain positive indefinitely. Individuals exposed to a partner with a diagnosis of primary or secondary syphilis within 3 months preceding the diagnosis may have incubating syphilis and should be treated even if serologic testing is negative. **See Cecil Essentials 107.**

Chancroid

Pφ Worldwide, chancroid is thought to be one of the most common causes of genital ulcer disease; however, this infection is much more common in the developing countries of Asia, Africa, and Latin America than in the United States. In the United States the disease has generally occurred in outbreaks in urban areas, often in association with the trading of sex for drugs, particularly crack cocaine.

The causative organism, *H. ducreyi*, gains entry through breaks in the epithelial surface during sexual contact with an individual with active infection. The ability of the organism to evade phagocytosis is thought to be important in pathogenesis. On histopathology, the ulcers have been shown to contain numerous CD4-positive T lymphocytes.

TP Typical lesions begin as a tender erythematous papule, which then becomes pustular; the pustule then ruptures to form an ulcerative lesion. There may be single or multiple lesions, and the lesions are painful. The ulcer base is described as granulomatous, frequently with a purulent exudate; the ulcer border is ragged but not indurated. Approximately half of the patients will have tender, enlarged inguinal lymph nodes, frequently unilateral, which may suppurate and drain (buboes).

Dx *H. ducreyi* is a fastidious organism that requires specialized media for growth and is therefore difficult to isolate in culture. DNA amplification techniques have been developed to aid in diagnosis but are not yet widely available. The CDC recommend that a clinical diagnosis of chancroid is appropriate in patients who have all of the following: (1) single or multiple painful genital ulcers; (2) no evidence of infection with *T. pallidum* by either dark field examination of exudate from the ulcer or serologic tests for syphilis performed at least 7 days after the appearance of the ulcer; (3) a typical clinical presentation and appearance of the ulcer; and (4) a negative test for the presence of HSV from the ulcer exudate.

Interpersonal and Communication Skills

The Five "Ps" for Sexual History

Taking a complete and accurate sexual history is an important skill for clinicians. It is imperative that clinicians feel comfortable speaking with patients in a way that is respectful and nonjudgmental so as to obtain correct information and to be effective in the delivery of information regarding risk reduction and prevention. The Sexually Transmitted Disease Treatment Guidelines from the CDC recommend an approach utilizing the **"Five Ps": partners, prevention of pregnancy, protection from STDs, practices, and past history of STDs.** Regarding partners, clinicians should ask patients, "Have you had sex with men, with women, or both?" They should ask patients to recall the number of sexual partners they have had in the past 2 months and the past 12 months, and also to provide an estimate of a lifetime number of partners. Clinicians should also question patients regarding what they (or their partner) are doing to prevent pregnancy and what they are doing to protect themselves from STDs and HIV infection. To understand for what types of infections the patient may be at risk, the clinician needs to ask about specific sexual practices including vaginal, anal, and oral sex. Patients are often more comfortable discussing their sexual history than inexperienced physicians in training are about asking the appropriate questions. This improves with practice and experience.

Professionalism

Maintain Confidentiality in Notifying Contacts of Patients with Transmissible Infections

When caring for a patient with an STD, it is important that the clinician ensure that patient confidentiality is maintained, while being aware of the laws regarding STD reporting and the importance of partner notification. Of the infections discussed in this chapter, syphilis, chancroid, and HIV infection are reportable in every state of the United States. Patients need to be aware that their infection must be reported and to receive assurance that these reports are kept confidential. Clinicians must encourage patients to inform sexual partners of their STD diagnosis and should make provisions for having their partners evaluated and treated. In most jurisdictions, the local health department can provide assistance to patients in contact tracing and partner notification, including assistance with anonymous notification. It is important that clinicians who manage patients with STDs address the infection from both the standpoint of the individual patient and the health of the public.

Systems-Based Practice

The Cost-Effectiveness of HIV Screening

In caring for patients with genital ulcer disease, it is important to address the issue of screening for HIV infection. Since September 2006, the CDC has recommended that HIV testing be offered to all individuals 13 to 64 years of age in all care settings including emergency departments, hospitals, and primary-care offices. In 2009 the American College of Physicians endorsed routine HIV screening for all patients 13 years of age and older. It is estimated that as many as 25% of HIV-infected adults in the United States are unaware of their HIV status. In addition to the risk to their own health, these individuals are an important source of transmission to others; it has been demonstrated that individuals who are aware of their HIV-positive status are more likely to modify their sexual practices to reduce the risk of transmission to partners. Several studies have suggested that at least a one-time screening of the entire U.S. population in this age range would be cost-effective.

Chapter 58
Vaginitis and Urethritis (Case 50)

Patricia D. Brown MD

Case: A 28-year-old woman presents acutely with complaints of discomfort in the vulvar region of 3 days, accompanied by pain with intercourse (dyspareunia). The patient complains of intense itching and burning in the vulvar area. She has noticed a small amount of thick, whitish-yellow discharge in her underwear; the discharge does not have any odor. She also complains of dysuria but denies urgency, frequency, or hesitancy; she has no lower abdominal pain or fever. The patient has no chronic medical illness and takes no regular medications except oral contraceptives. She was HIV-negative when tested during a routine visit for contraception 1 year ago. She is sexually active with a new (past 3 months) male partner who uses condoms inconsistently; she has had two additional partners in the preceding year. She states that her partner has no symptoms, but she is very concerned about the possibility of an STD. She has never been pregnant; her last menstrual period was 2 weeks ago and was normal.

- Cultures are generally not utilized in the diagnosis of vaginitis; however, microbiologic confirmation is required in patients with cervicitis and in men with urethritis; **non-culture-based (DNA amplification-based)** testing is most commonly utilized to confirm the diagnosis of gonorrhea (GC) or chlamydia. $78
- Any patient with an STD should be screened for other STDs, including screening for HIV. In light of the recent CDC recommendation that routine **HIV screening** should be offered to all patients in all health-care settings at least once, screening should be offered even if the final diagnosis is not an STD. $13

Clinical Entities	Medical Knowledge

Candida Vaginitis (Vulvovaginal Candidiasis)

Pφ *Candida* species (mainly *C. albicans*) can be part of the vaginal flora in asymptomatic women. Risk factors for symptomatic infection include antibiotic use, poorly controlled diabetes, and the use of oral contraceptives; however, the majority of women with vulvovaginal candidiasis (VVC) have no predisposing risk factor for infection. VVC is exceedingly common; it is estimated that almost 75% of women will have at least one episode in their lifetime.

TP The most common complaint of women with VVC is vulvar irritation, burning, and/or pruritus. Patients may complain of dysuria without other urinary tract symptoms, and dyspareunia. Discharge is typically not a prominent complaint; if present, it is typically scant. Examination of the vulvar area and the vaginal mucosa reveals erythema; linear ulcerations (fissures) and excoriations may be seen in the vulvar region. The presence of erythematous papules beyond the area of vulvar erythema (satellite lesions) is characteristic of candidal infection. Thick, clumped ("cottage cheese-like") discharge that is typically adherent to the vaginal mucosa is characteristic.

Dx The vaginal pH is normal (≤4.5), and the whiff test is negative. Microscopic examination of the saline wet mount will reveal leukocytes; microscopic examination of the KOH specimen reveals mycelia or budding yeast. There is no clear correlation between the severity of symptoms and the burden of organisms in women with VVC. In the presence of a typical clinical presentation, if fungal organisms are not visualized on the KOH preparation, a fungal culture should be obtained before the diagnosis is excluded.

Tx A number of topical antifungal agents (creams and suppositories) are available for the treatment of VVC; several are now available without prescription. A single 150-mg dose of oral fluconazole is also highly effective and may be preferred by many women because of ease of dosing and convenience.

Complicated VVC is defined as follows: (1) recurrent VVC (≥4 episodes per year); (2) severe symptoms or clinical findings; (3) pregnancy, poorly controlled diabetes, underlying immunosuppression; and (4) infection with a *Candida* species other than *C. albicans*. These patients should be treated with oral fluconazole every third day for three doses; patients with recurrent infection may also require long-term suppressive therapy. Only topical agents (for 7 days) are recommended for the treatment of pregnant women. **See Cecil Essentials 107.**

Trichomoniasis

Pφ Trichomoniasis, caused by *Trichomonas vaginalis*, a pear-shaped, motile protozoan, is generally a sexually transmitted infection with a variable (a few days to 1 month) incubation period. Nonvenereal transmission is also occasionally described. Mucosal damage (microulcerations, inflammation) is believed to be due to direct contact by the microorganism; attachment to host cells appears to be mediated by surface proteins. The organism attracts PMNs and activates the alternative complement pathway.

TP Women with trichomoniasis typically present with vulvovaginal irritation, pruritus, and/or soreness; profuse white or yellow discharge is common. Patients may have dysuria and dyspareunia; although trichomoniasis is not believed to cause ascending infection of the genital tract, 5% to 10% of women may complain of lower abdominal pain. Vulvar erythema may be present. On pelvic examination there is erythema of the vaginal walls and the cervix; punctuate hemorrhages of the cervix (colpitis macularis or strawberry cervix) are characteristic of this infection but can be visualized in only a very small proportion of women unless colposcopy is performed. Copious amounts of yellow to yellow-green discharge are typically present in the vaginal vault; the discharge is often frothy in appearance. Men with trichomoniasis are often asymptomatic. Symptomatic infection presents as urethritis; penile discharge is often quite scant.

Cervicitis/Urethritis

Pφ Mucopurulent cervicitis (MPC) in women and urethritis in men are most commonly caused by the sexually transmitted pathogens *N. gonorrhoeae* and *C. trachomatis*. In women, urethritis often occurs in conjunction with vaginitis, which may be due to any of the conditions reviewed above. *N. gonorrhoeae* organisms attach to mucosal epithelial cells via pili and outer membrane proteins and then penetrate into the submucosa eliciting an intense host inflammatory response, resulting in microabscess formation and sloughing of the epithelial surface. *Chlamydia* is an obligate intracellular organism. The extracellular infectious form (the elementary body) attaches to the host epithelial cell and enters via endocytosis; the organism then differentiates into its metabolically active form (reticulate body). Infected cells produce proinflammatory cytokines that elicit a host inflammatory response.

Herpes simplex may also cause cervicitis. Nongonococcal urethritis (NGU) can also be caused by *Trichomonas* and HSV; the potential role of other pathogens including *Mycoplasma genitalium*, *U. urealyticum*, and adenovirus has not yet been clearly established.

TP Women with MPC typically present with a complaint of purulent discharge. Intermenstrual bleeding, especially after intercourse, is common. Symptoms of vulvar irritation are absent, although patients may have dysuria. Lower abdominal pain or any signs of systemic toxicity (fever, nausea, vomiting) suggest ascending infection of the genital tract (pelvic inflammatory disease). On examination, the vulva and vaginal mucosa are normal in appearance; mucopurulent discharge is visualized emanating from the endocervical canal.

Men with urethritis present with dysuria (particularly with the first void in the morning) and penile discharge. If discharge is not readily apparent at the urethral meatus, attempts to "milk" the urethra (as described above under physical examination) should be made.

Dx The vaginal pH is often elevated (>4.5) in women with MPC, and the whiff test is negative. Increased numbers of leukocytes are seen on the wet mount. The diagnosis of GC should be confirmed by nucleic acid amplification testing (NAAT) of cervical samples. The presence of intracellular gram-negative diplococci on a Gram stain of cervical secretions is highly specific for gonorrhea, but the sensitivity is poor.

NAAT should be utilized to confirm the etiology of urethritis in men; NAAT can be performed on a sample of urethral discharge or a urine sample. The sensitivity of a Gram stain of urethral discharge for *N. gonorrhoeae* is much higher in men with symptomatic urethritis.

Tx Once a clinical diagnosis of MPC or urethritis in men is established, a decision must be made whether to treat empirically or to wait for the results of diagnostic testing. Patients who are unlikely to follow up for the results of diagnostic testing can be treated with single-dose regimens that cover both GC and chlamydia. Treatment options for GC include ceftriaxone 250 mg IM or cefixime 400 mg orally, each given as a single dose; ceftriaxone is preferred. Fluoroquinolones (ciprofloxacin, ofloxacin, levofloxacin) had been previously recommended for single-dose treatment of GC, but the increasing prevalence of fluoroquinolone resistance among GC isolates in the United States prompted the CDC to remove these agents from the list of preferred therapeutics. Because the prevalence of coinfection is high, patients with GC should also be treated for chlamydia. Treatment of chlamydia includes azithromycin 1 g orally as a single dose or doxycycline 100 mg orally twice daily for 7 days. Sexual partners must be referred for evaluation and treatment; azithromycin is preferred.

Men with persistent or recurrent symptoms should be evaluated to confirm objective evidence of urethritis. If compliance with treatment was questionable or repeat exposure to an untreated partner occurred, retreatment with the same regimen is reasonable. Otherwise the patient should be evaluated for trichomoniasis with a culture. If compliance with the initial treatment was likely and repeat exposure has not occurred, the CDC STD Treatment Guidelines recommend treatment with metronidazole or tinidazole 2 g orally as a single dose plus azithromycin 1 g orally as a single dose if azithromycin was not a component of the initial treatment regimen (it is thought that azithromycin may be more effective than doxycycline for treatment of *M. genitalium* infection). **See Cecil Essentials 107.**

Professionalism

Show Commitment to Professional Excellence

A patient may request that the physician provide treatment for vaginitis without examination (e.g., based on phone consultation). Although the importance of thorough examination in the management of patients has been stressed, some clinicians may also treat patients on an empirical basis even when they present to the office or clinic. This issue was recently addressed in a practice bulletin from the American College of Obstetrics and Gynecology (ACOG). Studies have shown that both self-diagnosis and symptoms-only (including telephone-based) diagnosis of vaginal complaints are **unreliable**. Patients who are already in the office should always be examined; patients requesting phone consultation should be asked to come in for further evaluation. A reliable patient who has had multiple previous confirmed episodes and who now has the same symptoms can be managed without examination, with the understanding that she must present for examination if symptoms do not respond to empirical therapy.

Systems-Based Practice

Directed Testing May Render Time- and Cost-Effective Care

Women with vaginal symptoms may present for care in settings where microscopy is not readily available. The ACOG practice bulletin for vaginitis addresses this issue. Important here is the determination of the pH of vaginal secretions. Patients with an elevated vaginal pH will need further testing for *Trichomonas* using a commercially available rapid test or culture. Various point-of-care tests have become available for the diagnosis of BV, but their exact place in management is currently uncertain. Rapid testing for the presence of *Candida* is not currently available, so a presumptive diagnosis will have to be made by history and examination findings, and confirmed by culture. However, if the clinician works in a setting where primary and/or acute care for women is provided, investing in a microscope is probably the most cost-effective option for the optimal management of patients with vaginal symptoms.

Chapter 59
Fever in the Hospitalized Patient (Case 51)

Patricia D. Brown MD

Case: A 56-year-old man was admitted to the hospital with 3 days of productive cough, fever, and chills. A chest radiograph revealed an extensive area of consolidation in the left lower lobe; because of hypoxia on presentation, he was admitted to the hospital for management of community-acquired pneumonia. The patient has no history of chronic medical illness but does have a 40-pack-year smoking history and a long-standing history of heavy alcohol use, drinking one pint of whiskey every few days for over 20 years. The patient was initially started on ceftriaxone and azithromycin; two sets of blood cultures obtained on admission grew *Streptococcus pneumoniae*, sensitive to penicillin. His antibiotics were changed to IV penicillin, and over the next 72 hours he slowly improved with resolution of fever and hypoxia, decreased cough, and good oral intake. The plan was to discharge him to home on hospital day 4 to complete a course of oral antibiotics; however, the patient developed a fever of 39.7°C.

Differential Diagnosis

Hospital-Acquired Infections	Complications/ Inadequate Treatment of Community-Acquired Pneumonia	Noninfectious Causes of Fever
Urinary tract infection (UTI)	Drug-resistant pathogen	(Sterile) IV-site phlebitis
Catheter-related bloodstream infection (BSI)	Parapneumonic effusion	Drug fever
Hospital-acquired pneumonia (HAP)	Empyema	DVT/pulmonary embolism
Clostridium difficile infection (CDI)		Alcohol withdrawal

It can be very difficult to distinguish symptomatic infection from asymptomatic bacteriuria in this setting; therefore, even in the presence of a positive urine culture, the diagnosis of symptomatic UTI as the etiology of fever should be considered only when other sources of infection have been excluded by careful clinical assessment. $19

IMAGING CONSIDERATIONS

→ HAP should be considered if new or worsening cough, dyspnea, or hypoxia occurs in association with fever; hypoxia would also raise the possibility of venous thromboembolic disease. A **chest radiograph** will document the presence of new or worsening infiltrates; thoracentesis should be performed if there is a pleural effusion to exclude the possibility of empyema. $45
→ If pulmonary embolism is a diagnostic consideration, **spiral CT or ventilation–perfusion scanning** can be utilized. $334, $316
→ Clinical suspicion for DVT can be evaluated by **duplex ultrasonography**. $107

Clinical Entities	Medical Knowledge

Hospital-Acquired Urinary Tract Infection

Pφ Like the vast majority of all UTIs, hospital-acquired infections are ascending infections due to pathogens that colonize the periurethral area and distal urethral meatus, and then gain entry to the urinary tract via the ascending route. Instrumentation of the urinary tract facilitates ascending infection. Infection may be confined to the bladder (cystitis) or ascend to involve the kidney (pyelonephritis).

MB Like all UTIs, the most common cause of health care–associated UTI is *Escherichia coli*. Depending on the length of hospitalization and prior antibiotic exposure, other pathogens that should be considered include other Enterobacteriaceae (*Klebsiella*, *Enterobacter*) and nosocomial gram-negative organisms such as *Serratia*, *Providencia*, *Citrobacter*, and *Pseudomonas*. *Enterococcus* species, including vancomycin-resistant enterococci (VRE), may also cause UTI in the hospital.

TP In noncatheterized patients the clinical presentation will be the same as that for community-acquired UTI; suprapubic tenderness, fever, leukocytosis, and/or other signs of systemic toxicity may be the only clinical findings in patients who have indwelling urinary catheters.

Dx The diagnosis of UTI should begin with a urinalysis (preferably with microscopic examination) to detect the presence of pyuria, followed by urine culture to confirm the microbiologic diagnosis. Patients with hospital-acquired UTI are at increased risk of antibiotic-resistant pathogens, so a urine culture with susceptibility testing should always be obtained, even if the urinalysis findings are strongly suggestive of UTI. As discussed above, the differentiation of asymptomatic bacteriuria and symptomatic UTI can be challenging, especially in patients with indwelling urinary catheters. Fever, leukocytosis, and other signs of systemic toxicity are suggestive of pyelonephritis rather than simple cystitis, and blood cultures should always be obtained to exclude concomitant bacteremia. Whether cystitis or pyelonephritis, hospital-acquired UTIs are always considered complicated infections.

Tx Increasing rates of resistance among *E. coli* in both the community and the health-care setting to TMP-SMX have been well described, raising concern regarding the appropriateness of this agent for empirical therapy of UTI in the hospital. Pending further information from susceptibility testing, fluoroquinolones (ciprofloxacin, levofloxacin) may be a better initial empirical choice in this setting. TMP-SMX may still be a reasonable initial empirical choice in patients who have been hospitalized for a short duration and have not received prior antibiotic therapy during the hospitalization; nitrofurantoin may be considered in patients with only cystitis. Patients with signs of sepsis require initial parenteral therapy; third-generation cephalosporins (ceftriaxone, cefotaxime) are reasonable initial empirical therapeutics; however, a Gram stain of the urine should be obtained to exclude the possibility of enterococcal infection, for which the treatment of choice would be ampicillin. Patients at risk for *Pseudomonas* infection, as well as those with signs of severe sepsis, should receive agents that provide broader coverage including coverage for *Pseudomonas* (cefepime, piperacillin–tazobactam); empirical coverage should be informed by local resistance data.

Hospital-Acquired Pneumonia

Pφ Like community-acquired pneumonias, the majority of HAPs are due to microaspiration of organisms that colonize the upper airways. In patients who are intubated (ventilator-associated pneumonia [VAP]), upper airway secretions may pool around the cuff of the endotracheal tube and are then aspirated during manipulation of the tube for suctioning or during positioning of the patient. HAP may also occur when the lungs are seeded hematogenously by BSI that originates from another site.

MB Pathogens that commonly cause community-acquired pneumonia may occur in patients with early-onset (within the first 4 days of hospitalization) HAP. Aerobic gram-negative bacilli (including *Pseudomonas aeruginosa*) and *S. aureus* must be considered possible pathogens in those patients with onset of infection after 4 days of hospitalization as well as those with risk factors for drug-resistant pathogens. These risk factors include the following: previous antimicrobial therapy, a known high frequency of resistant pathogens in the unit on which the patient is hospitalized, and immunosuppressive therapy or disease.

TP Fever, cough with sputum production, and worsening dyspnea are typical presenting features in patients with HAP. The clinical presentation may be more subtle in patients who are severely ill or debilitated, and in those with VAP. Focal findings on auscultation of the chest are helpful if present, but the absence of these findings is insufficient to exclude the possibility of pneumonia in patients with fever and respiratory symptoms.

Dx The diagnosis of HAP should always be confirmed by a chest radiograph that shows a new or worsening infiltrate. Radiographic interpretation may be challenging in patients with preexisting radiographic abnormalities such as pulmonary edema. Efforts should be made to obtain a sputum sample for Gram stain and culture before the institution of empirical antibiotic therapy; a sputum specimen should always be obtained via endotracheal suction from patients who are intubated, as a negative sputum Gram stain in a patient with no recent change in antibiotic therapy virtually excludes the diagnosis of VAP. Blood cultures should also be obtained in all patients in an attempt to confirm a microbial etiology of the infection, although blood cultures are positive in a minority of patients with HAP.

Tx Initial empirical antibiotic therapy must be selected based on the likelihood of resistant pathogens. For patients with early-onset pneumonia and no risk for drug-resistant pathogens, ceftriaxone plus a macrolide (such as azithromycin) or a respiratory fluoroquinolone (levofloxacin, moxifloxacin) can be used as initial therapy; those with late-onset infections or risk for drug-resistant pathogens will require more broad-spectrum coverage with an anti-pseudomonal β-lactam (cefepime, piperacillin-tazobactam, imipenem, or meropenem), in addition to an aminoglycoside or anti-pseudomonal fluoroquinolone, plus vancomycin or linezolid. Therapy should be reassessed based on culture results, and the narrowest spectrum agent that will still be effective should be continued. Seven days of therapy are sufficient for the majority of patients with HAP; 14 days of therapy are recommended for infections due to *Pseudomonas* or *Acinetobacter*. **See Cecil Essentials 22.**

Clostridium difficile Infection

Pφ *C. difficile* is found among the normal colonic flora in <5% of healthy individuals in the community, but >20% of individuals who are hospitalized may become colonized with this organism. When the normal colonic flora are disrupted by the use of antimicrobial therapy, toxogenic strains of *C. difficile* may multiply and produce two exotoxins, toxin A and toxin B. These toxins are highly cytotoxic via the disruption of the cytoskeleton of colonic mucosal cells, leading to mucosal injury and inflammation.

MB *C. difficile* is an anaerobic gram-positive bacillus. The organism forms spores that are resistant to antimicrobial therapy and frequently contaminate environmental surfaces, where they may serve as a source of nosocomial transmission. A new strain of *C. difficile* (the B1/Nap1 strain) has recently been recognized and appears to be responsible for epidemics of severe disease reported both in the United States and in other areas of the world.

Intervention
Sixty-seven hospitals participated in the study. The intervention consisted of ensuring the consistent use of five evidence-based procedures that reduce the risk of catheter-related BSI (use of proper hand hygiene, use of full-barrier precautions during insertion, cleansing of the skin with chlorhexidine, avoidance of the femoral site if possible, and prompt removal of catheters when no longer needed). The intervention included physician education regarding the evidence, a cart with all necessary supplies to support the intervention, a checklist to ensure consistent adherence to all the recommended procedures (coupled with empowerment of other members of the health-care team to stop the individual inserting the catheter in nonemergent situations if a step was omitted), discussion of catheter removal daily on rounds, and consistent feedback to providers regarding the numbers and rates of catheter-related BSIs.

Quality of evidence
Level II-2

Outcome/effect
Use of this relatively simple, evidence-based intervention resulted in a substantial (up to 66%) reduction in the incidence of catheter-related BSIs. This reduction was sustained throughout the 18-month study period.

Historical significance/comments
This study is significant in that the intervention was a simple one that relied on ensuring the consistent application of practices that are evidence-based utilizing a checklist to ensure that all steps were followed. Checklists to ensure that all steps in the multistep process are completed have been utilized in other settings where safety is of extreme importance (e.g., the airline industry) but have not been frequently utilized in the health-care setting.

Interpersonal and Communication Skills

Keep Inpatients Apprised of Ongoing Evaluations
Unexplained fever in a hospitalized patient can be frustrating for the patient as well as for the physician. It is important for the physician to keep the patient informed regarding the potential etiologies of fever and the rationale for the various diagnostic tests that are being performed. Patients are usually quite appreciative of frequent updates, which help to make uncertainty more bearable. In selected patients who are clinically stable and in whom common etiologies such as pneumonia, UTI, BSI, and DVT have been excluded, further evaluation may be continued in the outpatient setting, provided that careful follow-up can be arranged.

Professionalism

Respond Appropriately to Observed Breaches of Unsafe Medical Practices

The transmission of hospital-associated pathogens from one patient to another via the hands of health-care workers has been well established. However, observational surveys still show that compliance with recommendations regarding hand hygiene is still nowhere near 100% among health-care workers, and in some studies the lowest compliance rates are among physicians. Hand hygiene (soap and water with vigorous rubbing for at least 15 seconds or alcohol-based hand rubs) should be performed immediately before and immediately after any contact with the patient (including contact that involves touching only environmental surfaces). Strict compliance with this basic tenet of infection control is a professional imperative for all those who care for patients. Every member of the health-care team should be empowered to provide feedback to any individuals who are not compliant with these recommendations.

Systems-Based Practice

Reduce Hospital-Acquired Infections

It is estimated that hospital-acquired infections account for approximately 10,000 deaths per year in the United States, and a significant number of these infections are thought to be preventable. Reducing the incidence of hospital-acquired infection has become an important component of patient safety. The Centers for Medicare and Medicaid Services has announced that hospitals will no longer be reimbursed for the additional costs incurred as a result of the treatment of certain hospital-acquired infections that are considered to be potentially preventable. The most common hospital-acquired infection is UTI, and the majority of these are related to the use of indwelling urinary catheters. Physicians must ensure that urinary catheters are used only in those patients who have an accepted indication for catheterization. These include bladder outlet obstruction or other documented urinary retention, a diagnosis that requires an accurate assessment of urinary output, and incontinence imposing risk (perineal or sacral wound). The indication for catheterization should be documented, and the need for continued catheterization should be re-evaluated daily. Studies have shown that physicians are often unaware that their patients have an indwelling urinary catheter. For male patients whose indication for catheterization is not retention or bladder outlet obstruction, condom catheters have been shown to have a decreased risk of infection compared with indwelling urinary catheters.

Section XII
NEUROLOGIC
DISEASES

Section Editors
Michele Tagliati MD and
Stephen Krieger MD

Section Contents

60 Altered Mental Status (Case 52)
Nils Petersen MD

61 Dementia (Case 53)
Jessica L. Israel MD

62 Seizures (Case 54)
Julie Robinson-Boyer MD

63 Abnormal Movements (Case 55)
Joseph Rudolph MD and Michele Tagliati MD

64 Headache (Case 56)
Michelle Fabian MD and Jennifer Elboum MD

65 Dizziness and Vertigo (Case 57)
Lana Zhovtis Ryerson MD and Stephen Krieger MD

66 Weakness (Case 58)
Edward H. Yu MD and Maya Katz MD

Chapter 60
Altered Mental Status (Case 52)

Nils Petersen MD

Case: The patient is a 25-year-old man without significant past medical history. His girlfriend had called his private physician earlier this morning because he was confused and agitated overnight. He awakened her from sleep at around 2 AM after he fell over a chair and soon after urinated in the corner of their bedroom. He appeared confused and was complaining of a headache. He finally went back to sleep. This morning she was unable to awaken him, and he is warm to the touch.

Differential Diagnosis

Meningitis/encephalitis	Subarachnoid hemorrhage (SAH)	Trauma
Hypoglycemia	Intracranial hemorrhage	Intoxication

Speaking Intelligently

In evaluating a patient with altered mental status (AMS), determine whether the patient's level of consciousness is impaired, whether this is a disorder of thought content, and the time course of the illness. In derangements in level of consciousness that are acute and severe, it may be necessary to act faster to prevent permanent neurologic damage or even death. When assessing level of consciousness, it is essential to be able to very clearly pinpoint the patient's response to stimulus level; in this sense, it is more important to describe the patient's state of consciousness according to how he or she is acting or responding (e.g., sleepy, not responding to painful stimuli) than using nonspecific medical jargon such as "lethargic" or "confused." Such early, rapid assessments of severity and time course help to direct the rest of the examination, workup, and management.

PATIENT CARE

Clinical Thinking
- Consciousness is the state of full awareness of the self and one's relationship to the environment.

having the patient perform repetitive tasks like a series of digits and days of the week.

- ○ The key feature of an acute confusional state is inattention, which can manifest in three ways: distractibility, perseveration, and inability to focus on an ongoing stimulus. A distractible patient shifts attention from the examiner to another stimulus such as noise in the hallway. Perseveration is the repetition of phrases, answers, or tasks from previous questions.
- The essential elements of **language function** are comprehension, fluency, naming, repetition, reading, and writing. Fluent aphasia sometimes leads to the false impression of acute confusion; therefore, careful examination of language is important in every patient with AMS or acute confusional state.
- **Memory** is the ability to register, store, and retrieve memory. Loss of recent memory and the inability to retain new memories is a hallmark of dementia but is also frequently seen in delirium.
- **Remainder of neurologic exam:** In general, you should be as complete as possible in your neurologic exam, even in patients capable of only limited cooperation. In patients with severely impaired level of consciousness, you may not be able to reliably examine sensation, motor function, and coordination. The neurologic exam for stuporous or comatose patients should focus on brainstem function and the presence of other focal neurologic signs.
  - The **cranial nerve exam** for the comatose patient typically includes pupils and their response to light; gaze and oculocephalic reflex; response to caloric stimulation; breathing pattern; and corneal, cough, and gag reflexes. The **motor exam** in the comatose or stuporous patient is very different from that in the awake and cooperative patient and, instead of testing strength in different muscle groups, focuses on motor tone, reflexes, and overall motor response to painful stimulation.

Tests for Consideration

Diagnostic testing can be extremely helpful in many cases, but your clinical findings should guide your workup and not vice versa. As a result, there is no one algorithm for evaluating patients with AMS, and each case should be considered individually. The common indications and utility of various tests are discussed below.

- A **fingerstick glucose test** is more accurate than the glucose measurement on a complete metabolic profile and is very quick, easy, and cheap. It should be done first to check for either hypoglycemia or hyperglycemia, which both can cause altered consciousness and even mimic symptoms of stroke. Keep in mind that many patients with AMS receive a bolus of dextrose 50% in water (D50) by emergency medical services (EMS) before coming to the ED. $5

- **Laboratory studies:** A **complete blood count** (CBC) is commonly performed for elevated white blood cell (WBC) count in infections or low WBC count suggesting immunocompromised status or sepsis. Thrombocytopenia and AMS may result from thrombotic thrombocytopenic purpura (TTP). **Complete metabolic profile** may reveal important electrolyte abnormalities such as hyponatremia, hypoglycemia, hypocalcemia, hypercalcemia, or uremia. Acute changes in these values are more important than absolute numbers and are more likely to cause AMS. **Abnormal liver function tests** may also suggest hepatic encephalopathy. A **thyroid-stimulating hormone (TSH)** value does not come back as rapidly from the lab, but thyroid abnormalities can definitely cause altered consciousness in patients with either hyperthyroidism or hypothyroidism. $11, $12, $12, $24
- A **urine toxicology/drug screen** is always a good idea, especially in those with a psychiatric history or when polypharmacy is suspected. Remember that a blood alcohol concentration should be obtained in addition to the urine toxicology. $21
- **Chest radiograph and urinalysis** can be useful for confirming a source of infection (pneumonia or urinary tract infection [UTI]) because elderly people cannot always mount an immune response and this is a common cause of delirium. $45, $4
- An **electrocardiogram (ECG)** is important, especially because confusional states can sometimes be the only manifestation of an acute myocardial infarction. $27
- **Lumbar puncture (LP) with cerebrospinal fluid (CSF) analysis** is useful in both diagnosis of infection, SAH, and, rarely, leptomeningeal carcinomatosis. Keep in mind that the LP should be done before the introduction of antibiotics, because the results will be indispensable in tailoring your antimicrobial therapy. However, if you suspect that your patient has bacterial meningitis and there is a delay in performing the LP, emergent empirical antibiotics (and dexamethasone) should be administered before CSF analysis. Opening pressure should be measured and CSF sent for cell count and differential, Gram stain, and cultures, as well as glucose and protein concentrations. Further specific microbiology and nucleic acid amplification testing, such as polymerase chain reaction (PCR), can be pursued if other etiologies are suspected. $272
- **Electroencephalography (EEG)** can be used to assess for epileptiform (seizure) activity as in complex partial seizures of nonconvulsive status. It might also give clues in cases of toxic metabolic encephalopathy and herpes simplex encephalitis. $170

Dx Diagnosis is clinical, based on the above symptoms. CBC, blood cultures, chest radiograph, and urinalysis may be helpful in the initial approach.

Tx Treatment consists of antibiotics for any underlying illness and supportive care with or without symptomatic treatment with psychotropic medications for agitation. Remember that once patients have an in-hospital episode of delirium from any cause, their mortality significantly increases, so be aggressive in finding the source and initiate treatment. **See Cecil Essentials 96.**

Intracranial Hemorrhage (see also Chapter 64, Headache)

Pφ Epidural, subdural, or intraparenchymal bleeding in the brain leads to focal neurologic deficits by direct impact at the site of bleeding as well as by suddenly increasing intracranial pressure, thereby causing bilateral cerebral dysfunction. This, in turn, may cause an alteration in consciousness. Further swelling and mass effect might eventually lead to herniation and brain death, depending on the initial size of the hemorrhage.

TP Severe headache, focal neurologic deficits, and decreased level of consciousness can all be seen. Patients may also present with hypertension as either a cause or an effect of the hemorrhage.

Dx CT scan will reliably detect an acute intracranial hemorrhage.

Tx Neurosurgical intervention depends on localization of the hemorrhage (e.g., subdural vs. epidural vs. intraparenchymal), size of the hemorrhage, and presence of midline shift. Otherwise, supportive care is provided, with reversal of any anticoagulation and management of increased intracranial pressure and blood pressure. **See Cecil Essentials 127.**

Subarachnoid Hemorrhage (see also Chapter 64, Headache)

Pφ Sudden rupture of a saccular intracranial aneurysm with bleeding into the subarachnoid space causes cytokine release and inflammation that can diffusely impair brain metabolism as well as cause brain edema. Vasospasm may also occur within 3–7 days and result in acute ischemic stroke, causing further brain edema and worsened consciousness. In addition, SAH can cause acute hydrocephalus as CSF drainage is obstructed.

TP Symptoms consist of sudden onset of an extremely severe headache ("worst headache of my life"), with or without nuchal rigidity or impaired level of consciousness.

Dx CT scan usually reveals blood in the subarachnoid space, but if CT is negative and clinical suspicion is high, LP may show fresh blood or xanthochromia (yellow CSF from degraded red blood cells [RBCs]) in the case of a small hemorrhage.

Tx Cerebral angiogram is both diagnostic and therapeutic to find the source of bleeding and coil the aneurysm. Otherwise, supportive care is provided with reversal of any anticoagulation or antiplatelet therapy and management of increased intracranial pressure and blood pressure. Administration of IV calcium channel blockers can prevent vasospasm; occasionally aggressive neurosurgical intervention is necessary to treat hydrocephalus. **See Cecil Essentials 124.**

Metabolic Encephalopathy

Pφ Failure of different organ systems such as liver, kidneys, lungs, pancreas, thyroid, pituitary, or adrenal glands can lead to metabolic encephalopathy (brain dysfunction). Depending on the organ involved, this can be caused by accumulating toxins, electrolyte disturbances, changes in acid–base metabolism, endocrine effects, hypoxia, hypercapnia, or a combination of these factors. Eventually there may be to changes in neurotransmission or brain metabolism, brain edema, and decreased brain perfusion.

TP Metabolic derangements cause changes in level of consciousness without other focal neurologic signs. Depending on the severity of the metabolic abnormality, this can range from mild clouding of consciousness to stupor or coma. Sometimes the additive effect of multiple mild abnormalities can lead to severe encephalopathy.

Dx Clinical suspicion and examination will lead to the diagnosis, which is often confirmed with basic laboratory testing. Imaging with either CT or MRI will help to exclude other etiologies. An EEG may be helpful in showing diffuse cerebral dysfunction.

Tx The primary concern here consists of the ABCs; treatment of the underlying abnormality and supportive care are essential. **See Cecil Essentials 113.**

If there is no health-care proxy, it is imperative for the family to designate a point person with whom you will communicate primarily to prevent misunderstandings and repetitive discussions with different people. Be aware that some family members may react with anger, which is often a reflection of personal guilt. Remain calm and empathetic, and remember that you are there to provide your medical perspective. Thoughtful, honest, and clear communication goes a long way in guiding your care and preventing major missteps.

Professionalism

Assess Capacity and Respect Autonomy

Any physician is qualified to assess patient capacity, which is often at the crux of respecting the patient's decision making. In general, it is important to remember that capacity is situation-specific and that patients may have capacity to make some decisions but not others. The patient must have insight into his or her disease and be able to understand the risks and benefits of treatment options. It is perfectly acceptable to obtain consent or have conversations about treatment when the patient is lucid. Keep in mind that a person who has capacity will be consistent in his or her decision, so if you ask the patient about the same issue multiple times, the decision should remain the same. In some instances, however, such as cases of coma or stupor, it is very clear that patients lack capacity; therefore, it is always important to check whether patients have advance directives or a health-care proxy in place, as these are meant to be extensions of patient autonomy.

Systems-Based Practice

Stroke Protocol Is an Example of System-Based Coordination for Best Patient Care

The assessment of patients with suspected stroke is an emergency because of the limited therapeutic window for thrombolytic treatment; the stroke patient must be examined, evaluated, and then optimally treated with tissue plasminogen activator (t-PA) within 3 hours of onset. Although many patients are not candidates for TPA, it is of the utmost importance to evaluate them quickly and decide on appropriate management. To this end, the hospital-wide "code stroke" was developed to ensure that a patient is seen by a neurologist, has appropriate lab tests, and has a CT scan interpretation within 60 minutes of arriving at the hospital. Once a code stroke is called, the staff understands that this patient's workup becomes top priority. The code stroke has established a more efficient protocol for evaluating suspected stroke patients; previously, precious time was often wasted in the challenge to coordinate the required consultations, lab workup, and head imaging.

Chapter 61
Dementia (Case 53)

Jessica L. Israel MD

Case: The patient is a 76-year-old woman who managed a small restaurant with her husband for many years. He died 2 years ago, and now her son does most of the day-to-day work at the restaurant. She has a history of osteoarthritis and well-controlled diabetes mellitus. During the history and physical exam at the office visit, she is pleasant and cooperative. She tells you that she does not know why her son brought her to see you. She says she feels fine.

When you step out of the examination room, her son and his wife are waiting to talk with you. They tell you that they are worried about Mom and that she just hasn't been the same since her husband died. She now lives alone. She vehemently resists accepting any help and she argues with them if they try to help her. Her son has noticed that her pocketbook is full of bills that she hasn't paid and old receipts for things she bought many months ago. She has been forgetting appointments and sometimes even forgetting the names of their regular customers at the restaurant. She seems to repeat herself, asking the same question over and over. Some evenings, they believe, she doesn't bother to cook or eat dinner. They are very worried that she might have a problem with her memory.

Differential Diagnosis

Alzheimer disease	Vascular dementia	Lewy body dementia
Frontotemporal dementia	Mild cognitive impairment	Delirium
Depression		

- **Folstein Mini-Mental State Examination (MMSE):** This is the most commonly used test to assess cognitive function. It assesses multiple cognitive domains including orientation, recall, registration, calculation, attention, and visuospatial skills. The results of this test may be skewed by the level of education attained by the patient. Also, this test is difficult to administer to hospitalized patients because many of the questions are about orientation, and hospitalized patients often are not aware of their specific location within the hospital, even if there is no cognitive compromise. A score of less than 24, however, warrants further attention in the workup of dementia.
- The **clock-drawing test** assesses executive functioning and visuospatial skills. In this test the patient is asked to draw the face of a clock, including the numbers, and then to show the time as either 11 o'clock or 10 o'clock. If the evaluator then divides the clock into four quadrants, it is most common to find errors in the fourth quadrant, between 9 and 12 o'clock.
- The **mini-cog** is a combination of the clock-drawing test and the three-item recall section of the original MMSE. This combination has been recently evaluated and validated in older adults. It offers the advantage of allowing administration to patients whose native language is not English, or to those with less than a high school education. In general, because short-term memory is one of the earliest findings in demented patients, the three-item recall portion of this test is the single best screening tool. The patient is asked to repeat three words after hearing them and then to recall these words after 1 minute.

IMAGING CONSIDERATIONS

→ **CT scan of the head** (without contrast) is usually considered optional. However, it can be considered for patients with a post-acute change in their cognitive status (meaning that symptoms have occurred for <2 years). It may also be helpful for a patient with focal or asymmetric neurologic findings on examination, one who has had a recent fall or head injury, or one with the triad of symptoms that suggest a diagnosis of normal-pressure hydrocephalus (urinary incontinence, unsteady gait, and cognitive compromise). $334

→ **PET (positron emission tomography)** scan is not usually recommended but can be used if the diagnosis is unclear. A patient with Alzheimer disease shows characteristic parietal and temporal lobe abnormalities, while a patient with vascular dementia may show more widespread, irregular changes. $1037

| Clinical Entities | Medical Knowledge |

Alzheimer Disease

Pφ A diagnosis of Alzheimer disease can be confirmed at autopsy. The pathognomonic sign is an increased number of neuritic plaques in the cerebral cortex. These plaques are tortuous neuritic processes around a central amyloid core. There may also be neurofibrillary tangles, amyloid angiopathy, and granulovacuolar degeneration. Grossly, cerebral atrophy with ventricular dilatation is often present.

TP Alzheimer disease is a clinical diagnosis based on progressive memory loss and increasing inability to participate in activities of daily living (ADLs). Generally, motor and sensory functional compromise does not occur until late-stage disease. Memory impairment, particularly the inability to learn and recall new information, is the main symptom. Early-stage disease commonly presents with compromises in executive functioning skills and in judgment. Apraxia, aphasia, disorientation, and visuospatial abnormalities are also common.

Dx Rule out "reversible causes of dementia" (hypothyroidism, vitamin B_{12} deficiency, and neurosyphilis). Carefully test for evidence of concomitant depression. CT of the head, if obtained, should be normal or show atrophy. MMSE score of <24 is diagnostic. There will be impairment on the clock-drawing test and on three-item recall.

Tx Pharmacologic treatment includes the use of cholinesterase inhibitors (donepezil, rivastigmine, galantamine, and tacrine). These medications slow the breakdown of acetylcholine in the synaptic cleft. They slow the progression of the disease but are not curative. Some patients will experience a modest improvement in function and cognition. Cholinesterase inhibitors may also be helpful in controlling behavioral symptoms.

An *N*-methyl-D-aspartate antagonist (memantine) is also an indicated pharmacologic treatment in moderate-to-severe disease. It reduces glutamate-mediated excitotoxicity and is thought to be neuroprotective. Again, the medication is not curative but contributes to slowed disease progression, some modest improvement in cognitive function, and, possibly, behavioral control. **See Cecil Essentials 116.**

Delirium

Pφ Research on the neuropathology of delirium has examined alterations in many neurotransmitter systems, including acetylcholine, serotonin, dopamine, and γ-aminobutyric acid (GABA), as well as alterations in certain cytokines including tumor necrosis factor-α.

TP Delirium is very common in older adults. It is characterized by an acute change in mental status and a lack of attention. Delirium can present as an agitated change or a more hypoactive or quiet change.

Dx The Confusion Assessment Method (CAM) is the most clinically useful diagnostic tool, with >95% sensitivity and specificity. It requires an acute change in mental status or a fluctuating course, along with inattention, to make a diagnosis, along with either disorganized thinking or an altered level of consciousness.

Tx The treatment of delirium requires treatment of the underlying problem (e.g., electrolyte disturbance, untreated pain, or medication interactions). Occasionally, when the delirium threatens a patient's safety or dignity, low-dose antipsychotic medication may be needed. Modifying the risk factors that contribute to the development of delirium is also appropriate; these are very common in hospitalized patients (as a result of sleep deprivation, immobility, visual impairment, hearing impairment, and dehydration). **See Cecil Essentials 133.**

Depression

Pφ The pathophysiology of depression is related to disturbed neurotransmitter balance in serotonergic and noradrenergic systems. Various other neurohormonal systems have been implicated as well.

TP Symptoms at presentation may include difficulty with concentration or decision making, lack of motivation, loss of interest, apathy, sleep disturbance, psychomotor retardation, and impaired memory. Often symptoms overlap or appear very similar to those of patients with early dementia. The response to treatment often is what confirms the diagnosis. Depression has been referred to as a "pseudodementia." However, it is important to keep in mind that patients often present with concurrent depression and early-stage dementia and may require concurrent treatment for both these problems.

Dx A diagnosis of depression requires the presence of at least one core symptom that has lasted for >2 weeks with significant effect on the patient's everyday life and functioning; these core symptoms are loss of interest or pleasure, appetite change, weight loss, psychomotor agitation or retardation, energy loss, feelings of worthlessness or guilt, difficulty concentrating or making decisions, and recurrent thoughts of death or suicide. Older adults tend to present with more somatic, physical symptoms related to depression. Therefore, the diagnosis may be difficult because of the overlap of these symptoms with those of other physical illnesses. Using a geriatric depression scale questionnaire may be helpful.

Tx Treatment varies but may include administration of selective serotonin reuptake inhibitors, tricyclic antidepressants, or other antidepressants. Generally, the side effect profile and/or the possibility of drug–drug interactions with the patient's other medications will dictate the treatment. It may take as long as 3 months of treatment for the patient to begin to see a response to medication. Electroconvulsive therapy should be considered for patients with serious risk of suicide or poor oral intake related to their depression. **See Cecil Essentials 117, 133.**

ZEBRA ZONE

a. Creutzfeldt-Jakob disease: This is a spongiform encephalopathy associated with infective transmission via prions. Classic presentation of the disease includes dementia with myoclonus. An EEG may be helpful to establish the diagnosis, showing a characteristic spike-and-wave pattern. The disease is rapidly progressive, and many patients will die within a year of diagnosis.

Practice-Based Learning and Improvement: Evidence-Based Medicine

Title
Current pharmacologic treatment of dementia: a clinical practice guideline from the American College of Physicians and the American Academy of Family Physicians

Systems-Based Practice

Identify a Health-Care Proxy and Discuss End-of-Life Care

Dementia is a terminal illness, usually within 7 to 10 years of diagnosis. The medical literature supports the idea that patients with moderate dementia, even if they cannot make medical decisions themselves, can still clearly verbalize whom they trust to make medical decisions for them. Early in the course of treating a patient with dementia, it is important to help the patient appoint a health-care proxy. The physician should elicit from the patient and the patient's medical decision maker/family their personal ideas and expectations of the health-care system and should discuss the stages of the disease and the likely outcomes that can be anticipated. Many families find themselves in the hospital facing decisions about providing their loved ones with hydration, artificial nutrition, mechanical ventilation, and nursing home placement. End-of-life care in the hospital may significantly compromise patient dignity and comfort, and these discussions are best conducted in the outpatient setting. In addition, significant medical costs occur during the last weeks of a person's life, when hospital resources are often unwittingly invested in futile medical scenarios. Although advanced-care planning must be discussed within the context of a patient's particular belief systems, when presented with possible outcomes, many patients will choose to extend their home-care options and perhaps consider hospice, with an approach focused on comfort and dignity in the last stages of their illness. Currently, on average, patients are referred to hospice only in the last days of an illness. For patients who are declining and meet the criteria for advanced dementia earlier, referrals may be of tremendous benefit. Hospice offers an interdisciplinary approach (including physician, nurse, social worker, chaplain, volunteer services personnel, and physical therapists), attention to the caregivers, and even eventual bereavement support. With proper planning, goals of care can occur in the patient's home under realistic and well-supported expectations.

Suggested Readings

American Medical Association. Physician's guide to assessing and counseling older drivers. Available at: http://www.ama-assn.org/ama1/pub/upload/mm/433/older-drivers-guide.pdf.

American Psychiatric Association. Diagnostic and statistical manual of mental disorders. 4th ed. (DSM-IV). Washington, DC: American Psychiatric Association; 1994.

Inouye SK, van Dyke CH, Alessi CA, et al. Clarifying confusion: the Confusion Assessment Method: a new method for detection of delirium. Ann Intern Med 1990;113:941–948.

Peterson RC, Stevens JC, Ganguli M, et al. Practice parameter: early detection of dementia: mild cognitive impairment (an evidence-based review). Report of the Quality Standards Subcommittee of the American Academy of Neurology. Neurology 2001;56:1133–1142.

Chapter 62
Seizures (Case 54)

Julie Robinson-Boyer MD

Case: A 22-year-old woman was brought in by ambulance. She was at home sitting on the couch when her mother said that she became confused, her eyes rolled back, and then she fell to the floor and started shaking. She had been up late the night before studying for an exam. Upon arrival at the ED she was initially sleepy but then returned to her baseline mental status. During the episode she bit her tongue and had urinary incontinence. Her mother says she had a seizure once as a baby, associated with a fever. She had a normal birth history, normal development, and no prior medical problems. There is no family history of seizures.

Differential Diagnosis

Generalized tonic-clonic seizure	Simple partial seizure	Complex partial seizure
Psychogenic non-epileptic seizure (PNES)	Status epilepticus (SE)	

Speaking Intelligently

When encountering a patient with a suspected seizure, be sure the patient is stabilized. Then obtain a detailed history and perform a physical and neurologic examination. Consider the differential diagnosis of seizure versus other acute-onset neurologic events, such as syncope, stroke/transient ischemic attack (TIA), and migraine. It is important to find out if the patient has a prior history of seizures and is already being treated with antiepileptic drugs. If the episode is determined to be a seizure, then search for an acute cause, including metabolic abnormalities (hypoglycemia), fever or infection, intoxications (alcohol or drugs), organic lesions (tumor, stroke), and noncompliance with antiepileptic medications. A blood glucose level, blood counts, and electrolyte panels may be helpful in determining the cause of the seizure. In the ED setting, a non-contrast CT scan of the head is the initial imaging modality of choice. If meningitis is suspected, an LP should be performed, usually preceded by a CT scan of the head. Subsequently, you can pursue an MRI of the brain and EEG to complete the workup. The decision whether to treat with antiepileptic medications may vary depending on the characteristics of each individual case.

PATIENT CARE

Clinical Thinking

- Seizures are classified as either partial seizures (in which there is a focal or localized onset), generalized seizures (in which the seizure begins bilaterally), or special epileptic syndromes.
  - Partial seizures are further classified into **simple seizures** (when there is no alteration in consciousness) and **complex seizures** (when there is an alteration in consciousness).
  - Generalized seizures are separated into those that are truly generalized in onset (**primary generalized seizures**) from those that begin locally and then spread to become generalized (**secondarily generalized seizures**).
- Classification of seizures is important, because it allows the clinician to make predictions regarding the prognosis and to choose the best medication to treat that specific seizure type.
- A diagnosis of epilepsy is made when a patient has recurrent (two or more) seizures that are unprovoked.
- After a diagnosis of epilepsy is made, one must determine if the presentation fits known patterns of epilepsy syndromes.
- An **epilepsy syndrome** is a disorder characterized by similar seizure types, clinical features, neurologic abnormalities, and EEG pattern, with a somewhat predictable clinical course and response to antiepileptic drugs.
- Depending on the seizure classification or epilepsy syndrome, one can gain clues as to the underlying etiology of the seizure. Primary generalized epilepsies are most likely genetic or idiopathic, and are not associated with underlying structural abnormalities. On the other hand, partial seizures or secondarily generalized seizures are typically the result of an underlying brain lesion, such as congenital malformations, tumors, prior strokes, traumatic brain injury, or mesial temporal sclerosis.

History
- The history should include detailed questions regarding the characteristics of the seizure, including the prodrome(s), initial manifestations, pattern of evolution, postictal symptoms, level of consciousness, and associated bowel/bladder incontinence or tongue biting. If the patient loses consciousness during the seizure, a witness may be able to provide these details.
- The initial manifestations and pattern of evolution of the seizure can provide clues as to the localization of seizure onset. A history of a preceding aura is also important, as it provides a clue that the seizure is probably focal in origin, with the type of aura providing clues as to the location of the seizure focus. For example, a preceding epigastric aura suggests onset in the mesial temporal lobe.
- Additional information that should be obtained includes birth history; prior episodes of seizure; febrile seizure; history of head trauma, meningitis, or encephalitis; social history including alcohol and/or drug use; and a family history of epilepsy.

Physical Examination
- In adult patients the physical exam is usually unrevealing.
- A focal neurologic sign on exam, such as a hemiparesis, indicates an underlying brain lesion.
- In infants and children the physical exam is important, because one may find dysmorphic features or cutaneous abnormalities that may provide clues as to an underlying disease.

Tests for Consideration
- **Laboratory studies: Blood glucose**, **CBC**, and **electrolyte panel** (particularly sodium) should aid in the initial evaluation for a patient with seizure, to identify any acute cause. A **urine toxicology screen** and a **blood alcohol level** may be useful in the appropriate clinical setting. $7, $11, $12, $21, $15
- **EEG:** An EEG records electrical activity from the cerebral cortex and is the most sensitive tool for the diagnosis of epilepsy. It can provide support for the diagnosis of epilepsy, aids in epilepsy classification, and is valuable in determining the risk for seizure recurrence. A normal EEG, however, does not exclude the diagnosis of epilepsy. Sleep deprivation, photic stimulation, or hyperventilation can be used to increase the likelihood of recording EEG abnormalities. $170
- **LP:** Should be obtained, if the patient is febrile or has meningeal signs, to evaluate for evidence of CNS infection. $272
- **Cardiac stress tests, Holter monitors, tilt-table testing, or sleep studies:** May be indicated to evaluate some of the non-epileptic disorders. $297, $65, $298, $795

IMAGING CONSIDERATIONS

→ **Neuroradiology:** A brain imaging scan should be obtained to rule out the presence of organic lesions, including tumors, stroke, cysticercosis, mesial temporal sclerosis, or other structural abnormalities. **CT scanning** is easy to obtain, has widespread availability, and is usually the initial study of choice in the ED setting. Brain **MRI** provides increased sensitivity for lesions that would be missed by CT, such as mesial temporal sclerosis or small tumors. $334, $534

Clinical Entities	Medical Knowledge

Generalized Tonic-Clonic Seizure

Pφ Seizures result from a paroxysmal high-voltage electrical discharge of hyperexcitable neurons within an epileptogenic focus. Different mechanisms have been hypothesized to explain generalized seizures, including (1) an abnormal response of hyperexcitable cortical neurons to a normal thalamic input, (2) a primary subcortical abnormal trigger, and (3) an abnormal cortical innervation from subcortical structures.

TP A generalized seizure may be preceded by a **prodrome,** which consists of nonspecific premonitory symptoms for minutes to hours before the seizure, or an **aura,** which consists of the focal onset and helps localize the causative lesion within the cortex. A generalized seizure is characterized by a sudden loss of consciousness, with a **tonic phase** (bilateral stiffening, eyes open and rolled upward, loud vocalization, and incontinence) followed by a **clonic phase** (synchronous muscle jerking, tongue biting). The seizure is typically followed by a **postictal state,** at which time the patient is drowsy and confused.

Dx The EEG reveals generalized epileptiform discharges. The frequency and type (polyspike or spike-and-wave) of epileptiform discharges vary depending on the epilepsy type. Focal onset of discharges with spread to the bilateral hemispheres can be seen in secondarily generalized seizures. During the postictal phase, the EEG is generally slow and disorganized.

Tx Pharmacotherapy depends on the etiology and type of seizure, but in general valproic acid, lamotrigine, levetiracetam, topiramate, and zonisamide are considered broad-spectrum antiepileptic medications and are effective for primary and secondarily generalized seizures. Carbamazepine, oxcarbazepine, phenobarbital, phenytoin, tiagabine, gabapentin, and pregabalin are indicated for secondarily generalized seizures and may worsen some primary generalized seizures. **See Cecil Essentials 126.**

Simple Partial Seizure

Pφ Focal abnormal neuronal discharges without alteration of consciousness constitute this diagnosis.

TP Symptoms depend on the brain area where the abnormal neuronal discharge originates. Focal motor seizures originate from the frontal lobe. Typically head and eyes turn to the side opposite the seizure focus, which shows tonic contractions, possibly followed by clonic movements. A typical, albeit less common, presentation is the classic "Jacksonian march," characterized by the progressive involvement of muscle groups that follows the distribution of the homunculus along the motor cortex. When the epileptic focus is in the occipital lobe there may be unformed visual phenomena. Autonomic symptoms such as rising epigastric sensation, pallor, flushing, or pupillary changes may occur when the focus is in the temporal lobe, as well as automatisms, formed visual phenomena, and unpleasant odors or taste. Finally, abnormal sensory events can arise from a parietal lobe focus.

Dx Focal EEG abnormalities confirm the involvement of only one cerebral region or hemisphere.

Tx Medications indicated for simple partial seizures include carbamazepine, valproic acid, gabapentin, lamotrigine, topiramate, oxcarbazepine, zonisamide, levetiracetam, phenytoin, pregabalin, tiagabine, and phenobarbital. **See Cecil Essentials 126.**

Complex Partial Seizures

Pφ Focal onset of neuronal discharges with alteration of consciousness is diagnostic. Complex partial seizures typically originate from the temporal lobe and less frequently from the frontal lobe. They are usually associated with an acquired structural lesion such as a tumor or mesial temporal (hippocampal) sclerosis.

ZEBRA ZONE

a. **Syncope:** Transient loss of consciousness and loss of muscular tone that result from an acute global reduction in cerebral blood flow. Syncope has many diverse causes; a neurologic cause for syncope is found in fewer than 10% of cases. (See also Chapter 65, Dizziness and Vertigo, for a discussion of light-headedness and presyncope.)

b. **Sensory TIA:** Sensory symptoms with seizures are usually positive phenomena with tingling and paresthesias, whereas sensory TIAs typically present with a negative phenomenon such as numbness or loss of sensation. (See also Chapter 66, Weakness, for a discussion of TIA and stroke.)

c. **Migraine:** Basilar artery migraine is associated with episodes of confusion and even loss of consciousness, which may mimic a seizure. In children, migraine may present as cyclic vomiting. Positive visual phenomena occur in both migraine and occipital seizures. Typically the visual phenomena in a seizure are shorter lasting (<2 minutes) and patients see colors, whereas with migraine the symptoms last longer (>5 minutes) and patients typically see straight or jagged lines, scintillations, or black-and-white phenomena. (See also Chapter 64, Headache, for a discussion of migraine.)

d. **Hypoglycemia:** Most commonly presents with nonspecific complaints such as sweating, nausea, light-headedness, pallor, vomiting, abdominal pain, and hunger. Since the CNS functioning depends on glucose, cerebral symptoms also occur such as paresthesias, blurred vision, focal neurologic abnormalities, and/or seizures.

e. **Panic attacks:** Patients report palpitations, chest pain, shortness of breath, sweating, trembling, gastrointestinal discomfort, loss of control, feeling of choking, nausea, dizziness, paresthesias, chills, hot flashes, and intense fear, especially of dying. An attack usually lasts 5 to 30 minutes.

f. **Sleep disorders:** Narcolepsy–cataplexy syndrome consists of (1) narcolepsy, short sleep attacks; (2) cataplexy, sudden loss of muscle tone induced by changes in emotion; (3) sleep paralysis, episodes that occur during the transition between sleep and wakefulness, when a patient is awake but unable to move because of generalized hypotonia; and (4) hypnagogic hallucinations, vivid hallucinations that occur at the transition between sleep and wakefulness.

g. **Acute dystonic reaction:** Sustained involuntary muscle contractions in the face, neck, trunk, or extremities that occur shortly after the initiation of neuroleptic drug therapy. Treatment is effective, including discontinuing the offending agent and administration of benztropine.

Practice-Based Learning and Improvement: Evidence-Based Medicine

Title
A comparison of four treatments for generalized convulsive status epilepticus

Authors
Treiman DM, Meyers PD, Walton NY, et al.

Institution
Veterans Affairs Status Epilepticus Cooperative Study Group

Reference
N Engl J Med 1998;339:792–798

Problem
To determine the best initial drug treatment for generalized convulsive status epilepticus

Intervention
Three hundred eighty-four patients with overt generalized convulsive status epilepticus were randomized to one of four IV regimens: diazepam (0.15 mg/kg body weight) followed by phenytoin (18 mg/kg), lorazepam (0.1 mg/kg), phenobarbital (15 mg/kg), and phenytoin (18 mg/kg).

Quality of evidence
Level I

Outcome/effect
Treatment was considered successful if there was cessation of all motor and EEG seizure activity within 20 minutes after the beginning of drug infusion without return of seizure activity during the next 40 minutes. In patients with overt generalized status epilepticus, lorazepam was successful in 64.9% of patients who were assigned to receive it, phenobarbital in 58.2%, diazepam and phenytoin in 55.8%, and phenytoin in 43.6%. Lorazepam was significantly superior to phenytoin ($P = 0.002$). Lorazepam was not found to be more efficacious than phenobarbital or diazepam followed by phenytoin.

Chapter 63
Abnormal Movements (Case 55)

Joseph Rudolph MD and Michele Tagliati MD

Case: A 68-year-old man has been noticing a tremor in his right hand for the past year. The tremor began in his thumb, but it has spread to the entire hand and now his arm. It generally appears while he is watching television, walking, or is otherwise occupied, and lately it has been occurring more frequently. The shaking has been accompanied by a loss of dexterity of the same hand. He is finding it hard to button his left sleeve cuff and to tie his shoes. In addition, his wife has noticed a change in his gait. He seems to drag the right foot slightly when he takes a step, and he appears not to be able to walk as fast he used to. During the interview the patient's wife also comments that her sleep has been interrupted because the patient has had several outbursts of yelling and flailing of his arms and legs during his sleep. He adds that he has been having some wild dreams. Upon direct questioning, he also admits that he has not been able to smell his wife's cooking as well for the past 10 years.

Differential Diagnosis

Parkinson disease (PD)	Multiple system atrophy (MSA)	Progressive supranuclear palsy (PSP)
Essential tremor (ET)	Drug-related parkinsonism	Vascular parkinsonism

Speaking Intelligently

PD is the most common movement disorder. Despite its being a progressive, degenerative disease, a variety of treatments can help patients with PD to live a normal life span, with a greatly improved quality of life. In evaluating someone with possible PD, establish that he or she presents with the key clinical criteria. Specifically, look for tremor at rest, stiffness (rigidity), slowness of movement (bradykinesia), abnormalities of gait or balance (postural instability), and an overall development of these symptoms in a unilateral or at least asymmetric pattern. The patients may not be aware of some of the issues in which you are interested, but a spouse or family member may have noticed other problems. In addition, there are nonmotor symptoms of which lay people are unaware that are connected with PD but that become relevant and more disabling with disease progression. These include depression, anxiety, and cognitive dysfunction with slowed processing, but most functions are still generally intact, except for planning and judgment (frontal lobe symptoms), autonomic dysfunction including neurogenic bladder, erectile dysfunction, orthostatic hypotension, rapid eye movement (REM) behavior disorder (the seeming acting out of dreams), and loss of sense of smell. In more advanced cases a discussion with the caregiver assumes greater significance as specific issues that make it difficult to care for the patient but do not seem to be specifically part of the disease may come to light.

PATIENT CARE

Clinical Thinking
- PD appears in 12 to 20 of every 100,000 people per year, approaching a prevalence of 1 in 2000 people.
- Be aware of subtle symptoms or findings that may have been ignored by the patient or family but may be relevant to the diagnosis. For example, the patient may hold one arm slightly stiff while walking or may seem not to blink quite as frequently as one would expect in a healthy person.
- Early diagnosis and initiation of management with medications, dietary changes, and exercise may slow disease progression (although there is no true neuroprotective agent available).
- Stretching exercises may lower the risk of contractures, and exercising will keep the muscles active, minimizing the development of rigidity. Patient mobility is, of course, a significant issue for the patient as well as for the caregivers.

History
- Look for a collection of symptoms and signs that demonstrate loss of dexterity and flexibility.
- Does the patient recall loss of fine motor control, or perhaps muscle cramping in one limb?
- Is there difficulty swallowing with typically associated excess saliva pooling in the mouth?
- When the patient is walking, is one leg being dragged, or are there episodes of freezing (no obvious weakness, but seeming inability to move the legs, often occurring in doorways and approaching a chair or a crowd)?
- Does the patient cut his or her own food?
- Is there dizziness upon standing?

an MRI can be performed to rule out vascular parkinsonism or perhaps some of the "parkinson plus" conditions (e.g., multiple system atrophy, progressive supranuclear palsy, and dementia with Lewy bodies). PET scans can be used to delineate decreased activity in the basal ganglia, but they are expensive and not completely reliable. Clinical assessment via thorough history and examination, possibly including a standardized rating scale, is the usual method of diagnosis and subsequent monitoring.

Tx The mainstay of PD treatment is the exogenous replenishment of dopamine in the form of levodopa or dopamine agonists, although these medications affect primarily motor symptoms. Nonmotor symptoms generally require symptomatic treatment (blood pressure support for orthostatic hypotension or antidepressants for depression). Long-term care for a PD patient may become complicated, as patients may become less responsive to medication and develop fluctuations of their response to the medications. In addition, they may develop side effects, such as dyskinesias, which are coarse, choreic (writhing) involuntary movements. In the past decade, implantation of an electrical stimulator in the basal ganglia (known as deep brain stimulation [DBS]) has demonstrated excellent results in controlling the symptoms of moderate-to-severe PD. Other nonmedical modalities can be helpful, such as physical therapy, speech therapy, and behavioral therapy for gait difficulties, dysarthria, and psychiatric problems. **See Cecil Essentials 122.**

Multiple System Atrophy

Pφ MSA is characterized by the development of α-synuclein inclusions in glial cells of various regions of the brain, including substantia nigra pars compacta, locus ceruleus, putamen, inferior olive, pontine nuclei, cerebellar Purkinje cells, and intermediolateral columns. The degeneration may occur in different proportions, resulting in a spectrum of syndromes that vary based on the affected area. MSA-parkinsonism (MSA-P) involves mostly the degeneration of the striatonigral pathways. While it was originally thought that MSA affects presynaptic and postsynaptic dopaminergic neurons, patients with MSA-P may be responsive, at least in part, to levodopa therapy. MSA-cerebellar (MSA-C) mostly affects the olivocerebellar connections, with disproportionate involvement of the middle cerebellar peduncles. MSA-autonomic (MSA-A, also known as Shy-Drager syndrome) is characterized by the degeneration of the locus ceruleus, the dorsal motor nucleus of cranial nerve X, and the catecholamine-producing neurons of the ventrolateral medulla.

TP Although there are three variants of MSA, a typical patient may have components of all of them. MSA-C shows disproportionate ataxia, MSA-P includes parkinsonism, and MSA-A is primarily characterized by autonomic dysfunction, which may include orthostatic hypotension and bladder dysfunction. The presence of symptoms from two of these categories suggests a diagnosis of MSA.

Dx There is no definitive test for MSA, much as seen for PD. The diagnosis is clinical, and the probability of having MSA rises with an increased number of symptoms from an increased number of categories (autonomic dysfunction, parkinsonism, and cerebellar dysfunction).

Tx There is no disease-modifying treatment for MSA; treatment is symptomatic. Often parkinsonian patients have a limited response to levodopa and other dopaminergic agents. Autonomic dysfunction can be managed by giving vasoconstrictors and mineralocorticoids to increase blood pressure and using antispasmodics or catheters in the setting of urinary incontinence. Physical and speech therapies may also be useful. **See Cecil Essentials 122.**

Progressive Supranuclear Palsy

Pφ PSP is characterized by inclusion bodies similar to the neurofibrillary tangles of Alzheimer disease and composed of tau protein. Both neurons and glial cells are affected. Tufted astrocytes and globose tangles can be seen in the brainstem, particularly in the midbrain; the basal ganglia, particularly the subthalamic nucleus, substantia nigra, and globus pallidus; and in the cerebral cortex of the frontal lobes.

TP PSP usually manifests with early gait impairment or balance problems associated with falls. Eye movement abnormalities (slow saccades, vertical gaze palsy) are typical but may present late in the course. In addition, dysarthria and dysphagia commonly occur in PSP, as well as some degree of cognitive impairment. The dementia of PSP (as with all parkinsonian disorders) tends to be a subcortical dementia with loss of frontal functions, which include judgment and executive decision making. Thus, there tends to be a "dysexecutive syndrome" with mild behavioral abnormality. This is unlike Alzheimer disease, which tends to affect primarily memory or visuospatial recognition. Some PSP patients may exhibit typical parkinsonism, though with a poor response to levodopa.

Drug-Induced (Tardive) Parkinsonism

Pφ There are numerous therapeutic agents that can block dopamine synapses. For example, antipsychotics such as haloperidol are powerful blockers of dopamine D2 receptors. An understandable side effect of these medicines is the development of parkinsonian symptoms, including tremor, rigidity, and slowness of movement.

TP Neuroleptic-induced syndromes can develop acutely within hours or a few days, subacutely over several weeks, or after prolonged exposure to the dopamine blocker. When parkinsonism develops ≥6 months after exposure, the term "tardive" is used, implying a delayed onset. Drug-induced parkinsonism resembles idiopathic PD, with tremor, rigidity, and akinesia. Symptoms are usually (though not necessarily) bilateral and possibly reversible.

Dx Diagnosis is suspected through the history. Patients with tardive parkinsonism normally have a psychiatric history and a known history of neuroleptics intake. It is important to consider that patients, particularly when hospitalized, are administered drugs, the purpose of which they may be unaware. For example, an elderly person developing parkinsonian symptoms after being discharged from the hospital may have received haloperidol for agitation. Some antiemetic medications also have antidopaminergic activity (e.g., metoclopramide). Symmetrical symptom progression is often an element of drug-induced parkinsonism.

Tx Discontinuing the offending agent is the first step. On some occasions the patient has a significant psychiatric disease necessitating continuation of the antidopaminergic agent. The prescribing physician should be consulted to discuss other options, including use of atypical neuroleptics (e.g., clozapine, quetiapine). In some cases, even after the agent is removed the symptoms persist. In these cases patients should be treated the same as patients with regular PD. **See Cecil Essentials 122.**

ZEBRA ZONE

a. Dementia with Lewy bodies: Pathologically, this syndrome resembles PD in that affected cells have the same cytoplasmic inclusion bodies, known as Lewy bodies. In this case, however, the affected area may include the cerebral cortex, causing early cognitive impairment out of proportion to the accompanying motor symptoms, which usually include rigidity and bradykinesia more than tremor. There may be early development of visual hallucinations as well. Diagnostic workup should exclude Alzheimer disease and other dementias, but treatment includes therapy for dementia (including cholinesterase inhibitors) and for the parkinsonian symptoms.

b. **Spinocerebellar ataxias (SCAs):** This is a heterogeneous group of progressive ataxias caused by trinucleotide repeats. Patients present with various constellations of symptoms, including ataxia of gait and stance, limb movement ataxia, eye movement abnormalities, pyramidal tract signs, muscle atrophy, basal ganglia symptoms, bladder dysfunction, dysphagia, and dementia. While most of the SCAs do not typically present with parkinsonian findings, patients with SCA type 2 may have prominent parkinsonism in the absence of cerebellar signs. Age of presentation varies but is often within the first few decades of life.

c. **Wilson disease**, also known as hepatolenticular degeneration, is an autosomal-recessive disorder affecting copper binding, resulting in excessive copper buildup in the liver and brain. This results in basal ganglia dysfunction as well as behavioral and mental changes. Patients may present at an early age with tremor (more prominent in "wing-beating" position), rigidity, postural instability, dystonia, dysarthria, athetosis, and psychiatric problems such as depression, mania, or loss of impulse control. The hallmark finding is the Kayser-Fleischer ring, a brownish golden haze seen at the corneal rim, most visible on slit-lamp exam. MRI may show T_2 hypodensities in the superior colliculi and hyperdensities in the medial substantia nigra and tegmentum (resulting in a pattern resembling a panda's face). Treatment is with D-penicillamine, a copper-chelating agent, in early stages of the disease.

d. **Huntington disease** typically presents with chorea, slow saccades, and behavioral or cognitive changes, but in its juvenile form, parkinsonian symptoms may predominate. Rigidity, bradykinesia, resting tremor, dystonia, and ataxia may be present, as may seizures and myoclonus. HD is a trinucleotide-repeat disorder that is at this point untreatable. Chorea can be managed with dopamine-blocking or dopamine-depleting agents, but these may exacerbate the parkinsonian symptoms.

vital for the patient with PD (and the caregivers) to be aware of resources available for assistance and support. On the emotional level, there are support groups that meet in community centers and hospitals. Less well known is that there is an industry that has been developed to supply disabled patients with assistive devices. There are specially designed walking aids with wheels, seats, baskets, handbrakes, and enhanced swivel capacity. Some of these devices can project a horizontal line on the ground with a laser so as to provide a visual cue for the frozen patient. Kitchen utensils have been designed that do not require lifting or tilting, such as rocker knives and slant-bottomed bowls. There are innovations for dressing such as plastic sleeves to help slide on socks. Handlebars and poles can be installed in one's home for ease of transferring, and bathtubs, toilets, and staircases can be modified to improve navigability and safety. Physicians should be aware of these resources and refer patients to physical and occupational therapists for more detailed information.

Suggested Reading

Fahn S. A new look at levodopa based on the ELLDOPA study. J Neural Transm Suppl 2006;70:419–426.

Chapter 64
Headache (Case 56)

Michelle Fabian MD and Jennifer Elbaum MD

Case: The patient is a 42-year-old woman with a history of hypertension and polycystic ovarian syndrome who presented to the ED complaining of headache. The headache was severe enough that she called 911 and was brought in by ambulance. She described the pain as pulsating and located in the right frontal region, extending down into her neck. She vomited twice in the ambulance. She denied fever, chills, rash, weakness, numbness, changes in vision, or recent trauma. Her medications include oral contraceptives, a "blood pressure pill," and multivitamins. She reported a prior history of headaches but none so severe as to require medical advice. Her mother and aunt also have headaches, and there are no known neurologic diseases in her family.

Differential Diagnosis

Migraine	Meningitis	Mass lesion
Ruptured aneurysm/SAH	Pseudotumor cerebri	
Cluster headache	Temporal arteritis	

Speaking Intelligently

Headache is the most prevalent neurologic symptom, and most people not do see a doctor for their headaches because usually they are mild and infrequent. Fortunately, most headaches are benign conditions and fall into the category of primary headache disorders, such as tension, migraine, and cluster headaches. However, for the patients who experience these headaches on a regular basis, even "benign" headaches can be extremely disabling. Chronic headache sufferers experience a decline in their quality of life, with absences from work and the inability to participate in social activities; comorbid depression and anxiety are common. A small percentage of patients will experience "transformed" headaches that manifest as chronic daily headaches that are very difficult to treat. The approach to headache must begin by differentiating benign headaches from those that reflect underlying pathology that may be life-threatening.

PATIENT CARE

Clinical Thinking

- Since there is a very large differential diagnosis for headaches, it is helpful to think of headaches in three broad categories: acute, subacute, and chronic.
- New acute-onset headaches are concerning, as they suggest an acute event, such as an SAH or meningitis.
- Patients who report that they rarely have headaches but develop a sudden-onset severe headache should be evaluated emergently.
- Headache in the presence of neurologic signs and symptoms should immediately raise clinical suspicion for an intracranial process.
- Subacute-onset headache implies a slowly progressive process, such as a tumor or a vasculitis.
- Long-standing, recurrent headaches will usually be one of the primary headache disorders, and patients will often report that although the pain may be severe, "this is one of my typical migraines."

→ **Angiogram:** Visualizing the vasculature is important when considering a vasculitis, an aneurysm, or a venous sinus thrombosis. The gold-standard **conventional angiogram** is often not the test of choice, as it is invasive with potential procedural complications. Instead, a **CT angiogram**, **MR angiogram**, or MR venography (MRV) will usually be sufficient with minimal risk of adverse events. $3475, $338, $534

Clinical Entities	Medical Knowledge

Subarachnoid Hemorrhage

Pφ Rupture of a cerebral artery aneurysm leads to a sudden, dramatic increase in ICP. The subarachnoid space rapidly fills with blood. In severe hemorrhages, this blood may also leak into the intraventricular space or into the parenchyma. Both genetic and environmental factors predispose patients to formation of saccular aneurysms, the most common form of aneurysm. Saccular aneurysms tend to occur at arterial branch points, most commonly in the anterior communicating artery. Less common forms of aneurysms include mycotic aneurysms (formed by septic or neoplastic emboli that lodge in the arterial wall) and fusiform aneurysms.

TP Classically a patient with subarachnoid headache will experience an explosive, generalized headache that will often be described as "the worst headache of my life." Associated symptoms can include neck stiffness (usually), vomiting, photophobia, confusion, and loss of consciousness. Depending on whether there is parenchymal hemorrhage, the patient may also exhibit focal motor or sensory signs. Before aneurysmal rupture, patients are usually asymptomatic. However, they may present with a third-nerve palsy, which involves the pupil; the pupil will be asymmetrically enlarged and poorly reactive to light. This is caused by direct pressure from the aneurysm, most often from the posterior communicating artery, on the third-nerve fibers. This is an important syndrome not to be missed by the clinician because identification can be lifesaving.

Dx A noncontrast head CT scan has >90% sensitivity in SAH in the first 24 hours. If the head CT scan is negative but there is still a high suspicion for SAH, LP must be performed. LP typically reveals a high opening pressure, is grossly bloody with a very high RBC count, and is positive for xanthochromia—a yellow appearance to the supernatant.

Tx Initially, the most important treatment is to control blood pressure to decrease the chance of repeat bleeding. Antiepileptic drugs are administered to prevent seizures. At the same time, it is imperative to quickly identify the aneurysm that caused the hemorrhage. Once the aneurysm is identified and secured by either surgical or endovascular treatment, then traditionally triple-H therapy (hypertension, hypervolemia, hemodilution) is employed to prevent vasospasm. In addition, many patients require ventriculoperitoneal (VP) shunts if hydrocephalus develops. **See Cecil Essentials 119, 124.**

Acute Meningitis and Encephalitis

Pφ Meningitis is an infection of the arachnoid, the pia, and the subarachnoid space. Encephalitis is an infection of the brain parenchyma. When there are symptoms that seem to indicate infection of both meninges and brain, this is termed meningoencephalitis. CNS infections produce an intense inflammatory response. This response is often more detrimental than the pathogen itself and may lead to acute and chronic complications.

TP The two most common treatable life-threatening types of CNS infections seen are bacterial meningitis and herpes simplex virus (HSV) encephalitis. A patient with acute bacterial meningitis will typically present with severe generalized headache and neck stiffness. Fevers, chills, nausea, and vomiting are common. Level of consciousness may range from normal to confused or comatose. On exam, meningismus is prominent, although this sign may be absent in coma. Kernig and Brudzinski signs may also be present.

HSV encephalitis may have a similar presentation. There is usually fever, headache, and alteration in mental status. Patients can also exhibit prominent symptoms not often appreciated in meningitis, including olfactory hallucinations, aphasia, recurrent partial seizure, hemiparesis, and ataxia.

Mass Lesion

Pφ Brain, blood, and CSF are the three elements that reside in the finite space of the cranial vault. If a fourth element is introduced into this space, such as an intracranial mass, then the equilibrium between the preexisting elements is altered. Localized headache may be caused by distension of pain-sensitive structures. If the tumor continues to grow, there will be a rise in ICP, which may then cause generalized headache.

TP Patients with brain tumor will present in a variety of ways, including headache, seizure, or focal symptoms. Headaches from an intracranial mass can range from dull and constant to sharp and intermittent. Some patients will localize their headache to the approximate location of the mass; however, others will complain of generalized headaches. Patients will often describe headaches that awaken them from sleep. This is because lying in the recumbent position causes a transient increase in ICP. In the same manner other maneuvers that transiently increase ICP, such as coughing or straining, can worsen the headache. On exam there may be papilledema or focal signs referring to the mass.

Dx An intracranial mass is most readily identified with MRI. The addition of contrast can aid in elucidating what type of mass is present. If MRI is not available, CT can be used, but it is not as sensitive or informative. Further attempts to identify the mass noninvasively can be made using either MRI–single photon emission CT (MRI-SPECT) or PFT scan. However, most often a brain biopsy is necessary for definitive identification of the mass. The differential diagnosis of an intracranial mass should include brain abscess, which can have a similar presentation and appearance on imaging studies.

Tx Treatment of the intracranial mass is dependent on the type of tumor, its location, and the patient's clinical status. Patients who have clear signs of raised ICP are usually given corticosteroids to attempt to decrease the mass effect of the surrounding edema. In some cases, resection is attempted. Consultation with a neuro-oncologist and neurosurgeon is usually necessary. **See Cecil Essentials 127.**

Venous Sinus Thrombosis

Pφ Venous sinus thrombosis is the occlusion of an intracerebral venous sinus by thrombus. Sagittal, lateral, and cavernous sinuses are the most common sites for thrombosis. The thrombosis is presumably caused by a hypercoagulable state, whether that is from a genetic predisposition, medications such as oral contraceptives, an autoimmune process, the postpartum period, intracranial infection, or malignancy. Dehydration has also been implicated. Venous sinus thrombosis can lead to a host of complications such as venous infarction, seizure, and increased ICP.

TP Depending on the site of thrombosis, the presentation can vary. The superior sagittal sinus (SSS) is the most commonly affected sinus; patients with SSS thrombosis most often present with headache, which is usually constant and generalized, but can be located in the occipital region. Headache may be exacerbated by coughing, straining, or lying down. Patients with cavernous sinus thrombosis may also present with chemosis, exophthalmos, and ophthalmoplegia.

Dx Head CT both with and without contrast suggests the diagnosis, although it is by no means a sensitive test for this condition. MRV is the initial test of choice when venous sinus thrombosis is suspected. Further information can be gained by the more invasive conventional angiogram, although this is not always necessary. Once the diagnosis is confirmed, the cause of thrombosis should be pursued.

Tx Anticoagulation with either heparin or low-molecular-weight heparin is started when venous sinus thrombosis is diagnosed. Warfarin is usually titrated to therapeutic range for long-term therapy of at least 6 months and possibly longer depending on the cause. **See Cecil Essentials 124.**

Pseudotumor Cerebri

Pφ The cause of pseudotumor cerebri, also known as idiopathic intracranial hypertension (IIH), is not known. Theories include increased rate of CSF production, decreased rate of CSF absorption secondary to venous hypertension, slowed absorption of CSF by arachnoid villi, and increased brain volume due an increase both in intracranial blood volume and extravascular space. Pseudotumor is most commonly associated with obesity and menstrual irregularities. Other risk factors include excessive vitamin A ingestion, endocrine abnormalities, remote head trauma, and venous sinus thrombosis.

TP The headache in pseudotumor is most often constant and generalized; it may wake the patient up from sleep and worsens upon coughing or straining. There may be associated visual symptoms including blurring of vision, diplopia, or recurrent episodes of transient visual loss. In severe cases there may be complete visual loss. Exam can reveal papilledema and possibly retinal hemorrhage. There may be bilateral cranial nerve VI palsy. Visual fields may be constricted, and/or there may be an enlargement of the physiologic blind spot. More often, however, bedside visual testing will appear normal, and formal visual testing will have to be performed to identify abnormalities. The rest of the neurologic exam is normal.

Dx In a patient with headache and papilledema, neuroimaging with CT or MRI must be done initially to rule out a structural cause such as a mass lesion. Depending on the clinical scenario, MRV may also be appropriate. If neuroimaging proves unrevealing, LP is performed. Normal opening pressure is <180 mm H_2O in nonobese patients and <250 mm H_2O in obese patients. Thus, an opening pressure above these levels is diagnostic; however, these minimum thresholds for diagnosis may well be exceeded.

Tx On initial LP, when opening pressure is found to be elevated, a large-volume tap is performed in an attempt to decrease ICP. Acetazolamide, a carbonic anhydrase inhibitor that reduces CSF production, is typically administered. If symptoms persist, repeat LPs are performed. If this still proves unsuccessful (the patient still has symptoms or visual field testing shows worsening), either lumbar peritoneal shunt or optic nerve fenestration can be considered as surgical options for treatment. At the same time, it is imperative that the physician encourage aggressive attempts at weight loss, as this in itself may confer an improved prognosis. **See Cecil Essentials 119.**

Cluster Headache

Pφ The etiology of cluster headache is unknown. Some believe it is secondary to abnormal parasympathetic activity, mediated through the superior petrosal nerve and the sphenopalatine ganglion. Others have implicated the hypothalamus and its pathways because of the daily rhythmicity of attacks and their relationship to the circadian rhythm.

TP The headaches typically occur in "clusters," every day at the same time for a 4- to 6-week period, before remitting for months to years, when the cycle repeats. The pain, usually localized over one eye, is deep, stabbing, and unbearable. Prominent symptoms associated with cluster headache include ipsilateral ptosis, conjunctival injection and tearing, nasal stuffiness, and facial flushing. In contrast to the migraneur who prefers to lie in a quiet, dark environment, a cluster headache patient will often pace about until the pain stops. The headache will last between 15 minutes and 2 hours. Alcohol can trigger a headache in 70% of patients; however, if the patient is not in the midst of a cycle, alcohol has no effect.

Dx The diagnosis is made by a careful history and, if possible, observation during an attack.

Tx During an attack, cluster headache can be treated with 100% oxygen given by non-rebreather facial mask. With this treatment, the headache will usually resolve in 15 minutes. Other acute treatments include sumatriptan and intranasal lidocaine. Ergotamine can be effective in prevention of a single attack. To halt a cluster cycle, verapamil, lithium, and corticosteroids have all been used successfully. **See Cecil Essentials 119.**

Temporal Arteritis

Pφ Temporal arteritis is an autoimmune vasculitic syndrome of unknown cause that affects the superficial temporal artery exclusively in the majority of cases, and less commonly affects other larger arteries. It is thought that T cells invade the internal elastic lamina initially in response to an unknown antigen. Lymphokines are then released and attract monocytes, which carry out a full-thickness arterial invasion. In foci of inflammation there is frequent granuloma and giant cell formation. With progression of the disease, there is luminal proliferation causing stenosis of the artery and distal ischemia.

TP Patients with temporal arteritis usually present with increasingly severe, constant unilateral pain centered over the temporal artery. The pain can be dull, throbbing, or stabbing in character. Associated symptoms can include jaw claudication (pain with chewing), fatigue, anemia, and low-grade fever. If myalgias are a prominent feature, there may be coexistent polymyalgia rheumatica. The dreaded complication of temporal arteritis is visual loss due to involvement of the central retinal artery; this can occur with a prodrome of transient episodes of amaurosis fugax, or it can occur suddenly without warning. On exam a tender, nodular, enlarged, and erythematous superficial temporal artery may be present. If vision has been affected, it may manifest in abnormal visual fields, decreased visual acuity, or blindness. Otherwise the neurologic exam is usually normal.

Dx ESR is the initial test for temporal arteritis. While an ESR > 50 mm/hr is diagnostic, it is important to note that a normal ESR is seen in a minority of cases. In these cases, C-reactive protein (CRP) level may be more sensitive and should be checked. Temporal artery biopsy should then be performed for confirmation.

Tx The treatment for patients diagnosed with temporal arteritis is prednisone, usually starting at a dose of 40–60 mg daily. It should be started immediately, even before biopsy, especially in cases where impending visual loss is a concern. Patients may require a very slow taper over months, as symptoms may recur with a decrease in prednisone dose. **See Cecil Essentials 86, 119.**

ZEBRA ZONE

a. **Call-Fleming syndrome:** Also called reversible cerebral vasoconstriction, this is a recurrent thunderclap headache associated with extreme hypertension.

b. **Posterior reversible encephalopathy syndrome (PRES)** usually presents with headache, seizures, and confusion often associated with pregnancy, renal failure, or immunosuppression.

c. **Spontaneous CSF leak:** Severe headache with prominent orthostatic component. Also seen in the "post-LP" headache.

d. **Colloid tumor:** Mass lesion that can cause intermittent obstruction of the third ventricle with transient increase in ICP.

Practice-Based Learning and Improvement: Evidence-Based Medicine

Title
Treatment of migraine attacks with subcutaneous sumatriptan: first placebo-controlled study. The Subcutaneous Sumatriptan International Study Group

Authors
Visser WH, Ferrari MD, Bayliss EM, et al.

Institution
Department of Neurology, University Hospital Leiden, The Netherlands

Reference
Cephalalgia 1992;12:308–313

Problem
Migraine is a disabling condition for which there is a considerable need for better treatment.

Intervention
Randomized, double-blind, controlled trial comparing sumatriptan at three doses versus placebo in migraine

Quality of evidence
Level I

Outcome/effect
All doses of subcutaneous sumatriptan were significantly more effective than placebo. There was a dose–response effect with increasing efficacy at higher dose.

Historical significance/comments
This was the first large randomized controlled trial of sumatriptan treatment for migraine headache that showed the efficacy of triptans in this disorder.

Interpersonal and Communication Skills

Don't Allow the Electronic Medical Record (EMR) to Detract from Your Interpersonal Relationship
Use of the EMR is changing the physician–patient interactions to which we have become accustomed. As a medical community, we still await concretization of "best practices." The following five tips for using EMRs in your office practice have been modified from the blog referenced below:

1. **Use the EMR, and don't complain about it to the patient.** Let your patients know that you are using the EMR to help you take better care of them. If at times you struggle with an issue or face a learning-curve problem in starting up on the EMR, don't whine in front of the patient. If you tell patients the EMR is detracting from their care, with words or body language, they will believe you and will resent your allowing this to happen.

2. **Substitute voice contact for eye contact.** Involve the patient in your documentation process. Say "It's really important that I make an accurate note of the details of your headache pattern. This is going to be important in finding a solution to the problem." Then read aloud what you are typing as you enter the details.

3. **Tell patients how you make use of the strengths of your system.** If you use the system for recalls, reminders of services due, or electronic prescriptions, tell your patient how you are using these features to provide convenience.

4. **Try to find a reason to get the patient to look at something on the monitor with you.** In our patient with headache, perhaps you will review the MRI report with her. This helps the patient to see why you are looking at the monitor, and gives her confidence that the EMR lets you see data in a way that benefits her. Almost all patients want you to have the tools you need to take good care of them. If they see the EMR as a tool, just like a stethoscope or reflex hammer, they will feel good about their doctor making good use of that tool.

5. **Every visit requires a warm greeting and a warm closure.** Don't let the EMR get in the way of your physician–patient relationship. Greet the patient with physical and eye contact. A warm handshake and greeting starts any visit well. When the visit is over, you should again provide closure both physically and emotionally. This means eye contact, physical contact in an age- and gender-appropriate way, and some gesture to communicate that the visit is over. This has always been important but is even more so with the advent of EMRs; moreover, it can more easily be forgotten now, when we might be engrossed in hurrying to finish typing the assessment or plan and might skip the important closure of the visit.

Professionalism

Improve Access to Care to Decrease Emergency Department Visits
Patients with chronic headache syndromes account for a major portion of ED visits each year. In fact, in one study headache was the sixth most likely reason patients went to the ED. There are very effective preventative and symptomatic treatments for headache that could prevent many of these emergency visits. In an age in which EDs are overcrowded and understaffed, this would be extremely advantageous. However, because of lack of access to primary-care

doctors or to a neurologist, many patients do not receive proper prophylactic headache treatment. The result of this is that when they do experience a benign but severe headache, they have nowhere else to turn but to the ED. The burden that is placed on the health-care system is exacerbated by the suffering and loss of productivity experienced by a patient with headache who receives substandard treatment. All patients deserve equal access to the best treatments available, and it should be the mission of the medical profession to make sure that this occurs.

Systems-Based Practice

Criteria for Head Imaging: Costs, Benefits, and Potential Harms Must Be Considered

When a patient complains of chronic headaches, you must make a decision regarding the need to obtain an imaging study to investigate the possibility that the headache is secondary to an underlying structural abnormality. The vast majority of patients who come to the outpatient setting with a chronic headache syndrome have a primary headache disorder such as migraine and tension-type headaches. Routine performance of imaging on everyone with a headache not only is costly but also carries a risk of adverse events, such as allergic reactions to contrast dye. In addition, a number of incidental lesions that are not related to the headaches may be found on imaging studies but will surely cause significant anxiety to the patient. Yet, it is not uncommon for patients to come to the doctor fearing a brain tumor and needing the reassurance provided by an imaging study. Physicians, too, will find the knowledge gained from an imaging study reassuring in many cases. To help guide the decision, certain "red flags" should serve as indications to consider obtaining an imaging study, including (1) an unexplained abnormality on the neurologic examination, (2) headaches that worsen with Valsalva maneuver or awaken the patient from sleep, (3) new-onset headaches in an older person, and (4) progressively worsening headaches.

Suggested Readings

Bradley W, Darroff R, Fenichel G, Jankovic J, editors. Neurology in clinical practice. 5th ed. Philadelphia: Elsevier; 2008.

Frishberg BM, Rosenberg JH, Matchar DB. Evidence-based guidelines in the primary care setting: neuroimaging in patients with nonacute headache. US Headache Consortium. September 2000. Available from: http://www.aan.com/professionals/practice/pdfs/gl0088.pdf.

McCaig LF, Burt CW. National hospital ambulatory medical care survey: 2002 emergency department summary. Advance data from vital and health statistics; No. 340. Hyattsville, Maryland: National Center for Health Statistics; 2004.

Ropper A, Brown R. Adams and Victor's principles of neurology. 8th ed. New York: McGraw-Hill; 2005.

Rowland LP, editor. Merritt's neurology. 11th ed. Philadelphia: Lippincott Williams & Wilkins; 2005.

Chapter 65
Dizziness and Vertigo (Case 57)

Lana Zhovtis Ryerson MD *and Stephen Krieger* MD

Case: A 34-year-old woman presents to the ED with dizziness. She states that 2 days ago she began to feel a "spinning sensation" and was walking around "as though she were drunk." These symptoms worsened the day before admission, when she developed nausea and vomiting and had increasing difficulty walking. She has no significant past medical history. On exam she has beating nystagmus in all directions of gaze, worse when looking to the right. She has a slightly flattened right nasolabial fold. She has full strength and an intact sensory exam, but on coordination testing she has significant postural instability, as well as dysmetria in the right arm. She is unable to tandem walk, falling to the side.

Differential Diagnosis

Vertigo	Dizziness/presyncope/light-headedness
Benign paroxysmal positional vertigo (BPPV)	Orthostatic hypotension
Acute labyrinthitis/vestibular neuritis	Cardiac arrhythmia
Meniere disease	Vasovagal disorder
Cerebellar infarction or hemorrhage	Intoxication/medication side effects
Perilymphatic fistula	Anxiety

Speaking Intelligently

"Dizziness" refers to a variety of abnormal sensations relating to perception of the body's relationship to space. What can be difficult for both a patient and the physician is the subjectivity of the term dizziness; people use it to describe an array of abnormal sensations. Furthermore, patients may use different terms to describe the same kind of abnormal sensation, and one must clarify what patients are experiencing when beginning to characterize their symptoms.

Although prevalence studies vary in their definition of the symptom, dizziness is common in all age groups, and its prevalence increases modestly with age. While peripheral vestibular etiologies are among the most common causes, as many as 25% of patients with risk factors for stroke who present to the emergency medical setting with the combination of vertigo, nystagmus, and postural instability may have a stroke affecting the cerebellum.

For most patients the symptom of dizziness resolves spontaneously, but an important minority of patients can develop chronic, disabling symptoms. Patients with chronic dizziness may benefit from an approach aimed at identifying and managing treatable conditions, whether etiologic or contributory. This approach may include correcting visual impairment, improving muscle strength, adjusting medication regimens, identifying and treating psychological comorbidities such as anxiety and depression, and instructing patients on vestibular exercises.

PATIENT CARE

Clinical Thinking

- The first step in evaluating a patient with dizziness is to take a detailed history focusing on the meaning of the term "dizziness" to the patient and to classify his or her symptoms into vertigo as opposed to presyncopal light-headedness.
  - Vertigo is an illusory sensation of motion of either oneself or one's surroundings.
  - Presyncope is described as a light-headed, faint feeling, as though one were about to pass out, that is usually due to transient reduction of cerebral blood flow.
- If the symptoms are suggestive of vertigo, the next question that arises is whether the history and findings on examination are consistent with a central disorder such as hemorrhage/infarction of the cerebellum or a peripheral vestibular etiology such as benign positional vertigo or vestibular neuritis.
- It is vital that physicians are able to differentiate the two pathologic localizations, since central causes of acute vertigo, such as cerebellar hemorrhage and infarction, can be life-threatening and may require immediate intervention.

IMAGING CONSIDERATIONS

→ **Brain MRI** (with attention to the cerebellum and posterior fossa) is recommended when the examination of a patient with an acute vestibular syndrome yields findings suggestive of a central localization. Urgent imaging is also recommended when the onset of symptoms is sudden in a patient with prominent risk factors for stroke or when a new-onset headache accompanies the acute vertigo. $534

→ If prompt brain MRI is not available, **head CT** should be performed, with fine cuts through the cerebellum. $334

| Clinical Entities | Medical Knowledge |

Benign Paroxysmal Positional Vertigo

Pφ Otoliths, or calcium carbonate crystals, become dislodged from the utricle, one of the gravity-sensitive structures in the inner ear, and then migrate to the posterior semicircular canal, which is the most gravity-dependent structure in the vestibular labyrinths.

TP Classically, patients describe a brief spinning sensation brought on when turning in bed or tilting the head backward to look up or down. Each episode of vertigo lasts only 10–20 seconds. The initial onset of vertigo is often associated with nausea, with or without vomiting. The dizziness may be quite severe, so as to halt all activity during its duration.

Dx The diagnosis is generally made by eliciting the history of the episode, characterized by brief episodes of vertigo provoked by certain changes in head position such as rolling over in bed, bending over, and looking upward. The diagnosis can be confirmed with the Dix-Hallpike maneuver, for which the diagnostic criteria consist of typically rotatory nystagmus with the upper pole of the eye beating toward the dependent ear. The nystagmus typically begins after a latency of several seconds and is associated with a sensation of rotational vertigo. After the patient returns to the seated position, nystagmus is again observed, but the direction of nystagmus is reversed.

Tx The treatment currently recommended is the bedside canalith repositioning procedure (CRP), also known as the Epley maneuver. The purpose of the maneuver is to relocate free-floating debris from the posterior semicircular canal into the vestibule of the vestibular labyrinth, where it presumably adheres. The debris can be moved within the labyrinth noninvasively through a sequence of head orientations with respect to gravity.

Vestibular Neuritis

Pφ Although the pathophysiology is unclear, the condition is thought to result from a selective inflammation of the vestibular nerve and is presumably of viral origin.

TP Vestibular neuritis presents as rapid onset of severe, persistent vertigo, nausea, vomiting, and gait instability. Physical exam findings are consistent with an acute peripheral vestibular imbalance: spontaneous vestibular nystagmus and gait instability without a loss of the ability to ambulate. In pure vestibular neuritis, auditory function is preserved; when this syndrome is combined with unilateral hearing loss, it is called labyrinthitis.

Dx The diagnosis is based on the ability to clinically differentiate between peripheral and central causes of acute prolonged vertigo. ENG, if available, can document the unilateral vestibular loss.

Tx There is no established treatment for vestibular neuritis. Symptomatic therapy is typically used, with the main classes of drugs including antihistamines (meclizine, dimenhydrinate, promethazine), anticholinergic agents, antidopaminergic agents, and GABAergic agents (diazepam, clonazepam). These drugs do not eliminate but rather reduce the severity of vertiginous symptoms.

Meniere Disease

Pφ The disease is thought to be related to an increase in the volume of endolymph in the labyrinths (endolymphatic hydrops). The hydrops causes hearing loss by a direct effect on the sensory outer hair cells of the cochlea, but the sudden spells of vertigo are less well understood. Some cases appear to be related to mutations in the cochlin gene on chromosome 14q12–q13, with the disease showing genetic anticipation (i.e., becomes apparent at on earlier age as it is passed on to the next generation).

TP Patients present with recurring episodes of spontaneous episodic vertigo lasting for minutes to hours and usually associated with unilateral tinnitus, hearing loss, and a sensation of ear fullness. Acute attacks are characterized by severe vertigo, nausea, vomiting, and disabling imbalance. The attacks recur at intervals ranging from weeks to years.

Dx The diagnosis is made by obtaining the history of episodic vertigo associated with hearing loss and tinnitus, with family history helping to confirm the diagnosis. A low-frequency sensorineural hearing loss on audiometry and a unilateral reduced vestibular response on ENG help confirm the diagnosis.

Tx Diuretics and salt restriction are directed to reducing possible hydrops. Symptomatic relief may be obtained during acute attacks with drugs similar to those used for vestibular neuritis. In persistent, disabling, drug-resistant cases, surgical procedures such as endolymphatic shunting, labyrinthectomy, and vestibular nerve section can be helpful.

Cerebellar/Brainstem Infarct or Hemorrhage

Pφ The blood supply to the peripheral vestibular labyrinth and vestibular nerve, as well as the brainstem vestibular area and cerebellum, comes from the vertebrobasilar arterial system. Occlusion of one or more of the posterior circulation arteries due to embolism or atherosclerotic stenosis can produce cerebellar or brainstem vascular events.

TP Abrupt onset, history of TIAs, vascular disease, or significant other risk factors for stroke, usually associated with other neurologic symptoms, are diagnostic.

Dx On exam, spontaneous central-type nystagmus is seen with other associated signs of the lateral brainstem including Horner syndrome, facial numbness and weakness, hemiataxia, and dysarthria. MRI of brain shows infarction or hemorrhage in the medulla, pons, or cerebellum. Audiography may show ipsilateral hearing loss if the anterior cerebellar artery is involved.

Tx Patients with acute ischemic strokes may be offered IV tPA, intra-arterial tPA, or other clot-retrieving procedures depending on the institution and the time of onset of symptoms (for more details, see Chapter 66, Weakness). Within 72 hours after a cerebellar infarction, cerebellar swelling may develop that can compress the brainstem and produce obstructive hydrocephalus. Therefore, patients with cerebellar infarctions should be examined frequently in an ICU setting, and brain imaging should be repeated. If deterioration occurs, neurosurgical intervention may be warranted.

Perilymphatic Fistula

Pφ A perilymphatic fistula is an abnormal connection between the inner and middle ears that allows escape of perilymph fluid into the middle ear compartment. The episodic vertigo and/or hearing loss provoked by loud sounds occur because sound-induced pressure waves are abnormally distributed through the inner ear.

TP Signs suggesting this diagnosis include abrupt onset associated with a history of head trauma or sudden strain during heavy lifting, coughing, or sneezing, and possible association with chronic otitis or cholesteatoma.

Dx On physical exam, spontaneous, peripheral nystagmus associated with gait imbalance and unilateral hearing loss is noted. Possible perforation of the tympanic membrane may be noted. The most sensitive test for perilymph fistula is the vertigo and nystagmus induced by pressure in the external ear canal. ENG may show unilateral hypoexcitability; audiography may confirm the sensorineural hearing loss, and CT of the temporal bone may reveal associated skull fracture.

Tx The first step in treatment involves bed rest, head elevation, and avoidance of straining. Failure to resolve after several weeks of conservative therapy is an indication to consider a surgical patch.

ZEBRA ZONE

a. **Basilar artery migraine** is a rare form of migraine with aura, in which the auras consist of a combination of vertigo, dysarthria, tinnitus, diplopia, bilateral visual symptoms, bilateral paresthesias, and decreased level of consciousness. A migraine headache during or following the aura is required by current diagnostic criteria. MRI is often necessary to rule out other etiologies, with some patients having transient MRI abnormalities in the occipital cortex due to vasogenic edema.

b. **Acoustic neuromas (**or acoustic schwannomas) are Schwann cell–derived tumors commonly arising from the vestibular portion of the eighth cranial nerve and account for 80% to 90% of tumors involving the cerebellopontine angle. Symptoms associated with acoustic neuroma are due to cranial nerve involvement and cerebellar compression. Because the tumor grows slowly, the subtle imbalances in vestibular input are compensated by the CNS, and patients often do not experience disabling vertigo. Imbalance or a vague feeling of swaying may be the only manifestation of vestibular injury.

Practice-Based Learning and Improvement: Evidence-Based Medicine

Title
Short-term efficacy of Epley's manoeuvre: a double-blind randomized trial

Authors
von Brevern M, Seelig T, Radtke A, et al.

Institution
Neurologische Klinik, Charité, Campus Virchow-Klinikum, Berlin, Germany

Reference
J Neurol Neurosurg Psychiatr 2006;77:980–982

Problem
What maneuvers effectively treat posterior canal BPPV?

Intervention
Sixty-six patients with a diagnosis of BPPV based on a positive Dix-Hallpike maneuver compared a CRP with a sham procedure.

Quality of evidence
Level I

Outcome/effect
After 24 hours, 80% of treated patients were asymptomatic and had no nystagmus with the Dix-Hallpike maneuver, compared with 10% of sham patients. At this point, all patients in both the treatment and control groups with a persistently positive Dix-Hallpike maneuver underwent an Epley maneuver. Ninety-three percent of patients with BPPV from the original control group reported resolution of symptoms 24 hours after undergoing the procedure. By 1 week, 94% of patients in the original treatment group and 82% of patients in the original control group (all of whom underwent the maneuver at 24 hours) were asymptomatic.

Historical significance/comments
The Epley maneuver, or CRP, is used to clear the affected semicircular canal from mobile particles by a set of five successive head positions that are hand-guided by a therapist. At this time, two level I and three level II studies have demonstrated a short-term resolution of symptoms in patients treated in this way. As a result of the above-mentioned and other studies, the American Academy of Neurology released Level A recommendations for the CRP to be established as an effective and safe therapy that should be offered to patients of all ages with posterior semicircular canal BPPV.

Interpersonal and Communication Skills

Base Reassurance on Appropriate Medical Explanations
Although the symptoms of BPPV are extremely uncomfortable and will probably be frightening to the patient and his or her family, the disease does not usually portend serious neurologic impairment. Nonetheless, persons presenting with these symptoms will worry about having a very serious and debilitating illness. Simple reassurance must be accompanied by medical explanations based on an understanding of the patient's feelings, expectations, and ideas about causality. Reassurance that is perceived to have no real basis may be counterproductive. Failure to explore patients' ideas, expectations, and beliefs that underlie their concerns, and failure to validate those concerns using empathetic communication, can compromise the patient–physician relationship.

Professionalism

Uphold the Welfare of Patients Who Do Not Speak English
Dizziness and vertigo are complaints that are often evaluated in both the ED and outpatient settings, and their evaluation requires thorough clinical histories. Particularly in these high-volume environments, language barriers can be detrimental to optimal

providing effective care. Patients with diseases that cause weakness are often significantly disabled. An interdisciplinary team that includes rehabilitation specialists, neurosurgeons, pain specialists, and mental health professionals can be invaluable to the patient's recovery.

PATIENT CARE

Clinical Thinking

- Due to the huge scope of possible etiologies, the history and physical exam is essential in pinning down the most likely causes of weakness in a patient.
- Direct particular attention toward the progression and pattern of weakness, the onset and timing of weakness, and any associated symptoms, such as sensory abnormalities and speech difficulties.
- Categorizing the physical exam findings in a systematic manner allows for an anatomic localization of the disease process. A differential diagnosis can then be generated once the anatomic basis has been established.
- Correlating the presentation with the anatomic localization allows the clinician to formulate a working diagnosis.

History

- When a patient reports weakness, it can mean a variety of different things. For example, the patient may be feeling general malaise, or he or she may be referring to weakness of specific muscle groups. It is important to identify the location of the weakness, time of onset, duration and severity of the symptoms, and whether the weakness changes over the course of the day.
- Obtaining a history of any associated symptoms, such as any pain or sensory symptoms, is extremely important in narrowing down the differential diagnosis (numbness suggests neuropathy while pain suggests radiculopathy).
- The past medical history can identify risk factors for specific diseases (e.g., hypertension and diabetes are risk factors for stroke).
- Certain rare causes of weakness may be congenital (e.g., spinal muscular atrophy); therefore, a family history should be obtained.

Physical Examination

- The physical exam should focus on (1) gross observation for any abnormal or involuntary movements; (2) inspection of muscle bulk and tone; (3) palpation and percussion for tenderness and involuntary contractions; (4) muscle strength testing; (5) reflex testing (deep tendon reflexes and extensor plantar [Babinski] reflex); (6) sensory testing (particularly the pattern of deficits and any correlation with the site of weakness); and (7) cranial nerve involvement.

- Inspection of muscle bulk and tone can give clues as to whether the focus is lower motor neuron (atrophy and fasciculations) or upper motor neuron (increased tone, spasticity). Severe atrophy can also give clues to the time course and chronicity of weakness. Strength testing should be done systematically, comparing each major muscle group to the contralateral side. Subtle weakness can be detected with side-to-side comparison of limbs held against gravity (e.g., pronator drift). If indicated, checking the patient for muscle fatigue with simple repetitive exercise (e.g., maintaining abduction of the shoulder against resistance for 1 minute) can help identify neuromuscular junction disease (e.g., myasthenia gravis).
- Reflex testing is essential in differentiating lower motor neuron from upper motor neuron causes of weakness. Patients with upper motor neuron problems usually have hyperreflexia, whereas patients with lower motor neuron causes often have hyporeflexia. As with strength testing, comparison with the contralateral side is often helpful. Additional upper motor neuron findings include a positive Babinski reflex. Lower motor neuron findings are usually confined to atrophy of the weak limb or muscle, with hyporeflexia and possible fasciculations.

Tests for Consideration
- **Serum creatine kinase (CK):** CK elevation is classically seen in muscle damage from any cause, particularly inflammatory myopathies and glycogen storage diseases. Other causes of elevated CK include prolonged exercise, alcohol abuse, trauma, and hypothyroidism. $9
- **TSH:** TSH levels are elevated in patients with hypothyroidism and decreased in patients with hyperthyroidism. Some patients present with symmetrical proximal muscle weakness with associated myalgia (muscle pain), joint stiffness, and muscle enlargement (in weak muscles) consistent with a hypothyroid myopathy. Other patients present with proximal weakness with atrophy of the shoulder and pelvic girdle muscles, with heat intolerance and fatigue consistent with hyperthyroid myopathy. $24
- **Electrophysiology studies:** These include **nerve conduction studies (NCS)**, **needle electromyography (EMG)**, and **repetitive nerve stimulation (RNS)**. NCS assess the integrity of motor and sensory peripheral nerves by administering electrical pulses across the nerve being studied. Needle EMG involves insertion of a recording needle into muscle for assessment of underlying disease. Muscle activity at rest and with contraction is assessed for any pathologic patterns of abnormality. RNS is a modified NCS in which a nerve is repeatedly stimulated at a fixed frequency. A combination of these studies can help pinpoint the pathophysiologic mechanism of weakness to a peripheral nervous system process. $128

- **LP with CSF analysis:** Can help narrow the diagnosis.
  Relevant CSF studies are listed in the Clinical Entities section.
  Patients suspected of increased ICP should be fully evaluated
  with physical exam (including funduscopic exam to look for
  papilledema) and/or imaging studies before an LP to avoid the
  risk of cerebral herniation. $272
- **Biopsies** are rarely indicated in patients with
  weakness. Muscle biopsies may be helpful in
  differentiating different types of muscle disease.
  Nerve and skin biopsies, helpful in certain
  types of neuropathies, should be done on the
  affected site. $1190, $1321, $105

IMAGING CONSIDERATIONS

→ Imaging studies of the CNS are usually necessary.
→ A **CT scan** is a fast and inexpensive initial study that
  can help rule out most CNS causes of weakness. $334
→ An **MRI scan** should be performed if there are any
  abnormal findings on CT scan or if the history and/or
  physical exam raises suspicion of a CNS disease. $534

Clinical Entities   Medical Knowledge

Stroke

Pφ Pathologic changes include areas of necrosis in the brain due
to infarction that correlate with specific neurologic deficits.
Patients will usually have risk factors for atherosclerosis or
embolic disease, such as hypertension, diabetes mellitus,
hypercholesterolemia, coronary artery disease, peripheral artery
disease, and/or atrial fibrillation. Smoking and excess alcohol
intake, as well as a sedentary lifestyle and obesity, are also risk
factors for strokes.

TP Typical features include an acute onset of focal neurologic
deficits, which are usually unilateral. The location of the
weakness correlates to the areas of damage caused by the stroke.
Patients may have associated symptoms, including unilateral
sensory loss, as well as weakness in facial muscles leading to
difficulty with speaking or swallowing.

Dx The specific area of ischemia can be identified using CNS imaging
modalities, including CT and MRI.

Tx Treatment can be divided into management of acute events and prevention of further events. The thrombolytic agent, t-PA, should be administered to eligible patients who present within 3 hours of symptom onset. Stroke prevention should include antiplatelet agents such as acetylsalicylic acid (aspirin) or clopidogrel (Plavix). Anticoagulants such as warfarin (Coumadin) should be given to patients with risk factors for cardioembolic stroke such as atrial fibrillation. Cholesterol and blood pressure should be optimized with statin medications and antihypertensive agents, respectively. Optimal glucose management is important for diabetics. Patients should be encouraged to lead a healthy lifestyle, including a low-fat, low-cholesterol diet, regular exercise, and smoking cessation. **See Cecil Essentials 124.**

Transient Ischemic Attack

Pφ Because TIAs are reversible events, they cause no permanent pathologic changes. Patients will usually have a past medical history that includes risk factors for atherosclerosis and/or embolic disease.

TP TIAs are characterized by an acute onset of transient focal neurologic deficits caused by reversible ischemia. By definition, symptoms should last no longer than 24 hours, but typically they last for only a few minutes. TIAs are warning signs of future strokes.

Dx TIA is a clinical diagnosis that includes a history and physical exam consistent with a reversible focal neurologic deficit. CNS imaging studies should not show an acute stroke, as this would indicate infarction rather than a transient event.

Tx Treatment should focus on stroke prevention. This includes encouraging regular exercise and a low-fat, low-cholesterol diet. Medications include antiplatelet agents, as well as agents to optimize blood pressure and to manage cholesterol and glucose levels. **See Cecil Essentials 124.**

Multiple Sclerosis

Pφ Pathologically, patients with MS have multiple areas of demyelination and inflammation in the CNS that eventually form gliotic scars.

TP MS is the most common autoimmune inflammatory demyelinating disorder that affects the CNS. The typical age at onset of MS is 20–40 years, but the disease can also present in patients outside these age limits. There is an approximately 2:1 female predominance. Weakness can occur in any extremity or part of an extremity, depending on the site of the demyelinating lesion. Symptoms of an acute attack should last >24 hours. Patients often have associated symptoms based on the area of the CNS that is damaged. Since nerve conduction in demyelinated nerves slows down in warmth, patients may complain of worsening neurologic symptoms with increased temperatures, a condition called Uhthoff syndrome.

Dx The diagnosis of MS requires the dissemination of clinical events (and CNS lesions on MRI) that are separated by both time and space. CSF findings include elevated oligoclonal bands, IgG synthesis, and IgG index. In addition, some patients may have mildly elevated CSF protein and WBC counts.

Tx Treatment for MS includes the use of immunomodulatory medications. These disease-modifying medications are chronic treatments that prevent future exacerbations and delay the progression of the disease. They include interferon-β and glatiramer acetate, although immunosuppressive therapies such as mitoxantrone and natalizumab may be used for some refractory or progressive cases. IV methylprednisolone is used to treat acute exacerbations. An interdisciplinary team, including psychiatrists, social workers, physical therapists, and a dedicated nursing staff, is important in the treatment process. **See Cecil Essentials 129.**

Spinal Cord Injury

Pφ Pathologic changes will show the specific etiology of the spinal cord injury, which can include malignancy, osteoarthritis, trauma, infection, hemorrhage, or inflammation.

TP The site of weakness depends on the location of the spinal cord injury, with cervical spine disease affecting the upper and lower extremities, and thoracic and upper lumbar spine disease affecting the lower extremities. Since the spinal cord ends at L1–L2, lesions lower than this level affect the nerve roots and not the cord itself. Symptoms can have an acute or gradual onset, depending on the etiology of the injury. Patients will often have other associated symptoms, including pain, sensory loss, urinary/fecal incontinence or retention, and insidious gait abnormalities.

Dx Certain aspects of the history can be helpful in determining the etiology of the injury, including a history of cancer, bleeding diathesis, trauma, or osteoarthritis. Diagnostic studies such as CT scans and MRI scans will typically reveal the cause of the injury and should be done urgently when this diagnosis is suspected.

Tx Spinal cord injuries usually require urgent management to avoid irreversible neurologic deficits. Treatment may include surgery to prevent spinal cord compression from tumors, intervertebral disk herniations, abscesses, or hemorrhages. Radiation and/or corticosteroids should be offered to eligible patients with tumors compressing the spinal cord. Pain management is often critical in the care of these patients. Physical therapy should be offered after the acute management of a spinal cord injury to minimize permanent disability. **See Cecil Essentials 125.**

Peripheral Neuropathy

Pφ Peripheral nerve damage can be classified into two broad categories: lesions affecting the axons of the nerve (axonal) and lesions affecting the myelin sheath surrounding the axons (demyelinating). Neuropathies often have features of both types of damage depending on the etiology, but one type of damage typically predominates. The most common cause of diffuse, symmetrical sensory and motor neuropathy is diabetes mellitus. Less common causes include other metabolic, inherited, infective, inflammatory, toxic, and paraneoplastic diseases.

TP Age at presentation varies depending on etiology. Most patients with diabetic neuropathy present after several years of poor glycemic control. Weakness is typically preceded by several years of sensory abnormalities, including numbness, pain, and paresthesias. The onset is insidious and slowly progressive over years. Symptoms are invariably symmetrical and distal, with a "stocking–glove" distribution affecting the distal limbs and slowly ascending proximally over time. Characteristic weakness may include bilateral foot drop with a "slapping gait" due to limited dorsiflexion of the feet. Absent deep tendon reflexes, particularly distally and in the distribution of symptoms, are also characteristic.

Dx AChR antibodies are found in ~85% of cases. Myasthenic patients lacking AChR antibodies may have circulating antibodies specific to muscle-specific receptor tyrosine kinase (MuSK). RNS studies demonstrate a decremental muscle response to repeated stimulation, correlating with clinical findings of fatigue with exercise. The edrophonium test involves administration of acetylcholinesterase inhibitor (edrophonium chloride) in incremental doses followed by observation of the patient for an abrupt improvement in symptoms. All patients presenting with acquired myasthenia require CT of the chest to exclude the presence of a thymoma (present in 10% to 20% of myasthenic patients).

Tx Pharmacologic treatment includes symptomatic and immunosuppressant medications. Pyridostigmine bromide (Mestinon) is the first-line cholinesterase inhibitor for alleviation of weakness and fatigue. Prednisone is the first choice for immunosuppressant therapy and is indicated when symptoms are not adequately controlled by cholinesterase inhibitors. **See Cecil Essentials 132.**

Myopathy

Pφ Myopathies are a broad group of disorders causing impairment in the function and/or structure of skeletal muscle. Pathophysiology is determined by whether the cause is hereditary (i.e., muscular dystrophy) or acquired (i.e., inflammatory myopathies). Myopathic features on muscle biopsy include possible inflammatory infiltration and/or atrophy in clinically weak muscles.

TP Age at presentation is variable. Symmetrical proximal weakness without sensory symptoms always warrants investigation for myopathy. The most common myopathic condition encountered in adults is inclusion body myositis (IBM), which is characterized by slowly progressive proximal and distal weakness generally after the age of 50 years. The hallmark of IBM is early weakness and atrophy of the quadriceps, forearms, and ankle dorsiflexors. Polymyositis and dermatomyositis also manifest as symmetrical proximal muscle weakness; cutaneous manifestations of dermatomyositis (i.e., Gottron papules or periorbital heliotrope rash) may precede the onset of muscle disease. Different myopathies preferentially affect different muscle groups, making categorization of the pattern of weakness imperative in diagnosing these conditions.

Dx Serum CK is elevated in most patients with muscle disease. Electrophysiologic studies confirm the clinical diagnosis by revealing myopathic features on needle EMG. Muscle biopsy of a clinically weak muscle can also help confirm the diagnosis. In addition, it can also help pinpoint the etiology of muscle disease by revealing characteristic histologic features. Molecular genetic testing can also be performed if a hereditary condition is suspected (e.g., dystrophin in Duchenne muscular dystrophy).

Tx Management is determined by the cause of the disease. Acquired inflammatory myopathies may respond to immunomodulating therapy such as corticosteroids (prednisone). Immunosuppressive therapy (e.g., methotrexate, azathioprine, or IV immunoglobulin) can be employed as a second-line intervention if the disease is refractory to steroids. IBM responds poorly to immunosuppressive therapy. All patients with muscle disease require physical and occupational therapy to help maintain and build strength. **See Cecil Essentials 131.**

ZEBRA ZONE

a. **Amyotrophic lateral sclerosis (ALS, Lou Gehrig disease, motor neuron disease):** Progressive degeneration of the anterior horn cells causes asymmetric weakness with atrophy and fasciculations in skeletal muscles of the face, pharynx, thorax, and limbs. Lower motor neuron weakness is always coupled with upper motor neuron signs, such as hyperreflexia with Babinski signs. This degenerative disease is associated with very high mortality, and most patients succumb to respiratory compromise due to progressive weakness of the pharynx and loss of airway protection.

b. **Neurosarcoidosis:** Sarcoidosis is an inflammatory granulomatous disorder that can affect the central and/or peripheral nervous systems. Five percent of patients with sarcoidosis will have a neurologic manifestation of the disease. The most common age at onset is during the fourth or fifth decade of life. Diagnostic aids include MRI, electrophysiology studies, and laboratory studies (including CSF analysis and serum angiotensin-converting enzyme [ACE] levels). Symptomatic muscle, nerve, or brain biopsy can help confirm the diagnosis. Treatment is primarily with steroids and immunosuppression.

Systems-Based Practice

Practice Guidelines Facilitate Process Improvement

Quality improvement initiatives provide guidelines for improving health-care access, delivery, and management. The American Stroke Association's (ASA) Get with the Guidelines (GWTG) initiative was designed to help ensure continuous quality improvement of acute-stroke treatment and ischemic-stroke prevention. This initiative is practiced in all designated Primary Stroke Centers and helps ensure that stroke patients at these institutions are treated and discharged appropriately according to current best-practice guidelines. Designated GWTG coordinators at each stroke center are responsible for ascertaining whether acute-stroke patients are diagnosed quickly and treated in accordance with these guidelines, such as quick delivery of t-PA to patients fulfilling appropriate criteria. Following acute treatment, GWTG also involves care team protocols following hospital discharge to ensure that patients are monitored appropriately (e.g., cholesterol management and dysphagia screening).

Index

Note: Page numbers followed by f refer to figures; page numbers followed by t refer to tables; page numbers followed by b refer to boxes.

A
AAVRT (antidromic atrioventricular reentrant/reciprocating tachycardia), 111b–112b
Abbreviations, and medical errors, 536–537
ABCDE, of melanoma, 451
Abdominal examination
  for arrhythmias, 106
  for chest pain, 69
  for constipation, 325
  for jaundice, 348
  for testicular mass, 433
Abdominal pain, 281–293
  due to acute intermittent porphyria, 289
  due to acute mesenteric ischemia, 288b–289b
  algorithmic evaluation of, 291b–292b
  due to appendicitis, 282, 286b
  case on, 281
  due to celiac artery compression syndrome, 289
  due to cholecystitis, 283b–284b
  due to choledocholithiasis, 284b–285b
  clinical entities for, 283b–289b
  differential diagnosis of, 281b
  due to diverticulitis, 282, 285b
  due to functional disorders, 291
  due to hereditary angioedema, 289
  jaundice with, 347
  location of, 282
  due to pancreatitis, 286b–288b
    nutrition support for, 290
  patient care for, 282
    clinical thinking in, 282
    discussion of bowel habits in, 290–291
    history in, 282
    imaging considerations in, 283b
    physical examination in, 282
    tests for consideration in, 282
  due to perforated viscus, 283b
  during pregnancy, 292
  speaking intelligently on, 281b
  zebra zone for, 289b
Abdominal radiographs
  for abdominal pain, 283b
  for constipation, 326b

Abdominal tenderness
  constipation with, 325
  with nausea and vomiting, 296
Abdominal ultrasound
  for abdominal pain, 291
  for jaundice, 350b
ABG (arterial blood gas)
  for acid-base disorders, 222
  for dyspnea, 147
  for polyuria and polydipsia, 500
ABO incompatibility, 387
Abscess
  epidural, 42
  skin and soft-tissue, 609b–610b
Abuse, and GI complaints, 345
ACABS (acute community-acquired bacterial sinusitis), 620b, 623
Acanthosis nigricans, paraneoplastic, 485
Access to care
  in community, 231
  and emergency department visits, 724–725
  physician as patient advocate for, 749
Accountable Care Organizations (ACOs), 565
ACE (angiotensin-converting enzyme), serum concentration of, 399
ACE (angiotensin-converting enzyme) inhibitors, for hypertension
  essential, 128b–131b
  due to renal disease, 132b
Acetylcholine receptor (AChR) antibodies, in myasthenia gravis, 745b–746b
Achalasia
  dysphagia due to, 307b
  pseudo-, 307b
Acid, 220
Acid-base disorder(s), 219–232
  anion gap in, 220–221
  case on, 219
  clinical entities for, 223b–229b
  compensation in, 220
  contraction alkalosis as, 228b–229b
  differential diagnosis of, 219b
  expected changes in, 221t
  due to GI loss of HCO_3, 227b–228b
  ketoacidosis as, 225b–226b

Acid-base disorder(s) *(Continued)*
  lactic acidosis as, 224b–225b
  due to methanol and ethylene glycol
    poisoning, 223b–224b
    fomepizole for, 230
  due to milk-alkali syndrome, 229b
  mixed, 220
  patient care for, 220
    clinical thinking in, 220–221
    history in, 221
    physical examination in, 221–222
    stepwise approach to, 220–221
    tests for consideration in, 222
  renal tubular acidosis as, 228b
  due to salicylate intoxication, 227b
  speaking intelligently on, 219b–220b
  due to uremia, 226b
  due to ureteral diversion, 230
  zebra zone for, 230b
Acid-base status, for electrolyte disorders,
    234
Acidosis
  lactic, 224b–225b
  metabolic, 220, 221t
    due to salicylate intoxication,
      227b
    due to uremia, 226b
    due to ureteral diversion, 230
  renal tubular, 228b
  respiratory, 220, 221t
Acid-peptic disease, nausea and vomiting
    due to, 293b–294b
ACOs (Accountable Care Organizations),
    565
Acoustic neuroma, 734
Acoustic schwannoma, 734
Acquired cystic kidney disease, 270, 273b
Acral lentiginous melanoma, 453b–454b
Acromegaly, hypertension due to, 139
ACS. *See* Acute coronary syndrome (ACS).
ACTH (adrenocorticotropic hormone) excess
  Cushing syndrome due to, 523b–524b
  weight gain and obesity due to,
    521–522, 523b–524b
Actinic keratosis, 455b
Activated partial thromboplastin time
    (aPTT), for excessive bleeding or
    clotting, 390
Active surveillance, for prostate cancer,
    423
Activities of daily living (ADLs), with
    Parkinson disease, 709–710
Activity-based cost accounting, 346
Acute bronchitis, 159b–160b, 621b
Acute colonic pseudo-obstruction,
    329b–330b
Acute community-acquired bacterial
    sinusitis (ACABS), 620b, 623
Acute confusional state. *See* Altered mental
    status (AMS).

Acute coronary syndrome (ACS), 67–68
  door-to-balloon time for, 71b–72b, 80
  myocardial infarction as
    non–ST-elevation, 67, 72b
    ST-elevation, 67, 71b–72b
  side conversations during procedures for,
    79
  unstable angina as, 67, 73b
Acute dystonic reaction, 695
Acute inflammatory demyelinating
    polyneuropathy (AIDP), 744b–745b
Acute intermittent porphyria (AIP),
    abdominal pain due to, 289
Acute interstitial nephritis (AIN), 206b
Acute kidney injury (AKI), 199–210
  due to acute intermittent nephritis, 206b
  due to acute tubular necrosis, 206b–207b
  case on, 199
  clinical entities for, 203b–207b
  due to contrast-induced nephropathy,
    210
  defined, 199b–200b
  differential diagnosis of, 199b
  drug-induced, 208b
  due to glomerulonephritis, 205b
  due to heart failure, 203b–204b
  hemodialysis for
    allocation of finite resources of, 210
    risks and benefits of, 209
  due to hemolytic uremic syndrome,
    204b–205b
  models for prognostic stratification and
    risk adjustment with, 208
  patient care for, 200
    clinical thinking in, 200
    history in, 200–201
    imaging considerations in, 202b
    physical examination in, 201
    tests for consideration in, 201
  speaking intelligently on, 199b–200b
  due to thrombotic thrombocytopenic
    purpura, 204b–205b
  due to urinary tract obstruction, 207b
  due to volume depletion, 203b
  zebra zone for, 208b
Acute leukemia, with peripheral
    pancytopenia, 376
Acute mesenteric ischemia, 288b–289b
Acute myelogenous leukemia (AML), 376,
    379b–380b
  prophylactic platelet transfusions for,
    385
Acute renal failure (ARF), prognostic
    stratification and risk adjustment
    models for, 208
Acute retroviral syndrome, rash due to, 601
Acute tubular necrosis (ATN), 206b–207b
Acyclovir
  for genital herpes, 628b–629b
  for varicella zoster virus, 597b–598b

Addison disease, hypoglycemia due to, 514b–515b

Adenitis, cervical, 442b–443b

Adenoma(s)
adrenal
aldosterone-secreting, 462b
cortisol-secreting, 461b–462b
metanephric, 276
pituitary, 545b–546b

ADH (antidiuretic hormone)
in diabetes insipidus, 503b–504b
syndrome of inappropriate secretion of, paraneoplastic, 485, 488b–489b

Adjuvant chemotherapy, for breast cancer, 416b–418b

ADLs (activities of daily living), with Parkinson disease, 709–710

Adnexal mass, incidentally discovered, 464b–465b

Adrenal adenoma
aldosterone-secreting, 462b
cortisol-secreting, 461b–462b, 524

Adrenal hyperplasia, micronodular, weight gain and obesity due to, 524

Adrenal imaging, for hypertension, 128b

Adrenal insufficiency
hypoglycemia due to, 514b–515b
weight loss due to, 535

Adrenal mass, incidentally discovered, 460b–461b
aldosterone-secreting, 462b
benefits and risks of testing for, 469
cortisol-secreting, 461b–462b
evidence-based medicine on, 467
pheochromocytoma as, 463b
primary adrenocortical adenocarcinoma as, 463b–464b

Adrenocortical adenocarcinoma, incidentally discovered, 463b–464b

Adrenocorticotropic hormone (ACTH) excess
Cushing syndrome due to, 523b–524b
weight gain and obesity due to, 521–522, 523b–524b

Advance directive, talk with family with no, 673–674

Advancing Medical Professionalism to Improve Health Care, 7

Aeromonas hydrophila, skin and soft tissue infections with, 613

Afibrinogenemia, 394

Agnogenic myeloid metaplasia (AMM)
pancytopenia due to, 383b–384b
peripheral smear of, 362

AIDP (acute inflammatory demyelinating polyneuropathy), 744b–745b

AIN (acute interstitial nephritis), 206b

AIP (acute intermittent porphyria), abdominal pain due to, 289

Air, on chest radiographs, 188, 189f

Airway, with altered mental status, 665

AKA (alcoholic ketoacidosis), 225b–226b

AKI. See Acute kidney injury (AKI).

Alcohol intoxication, altered mental status due to, 669b

Alcohol use, and osteoporosis, 555

Alcohol withdrawal, altered mental status due to, 669b

Alcoholic hypoglycemia, 512b–513b

Alcoholic ketoacidosis (AKA), 225b–226b

Alcoholism
hypertension secondary to, 133b–134b
screening for, 31b

Aldosterone-secreting adrenal mass, incidentally discovered, 462b

Aldosteronism, primary, hypertension due to, 135b

Alendronate, for fracture risk reduction with osteoporosis, 563

Alkaline phosphatase
and fragility fracture, 556
in jaundice, 349t

Alkalosis
contraction, 228b–229b
metabolic, 220, 221t
hypertension with, 135b
due to milk-alkali syndrome, 229b
volume contraction and, 228b–229b
respiratory, 220, 221t

Allergic contact dermatitis, 51

Allergic rhinitis, 54b

Allergy, medication, 603

Alpha fetoprotein, with jaundice, 349

Alport syndrome, 248b–249b

ALS (amyotrophic lateral sclerosis), 747

Altered mental status (AMS), 663–675
assessing capacity and respecting autonomy with, 674
case on, 663
clinical entities for, 668b–671b
differential diagnosis of, 663b
due to intoxication or substance withdrawal, 669b
due to intracranial hemorrhage, 670b
due to leptomeningeal carcinomatosis, 672
due to meningitis/encephalitis, 668b
due to metabolic encephalopathy, 671b
due to paraneoplastic limbic encephalitis, 672
patient care for, 663
clinical thinking in, 663–664
history in, 664–665
imaging considerations in, 668b
physical examination in, 665–666
talking to family about, 673–674
tests for consideration in, 666
prevention in hospitalized older patients of, 672
speaking intelligently on, 663b
stroke protocol for, 674–675

Altered mental status (AMS) *(Continued)*
  due to subarachnoid hemorrhage,
    670b–671b
  due to systemic infection, 669b–670b
  due to thrombotic thrombocytopenic
    purpura, 672
  zebra zone for, 672b
Alzheimer disease, 679b
  apolipoprotein E*4 in, 677
Ambulatory internal medicine
  common problems in, 35–56
  complex problems in, 56–62
  interpersonal and communication skills
    in, 21–22
  medical knowledge in, 20–21
  patient care in, 19–20
  practice-based learning and improvement
    in, 21
  preventive medicine in, 24–35
  professionalism in, 22–23
  systems-based practice in, 23
  tips for learning in clerkship for, 19–24
Amenorrhea, 538–552
  algorithmic process for diagnosis of,
    552
  due to androgen-secreting tumors, 550
  due to Asherman syndrome, 550
  case on, 538
  clinical entities for, 542b–549b
  consulting with nonphysician members
    of interdisciplinary team for, 552
  defined, 539b
  differential diagnosis of, 539b
  due to hyperthyroidism, 547b
  hypothalamic, 542b–543b
  due to hypothyroidism, 546b
  due to Kallmann syndrome, 550
  due to nonclassical congenital adrenal
    hyperplasia, 550
  patient care for, 539
    clinical thinking in, 539–540
    history in, 540
    imaging considerations in, 542b
    physical examination in, 540–541
    tests for consideration in, 541
  due to pituitary adenoma, 545b–546b
  due to polycystic ovarian syndrome,
    547b–548b
    diagnostic criteria and long-term
      health risks of, 551
  primary, 539b, 540
  due to primary ovarian insufficiency,
    548b–549b
  due to prolactinoma, 543b–544b
  secondary, 539b, 540
  speaking intelligently on, 539b
  tailoring encounter to individual with,
    551–552
  zebra zone for, 550b
Americans with Disabilities Act, 592

AML (acute myelogenous leukemia), 376,
    379b–380b
  prophylactic platelet transfusions for, 385
AMM (agnogenic myeloid metaplasia)
  pancytopenia due to, 383b–384b
  peripheral smear of, 362
Ampullary cancer, jaundice due to, 355
AMS. *See* Altered mental status (AMS).
Amylase
  with jaundice, 349
  with nausea and vomiting, 296
  with polyuria and polydipsia, 500
Amyloidosis, edema due to, 215b
Amyotrophic lateral sclerosis (ALS), 747
ANA (antinuclear antibody) test, for
    chronic joint paint, 580
Androgen deprivation therapy
  bone loss due to, 554
  for prostate cancer, 423
Androgen-secreting tumors, amenorrhea
    due to, 550
Anemia
  aplastic, 376, 378b–379b
  of chronic disease, 47b
  contemporary approach to diagnosis of,
    48
  hemolytic
    autoimmune, 373–374
    microangiopathic, 372–373, 373f
  iron deficiency, 47b
  macrocytic, 45b
  megaloblastic, 376, 380b–381b
  microcytic, 45b
  normocytic, 45b
  sideroblastic, 48
Angina
  intestinal, 288b–289b
  stable, 67
  unstable, 67, 73b
  variant or Prinzmetal, 77
Angiodysplasia, GI bleeding due to,
    315b–316b
Angioedema, hereditary, abdominal pain
    due to, 289
Angiographer, perspective of, 82–86, 84f
Angiography
  for GI bleeding, 314b, 322–323
  for headache, 713b–714b
  interpretation of, 86
Angiomyolipoma, renal, 270, 275b
Angiotensin II receptor blockers (ARBs),
    for hypertension
  essential, 128b–131b
  due to primary renal disease, 132b
Angiotensin-converting enzyme (ACE),
    serum concentration of, 399
Angiotensin-converting enzyme (ACE)
    inhibitors, for hypertension
  essential, 128b–131b
  due to renal disease, 132b

Anion gap, 220–221
  urine, 222
Ankle-brachial index, with polyuria and
    polydipsia, 501
Ankylosing spondylitis, 585b–587b
Anorexia nervosa
  amenorrhea due to, 542b–543b
  weight loss due to, 534b–535b
Anteroposterior (AP) view, 189
Antibiotics
  indiscriminate use of, 345
  for upper respiratory tract infections,
    617, 624–625
Anticoagulation, for atrial fibrillation,
    115–116
Anti–cyclic citrullinated protein (anti-CCP),
    for chronic joint paint, 580
Antidiuretic hormone (ADH)
  in diabetes insipidus, 503b–504b
  syndrome of inappropriate secretion of,
    paraneoplastic, 485, 488b–489b
Antidromic atrioventricular reentrant (or
    reciprocating) tachycardia (AAVRT),
    111b–112b
Anti–glomerular basement membrane
    (anti-GBM) antibody disease,
    hemoptysis due to, 172b–173b
Antihypertensive medications
  for essential hypertension, 128b–131b
  for hypertensive crisis, 128b–131b
Antinuclear antibody (ANA) test, for
    chronic joint paint, 580
Antiphospholipid antibody syndrome,
    583b–585b
Anuria, 200
Aorta, on chest radiographs, 193–194
Aortic coarctation, hypertension due to,
    139
Aortic dissection, chest pain due to,
    73b
Aortic stenosis (AS), congestive heart
    failure due to, 93b–94b
AP (anteroposterior) view, 189
Aplastic anemia, 376, 378b–379b
Apolipoprotein E*4 (APOE*4), in dementia,
    677
Appearance, 9
  with arrhythmias, 106
  with hypertension, 126
  with nausea and vomiting, 296
Appendicitis, 282, 286b
aPTT (activated partial thromboplastin
    time), for excessive bleeding or
    clotting, 390
ARBs (angiotensin receptor blockers), for
    hypertension
  essential, 128b–131b
  due to primary renal disease, 132b
Architectural distortion, in breast mass,
    413, 413f

Aredia (pamidronate), for hypercalcemia of
    malignancy, 486b–488b, 491–493
ARF (acute renal failure), prognostic
    stratification and risk adjustment
    models for, 208
Arrhythmia(s), 103–116
  atrial fibrillation/atrial flutter as,
    108b–109b
    coordinating care in outpatient
      setting for, 115–116
    informed decisions by patient on use
      of anticoagulation for, 115
    patient access to health care and
      follow-up for, 115
    rate control vs. rhythm control for,
      114
  atrioventricular nodal reentrant
      tachycardia (junctional reciprocating
      tachycardia) as, 110b–111b
  atrioventricular reentrant (or
      reciprocating) tachycardia as,
      111b–112b
  case on, 103
  clinical entities for, 108b–113b
  comorbidities with, 105
  differential diagnosis of, 104b
  multifocal atrial tachycardia as, 110b
  patient care for, 105
    clinical thinking in, 105–106
    history in, 104, 106
    imager's initial algorithm in, 107b
    physical examination in, 106–107
    tests for consideration in, 107
  signs associated with, 104
  speaking intelligently on, 104b–105b
  in tachycardia-bradycardia syndrome,
    113
  torsades de pointes as, 113
  ventricular tachycardia as, 112b–113b
  zebra zone for, 113b
Arterial blood gas (ABG)
  for acid-base disorders, 222
  for dyspnea, 147
  for polyuria and polydipsia, 500
Arteriovenous malformation (AVM)
  GI bleeding due to, 315b–316b
  solitary pulmonary nodule due to,
    184b
Arteritis, temporal, headache due to, 38,
    721b–722b
Arthritis
  enteropathic, 585b–587b
  functional history for, 591
  osteo-, 580, 581b–582b
  psoriatic, 585b–587b
  reactive, 585b–587b
  rheumatoid, 582b–583b
    cardiovascular morbidity and mortality
      in women with, 591
    physical examination for, 580

Blood urea nitrogen/creatinine (BUN/Cr) ratio, for acute kidney injury, 201–202
Bloodstream infection (BSI), catheter-related, 652b–653b, 657
BMP. *See* Basic metabolic panel (BMP).
BNP (brain natriuretic peptide)
  for congestive heart failure, 92
  for dyspnea, 147
  for weight loss, 532
Body mass index (BMI), 30b
  for weight gain and obesity, 521
Bone(s), on chest radiographs, 188, 189f, 194
Bone marrow aspiration and biopsy
  for excessive bleeding or clotting, 390
  for lymphadenopathy, 399
  for neck mass, 441
  for pancytopenia, 376
Bone marrow disorders, complex discussions about, 385–386
Bone metastases
  back pain due to, 426b
  fragility fracture due to, 563
Book, structure of, 3–4
Bordetella pertussis, 621b, 623
Borrelia burgdorferi, 598b–599b
Bouchard nodes, 581b–582b
Bowel habits, discussion of, 290–291
Bowel sounds, absent, 282
BP. *See* Blood pressure (BP).
BPH (benign prostatic hypertrophy), 264b
BPPV. *See* Benign paroxysmal positional vertigo (BPPV).
Brachytherapy, for prostate cancer, 423
Bradycardia, 119
Brain imaging, for hypertension, 128b
Brain metastases, increased intracranial pressure due to, 479
Brain natriuretic peptide (BNP)
  for congestive heart failure, 92
  for dyspnea, 147
  for weight loss, 532
Brain tumor, headache due to, 718b
Brainstem infarct or hemorrhage, vertigo due to, 732b–733b
BRCA1 and *BRCA2* genes, 420
Breast
  fat necrosis of, 419
  hematoma of, 419
  trauma to, 419
Breast biopsy, 414
  core needle, 414
  excisional, 414
  fine-needle aspiration, 414
  stereotactic, 414
Breast cancer, 416b–418b
  estimating risk of, 26b–27b
  family history of, 420
  male, 419

Breast cancer *(Continued)*
  mammography of, 412–413, 412f
  management of, 416b–418b
  due to metastatic deposits, 419
  National Surgical Breast and Bowel Project for, 419b–420b
  screening for, 26b–27b
Breast conservation therapy, 416b–418b
Breast cyst, 415b
Breast Imaging Reporting and Data System (BI-RADS), 411b, 412t, 421
Breast mass, 409–414
  access to care for, 421
  benign
    due to benign breast nodularity, 415b–416b
    due to cyst, 415b
    due to fibroadenoma, 414b–415b
    mammography of, 411
    due to trauma, 419
  biopsy of, 414
    core needle, 414
    excisional, 414
    fine-needle aspiration, 414
    stereotactic, 414
  case on, 409
  clinical entities for, 414b–418b
  differential diagnosis of, 409b
  malignant, 416b–418b
    family history of, 420
    in male, 419
    mammography of, 412–413, 412f
    due to metastatic deposits, 419
    National Surgical Breast and Bowel Project for, 419b–420b
  mammography of
    architectural distortion in, 413, 413f
    benign, 411
    bilateral screening, 411b
    BI-RADS assessment for, 411b, 412t, 421
    calcifications in, 413, 413f
    diagnostic, 411b
    malignant, 412–413, 412f
  patient care for, 409–410
    clinical thinking in, 409–410
    history in, 410
    imaging considerations in, 411b
    physical examination in, 410
  due to phyllodes tumor, 419
  speaking intelligently on, 409b
  triple test for, 409b
  zebra zone for, 419b
Breast nodularity, benign, 415b–416b
Breast self-exam (BSE), 26b–27b
Bromocriptine, for prolactinoma, 543b–544b
Bronchiectasis, 162b
Bronchitis, acute, 159b–160b, 621b
Bronchogenic cyst, 184b

Bronchoscopy, of solitary pulmonary nodule, 181

Brudzinski sign, headache with, 713

BSE (breast self-exam), 26b–27b

BSI (bloodstream infection), catheter-related, 652b–653b, 657

Buboes, in chancroid, 631b–632b

BUN (blood urea nitrogen), with polyuria and polydipsia, 500

BUN/Cr (blood urea nitrogen/creatinine) ratio, for acute kidney injury, 201–202

Burnout, prevention of, 430

"Butterfly rash," 583b–585b

BV (bacterial vaginosis), 640b–641b

C

CA 19-9, with jaundice, 349

Cabergoline, for prolactinoma, 543b–544b

CAD (coronary artery disease)
aspirin for prevention of, 29b
congestive heart failure due to, 91–92
patient education on risk factor modification for, 79

CAH (congenital adrenal hyperplasia), nonclassical, amenorrhea due to, 550

Cairo-Bishop definition, of tumor lysis syndrome, 474b–476b

Calcifications, in breast mass, 413, 413f

Calcium
in acid-base disorders, 222
for hypocalcemia, 240b
and osteoporosis, 554, 556, 558b–559b
with polyuria and polydipsia, 500

Calcium disorder(s)
history for, 234
hypercalcemia as, 241b–242b
hypocalcemia as, 240b

Calcium stones, 251b–252b, 265b–266b

Call-Fleming syndrome, 722

CAM (Confusion Assessment Method), 682b

CA-MRSA (community-associated methicillin-resistant *Staphylococcus aureus*), 609b–610b, 614–615

Canalith repositioning procedure (CRP), 730b–731b, 734

Cancer. *See* Oncologic disease(s).

Cancer patients, emergencies in. *See* Oncologic emergencies.

Candida albicans, vulvovaginitis due to, 261b–262b

Candida vaginitis, 638b–639b, 644

Candidiasis, vulvovaginal, 638b–639b, 644

Capacity, with altered mental status, 674

Capitation payment, 154

Capnocytophaga canimorsus, cellulitis due to, 608b–609b

Carcinoid syndrome, diarrhea due to, 343

Carcinomatosis, leptomeningeal, 672

Cardiac auscultation
for arrhythmias, 106
for chest pain, 69
for hypertension, 126

Cardiac catheterization
for congestive heart failure, 93
door-to-balloon time for, 71b–72b, 80
side conversations during, 79

Cardiac causes, of chest pain, 65b

Cardiac chamber size, on ECG, 122

Cardiac disease
and edema, 212
risk stratification for, 68

Cardiac markers
for arrhythmias, 107
for chest pain, 69

Cardiac silhouette, 193, 194f

Cardiac syndrome X, 77

Cardiomyopathy
dilated, 97b–98b
hypertrophic, 98b–99b
ischemic, 95b–96b
peripartum, 100
restrictive, 99b
stress-induced (tako-tsubo), 77

Cardiovascular disease
chest pain due to, 65–81
congestive heart failure as, 90–103
coronary angiography for, 81–89
electrocardiogram for, 117–123
hypertension as, 123–142
palpitations and arrhythmias as, 103–116

Caregiver
of patient with dementia, 684–685
of patient with Parkinson disease, 709

Carotid bruits
with arrhythmias, 106
with chest pain, 69
with hypertension, 126–127

Case payment, 154

Catecholamines, in pheochromocytoma, 463b

Catheter(s), for coronary angiograms, 86–87

Catheter-related bloodstream infections, 652b–653b, 657

Cavernous sinus thrombosis, 623

Cavity, in chest radiographs, 190–191, 191f

CBC. *See* Complete blood count (CBC).

CCP (cyclic citrullinated peptide) antibodies, for chronic joint paint, 580

CDI (*Clostridium difficile* infection)
diarrhea due to, 337, 345, 655b–656b
fever in hospitalized patient due to, 649, 655b–656b

Cefixime, for gonococcal urethritis, 642b–643b

CMP. *See* Comprehensive metabolic panel (CMP).
Coagulation tests
  for arrhythmias, 107
  for chest pain, 70
Coarctation of aorta, hypertension due to, 139
Cobalamin deficiency, megaloblastic anemia due to, 380b–381b
COBRA (Consolidated Omnibus Budget Reconciliation Act), 311
Cocaine abuse, hypertension secondary to, 133b–134b
Coccidioidomycosis
  rash due to, 602
  solitary pulmonary nodule due to, 183b
Cognitive impairment, mild, 681b
Cold, common, 619b
Colic, biliary, 284b–285b
Colitis
  collagenous, 343
  ischemic, 342b
  lymphocytic, 343
  microscopic, 343
  ulcerative
    diarrhea due to, 339b–340b
    enteropathic arthritis in, 585b–587b
Collagenous colitis, 343
Colloid tumor, 722
Colonic pseudo-obstruction, acute, 329b–330b
Colonoscopy, 27b–28b
  for constipation, 325
  for GI bleeding, 314
  polypectomy during, 330, 332
  preparation for, 331, 332f
  for weight loss, 532b
Colorectal cancer
  colonoscopy for prevention of, 330–331
  constipation due to, 327b
  GI bleeding due to, 319b
  screening for, 27b–28b, 334
Colpitis macularis, 639b–640b
Coma. *See* Altered mental status (AMS).
Common cold, 619b
Communication skills. *See* Interpersonal and communication skills.
Community, access to care in, 231
Community education, on pigmented skin lesions, 459
Community-associated methicillin-resistant *Staphylococcus aureus* (CA-MRSA), 609b–610b, 614–615
Competency(ies), 5–7, 12–13
  defined, 5
  history of, 6
  interpersonal and communication skills as, 6, 12
  medical knowledge as, 6, 12
  patient care as, 6, 12

Competency(ies) *(Continued)*
  practice-based learning and improvement as, 6, 12
  professionalism as, 6, 13
  self-assessment form for, 15b
  vs. structure- and process-based education, 5–6
  systems-based practice as, 6, 13
Complete blood count (CBC)
  for altered mental status, 667
  for arrhythmias, 107
  for chest pain, 70
  for chronic joint pain, 580
  for constipation, 325
  for diarrhea, 337
  for dyspnea, 146
  elevated. *See* Elevated blood counts.
  for excessive bleeding or clotting, 389
  for hypertension, 127
  for jaundice, 349
  for nausea and vomiting, 296
  for neutropenia, 473
  for paraneoplastic syndromes, 486
  for pigmented skin lesions, 451
  for polyuria and polydipsia, 500
  for weight loss, 532
Complex discussions, with patient, 385–386
Complex problems, 56–62
  case on, 56
  financial issues with, 60
  helping patients obtain their medications with, 61
  medication reconciliation with, 60
  patient care for, 58–59
    clinical thinking in, 58
    follow-up in, 59
    history in, 58–59
    physical examination in, 59
    tests for consideration in, 59
  problem list for, 56b
  speaking intelligently on, 57b
Compliance, determining likelihood of, 140
Comprehensive metabolic panel (CMP)
  for altered mental status, 667
  for diarrhea, 337
  for GI bleeding, 314
  for nausea and vomiting, 296
  for paraneoplastic syndromes, 486
  for weight loss, 532
Compression fracture, back pain due to, 42, 426b–427b
Computed tomography (CT)
  for abdominal pain, 283b, 292
  for altered mental status, 668b
  for amenorrhea, 542b
  for chest pain, 70b
  for constipation, 326b
  for cough, 157b
  for dementia, 678b

Computed tomography (CT) *(Continued)*
for dyspnea, 147b
for dysuria, 258b
for excessive bleeding or clotting, 390b
of fragility fracture, 556b–558b
for headache, 713b–714b
for hematuria, 247b
of incidentally detected mass, 467
for jaundice, 350b
for malignant melanoma, 452b
for nausea and vomiting, 297b
of neck mass, 442
for oncologic emergencies, 474b
of renal mass, 271b
for skin and soft tissue infections, 607b
of solitary pulmonary nodule, 180
of testicular mass, 434b
for weakness, 740b
Computed tomography (CT) colonography,
27b–28b
Computed tomography (CT) urography, for
renal mass, 271b
Computed tomography/positron emission
tomography (CT/PET), for malignant
melanoma, 452b
Computerized provider order entry (CPOE)
system, 44
Confidentiality, 10, 176, 357, 518–519
with biopsy results, 311
with sexually transmitted infections,
634
with telephone calls, 492
Confusion. *See* Altered mental status
(AMS).
Confusion Assessment Method (CAM),
682b
Congenital adrenal hyperplasia (CAH),
nonclassical, amenorrhea due to,
550
Congestive heart failure (CHF), 90–103
acute kidney injury due to, 203b–204b
due to aortic stenosis, 93b–94b
due to cardiomyopathy
dilated, 97b–98b
hypertrophic, 98b–99b
ischemic, 95b–96b
peripartum, 100
restrictive, 99b
case on, 90
due to Chagas disease, 100
clinical entities for, 93b–100b
due to coronary artery disease, 91–92
diastolic, 97b
differential diagnosis of, 90b
discussing prognosis and compliance
with therapy for, 101–102
left-sided, 92
due to mitral regurgitation, 94b–95b
monitoring compliance with core
measures for, 102

Congestive heart failure (CHF) *(Continued)*
patient care for, 91
clinical thinking in, 91
history in, 91–92
imaging considerations in, 93b
physical examination in, 92
tests for consideration in, 92
prophylactic implantation of defibrillator
for, 101b
due to pulmonary hypertension,
99b–100b
right-sided, 92
speaking intelligently on, 90b–91b
weight loss due to, 533b
zebra zone for, 100b
Consciousness, 663
level of, 665
Consent, informed, 358, 447
Consolidated Omnibus Budget
Reconciliation Act (COBRA), 311
Consolidation, on chest radiographs, 191,
192f
Constipation, 324–334
due to acute colonic pseudo-obstruction
(Ogilvie syndrome), 329b–330b
case on, 324
clinical entities for, 326b–330b
due to colon cancer, 327b
colonoscopy for prevention of,
330–331
screening for, 334
differential diagnosis of, 324b
due to Hirschsprung disease, 330
due to impaction, 325, 328b,
333–334
due to intussusception, 330
due to irritable bowel syndrome,
326b–327b
medication-related, 328b–329b
patient care for, 324–325
clinical thinking in, 324–325
history in, 325
imaging considerations in, 326b
physical examination in, 325
tests for consideration in, 325
speaking intelligently on, 324b
due to volvulus, 325, 329b
zebra zone for, 330b
Consultation, informing patients and
families about, 481
Contraction alkalosis, 228b–229b
Contrast agent, water-soluble, for adhesive
small bowel obstruction, 302
Contrast-induced nephropathy (CIN), 210
COPD. *See* Chronic obstructive pulmonary
disease (COPD).
Core measures, monitoring compliance
with, 102
Core needle biopsy, of breast mass, 414
Coronary anatomy, 81–82, 82f

Coronary angiography, 81–89
  angiographer's perspective during,
    82–86, 84f
  basic coronary anatomy for, 81–82, 82f
  catheters for, 86–87
  equipment for, 81
  goal of, 81
  indications for, 81
  interpretation of
    exercises on, 87–89, 87f–89f
    helpful clues for, 86
  medical knowledge on, 81
  projections (views) in, 82–86, 84f
    LAO cranial, 86, 86f
    LAO straight, 85, 85f
    RAO caudal, 85, 85f
    RAO cranial, 84, 85f
  thinking like an interventional
    cardiologist with, 86–89
Coronary arteries
  anatomy of, 81–82, 82f
  angiographic views of, 82–86, 84f
Coronary artery disease (CAD)
  aspirin for prevention of, 29b
  congestive heart failure due to, 91–92
  patient education on risk factor
    modification for, 79
Coronary heart disease, risk stratification
    for, 66
Cortisol deficiency, hypoglycemia due to,
    514b–515b
Cortisol levels
  for Cushing syndrome, 524
  for electrolyte disorders, 234
  for weight gain and obesity, 522
Cortisol-secreting adrenal mass
  incidentally discovered, 461b–462b
  weight gain and obesity due to, 524
Cost(s), direct vs. indirect, 346
Cost accounting, activity-based, 346
Costophrenic angles, on chest radiographs,
    193, 193f
Cough, 155–166
  acute, 155b, 156
  due to acute bronchitis, 159b–160b
  due to allergic rhinitis, 54b
  due to aspiration pneumonitis, 164
  due to asthma, 53b
  due to bronchiectasis, 162b
  cases on, 52–53, 155
  chronic, 155b, 156
  clinical entities for, 53b–54b,
    157b–163b
  due to cystic fibrosis, 162b–163b
  differential diagnosis of, 52b, 155b
  evidence-based medicine on, 55
  due to gastroesophageal reflux disease,
    54b
  due to head and neck cancer, 54
  due to influenza, 161b

Cough (Continued)
  patient care for, 52–53, 156
    clinical thinking in, 52, 156
    history in, 53, 156
    imaging considerations in, 157b
    physical examination in, 53, 156
    tests for consideration in, 53, 156
  due to pertussis, 54
  due to pneumonia, 157b–159b
    determining patients' wishes regarding
      mechanical ventilation for, 165
    evidence-based practice guidelines for,
      165
    prediction rule to identify low-risk
      patients with, 164
    preempting future anxieties by
      discussion natural course of,
      164–165
  due to pulmonary embolus, 54
  red flags with, 53
  speaking intelligently on, 155b
  due to tuberculosis, 160b
  zebra zone for, 54b, 164b
Counter-regulatory hormone deficiency,
    hypoglycemia due to, 514b–515b
Courvoisier sign, 354b
Cowden disease, 490
C-peptide level, with polyuria and
    polydipsia, 501
CPOE (computerized physician order entry)
    system, 44
CPPD deposition disease, 574b
  history of, 570
  physical examination for, 570
Cranial nerve exam, for altered mental
    status, 666
Creatine kinase (CK), for weakness, 739
Creatine kinase–isoenzyme B (CK-MB), for
    chest pain, 67, 69
Creatinine, serum
  for edema, 212
  for polyuria and polydipsia, 500
Crescent formation, in glomerulonephritis,
    205b
CREST syndrome, 588b–590b
Creutzfeldt-Jakob disease, 683
Crohn disease
  diarrhea due to, 339b–340b
  enteropathic arthritis in, 585b–587b
  maintenance infliximab for, 344
CRP (canalith repositioning procedure),
    730b–731b, 734
Cryptococcus neoformans
  rash due to, 602
  skin and soft tissue infections with, 613
Crystalluria, in acid-base disorders, 223
CSF. See Cerebrospinal fluid (CSF).
CT. See Computed tomography (CT).
CTIN (chronic tubulointerstitial nephritis),
    249b

Cultural differences, barriers posed by, 303

CURB-65, for pneumonia, 157b–159b

Cushing syndrome
and fragility fracture, 556
hypertension due to, 137b–138b
osteoporosis due to, 559b–560b
pituitary, 524
subclinical, 461b–462b
weight gain and obesity due to, 521–522, 523b–524b

CVC (central venous catheter), bloodstream infection related to, 652b–653b

CVP (central venous pressure), for acute kidney injury, 201

Cyclic citrullinated peptide (CCP) antibodies, for chronic joint paint, 580

Cyclic vomiting syndrome, 301

Cyst
breast, 415b
bronchogenic, 184b
ovarian, 464b–465b

Cystic fibrosis (CF), 162b–163b

Cystic kidney disease, acquired, 270, 273b

Cystic pattern, on chest radiographs, 193

Cystine stones, 251b–252b, 265b–266b

Cystitis
dysuria due to, 260b
evidence-based medicine for, 267
hematuria due to, 252b–253b
hospital-acquired, 650b–652b

Cystoscopy
for dysuria, 258
for hematuria, 247

D

DAH (diffuse alveolar hemorrhage) syndromes, 172b–173b

Dasatinib, for chronic myelogenous leukemia, 367

"DASH" diet, for essential hypertension, 128b–131b

DBP (diastolic blood pressure), 125

DBS (deep brain stimulation), for Parkinson disease, 701b–702b

dcSSc (diffuse cutaneous systemic sclerosis), 588b–590b

D-Dimer test
for dyspnea, 147
for excessive bleeding or clotting, 390
for pulmonary embolism, 74b–75b

Decision makers, identifying, 231

Decision making, physician-patient joint, 468

Decubitus view, 189

Deep brain stimulation (DBS), for Parkinson disease, 701b–702b

"Defensive medicine," 303–304

Defibrillator implantation, for myocardial infarction and reduced ejection fraction, 101b

Delirium. See also Altered mental status (AMS).
dementia due to, 682b
prevention in hospitalized older patients of, 672

Dementia, 675–687
due to Alzheimer disease, 679b
care for caregiver of patient with, 684–685
case on, 675
clinical entities for, 679b–683b
due to Creutzfeldt-Jakob disease, 683
defined, 676
due to delirium, 682b
due to depression, 682b–683b
differential diagnosis of, 675b
driving evaluation for, 685
frontotemporal, 681b
health care proxy and end-of-life care for, 686
Lewy body, 680b–681b
movement abnormalities due to, 706–707
due to mild cognitive impairment, 681b
patient care for, 676
clinical thinking in, 676
history in, 676–677
imaging considerations in, 678b
physical examination in, 677
tests for consideration in, 677
pharmacologic treatment of, 683
pseudo-, 682b–683b
speaking intelligently on, 676b
vascular, 680b
zebra zone for, 683b

Densities, on chest radiographs, 188, 189f

Depression
in caregiver of patient with dementia, 684–685
dementia due to, 682b–683b
screening for, 31b

Dermatitis
allergic contact, 51
atopic, 50b, 51
nummular, 51
seborrheic, 50b

Dermatomyositis
paraneoplastic, 485
weakness due to, 746b–747b

Desquamative inflammatory vaginitis (DIV), 644

Device makers, disclosing relationship with, 102

Dexamethasone, for spinal cord compression, 476b–477b

Dexamethasone suppression test
  for Cushing syndrome, 524
  for weight gain and obesity, 522
DGI (disseminated gonococcal infection)
  rash due to, 600b–601b
  septic arthritis due to, 572b–573b
Diabetes insipidus (DI), 236b–237b
  history of, 499
  polyuria and polydipsia due to,
      503b–504b
Diabetes mellitus
  atherosclerosis in, 139
  gestational, 503b
  hypoglycemia with
    due to counter-regulatory hormone
        deficiency, 514b–515b
    in hospitalized patients, 517
    due to medications, 510b–511b
    proactive communicating regarding
        possible episodes of, 518
  patient care for, 498, 506
    clinical thinking in, 498
    empowering patients to manage their
        disease in, 506
    evidence-based medicine for, 505
    history in, 498–499
    involving families in, 506
    physical examination in, 499
    tests for consideration in, 499
  screening for, 29b
  type 1 (insulin-dependent), 498, 501b
  type 2 (non–insulin-dependent), 498,
      502b–503b
Diabetes-related nausea and vomiting,
      293b–294b
Diabetic diarrhea, 343
Diabetic enteropathy, 343
Diabetic foot infections, 612b–613b,
      614–615
Diabetic ketoacidosis (DKA), 225b–226b
  clinical thinking on, 498
  history of, 498–499
  hyperkalemia in, 500
  phosphorus in, 500
  physical examination in, 499
  treatment of, 225b–226b, 501b
Diabetic nephropathy, edema due to, 216b,
      217
Diabetic neuropathy, 743b–744b
Diagnosis-related groups (DRGs), 506
Diagnostic test, patient refusal of, 255
Dialysis
  allocation of finite resources of, 210
  permitting or restricting access to, 218
  risks and benefits of, 209
Diarrhea, 334–346
  and abuse, 345
  due to carcinoid syndrome, 343
  case on, 334–335
  clinical thinking in, 335–336
  clinical entities for, 338b–342b

Diarrhea (Continued)
  due to Clostridium difficile, 337, 345,
      655b–656b
  due to colitis
    ischemic, 342b
    microscopic, 343
    ulcerative, 339b–340b
  diabetic, 343
  differential diagnosis of, 335b
  factitious, 336, 343
  functional, 340b–341b
  infectious, 338b–339b
  due to inflammatory bowel disease,
      339b–340b
    evidence-based medicine for, 344
  due to irritable bowel syndrome,
      340b–341b
  due to malabsorption, 341b–342b
  medication-induced, 336
  patient care for, 335
    clinical thinking in, 335–336
    history in, 336
    physical examination in, 336–337
    tests for consideration in, 337
  speaking intelligently on, 335b
  zebra zone for, 343b
Diastolic blood pressure (DBP), 125
Diastolic heart failure, 97b
DIC (disseminated intravascular
      coagulation), 391b
Diet(s), 31b
  for diabetes mellitus type 2,
      502b–503b
  for electrolyte disorders, 243
  for essential hypertension, 128b–131b
  for weight gain and obesity, 523
Dieulafoy lesion, 320
Differential count
  for neutropenia, 473
  for paraneoplastic syndromes, 486
Difficult patients, 141
Diffuse alveolar hemorrhage (DAH)
      syndromes, 172b–173b
Diffuse cutaneous systemic sclerosis
      (dcSSc), 588b–590b
Diffuse findings, on chest radiographs,
      191–193
Diffuse parenchymal lung disease, 152b
Dilantin (phenytoin)
  bone loss due to, 554
  for status epilepticus, 692b–693b
Dilated cardiomyopathy, 97b–98b
Diphtheria, 623
Direct costs, 346
Dirofilariasis, solitary pulmonary nodule due
      to, 182b
Disabled, legal provision for treatment of,
      592
Disc herniation, 41b
Discoid lupus, 583b–585b

Disease-modifying antirheumatic drugs (DMARDs), for rheumatoid arthritis, 582b–583b
Disopyramide, hypoglycemia due to, 511b–512b
Disseminated gonococcal infection (DGI) rash due to, 600b–601b
   septic arthritis due to, 572b–573b
Disseminated intravascular coagulation (DIC), 391b
DIV (desquamative inflammatory vaginitis), 644
Diverticulitis, 282, 285b
Diverticulosis, 316b–317b
Diverticulum(i)
   defined, 316b–317b
   Zenker, 301
Dix-Hallpike maneuver, 729f
Dizziness, 726–736
   due to acoustic neuroma, 734
   due to basilar artery migraine, 734
   due to benign paroxysmal positional vertigo, 730b–731b, 734–735
   case on, 726
   due to cerebellar/brainstem infarct or hemorrhage, 732b–733b
   clinical entities for, 730b–733b
   defined, 727b
   differential diagnosis of, 726b
   due to Meniere disease, 731b–732b
   and nystagmus, 728t
   patient care for, 727
      clinical thinking in, 727
      history in, 728
      imaging considerations in, 730b
      physical examination in, 728, 729f
      tests for consideration in, 729
   due to perilymphatic fistula, 733b
   speaking intelligently on, 727b
   due to vestibular neuritis, 731b
   zebra zone for, 734b
DKA. See Diabetic ketoacidosis (DKA).
DMARDs (disease-modifying antirheumatic drugs), for rheumatoid arthritis, 582b–583b
Do Not Intubate (DNI) order, 165
Donovanosis, 632
Door-to-balloon time, 71b–72b, 80
Dopamine agonists
   for Parkinson disease, 701b–702b
   for prolactinoma, 543b–544b
Double-contrast barium enema, for colorectal cancer screening, 27b–28b
Doxycycline, for chlamydia, 642b–643b
DRGs (diagnosis-related groups), 506
Driving evaluation, for dementia, 685
Driving restrictions, with seizures, 697
Drug(s). See also Medication(s).
Drug intoxication, altered mental status due to, 669b

Drug manufacturers, disclosing relationship with, 102
Drug withdrawal, altered mental status due to, 669b
Drug-induced parkinsonism, 706b
   vs. Parkinson disease, 701b–702b
Drug-induced thrombocytopenia, 392b
Dual-energy x-ray absorptiometry (DXA) scan, 29b
   for fragility fracture, 556b–558b
   for patients at risk for osteoporosis, 564–565
Duodenal cancer, jaundice due to, 355
Duodenal ulcers, 314b–315b
"Dysexecutive syndrome," in progressive supranuclear palsy, 703b–704b
Dysfibrinogenemia, 394
Dysnatremia(s)
   history for, 233
   hypernatremia as, 236b–237b
   hyponatremia as, 235b–236b
Dysphagia, 305–311
   due to achalasia, 307b
   due to Barrett esophagus, 311
   case on, 305
   clinical entities for, 307b–309b
   differential diagnosis of, 305b
   due to eosinophilic esophagitis, 308b–309b
   due to esophageal cancer, 307b–308b
      evidence-based medicine for, 310
      patient confidentiality with, 311
      prognosis with, 310–311
   patient care for, 306
      clinical thinking in, 306
      history in, 306
      physical examination in, 306
      tests for consideration in, 306
   due to peptic stricture, 309b
   due to Schatzki ring (esophageal ring), 309b
   speaking intelligently on, 306b
Dyspnea, 145–154
   due to asthma, 149b
   case on, 145
   clinical entities for, 148b–152b
   due to COPD or emphysema, 149b–150b
      hospital reimbursement for, 154
      salmeterol and fluticasone propionate for, 152
   differential diagnosis of, 145b
   due to interstitial lung disease, 152b
   patient care for, 146
      clinical thinking in, 146
      history in, 146
      imaging considerations in, 147b
      physical examination in, 146
      tests for consideration in, 146
   due to pleural effusion, 151b
   due to pneumothorax, 151b

Dyspnea *(Continued)*
    due to pulmonary edema, 148b–149b
    due to pulmonary embolism, 148b
    due to sleep apnea, 150b
    smoking cessation for, 153
    speaking intelligently on, 145b
Dystonic reaction, acute, 695
Dysuria, 256–268
    due to Behcet syndrome, 266
    due to benign prostatic hypertrophy,
        264b
    case on, 256
    clinical entities for, 259b–266b
    due to cystitis, 260b
        evidence-based medicine on, 267
    differential diagnosis of, 256b
    due to epididymo-orchitis, 263b
    due to nephrolithiasis, 265b–266b
    patient care for, 256–258
        clinical thinking in, 256–257
        history in, 257, 267–268
        imaging considerations in, 258b
        physical examination in, 257–258
        psychological, 268
        tests for consideration in, 258
    due to prostatitis, 262b–263b
    due to pyelonephritis, 260b–261b
    due to sexually transmitted infection,
        268
    speaking intelligently on, 256b
    due to urethral diverticulum, 265b
    due to urethral stricture, 264b–265b
    due to urethritis, 259b
    due to vulvovaginitis, 261b–262b
    zebra zone for, 266b

E
Early Lung Cancer Action Program (ELCAP),
    185
EBV (Epstein-Barr virus), lymphadenopathy
    due to, 401b
ECG. *See* Electrocardiogram (ECG).
Echocardiography
    for arrhythmias, 107b
    for chest pain, 70b
    for dyspnea, 147b
    for edema, 213b
    for hypertension, 127, 128b
Ecthyma gangrenosum, 601–602
Eczema, atopic *vs.* non-atopic, 51
Edema, 211–218
    due to amyloidosis, 215b
    case on, 211
    clinical entities for, 213b–216b
    due to diabetic nephropathy, 216b, 217
    differential diagnosis of, 211b
    due to focal segmental
        glomerulosclerosis, 214b
    due to light-chain deposition disease,
        216

Edema *(Continued)*
    due to membranous nephropathy,
        214b–215b
    due to minimal-change disease,
        213b–214b
    patient care for, 211
        clinical thinking in, 211–212
        history in, 212
        imaging considerations in, 213b
        physical examination in, 212
        tests for consideration in, 212
    pulmonary, 148b 149b
    renal diseases and, 212
    due to systemic lupus erythematosus,
        216
    zebra zone for, 216b
Edrophonium chloride test, for myasthenia
    gravis, 745b–746b
EEG (electroencephalogram)
    for altered mental status, 667
    for seizures, 689
EGD (esophagogastroduodenoscopy)
    for GI bleeding, 314
    for nausea and vomiting, 296
EHR (electronic health record), 44
    and physician-patient relationship,
        723–724
Eikenella corrodens, cellulitis due to,
    608b–609b
Ejection fraction, reduced, defibrillator
    implantation for, 101b
ELCAP (Early Lung Cancer Action Program),
    185
Electrocardiogram (ECG)
    for arrhythmias, 107
    for chest pain, 69
    for congestive heart failure, 92
    for dyspnea, 147
    for hypertension, 127
    indications for, 117
    interpretation of, 117–123
        axis in, 121–122
        evidence of ischemia, injury, or
            infarction in, 122–123
        hypertrophy and chamber size in, 122
        narrative description in, 123, 123f
        rate in, 119
        rhythm in, 119–121, 120f–121f
        systematic approach for, 117–123,
            118f
    for nausea and vomiting, 296
Electroencephalogram (EEG)
    for altered mental status, 667
    for seizures, 689
Electrolyte(s)
    stool, with diarrhea, 338
    urine, in acid-base disorders, 222
Electrolyte disorder(s), 232–244
    access to care for, 243–244
    case on, 232

Electrolyte disorder(s) *(Continued)*
clinical entities for, 235b–242b
diet and nutrition for, 243–244
differential diagnosis of, 232b
due to familial hypokalemic periodic
paralysis, 242
home phlebotomy for, 243–244
hypercalcemia as, 241b–242b
hyperkalemia as, 238b–239b
hypernatremia as, 236b–237b
and central pontine myelinolysis, 242
hypocalcemia as, 240b
hypokalemia as, 237b–238b
hyponatremia as, 235b–236b
patient care for, 233
clinical thinking in, 233
history in, 233–234
physical examination in, 234
tests for consideration in, 234
speaking intelligently on, 233b
zebra zone for, 242b
Electromyography (EMG), for weakness,
739
Electronic health record (EHR), 44
and physician-patient relationship,
723–724
Electronic medical record (EMR). *See*
Electronic health record (EHR).
Electrophysiology studies, for weakness,
739
Elevated blood counts, 361–367
case on, 361
due to chronic myelogenous leukemia,
364b–365b
clinical entities for, 363b–365b
differential diagnosis of, 361b
due to erythrocytosis, 365
due to essential thrombocytosis, 364b
due to granulocytosis, 365
patient care for, 361
clinical thinking in, 361–362
history in, 362
physical examination in, 362
tests for consideration in, 362
due to polycythemia vera, 363b
low-dose aspirin for, 366
speaking intelligently on, 361b
due to thrombocytosis, 365
zebra zone for, 365b
EM (erythema migrans), 598b–599b
E-mail, communication via, 33–34
Embolism, pulmonary
chest pain due to, 74b–75b
cough due to, 54
dyspnea due to, 148b
hemoptysis due to, 174b–175b
Emergencies, oncologic. *See* Oncologic
emergencies.
Emergency department visits, improve
access to care to decrease, 724–725

Emergency Medical Treatment & Labor Act
(EMTALA), 527–528
Emergency medicine physician, for acute
joint pain, 577
Emergency services, ensuring access to,
527–528
Emergency supply, of medications, 61
EMG (electromyography), for weakness,
739
Emphysema, 149b–150b
EMR (electronic medical record). *See*
Electronic health record (EHR).
EMTALA (Emergency Medical Treatment &
Labor Act), 527–528
Encephalitis
altered mental status due to, 668b
headache due to, 715b–716b
paraneoplastic limbic, 672
Encephalopathy
metabolic, 671b
posterior reversible, 722
Endocarditis, bacterial, 172b–173b
Endocrine disease(s)
amenorrhea as, 538–552
fragility fracture as, 553–565
hypoglycemia as, 507–519
hypoglycemia due to, 514b–515b
osteoporosis due to, 555
polyuria and polydipsia as, 497–507
weight gain and obesity as, 519–528
weight loss as, 529–538
End-of-life care, for dementia, 686
Endoscopic evaluation, for diarrhea, 338
Endoscopic retrograde
cholangiopancreatography (ERCP),
for jaundice, 350b
Endoscopic ultrasound (EUS)
for dysphagia, 307
for jaundice, 350b
Enteropathic arthritis, 585b–587b
Enthesitis, due to seronegative
spondyloarthropathy, 585b–587b
Eosinophil(s)
on peripheral smear, 369
urine, for acute kidney injury, 202
Eosinophilic esophagitis, 308b–309b
Epididymo-orchitis
dysuria due to, 263b
testicular mass due to, 436
Epidural abscess, back pain due to, 42
Epilepsy. *See also* Seizures.
diagnosis of, 688
Epilepsy syndrome, 688
Epinephrine deficiency, hypoglycemia due
to, 514b–515b
Epley maneuver, 730b–731b, 734
Epstein-Barr virus (EBV), lymphadenopathy
due to, 401b
ER (estrogen receptor), in breast cancer,
416b–418b

ERCP (endoscopic retrograde cholangiopancreatography), for jaundice, 350b
Ergocalciferol, for osteomalacia, 560b–561b
Erysipelas, 609b
Erythema, with skin and soft tissue infections, 606–607
Erythema migrans (EM), 598b–599b
Erythrocyte sedimentation rate (ESR), for weight loss, 532
Erythrocytosis, 365
Erythromycin, for chancroid, 631b–632b
Esophageal cancer
  dysphagia due to, 307b–308b
  evidence-based medicine for, 310
  patient confidentiality with, 311
  prognosis with, 310–311
Esophageal disease, chest pain due to, 76b
Esophageal dysphagia. See Dysphagia.
Esophageal manometry, 306
Esophageal ring, 309b
Esophagitis, eosinophilic, 308b–309b
Esophagogastric varices, 318b
Esophagogastroduodenoscopy (EGD)
  for GI bleeding, 314
  for nausea and vomiting, 296
Esophagus, Barrett
  dysphagia due to, 311
  and esophageal cancer, 307b–308b
ESR (erythrocyte sedimentation rate), for weight loss, 532
Essential thrombocytosis (ET)
  elevated blood count due to, 364b
  history of, 362
  physical examination for, 362
  tests for consideration in, 363
Essential tremor (ET), 704b–705b
  vs. Parkinson disease, 700
Estradiol level, for amenorrhea, 541, 552
Estrogen deficiency, osteoporosis due to, 554
Estrogen level, for amenorrhea, 541, 552
Estrogen receptor (ER), in breast cancer, 416b–418b
ET (essential thrombocytosis). See Essential thrombocytosis (ET).
ET (essential tremor), 704b–705b
  vs. Parkinson disease, 700
Ethanol-induced hypoglycemia, 512b–513b
Ethylene glycol poisoning, acid-base disorders due to, 223b–224b
EUS (endoscopic ultrasound)
  for dysphagia, 307
  for jaundice, 350b
Evidence-based practice guidelines, 165
Excessive bleeding or clotting, 387–396
  due to acquired factor VIII deficiency, 392b
  due to acquired qualitative platelet disorders, 394

Excessive bleeding or clotting (Continued)
  due to acquired von Willebrand syndrome, 394
  due to afibrinogenemia or dysfibrinogenemia, 394
  case on, 387
  clinical entities for, 390b–393b
  conversations with patients about, 395
  differential diagnosis of, 388b
  due to disseminated intravascular coagulation, 391b
  due to drug-induced thrombocytopenia, 392b
  due to immune thrombocytopenic purpura, 390b–391b
  medication reconciliation with, 396
  due to other clotting factor inhibitors, 394
  patient care for, 388
    clinical thinking in, 388–389
    history in, 389
    imaging considerations in, 390b
    physical examination in, 389
    tests for consideration in, 389
  patient's right to refuse treatment for, 395
  due to platelet aggregation disorders, 394
  due to psychogenic purpura, 394
  speaking intelligently on, 388b
  due to thrombotic thrombocytopenic purpura, 393b
    plasma exchange vs. plasma infusion for, 394
  due to vitamin K deficiency, 393b
  zebra zone for, 394b
Excision margins, for malignant melanoma, 457
Excisional biopsy
  of breast mass, 414
  of pigmented skin lesions, 451
Excisional lymph node biopsy, for lymphadenopathy, 399
Exercise, 31b
  for diabetes mellitus type 2, 502b–503b
  for weight gain and obesity, 523
External-beam radiation therapy, for prostate cancer, 423
Extremity examination
  for arrhythmias, 107
  for chest pain, 69

F
Factitious hypoglycemia, 509, 515b–516b
Factor VIII deficiency, acquired, 392b
Famciclovir
  for genital herpes, 628b–629b
  for varicella zoster virus, 597b–598b
Familial hypokalemic periodic paralysis, 242

Family history
 of breast cancer, 420
 of hypertension, 126
Family Medical Leave Act, 592
Family members
 anticipating disagreements among, 231
 caring for, 186, 537
Fasciitis, necrotizing, 611b
Fasting blood glucose, for diabetes
  mellitus, 498
Fasting glucose, 29b
Fasting lipid profile, 29b
Fasting plasma glucose, for polyuria and
  polydipsia, 499
Fat malabsorption, diarrhea due to,
  341b–342b
Fat necrosis, of breast, 419
Fatigue
 due to anemia
  of chronic disease, 47b
  contemporary approach to diagnosis
   of, 48
  iron deficiency, 47b
  macrocytic, 45b
  microcytic, 45b
  sideroblastic, 48
 case study on, 45–46
 clinical entities for, 47b
 differential diagnosis of, 45b
 patient care for, 46
  clinical thinking in, 46
  history in, 46
  physical examination in, 46
  tests for consideration in, 46
 speaking intelligently on, 45b
 due to thalassemia, 48
 zebra zone for, 48b
FDG-PET (18-fluorodeoxyglucose positron
   emission tomography), of solitary
   pulmonary nodule, 180
FDPs (fibrin degradation products), for
   excessive bleeding or clotting, 390
Fecal impaction, constipation due to, 325,
  328b, 333–334
Fecal leukocytes, for diarrhea, 337
Fecal occult blood testing (FOBT), 27b–28b
Feedback, 11
Female athlete triad, 542b–543b
FE$_{Na}$ (fractional excretion of sodium), for
   acute kidney injury, 202
Fever
 in cancer patient, 471, 471b
  neutropenic, 473, 477b–479b
 in hospitalized patient, 647–660
  case on, 647
  due to catheter-related bloodstream
   infection, 652b–653b, 657
  clinical entities for, 650b–656b
  clinical thinking on, 648

Fever *(Continued)*
  due to *Clostridium difficile* infection,
   649, 655b–656b
  differential diagnosis of, 647b
  history of, 648–649
  due to hospital-acquired pneumonia,
   650b, 654b–655b
  due to hospital-acquired UTI,
   649–650, 650b–652b
  imaging considerations for, 650b
  keeping patients apprised of ongoing
   evaluations for, 658
  due to malignant hyperthermia, 657
  due to neuroleptic malignant
   syndrome, 657
  patient care for, 648
  physical examination for, 649
  due to serotonin syndrome, 657
  speaking intelligently on, 648b
  tests for consideration for, 649
  zebra zone for, 657b
FHA (functional hypothalamic amenorrhea),
  542b–543b
Fiberoptic bronchoscopy, for hemoptysis,
  168
Fibrin degradation products (FDPs), for
   excessive bleeding or clotting, 390
Fibroadenoma, 414b–415b
Fibroma
 neck mass due to, 444b–445b
 solitary pulmonary nodule due to, 184b
Fibromyalgia, 587b–588b
Financial issues, 60
Fine-needle aspiration (FNA) biopsy
 of breast mass, 414
 of neck mass, 441, 446
Finger-stick blood glucose
 for altered mental status, 666
 for hypertension, 127
 for polyuria and polydipsia, 499
Flexible sigmoidoscopy, for constipation,
  325
Fluconazole, for vulvovaginal candidiasis,
  644
Fluid, on chest radiographs, 188, 189f
18-Fluorodeoxyglucose positron emission
   tomography (FDG-PET), of solitary
   pulmonary nodule, 180
Fluoroquinolones, hypoglycemia due to,
  511b–512b
Fluticasone propionate, for COPD, 152
FNA (fine-needle aspiration) biopsy
 of breast mass, 414
 of neck mass, 441, 446
FOBT (fecal occult blood testing), 27b–28b
Focal segmental glomerulosclerosis (FSGS),
  214b
Folic acid deficiency, 380b–381b
Follicle-stimulating hormone (FSH) level,
   for amenorrhea, 541, 552

Folliculitis, due to *Pseudomonas* species, 613
Folstein Mini-Mental State Examination, for dementia, 678
Fomepizole, for methanol poisoning, 230
Foot infections, diabetic, 612b–613b, 614–615
Foot ulcers, diabetic, 612b–613b, 614–615
Foreign bodies, on chest radiographs, 194–195
Fosphenytoin, for status epilepticus, 692b–693b
FOUR score, 665
Fractional excretion of sodium (FE$_{Na}$), for acute kidney injury, 202
Fracture(s), compression, 42, 426b–427b
Fragility fractures, 553–565
  case on, 553
  clinical entities for, 558b–562b
  differential diagnosis of, 553b
  due to metastatic cancer to bone, 563
  due to multiple myeloma, 562b
  due to osteogenesis imperfecta, 563
  due to osteomalacia, 560b–561b
  due to osteoporosis
    alendronate for risk reduction for, 563
    identification and treatment of patients at risk for, 564–565
    primary, 558b–559b
    secondary to medical conditions, 559b–560b
  due to Paget disease, 561b–562b
  patient care for, 554
    clinical thinking in, 554
    history in, 554–555
    imaging considerations in, 556b–558b
    physical examination in, 555
    tests for consideration in, 555
  patient education on, 564
  speaking intelligently on, 553b
  zebra zone for, 563b
Free thyroxine (free T$_4$)
  for amenorrhea, 552
  for weight loss, 532
Frontotemporal dementia, 681b
FSGS (focal segmental glomerulosclerosis), 214b
FSH (follicle-stimulating hormone) level, for amenorrhea, 541, 552
Functional bowel disease, 291
Functional diarrhea, 340b–341b
Functional history, for arthritis, 591
Functional hypothalamic amenorrhea (FHA), 542b–543b
Funduscopic exam, for chest pain, 68
Fungal pathogens
  lymphadenopathy due to, 442
  rash due to, 602

G
GABHS (group A β-hemolytic streptococcus), pharyngitis due to, 621b–622b
GAD (glutamic acid decarboxylase) antibodies, with polyuria and polydipsia, 501
Gallbladder inflammation, 283b–284b
Gallstone(s)
  abdominal pain due to, 284b–285b
  acute pancreatitis due to, 286b–288b
  jaundice due to, 352b
Gallstone ileus, 301
Gangrene, gas, 613
Gardner syndrome, 490
Gardnerella vaginalis, 640b–641b
Gas gangrene, 613
Gastric antral vascular ectasia (GAVE) syndrome, 320
Gastric cancer, GI bleeding due to, 319b–320b
Gastric emptying, for nausea and vomiting, 297b
Gastric ulcers, 314b–315b
Gastroenteritis, 293b–294b, 297b–298b
Gastroesophageal reflux disease (GERD)
  chest pain due to, 76b
  cough due to, 54b
  dysphagia due to, 309b
Gastrointestinal (GI) bleeding, 312–323
  due to arteriovenous malformation, 315b–316b
  case on, 312
  clinical entities for, 314b–320b
  due to colon cancer, 319b
  due to Dieulafoy lesion, 320
  differential diagnosis of, 312b
  due to diverticulosis, 316b–317b
  due to esophagogastric varices, 318b
  due to gastric antral vascular ectasia syndrome, 320
  due to gastric cancer, 319b–320b
  due to hemorrhoids, 317b
  due to Mallory-Weiss tear, 320
  patient care for, 312
    clinical thinking in, 312–313
    history in, 313
    imaging considerations in, 314b
    multidisciplinary, 321
    nasogastric tube in, 313
    nonjudgmental, 322
    physical examination in, 313
    tests for consideration in, 313
  due to peptic ulcer disease, 314b–315b
  evidence-based medicine for, 320
  speaking intelligently on, 312b
  time-efficient systems-based approach to diagnosis of, 322–323
  zebra zone for, 320b

Gastrointestinal (GI) disease
  abdominal pain as, 281–293
  chest pain due to, 65b
  constipation as, 324–334
  diarrhea as, 334–346
  esophageal dysphagia as, 305–311
  gastrointestinal bleeding as, 312–323
  jaundice as, 346–358
  nausea and vomiting as, 293–305
Gastroparesis, 300b–301b
Gatifloxacin, hypoglycemia due to,
    511b–512b
Gaucher disease, 384
GAVE (gastric antral vascular ectasia)
    syndrome, 320
GBS (Guillain-Barré syndrome),
    744b–745b
GC infection. *See* Gonococcal (GC)
    infection.
Genetic testing, for weight gain and
    obesity, 522
Genital herpes, 627, 628b–629b, 633
Genital ulcers, 625–635
  case on, 625–626
  due to chancroid, 631b–632b
  clinical entities for, 628b–632b
  differential diagnosis of, 626b
  due to granuloma inguinale
    (donovanosis), 632
  due to herpes simplex virus, 627,
    628b–629b, 633
  HIV screening for, 635
  due to lymphogranuloma venereum, 627,
    632
  noninfectious etiologies of, 632
  patient care for, 626
    clinical thinking in, 626–627
    confidentiality in, 634
    history in, 627, 634
    physical examination in, 627
    tests for consideration in, 627
  speaking intelligently on, 626b
  due to syphilis, 627, 630b–631b
  zebra zone for, 632b
GERD (gastroesophageal reflux disease),
    chest pain due to, 76b
Germ cell tumors, nonseminomatous, 434,
    435b–436b
German measles, 601
Gestational diabetes mellitus, 503b
Get with the Guidelines (GWTG), 750
GI. *See* Gastrointestinal (GI).
Giant hairy nevus, 456
Gifts, from patients, 154
Gilbert syndrome, 348
Glasgow Coma Scale, 665
Gleason score, 422–423
Glomerulonephritis (GN)
  acute kidney injury due to, 205b
  post-streptococcal, 172b–173b

Glomerulosclerosis, focal segmental, 214b
Glucagon deficiency, hypoglycemia due to,
    514b–515b
Glucocorticoid excess
  bone loss due to, 554
  hypertension due to, 137b–138b
  obesity due to, 521–522, 523b–524b
  osteoporosis due to, 559b–560b
Glucose
  fasting, 29b
    for diabetes mellitus, 498
    for polyuria and polydipsia, 499
  finger-stick
    for altered mental status, 666
    for hypertension, 127
    for polyuria and polydipsia, 499
  random plasma, for polyuria and
    polydipsia, 499
Glutamic acid decarboxylase (GAD)
    antibodies, with polyuria and
    polydipsia, 501
Glycosylated hemoglobin, for polyuria and
    polydipsia, 499–500
GN (glomerulonephritis)
  acute kidney injury due to, 205b
  post-streptococcal, 172b–173b
Gonococcal (GC) infection
  cervicitis/urethritis due to, 642b–643b
  disseminated
    rash due to, 600b–601b
    septic arthritis due to, 572b–573b
  septic arthritis due to, 571, 572b–573b,
    576–577
Goodpasture syndrome, 172b–173b
Gottron papules, 485
Gout, 573b–574b
  history of, 570
  physical examination for, 570
  pseudo-
    history of, 570
    physical examination for, 570
Gram-negative organisms, cellulitis due to,
    608b–609b
Granulocytosis, 365
Granuloma inguinale, 632
Granulomatosis, Wegener, 172b–173b
Graves disease
  amenorrhea due to, 547b
  weight loss due to, 534b
Grieving, for patients, 430
Group A β-hemolytic streptococcus
    (GABHS), pharyngitis due to,
    621b–622b
Group A streptococcus, erysipelas due to,
    609b
Group B streptococcus, cellulitis due to,
    608b–609b
Growth hormone deficiency
  hypoglycemia due to, 514b–515b
  weight gain and obesity due to, 526

Guillain-Barré syndrome (GBS), 744b–745b
GWTG (Get with the Guidelines), 750

H
HA (hypothalamic amenorrhea), 542b–543b
Haemophilus ducreyi, 631b–632b
Haemophilus influenzae
  acute community-acquired bacterial sinusitis due to, 620b
  otitis media due to, 622b–623b
Hamartoma, solitary pulmonary nodule due to, 182b–183b
Hand hygiene, in infection control, 659
HAP (hospital-acquired pneumonia), 650b, 654b–655b
Hashimoto thyroiditis, 524b–525b
HCAPS (Hospital Consumer Assessment of Healthcare Providers and Systems), 736
HCG (human chorionic gonadotropin), with nausea and vomiting, 296
HCM (hypertrophic cardiomyopathy), 98b–99b
HCO₃- (bicarbonate)
  in acid-base disorders, 222
  GI loss of, 227b–228b
  with polyuria and polydipsia, 500
HDL (high-density lipoprotein) level, screening for, 29b
Head and neck cancer
  cough due to, 54
  human papillomavirus and, 440
  squamous cell carcinoma as, 443b
Headache(s), 710–726
  acute-onset, 711
  due to Call-Fleming syndrome, 722
  case on, 35–38, 710
  clinical entities for, 37b–38b, 714b–722b
  cluster, 37b, 720b–721b
  due to colloid tumor, 722
  differential diagnosis of, 35b, 711b
  evidence-based medicine on, 38
  long-standing recurrent, 711
  due to mass lesion, 718b
  due to meningitis and encephalitis, 715b–716b
  migraine, 37b–38b, 716b–717b
    basilar artery, 734
    evidence-based medicine on, 38, 722
    vs. seizures, 694
  patient care for, 36–38, 711
    clinical thinking in, 36, 711
    history in, 36, 712
    imaging considerations in, 713b–714b, 725
    physical examination in, 36, 712–713
    tests for consideration in, 36–38, 713

Headache(s) *(Continued)*
  due to posterior reversible encephalopathy syndrome, 722
  practice-based learning and improvement for, 38b–39b
  primary *vs.* secondary, 35b
  due to pseudotumor cerebri, 719b–720b
  speaking intelligently on, 36b, 711b
  due to spontaneous CSF leak, 722
  subacute-onset, 711
  due to subarachnoid hemorrhage, 38, 714b–715b
  due to temporal arteritis, 38, 721b–722b
  tension, 37b
  due to venous sinus thrombosis, 719b
  zebra zone for, 38b, 722b
Health Insurance Portability and Accountability Act (HIPAA), 33–34, 176, 357, 518–519
Healthcare proxy, for dementia, 686
Heart failure
  congestive. *See* Congestive heart failure (CHF).
  diastolic, 97b
Heart rate, 119
Heart rhythm, 119–121, 120f–121f
Heart silhouette, 193, 194f
Heart sounds, 106
Heberden nodes, 581b–582b
Heliotrope rash, 485
Hemangioma, neck mass due to, 444b–445b
Hematemesis, 312b
Hematocele, 436
Hematochezia, 312b
Hematocrit
  for excessive bleeding or clotting, 389
  for GI bleeding, 313
Hematologic disease
  elevated blood counts due to, 361–367
  excessive bleeding or clotting due to, 387–396
  lymphadenopathy and splenomegaly due to, 396–406
  pancytopenia due to, 375–387
  peripheral smear for, 368–374
Hematoma, of breast, 419
Hematuria, 244–255
  due to Alport syndrome, 248b–249b
  associated symptoms with, 246
  case on, 244
  due to chronic tubulointerstitial nephritis, 249b
  cigarette smoking and, 246
  clinical entities for, 247b–253b
  due to cystitis, 252b–253b
  degree of, 246
  differential diagnosis of, 245b
  evidence-based medicine on, 254b
  family history for, 246

Hematuria *(Continued)*
due to hyperuricosuria and
hypercalciuria, 254
due to IgA nephropathy, 247b–248b
due to nephrolithiasis, 251b–252b
due to papillary necrosis, 253b
patient care for, 245
clinical thinking in, 245
history in, 246
imaging considerations in, 247b
physical examination in, 246
tests for consideration in, 246
due to polycystic kidney disease,
249b–250b
recent skin infections or URIs and, 246
due to sickle cell disease, 254
speaking intelligently on, 245b
toxin exposure and, 246
due to transitional cell carcinoma,
250b–251b
zebra zone for, 254b
Hemidiaphragms, on chest radiographs, 193
Hemodialysis
allocation of finite resources of, 210
permitting or restricting access to, 218
risks and benefits of, 209
Hemoglobin
for excessive bleeding or clotting, 389
with GI bleeding, 313
glycosylated, for polyuria and polydipsia,
499–500
Hemoglobin A_{1c} (HgA_{1c}), 29b
for polyuria and polydipsia, 499–500
Hemoglobinuria, paroxysmal nocturnal, 384
Hemolytic anemia
autoimmune, 373–374
microangiopathic, 372–373, 373f
Hemolytic transfusion reaction, 387
Hemolytic uremic syndrome (HUS),
204b–205b
Hemoptysis, 166–177
due to aspergilloma (mycetoma),
171b–172b
case on, 166
clinical entities for, 168b–175b
cryptogenic, 175
defined, 166b–167b
differential diagnosis of, 166b
and communication priorities, 176
due to diffuse alveolar hemorrhage
syndromes, 172b–173b
intensivists in ICU for, 176–177
due to lung cancer, 170b–171b
massive, 167
patient care for, 167
clinical thinking in, 167
history in, 167
imaging considerations in, 168b
physical examination in, 167
tests for consideration in, 168

Hemoptysis *(Continued)*
patient confidentiality with, 176
due to pulmonary embolism, 174b–175b
speaking intelligently on, 166b–167b
due to tuberculosis, 168b–169b
Hemorrhage
intracranial, 670b
subarachnoid
altered mental status due to,
670b–671b
headache due to, 38, 714b–715b
Hemorrhagic bullous cellulitis, 613
Hemorrhoids, 317b
Hepatic mass, incidentally discovered, 466b
Hepatitis
jaundice due to, 350b–351b
pancytopenia due to, 384
Hepatobiliary iminodiacetic acid (HIDA)
scan, for abdominal pain, 292
Hepatocellular causes, of jaundice, 347b,
348–349
Hepatolenticular degeneration, 707
HER2/neu status, in breast cancer,
416b–418b
Hereditary angioedema, 289
Hereditary spherocytosis, 374, 374f
Hernia, inguinal, 432b
Herpes, genital, 627, 628b–629b, 633
Herpes simplex virus (HSV)
cervicitis and urethritis due to,
642b–643b
genital ulcers due to, 627, 628b–629b,
633
Herpes simplex virus (HSV) encephalitis,
headache due to, 715b–716b
Herpes zoster, 597b–598b
Herpes zoster vaccine, 30b–31b, 602
Heterophile antibody test, for
lymphadenopathy and splenomegaly,
398
HgA_{1c} (hemoglobin A_{1c}), 29b
for polyuria and polydipsia, 499–500
HHM (humoral hypercalcemia of
malignancy), 486b–488b
HIDA (hepatobiliary iminodiacetic acid)
scan, for abdominal pain, 292
High-density lipoprotein (HDL) level,
screening for, 29b
HIPAA (Health Insurance Portability and
Accountability Act), 33–34, 176,
357, 518–519
Hirschsprung disease, 330
Histoplasma capsulatum, solitary pulmonary
nodule due to, 184b
Histoplasmosis, rash due to, 602
HIV. *See* Human immunodeficiency virus
(HIV).
Hodgkin lymphoma
lymphadenopathy due to, 399b–400b
neck mass due to, 444b

Home phlebotomy, 243–244

Hormonal therapy, for prostate cancer, 423

Hospice
    for dementia, 686
    for metastatic cancer, 430–431

Hospital Consumer Assessment of
        Healthcare Providers and Systems
        (HCAPS), 736

Hospital reimbursement, for COPD, 154

Hospital-acquired infections
    catheter-related bloodstream infections
        as, 652b–653b, 657
    with Clostridium difficile, 649, 655b–656b
    pneumonia as, 650b, 654b–655b
    reduction of, 659
    UTIs as, 649–650, 650b–652b

Hospital-acquired pneumonia (HAP), 650b,
        654b–655b

HPV (human papillomavirus), and head and
        neck cancer, 440

11β-HSD2 (11β–hydroxysteroid
        dehydrogenase type 2) deficiency,
        hypertension due to, 135b

HSV (herpes simplex virus)
    cervicitis and urethritis due to,
        642b–643b
    genital ulcers due to, 627, 628b–629b,
        633

HSV (herpes simplex virus) encephalitis,
        headache due to, 715b–716b

Human chorionic gonadotropin (HCG), with
        nausea and vomiting, 296

Human immunodeficiency virus (HIV), 402b
    evidence-based medicine for, 403
    lymphadenopathy due to, 402b
    pancytopenia due to, 384
    rash due to, 601
    RNA testing for, 398–399
    screening for, 635
    testing for, 29b, 33
    weight loss with
        case on, 529
        differential diagnosis of, 529b
        oxandrolone for, 536

Human papillomavirus (HPV), and head and
        neck cancer, 440

Humoral hypercalcemia of malignancy
        (HHM), 486b–488b

Huntington disease, 707

HUS (hemolytic uremic syndrome),
        204b–205b

Hydrocele, 432b

11β-Hydroxysteroid dehydrogenase type 2
        (11βHSD2) deficiency, hypertension
        due to, 135b

Hypercalcemia, 241b–242b
    of malignancy, 486b–488b
    case on, 483
    costs and benefits of medications for,
        492–493

Hypercalcemia (Continued)
    differential diagnosis of, 483b
    evidence-based medicine for, 491
    physical examination for, 485
    polyuria and polydipsia due to, 504b

Hypercalciuria, hematuria due to, 254

Hypercortisolism
    in Cushing syndrome, 523b–524b
    subclinical, 461b–462b

Hyperglycemia
    clinical entities for, 501b–504b
    clinical thinking on, 498
    history of, 498–499
    physical examination for, 499
    tests for consideration with, 499

Hyperinsulinism. See Hypoglycemia.

Hyperkalemia, 238b–239b
    with polyuria and polydipsia, 500
    in tumor lysis syndrome, 474b–476b

Hyperleukocytosis, 479

Hypernatremia, 236b–237b

Hyperparathyroidism
    and fragility fracture, 555–556
    hypercalcemia due to, 241b–242b
    hypertension due to, 138b
    osteoporosis due to, 559b–560b

Hyperphosphatemia, in tumor lysis
        syndrome, 474b–476b

Hyperprolactinemia, amenorrhea due to,
        543b–544b

Hypertension, 123–142
    due to acromegaly, 139
    due to alcoholism and substance abuse,
        133b–134b
    due to aldosteronism and other
        mineralocorticoid excess states,
        135b
    and atherosclerosis in diabetes, 139
    case on, 123–124
    clinical entities for, 128b–138b
    due to coarctation of aorta, 139
    complications of, 128b–131b
    cost-effectiveness of treatment of, 141
    due to Cushing syndrome and
        glucocorticoid excess, 137b–138b
    definition of, 124–125
    determining likelihood of compliance
        with, 140
    differential diagnosis of, 124b
    difficult patients with, 141
    essential, 128b–131b
    hypertensive crisis with, 128b–131b
    with hypokalemia and metabolic
        alkalosis, 135b
    iatrogenic, 133b
    idiopathic intracranial, 719b–720b
    due to impaired autonomic reflexes and
        autonomic dysfunction, 139
    "masked," 128b–131b
    due to obesity, 136b

Hypertension *(Continued)*
due to other endocrine diseases, 138b
patient care for, 124
clinical thinking in, 124–125
history in, 125–126
imaging considerations in, 128b
physical examination in, 126–127
tests for consideration in, 127
due to pheochromocytoma, 134b
pre-, 125
due to primary (parenchymal) renal
disease, 132b
pseudo-, 126
pulmonary, 99b–100b
due to renovascular disease, 136b–137b
screening for, 30b
due to sleep apnea, 136b
speaking intelligently on, 124b
symptoms of, 128b–131b
"white coat," 128b–131b
zebra zone for, 139b
Hypertensive emergencies, 128b–131b
Hyperthermia, malignant, 657
Hyperthyroidism
amenorrhea due to, 547b
hypertension due to, 138b
osteoporosis due to, 559b–560b
radioactive iodine for, 538
weight loss due to, 534b
Hypertrophic cardiomyopathy (HCM),
98b–99b
Hypertrophy, on ECG, 122
Hyperuricemia, in tumor lysis syndrome,
474b–476b
Hyperuricosuria, 254
Hyperviscosity, 479
Hypocalcemia, 240b
in tumor lysis syndrome, 474b–476b
Hypocaloric diets, for weight gain and
obesity, 523
Hypoglycemia, 507–519
alcoholic, 512b–513b
case on, 507
due to cervical cancer, 516
clinical entities for, 510b–516b
due to counter-regulatory hormone
deficiency, 514b–515b
with diabetes
due to counter-regulatory hormone
deficiency, 514b–515b
in hospitalized patients, 517
due to medications, 510b–511b
proactive communicating regarding
possible episodes of, 518
differential diagnosis of, 508b
vs. seizures, 694
factitious, 509, 515b–516b
fasting, 509
due to insulin-secreting tumors
(insulinomas), 513b–514b

Hypoglycemia *(Continued)*
medication-induced
in diabetic patients, 510b–511b
due to factitious administration of
hypoglycemic agents, 509,
515b–516b
in nondiabetic patients, 511b–512b
due to non–insulin-secreting tumors,
514b
patient care for, 508
clinical thinking in, 508–509
history in, 509
physical examination in, 509
tests for consideration in, 510
due to pheochromocytoma, 516
reactive, 508–509
speaking intelligently on, 508b
zebra zone for, 516b
Hypoglycemic agents
for diabetes mellitus type 2,
502b–503b
factitious administration of, 509,
515b–516b
Hypokalemia, 237b–238b
hypertension with, 135b
with polyuria and polydipsia, 500
Hypokalemic periodic paralysis, familial,
242
Hyponatremia, 235b–236b
in malignancy, 483, 483b, 488b–489b
with polyuria and polydipsia, 500
Hypoparathyroidism, hypocalcemia due to,
240b
Hypotension, with altered mental status,
665
Hypothalamic amenorrhea (HA),
542b–543b
Hypothyroidism
amenorrhea due to, 546b
dementia due to, 677
hypertension due to, 138b
weight gain and obesity due to,
524b–525b

I
IADL (instrumental activities of daily
living), in dementia, 676–677
IBD (inflammatory bowel disease)
diarrhea due to, 339b–340b
evidence-based medicine for, 344
IBM (inclusion body myositis),
746b–747b
IBS (irritable bowel syndrome)
constipation due to, 326b–327b
diarrhea due to, 340b–341b
ICD (implantable cardioverter-defibrillator),
101
ICP (intracranial pressure) increase
due to brain metastases, 479
headache with, 712

IDDM (insulin-dependent diabetes mellitus), 498, 501b
Identification, patient, 592
Idiopathic intracranial hypertension (IIH), 719b–720b
IgA (immunoglobulin A) nephropathy, 247b–248b
ILD (interstitial lung disease), 152b
Ileus, 293b–294b
  gallstone, 301
  postoperative, 299b–300b
Imatinib, for chronic myelogenous leukemia, 367
Immune thrombocytopenic purpura (ITP), 390b–391b
Immunization, 30b–31b
Immunoglobulin A (IgA) nephropathy, 247b–248b
Impaction, 325, 328b, 333–334
Impaired physician, 43–44
Implantable cardioverter-defibrillator (ICD), 101
Incidentally discovered mass lesions, 459–470
  adrenal, 460b–461b
    aldosterone-secreting, 462b
    benefits and risks of testing for, 469
    cortisol-secreting, 461b–462b
    evidence-based medicine on, 467
    pheochromocytoma as, 463b
    primary adrenocortical adenocarcinoma as, 463b–464b
  case on, 459
  clinical entities for, 460b–467b
  differential diagnosis of, 459b
  hepatic, 466b
  ovarian, 464b–465b
  patient care for, 460
    clinical thinking in, 460
    history and physical examination in, 460
    physician-patient joint decision making on, 468
    primacy of patient welfare in, 469
    risks and benefits of testing for, 469
  renal, 465b–466b
  solitary pulmonary nodule as, 466b–467b
    delivering unexpected news about, 185–186
    standardized follow-up for, 186, 187t
  speaking intelligently on, 460b
Incidentaloma. See Incidentally discovered mass lesions.
Inclusion body myositis (IBM), 746b–747b
Indirect costs, 346
Infection(s)
  altered mental status due to, 669b–670b
  diabetic foot, 612b–613b, 614–615
  fever in hospitalized patient due to, 647–660

Infection(s) (Continued)
  genital ulcers due to, 625–635
  hospital-acquired
    catheter-related bloodstream, 652b–653b, 657
    with Clostridium difficile, 649, 655b–656b
    pneumonia as, 650b, 654b–655b
    reduction of, 659
    UTIs as, 649–650, 650b–652b
  presenting with rash, 595–604
    accurate documentation of medical information for, 603
    due to bacterial pathogens, 601–602
    case on, 595
    clinical entities for, 597b–601b
    clinical thinking on, 596
    differential diagnosis of, 595b
    due to disseminated gonococcal infection, 600b–601b
    due to fungal pathogens, 602
    history of, 596
    due to Lyme borreliosis, 598b–599b
    due to medication allergy, 603
    patient care for, 596
    physical examination for, 596–597
    punch biopsy for, 604
    due to Rocky Mountain spotted fever, 599b–600b
    speaking intelligently on, 595b–596b
    tests for consideration for, 597
    due to varicella zoster virus, 597b–598b, 602
    due to viral pathogens, 601
    zebra zone for, 601b–602b
  sexually transmitted. See Sexually transmitted diseases (STDs).
  skin and soft-tissue, 604–615
  upper respiratory tract, 616–625
  vaginitis and urethritis due to, 635–646
Infection control, hand hygiene in, 659
Infectious lymphadenopathy, neck mass due to, 442b–443b
Infiltrating ductal carcinoma, 416b–418b
Inflammatory bowel disease (IBD)
  diarrhea due to, 339b–340b
  evidence-based medicine for, 344
Inflammatory lymphadenopathy, 442b–443b
Inflammatory spondyloarthropathies, 42
Infliximab, for Crohn disease, 344
Influenza, 161b
  diagnosis of, 618, 619b
  treatment of, 617, 619b
Influenza vaccine, 30b–31b
Informed consent, 358, 447
Informed decisions, assisting patients in making, 115
Inguinal exam, for testicular mass, 433
Inguinal hernia, 432b

INR. *See* International normalized ratio
(INR).
Inspiration, on chest radiographs, 189–190
Instrumental activities of daily living
(IADL), in dementia, 676–677
Insulin
for diabetes mellitus
type 1, 501b
type 2, 502b–503b
hypoglycemia due to, 510b–511b
Insulin-dependent diabetes mellitus
(IDDM), 498, 501b
Insulinoma, 513b–514b
Insulin-secreting tumors, 513b–514b
Intensivists, 176–177
Interdisciplinary team, coordinating care
of, 577
Interferon-γ release assay, for neck mass,
441
Interlobular pleural effusion, 184b
Internal Medicine Clerkship
appearance in, 9
confidentiality in, 10
duties during, 8–10
feedback during, 11
goals of, 8
learning effectively on, 10–11
teamwork in, 9–10
timeliness in, 9
tips for, 8–11
International normalized ratio (INR)
for atrial fibrillation, 115–116
for GI bleeding, 314
for jaundice, 349
for pigmented skin lesions, 451
Internet, communication via, 33–34
Interpersonal and communication skills, 6,
13
Interstitial lung disease (ILD), 152b
Intestinal angina, 288b–289b
Intoxication, altered mental status due to,
669b
Intracranial hemorrhage, 670b
Intracranial hypertension, idiopathic,
719b–720b
Intracranial mass, headache due to, 718b
Intracranial pressure (ICP) increase
due to brain metastases, 479
headache with, 712
Intraductal papillary mucinous neoplasm
(IPMN), 355
Intravenous pyelogram (IVP), for
hematuria, 247b
Intrinsic renal disease, 199b–200b, 201
Intubation, determining patients' wishes
regarding, 165
Intussusception
constipation due to, 330
nausea and vomiting due to, 301
Invasive ductal carcinoma, 416b–418b

Invasive lobular carcinoma, 416b–418b
IPMN (intraductal papillary mucinous
neoplasm), 355
Iron deficiency anemia, 47b
Irritable bowel syndrome (IBS)
constipation due to, 326b–327b
diarrhea due to, 340b–341b
Ischemic cardiomyopathy, 95b–96b
Ischemic colitis, 342b
Ischemic strokes, in women, aspirin for
prevention of, 29b
Islet cell tumors, 513b–514b
ITP (immune thrombocytopenic purpura),
390b–391b
IVP (intravenous pyelogram), for
hematuria, 247b

J
Jacksonian march, 691b
JAK2 V617F, in polycythemia vera, 363,
363b
Jaundice, 346–358
with abdominal pain, 347
due to autoimmune pancreatitis, 355
due to benign stricture, 353b–354b
case on, 346
due to cholangitis, 353b
due to choledocholithiasis, 352b
due to cirrhosis, 351b–352b
clinical entities for, 350b–354b
differential diagnosis of, 347b
extrahepatic causes of, 347b
due to Gilbert syndrome, 348
hepatocellular causes of, 347b, 348–349
informed consent for procedures for, 358
due to intraductal papillary mucinous
neoplasm, 355
obstructive causes of, 347b, 348–349
due to other periampullary tumors, 355
due to pancreatic adenocarcinoma, 354b
delivering news of, 356–357
patient care for, 347
clinical thinking in, 347
history in, 347–348
imaging considerations in, 350b
physical examination in, 348
tests for consideration in, 348, 349t
due to sarcoidosis, 355
due to sepsis, 355
and severity of liver disease, 355
speaking intelligently on, 347b
zebra zone for, 355b
Joint pain
acute, 569–577
case on, 569
clinical entities for, 571b–575b
clinical thinking on, 570
coordinating care of interdisciplinary
team for, 577

Joint pain *(Continued)*
  differential diagnosis of, 569b
  evidence-based medicine for,
    575b–576b
  due to gonococcal arthritis, 571,
    572b–573b, 576–577
  due to gout, 570, 573b–574b
  history of, 570
  due to nongonococcal septic arthritis,
    571b–572b
  obtaining sexual history for, 576–577
  due to oxalate crystal deposition in
    chronic renal failure, 575
  patient care for, 570
  physical examination for, 570
  due to pseudogout/CPPD deposition,
    570, 574b
  due to rarer forms of septic arthritis,
    575
  speaking intelligently on, 569b
  tests for consideration for, 571
  due to viral arthritis, 575b
  zebra zone for, 575b
  chronic, 578–592
    due to adult-onset Still disease, 590
    case on, 578
    clinical entities for, 581b–590b
    clinical thinking on, 578–579
    differential diagnosis of, 578b
    due to fibromyalgia, 587b–588b
    functional history for, 591
    history of, 579
    imaging considerations for, 581b
    due to osteoarthritis, 580, 581b–582b
    patient care for, 578
    physical examination for, 580
    due to rheumatoid arthritis, 580,
      582b–583b, 591
    due to sarcoidosis, 590
    due to seronegative
      spondyloarthropathies, 585b–587b
    speaking intelligently on, 578b
    due to systemic lupus erythematosus,
      583b–585b
    due to systemic sclerosis, 588b–590b
    tests for consideration for, 580
    zebra zone for, 590b
Joint replacement, patient identification
  for, 592
Junctional reciprocating tachycardia,
  110b–111b
Junctionally generated rhythm, 119

K
Kallmann syndrome, 550
Karyotype analysis, for amenorrhea, 541
Kayser-Fleischer ring, 707
KCl (potassium chloride), for hypokalemia,
  237b–238b
Keratoacanthoma, 456

Keratosis(es)
  actinic, 455b
  seborrheic, paraneoplastic, 486
Kernig sign, headache with, 713
Ketoacidosis, 225b–226b
  alcoholic, 225b–226b
  diabetic, 225b–226b
    clinical thinking on, 498
    history of, 498–499
    hyperkalemia in, 500
    phosphorus in, 500
    physical examination for, 499
    treatment of, 225b–226b, 501b
Ketones
  in acid-base disorders, 222
  in polyuria and polydipsia, 500
Kidney, medullary sponge, 270, 273b–274b
Kidney disease. *See* Renal disease(s).
Kidney injury, acute. *See* Acute kidney
  injury (AKI).
Kidney stones
  dysuria due to, 265b–266b
  hematuria due to, 251b–252b
Klatskin tumor, 355
Klebsiella granulomatis, 632
Koilonychia, 46

L
Lactic acidosis, 224b–225b
Lactobacillus, in vaginal flora, 640b–641b
Lactose intolerance, diarrhea due to,
  341b–342b
LAD (left anterior descending) artery
  anatomy of, 81–82, 82f
  angiographic views of, 83, 84f–85f
Lambert-Eaton myasthenic syndrome
  (LEMS), 485, 489b–490b
Language barriers, 735–736
Language function, with altered mental
  status, 666
Laryngoscopy, for neck mass, 441
Lateral view, 189
Laxative abuse, diarrhea due to, 336, 343
LBP (low back pain). *See* Back pain.
lcSSc (limited cutaneous systemic
  sclerosis), 588b–590b
Learning, during clerkship, 10–11
Left anterior descending (LAD) artery
  anatomy of, 81–82, 82f
  angiographic views of, 83, 84f–85f
Left circumflex (LCX) artery
  anatomy of, 81–82, 82f
  angiographic views of, 83, 84f–85f
Left main coronary artery
  anatomy of, 81–82, 82f
  angiographic views of, 83, 84f
Left-sided heart failure, 92
Leg weakness, in cancer patient, 471, 471b
Legal provision, for treatment of disabled,
  592

Leishmaniasis, visceral, 384
LEMS (Lambert-Eaton myasthenic syndrome), 485, 489b–490b
Lentigo maligna, 453b–454b
Leptin deficiency, weight gain and obesity due to, 526
Leptomeningeal carcinomatosis, 672
Leukemia
  acute, with peripheral pancytopenia, 376
  acute myelogenous
    pancytopenia due to, 376, 379b–380b
    prophylactic platelet transfusions for, 385
  chronic myelogenous, 364b–365b
    clinical trials of tyrosine kinase inhibitors for, 367
    elevated blood count due to, 364b–365b
    history of, 362
    imatinib and dasatinib for, 367
    physical examination for, 362
    prognosis for, 366–367
    tests for consideration in, 362–363
Leukostasis, 479
Levine sign, 66
Levodopa, for Parkinson disease, 701b–702b, 708
Lewy body dementia, 680b–681b
  movement abnormalities due to, 706–707
LFTs. See Liver function tests (LFTs).
LGV (lymphogranuloma venereum), 627, 632
LH (luteinizing hormone) level, for amenorrhea, 541, 552
Licorice, hypertension due to, 135b
Lifelong learning, 405
Light-chain deposition disease, 216
Limbic encephalitis, paraneoplastic, 672
Limited cutaneous systemic sclerosis (lcSSc), 588b–590b
Lipase
  with jaundice, 349
  with nausea and vomiting, 296
  with polyuria and polydipsia, 500
Lipid(s), with polyuria and polydipsia, 501
Lipid panel, 29b
  for hypertension, 127
Lipoma, neck mass due to, 444b–445b
Liver disease
  chronic
    GI bleeding due to, 313
    signs of, 348
  and edema, 212
  prognostic criteria for, 355
Liver function tests (LFTs)
  for abdominal pain, 282
  for altered mental status, 667
  for arrhythmias, 107
  for chest pain, 70

Liver function tests (LFTs) (Continued)
  for edema, 212
  for jaundice, 348–349
Lofgren triad, 590
Lorazepam, for status epilepticus, 692b–693b
Lou Gehrig disease, 747
Low back pain (LBP). See Back pain.
Lumbar puncture (LP)
  for altered mental status, 667
  for headache, 713
  for seizures, 689
  for weakness, 740
Lumpectomy, 416b–418b
Lung cancer
  Early Lung Cancer Action Program for, 185
  hemoptysis due to, 170b–171b
  palliative care for, 428
  solitary pulmonary nodule due to, 181b–182b
Lung cavity, on chest radiographs, 190–191, 191f
Lung fields, on chest radiographs, 190
Lupus, discoid, 583b–585b
Lupus erythematosus, systemic, 583b–585b
  chronic joint pain due to, 583b–585b
  edema due to, 216
  pancytopenia due to, 384
Lupus nephritis, membranous, 583b–585b
Luteinizing hormone (LH) level, for amenorrhea, 541, 552
Lyme borreliosis, 598b–599b
Lyme disease, 598b–599b
Lymph node biopsy
  excisional, for lymphadenopathy, 399
  sentinel, for malignant melanoma, 451
Lymphadenopathy and splenomegaly, 396–406
  due to autoimmune diseases, 403
  case on, 396
  clinical entities for, 399b–402b
  critical laboratory results for, 406
  differential diagnosis of, 397b
  due to Hodgkin lymphoma, 399b–400b
    evidence-based medicine for, 403
  due to malignant diseases, 403
  due to mononucleosis/Epstein-Barr virus, 401b
  with nausea and vomiting, 296
  neck mass due to infectious or inflammatory, 442b–443b
  due to non-Hodgkin lymphoma, 400b–401b
  due to other infections, 403
  patient care for, 397
    clinical thinking in, 397–398
    history in, 398
    physical examination in, 398
    tests for consideration in, 398

Lymphadenopathy and splenomegaly
(Continued)
due to primary HIV infection, 402b
due to sarcoidosis, 401b–402b
speaking intelligently on, 397b
due to storage diseases, 403
zebra zone for, 403b
Lymphocytes, on peripheral smear, 368
Lymphocytic colitis, 343
Lymphogranuloma venereum (LGV), 627,
632
Lymphoma(s)
aggressive, 444
highly aggressive, 444
Hodgkin
lymphadenopathy due to, 399b–400b
neck mass due to, 444b
indolent, 444
non-Hodgkin
lymphadenopathy due to, 400b–401b
neck mass due to, 444b

M
Macrocytic anemia, 45b
Magnetic resonance
cholangiopancreatography (MRCP),
350b
Magnetic resonance imaging (MRI)
for altered mental status, 668b
for amenorrhea, 542b
for back pain in cancer patient, 425b
of breast mass, 411b
for congestive heart failure, 93b
for dizziness or vertigo, 730b
for dysuria, 258b
for excessive bleeding or clotting, 390b
of fragility fracture, 556b–558b
for headache, 713b–714b
for jaundice, 350b
for movement abnormalities, 701b
for oncologic emergencies, 474b
of renal mass, 271b
for skin and soft tissue infections, 607b
of testicular mass, 434b
for weakness, 740b
Major depressive disorder, in caregiver of
patient with dementia, 684–685
Malabsorption, 341b–342b
Malassezia, seborrheic dermatitis due to,
50b
Male breast cancer, 419
Malignancy. See also Oncologic disease(s).
hypercalcemia of, 241b–242b
case on, 483
costs and benefits of medications for,
492–493
differential diagnosis of, 483b
evidence-based medicine for, 491
physical examination for, 485
Malignant hyperthermia, 657

Malignant melanoma, 453b–454b
ABCDE of, 451
excision margins for, 457
imaging considerations for, 452b
sentinel lymph node biopsy for, 451
wide local excision for, 451
Mallory-Weiss tear, 320
Mammography, 26b–27b
architectural distortion on, 413, 413f
of benign mass, 411
bilateral screening, 411b
BI-RADS assessment for, 411b, 412t, 421
calcifications in, 413, 413f
diagnostic, 411b
for low-income or uninsured women, 421
of malignant mass, 412–413, 412f
for weight loss, 532b
Mass lesion, headache due to, 718b
Mastectomy, 416b–418b
MAT (multifocal atrial tachycardia), 110b
MDS (myelodysplastic syndrome), 376,
382b–383b
Measles, 601
Mechanical ventilation, determining
patients' wishes regarding, 165
Mediastinitis, 76b
Medicaid, 61, 448
Medical decision making, practice
guidelines in, 55–56
Medical errors
abbreviations and, 536–537
maintaining honesty in face of, 577
Medical home, patient-centered, 231–232
Medical jargon, in communication with
patient, 405
Medical knowledge, 6, 12
Medical oncologist, 432b
Medicare, 506–507
Medication(s). See also Drug(s).
helping patients to obtain, 61
identification of, 57b
Medication allergy, 603
Medication errors, 519
Medication reconciliation, 60, 396
Medication-induced acute kidney injury,
208b
Medication-induced constipation,
328b–329b
Medication-induced diarrhea, 336
Medication-induced hypertension, 133b
Medication-induced hypoglycemia
in diabetic patients, 510b–511b
due to factitious administration of
hypoglycemic agents, 509,
515b–516b
in nondiabetic patients, 511b–512b
Medication-induced nausea and vomiting,
293b–294b
Medication-induced osteoporosis, 554
Medication-induced rash, 603

Medullary sponge kidney (MSK) disease, 270, 273b–274b

Megaloblastic anemia, 376, 380b–381b

Melanocortin 4 receptor mutations, weight gain and obesity due to, 526

Melanocytic nevi, benign, 456b

Melanoma, 453b–454b
  ABCDE of, 451
  acral lentiginous, 453b–454b
  excision margins for, 457
  imaging considerations for, 452b
  lentigo maligna type of, 453b–454b
  nodular, 453b–454b
  sentinel lymph node biopsy for, 451
  superficial spreading, 453b–454b
  wide local excision for, 451

Melena, 312b

Memantine, for Alzheimer disease, 679b

Membranous lupus nephritis, 583b–585b

Membranous nephropathy, 214b–215b

Memory, with altered mental status, 666

Meniere disease, 731b–732b

Meningismus, 712

Meningitis
  altered mental status due to, 668b
  headache due to, 715b–716b

Meningococcal vaccine, 30b–31b

Meningococcemia, 601–602

Menstrual period, and seizures, 696

Mental status, altered. *See* Altered mental status (AMS).

Mental status examination (MSE), 665–666

Mesenteric ischemia
  acute, 288b–289b
  chronic, 288b–289b

Metabolic acidosis, 220, 221t
  due to salicylate intoxication, 227b
  due to uremia, 226b
  due to ureteral diversion, 230

Metabolic alkalosis, 220, 221t
  hypertension with, 135b
  due to milk-alkali syndrome, 229b
  volume contraction and, 228b–229b

Metabolic encephalopathy, 671b

Metabolic panel
  for acid-base disorders, 222
  for acute kidney injury, 201–202
  for altered mental status, 667
  for arrhythmias, 107
  for back pain in cancer patient, 425
  for chest pain, 69–70
  for chronic joint pain, 580
  for constipation, 325
  for diarrhea, 337
  for GI bleeding, 314
  for hematuria, 247
  for hypertension, 127
  for jaundice, 349
  for nausea and vomiting, 296
  for paraneoplastic syndromes, 486

Metabolic panel *(Continued)*
  for renal mass, 271
  for tumor lysis syndrome, 473
  for weight loss, 532

Metanephric adenomas, 276

Metanephrines, in pheochromocytoma, 463b

Metastasis(es)
  to bone
    back pain due to, 426b
    fragility fracture due to, 563
  to breast, 419
  case on, 423
  clinical entities for, 426b–427b
  differential diagnosis of, 424b, 426b–427b
  palliative care and hospice for, 428b, 430–431
  patient care for, 424
    clinical thinking in, 424
    history in, 424–425, 428–429, 429f
    imaging considerations in, 425b
    physical examination in, 425
    tests for consideration in, 425
  to skin, 456
  from testicular mass, 432b

Methanol poisoning
  acid-base disorders due to, 223b–224b
  fomepizole for, 230

Methicillin-resistant *Staphylococcus aureus* (MRSA), 609b–610b, 614–615

Metoprolol, for acute myocardial infarction, 78

Metronidazole
  for bacterial vaginosis, 640b–641b
  for trichomoniasis, 639b–640b
  for urethritis, 642b–643b

MI. *See* Myocardial infarction (MI).

Microalbumin-to-creatinine ratio, for polyuria and polydipsia, 500

Microangiopathic hemolytic anemia, 372–373, 373f

Microcytic anemia, 45b

Microscopic colitis, 343

Microscopic polyarteritis, 172b–173b

Midnight salivary cortisol, for weight gain and obesity, 522

Migraine headache, 37b–38b, 716b–717b
  basilar artery, 734
  evidence-based medicine on, 38, 722
  vs. seizures, 694

Mild cognitive impairment, 681b

Milk-alkali syndrome, 229b

Mineralocorticoid excess, hypertension due to, 135b

Mini-cog, for dementia, 678

Minimal-change disease, 213b–214b

Mini-Mental State Examination (MMSE), for dementia, 678

Mitral regurgitation (MR), congestive heart failure due to, 94b–95b

Mobiluncus, bacterial vaginosis due to, 640b–641b
Monocytes, on peripheral smear, 369
Monogenic obesity, 526
Mononucleosis, 401b
Monosodium urate crystals, in gout, 573b–574b
Moraxella catarrhalis
  acute community-acquired bacterial sinusitis due to, 620b
  otitis media due to, 622b–623b
Motor exam, for altered mental status, 666
Motor neuron disease, 747
Movement abnormalities, 698–710
  case on, 698
  clinical entities for, 701b–706b
  due to dementia with Lewy bodies, 706–707
  differential diagnosis of, 698b
  due to essential tremor, 704b–705b
  due to Huntington disease, 707
  due to multiple system atrophy, 702b–703b
  due to Parkinson disease, 701b–702b
    dignity and respect for patients with, 709
    family caregivers for, 709
    levodopa for, 708
    support groups and assistive devices for, 709–710
  due to parkinsonism
    drug-induced (tardive), 706b
    vascular, 705b
  patient care for, 699
    clinical thinking in, 699
    history in, 699–700
    imaging considerations in, 701b
    physical examination in, 700
    tests for consideration in, 700
  due to progressive supranuclear palsy, 703b–704b
  speaking intelligently on, 698b–699b
  due to spinocerebellar ataxias, 707
  due to Wilson disease, 707
  zebra zone for, 706b–707b
MPC (mucopurulent cervicitis), 642b–643b
MPDs. *See* Myeloproliferative disorders (MPDs).
MR (mitral regurgitation), congestive heart failure due to, 94b–95b
MRCP (magnetic resonance cholangiopancreatography), 350b
MRI. *See* Magnetic resonance imaging (MRI).
MRSA (methicillin-resistant *Staphylococcus aureus*), 609b–610b, 614–615
MS (multiple sclerosis), 741b–742b
MSA (multiple system atrophy), 702b–703b

MSE (mental status examination), 665–666
MSK (medullary sponge kidney) disease, 270, 273b–274b
Mucopurulent cervicitis (MPC), 642b–643b
Multidisciplinary care, 321
Multifocal atrial tachycardia (MAT), 110b
Multiple myeloma, fragility fracture due to, 562b
Multiple sclerosis (MS), 741b–742b
Multiple system atrophy (MSA), 702b–703b
Muscle biopsy, for weakness, 740
Musculoskeletal exam, for back pain in cancer patient, 425
Musculoskeletal low back pain, 427b
Myasthenia gravis, 745b–746b
Mycetoma, hemoptysis due to, 171b–172b
Mycobacteria, atypical, skin and soft tissue infections with, 613
Mycobacterium marinum, skin and soft tissue infections with, 613
Mycoplasma hominis, bacterial vaginosis due to, 640b–641b
Myeloblasts, on peripheral smear, 369
Myelodysplastic syndrome (MDS), 376, 382b–383b
Myelofibrosis, 383b–384b
Myeloma, multiple, fragility fracture due to, 562b
Myeloproliferative disorders (MPDs)
  patient care for, 361
    clinical thinking in, 361–362
    history in, 362
    physical examination in, 362
  prognosis for, 366–367
Myocardial infarction (MI)
  defibrillator implantation for, 101b
  door-to-balloon time for, 71b–72b, 80
  on ECG, 122
  evidence-based medicine on, 78
  non-ST-elevation (NSTEMI), 67, 72b
  ST-elevation (STEMI), 67, 71b–72b
Myocardial ischemia, on ECG, 122
Myopathy, 746b–747b

N
NAAT (nucleic acid amplification testing), for gonococcus, 642b–643b
Narcolepsy-cataplexy syndrome, *vs.* seizures, 694
Nasogastric (NG) lavage, for GI bleeding, 322–323
Nasogastric (NG) tube
  for GI bleeding, 313
  for nausea and vomiting, 303
National Board of Medical Examiners (NBME) Shelf Examination in Medicine, 8
National Surgical Adjuvant Breast and Bowel Project (NSABP), 419b–420b

Nausea and vomiting, 293–305
due to acid-peptic disease, 293b–294b
due to bezoars, 301
case on, 293
clinical entities for, 297b–301b
due to cyclic vomiting syndrome, 301
diabetes-related, 293b–294b
differential diagnosis of, 293b–294b
due to gastroenteritis, 293b–294b,
297b–298b
due to gastroparesis, 300b–301b
due to ileus, 293b–294b
gallstone, 301
postoperative, 299b–300b
due to intussusception, 301
medication-related, 293b–294b
patient care for, 294–296
clinical thinking in, 294–295
compassion in, 303
history in, 295
imaging considerations in, 297b
nasogastric tube in, 303
physical examination in, 295–296
tests for consideration in, 296
unnecessary, 303–304
due to small bowel obstruction,
293b–294b, 298b–299b
water-soluble contrast agent for, 302
speaking intelligently on, 294b
due to superior mesenteric artery
syndrome, 301
zebra zone for, 301b
due to Zenker diverticulum, 301
NBME (National Board of Medical
Examiners) Shelf Examination in
Medicine, 8
NCSs (nerve conduction studies), 739
Neck mass, 439–448
due to benign neoplasms and congenital
anomalies, 444b–445b
case on, 439
clinical entities for, 442b–446b
differential diagnosis of, 439b
due to infectious or inflammatory
lymphadenopathy, 442b–443b
due to lymphoma (Hodgkin and
non-Hodgkin), 444b
patient care for, 440
clinical thinking in, 440
evidence-based medicine on, 446
history in, 440
imaging considerations in, 442b
Medicaid reimbursement for, 448
physical examination in, 441
practice guidelines on, 447–448
tests for consideration in, 441
speaking intelligently on, 439b–440b
due to squamous cell carcinoma of head
and neck, 443b
due to thyroid cancer, 445b–446b

Necrotizing fasciitis, 611b
Neisseria gonorrhoeae
mucopurulent cervicitis due to,
642b–643b
rash due to, 600b–601b
septic arthritis due to, 572b–573b
urethritis due to, 259b, 642b–643b
Nephritis
acute interstitial, 206b
chronic tubulointerstitial, 249b
membranous lupus, 583b–585b
Nephrolithiasis
dysuria due to, 265b–266b
hematuria due to, 251b–252b
Nephropathy
contrast-induced, 210
diabetic, 216b, 217
membranous, 214b–215b
Nephrotic syndrome, 211b, 213
Nerve conduction studies (NCSs), 739
Neuralgia, postherpetic, 597b–598b, 602
Neuroleptic malignant syndrome, 657
Neurologic abnormalities, with nausea and
vomiting, 296
Neurologic disease
abnormal movements as, 698–710
altered mental status as, 663–675
dementia as, 675–687
dizziness and vertigo as, 726–736
headache as, 710–726
seizures as, 687–697
weakness as, 737–750
Neurologic examination
for arrhythmias, 107
for back pain in cancer patient, 425
for chest pain, 69
Neuroma
acoustic, 734
neck mass due to, 444b–445b
Neurosarcoidosis, 747
Neurosyphilis, 677
Neutropenic fever, 477b–479b
history of, 473
outpatient treatment of, 481–482
patient education about, 481
physical examination for, 473
Neutrophils, on peripheral smear, 369, 369f
Nevus(i)
atypical, 455b
benign, 456b
giant hairy, 456
of Ota and Ito, 456
Spitz, 456
NG (nasogastric) lavage, for GI bleeding,
322–323
NG (nasogastric) tube
for GI bleeding, 313
for nausea and vomiting, 303
NGU (nongonococcal urethritis),
642b–643b

NHL (non-Hodgkin lymphoma)
   lymphadenopathy due to, 400b–401b
   neck mass due to, 444b
NIDDM (non–insulin-dependent diabetes
      mellitus), 498, 502b–503b
Nil disease, 213b–214b
Nitroglycerin, for STEMI, 71b–72b
N-methyl-D-aspartate antagonist, for
      Alzheimer disease, 679b
Nodular melanoma, 453b–454b
Nodular pattern, on chest radiographs, 192,
      192f
Non–English-speaking patients, 735–736
Nongonococcal septic arthritis,
      571b–572b
Nongonococcal urethritis (NGU),
      642b–643b
Non-Hodgkin lymphoma (NHL)
   lymphadenopathy due to, 400b–401b
   neck mass due to, 444b
Non–insulin-dependent diabetes mellitus
      (NIDDM), 498, 502b–503b
Non–insulin-secreting tumors, hypoglycemia
      due to, 514b
Non–islet cell tumors, hypoglycemia due
      to, 514b
Nonjudgmental demeanor, 322
Nonseminomatous germ cell tumors
      (NSGCTs), 434, 435b–436b
Non–small cell lung cancer (NSCLC),
      170b–171b
   metastatic, 428
Non–ST-elevation myocardial infarction
      (NSTEMI), 67, 72b
Normocytic anemia, 45b
NSABP (National Surgical Adjuvant Breast
      and Bowel Project), 419b–420b
NSGCTs (nonseminomatous germ cell
      tumors), 434, 435b–436b
Nuclear bone scan, for fragility fracture,
      556b–558b
Nuclear imaging, for chest pain, 70b
Nucleated red blood cells, on peripheral
      smear, 371, 372f
Nucleic acid amplification testing (NAAT),
      for gonococcus, 642b–643b
Nummular dermatitis, 51
Nutrition
   for acute pancreatitis, 290
   for electrolyte disorders, 243–244
Nystagmus, 728t

O
OAVRT (orthodromic atrioventricular
      reentrant/reciprocating tachycardia),
      111b–112b
Obesity. See Weight gain and obesity.
Obstruction series, for nausea and
      vomiting, 297b
Occult blood, with diarrhea, 337

OCPs (oral contraceptive pills)
   for polycystic ovarian syndrome,
      547b–548b
   and seizures, 696
Ogilvie syndrome, constipation due to,
      329b–330b
25-OH vitamin D, for fragility fracture, 555
Oliguria, 200
OM (otitis media), 622b–623b
Omeprazole, for peptic ulcers, 320
Oncologic disease(s)
   breast mass as, 409–414
   incidentally discovered mass lesions as,
      459–470
   neck mass as, 439–448
   oncologic emergencies in, 470–482
   paraneoplastic syndrome as, 483–493
   pigmented skin lesions as, 449–459
   prostate mass as, 421–431
   testicular mass as, 431–439
   weight loss due to, 533b
Oncologic emergencies, 470–482
   clinical entities for, 474b–479b
   consultation for, 481
   fever as, 471, 471b
      neutropenic, 477b–479b
   hypercalcemia as, 479
   hyperleukocytosis and leukostasis as,
      479
   hyperviscosity as, 479
   increased intracranial pressure as, 479
   low back pain and leg pain as, 471–473,
      471b
   outpatient treatment for, 481–482
   patient care for, 472
      clinical thinking in, 472
      history in, 472–473
      physical examination in, 473
      tests for consideration in, 473
   patient education on, 481
   renal failure as, 470, 470b
   speaking intelligently on, 471b–472b
   spinal cord compression as, 472–473,
      476b–477b
      direct decompressive surgical resection
         for, 480
   superior vena cava syndrome as, 479
   tumor lysis syndrome as, 472–473,
      474b–476b
   zebra zone for, 479b
Oncologist, medical, 432b
Open biopsy, of neck mass, 441
Oral contraceptive pills (OCPs)
   for polycystic ovarian syndrome,
      547b–548b
   and seizures, 696
Orlistat, for weight gain and obesity, 523
Orthodromic atrioventricular reentrant (or
      reciprocating) tachycardia (OAVRT),
      111b–112b

Orthopedic surgeon, for acute joint pain, 577
Oseltamivir, for influenza, 619b
Osmolality
    with acid-base disorders, 222–223
    with polyuria and polydipsia, 500
Osmolar gap, in acid-base disorders, 222–223
Osteoarthritis, 580, 581b–582b
Osteogenesis imperfecta, 563
Osteomalacia, 560b–561b
Osteomyelitis
    back pain due to, 427b
    due to diabetic foot ulcers, 612b–613b
Osteoporosis
    compression fracture due to, 426b–427b
    fragility fractures due to
        alendronate for risk reduction for, 563
        case on, 553
        identification and treatment of patients at risk for, 564–565
        primary, 558b–559b
        secondary to medical conditions, 559b–560b
        speaking intelligently on, 553b
    medication-induced, 554
    patient care for, 554
        clinical thinking in, 554
        history in, 554–555
        imaging considerations in, 556b–558b
        physical examination in, 555
        tests for consideration in, 555
    screening for, 29b
Otitis media (OM), 622b–623b
Outpatient primary care. See Ambulatory internal medicine.
Ova, with diarrhea, 338
Ovarian cancer, incidentally discovered, 464b–465b
Ovarian cyst, incidentally discovered, 464b–465b
Ovarian insufficiency, primary, 548b–549b
Ovarian mass, incidentally discovered, 464b–465b
Oxalate crystal deposition, arthritis due to, 575
Oxandrolone, for HIV-associated weight loss, 536
Oxygenation, with altered mental status, 665

P
P waves, 118, 118f
PA (posteroanterior) view, 189
PAC (plasma aldosterone concentration), for adrenal mass, 462b
Paget disease, fragility fracture due to, 561b–562b
Pain assessment, PQRST method of, 712

Pain history, 424, 428–429, 429f
Pain scales, 429, 429f
Palliative care, for metastatic cancer, 428, 430–431
Palpitations, 103–116
    due to atrial fibrillation/atrial flutter, 108b–109b
        coordinating care in outpatient setting for, 115–116
        informed decisions by patient on use of anticoagulation for, 115
        patient access to health care and follow-up for, 115
        rate control vs. rhythm control for, 108b–109b, 114
    due to atrioventricular nodal reentrant tachycardia (junctional reciprocating tachycardia), 110b–111b
    due to atrioventricular reentrant (or reciprocating) tachycardia, 111b–112b
    case on, 103
    clinical entities for, 108b–113b
    comorbidities with, 105
    differential diagnosis of, 104b
    due to multifocal atrial tachycardia, 110b
    patient care for, 105
        clinical thinking in, 105–106
        history in, 104, 106
        imager's initial algorithm in, 107b
        physical examination in, 106–107
        tests for consideration in, 107
    speaking intelligently on, 104b–105b
    due to tachycardia-bradycardia syndrome, 113
    due to torsades de pointes, 113
    due to ventricular tachycardia, 112b–113b
    zebra zone for, 113b
Pamidronate (Aredia), for hypercalcemia of malignancy, 486b–488b, 491–493
Pancreatic adenocarcinoma, jaundice due to, 354b
Pancreatitis
    abdominal pain due to, 286b–288b
    autoimmune, 355
    nutrition support for, 290
Pancytopenia, 375–387
    acute leukemia with peripheral, 376
    due to acute myelogenous leukemia, 376, 379b–380b
        prophylactic platelet transfusions for, 385
    due to aplastic anemia, 376, 378b–379b
    bone marrow biopsy for, 376
    case on, 375
    clinical entities for, 378b–384b
    complex discussions about, 385–386
    differential diagnosis of, 375b

Pancytopenia *(Continued)*
  due to Gaucher disease, 384
  due to hemolytic transfusion reaction,
    387
  due to hepatitis A, B, and C, 384
  due to HIV, 384
  due to megaloblastic anemia, 376,
    380b–381b
  due to myelodysplastic syndromes, 376,
    382b–383b
  due to myelofibrosis, 383b–384b
  due to paroxysmal nocturnal
    hemoglobinuria, 384
  patient care for, 376
    clinical thinking in, 376–377
    history in, 377
    physical examination in, 377
    tests for consideration in, 378
  due to sarcoidosis, 384
  speaking intelligently on, 375b
  stem cell transplant for, 386
  due to systemic lupus erythematosus,
    384
  due to visceral leishmaniasis, 384
  zebra zone for, 384b
Panic attacks, *vs.* seizures, 694
Pap smear, 28b
Papillary necrosis, hematuria due to,
    253b
Papilledema, due to pseudotumor cerebri,
    719b–720b
Paraneoplastic limbic encephalitis, altered
    mental status due to, 672
Paraneoplastic syndromes, 483–493
  clinical entities for, 486b–490b
  Cowden disease as, 490
  delivering news of, 492
  dermatomyositis as, 485
  Gardner syndrome as, 490
  hypercalcemia as, 486b–488b
    case on, 483
    costs and benefits of medications for,
      492–493
    differential diagnosis of, 483b
    evidence-based medicine for, 491
  hyponatremia as, 483, 483b, 488b–489b
  Lambert-Eaton myasthenic syndrome as,
    485, 489b–490b
  patient care for, 484
    clinical thinking in, 484–485
    history in, 485
    imaging considerations in, 486b
    physical examination in, 485–486
    tests for consideration in, 486
  SIADH as, 485, 488b–489b
  speaking intelligently on, 484b
  Sweet syndrome as, 490
  weakness as, 484, 484b, 489b–490b
  zebra zone for, 490b
Parasites, diarrhea due to, 338

Parathyroid hormone (PTH)
  in calcium homeostasis, 240b
  and fragility fracture, 555–556
  in hypercalcemia of malignancy,
    486b–488b
  with polyuria and polydipsia, 500
Parathyroid hormone–related protein
    (PTHrP), in hypercalcemia of
    malignancy, 486b–488b
Parkinson disease (PD)
  clinical thinking on, 699
  dignity and respect for patients with,
    709
  vs. essential tremor, 700
  family caregivers for, 709
  history of, 699–700
  imaging considerations for, 701b
  levodopa for, 708
  movement abnormalities due to,
    701b–702b
  physical examination for, 700
  vs. secondary parkinsonism, 701b–702b
  speaking intelligently on, 698b–699b
  support groups and assistive devices for,
    709–710
  tests for consideration for, 700
"Parkinson plus" conditions, 701b–702b
Parkinsonism
  drug-induced (tardive), 706b
  vs. Parkinson disease, 701b–702b
  vascular, 705b
Paroxysmal nocturnal hemoglobinuria,
    384
Partial thromboplastin time (PTT), for
    pigmented skin lesions, 451
Partnership for Prescription Assistance
    (PPARx), 61
Pasteurella multocida, cellulitis due to,
    608b–609b
Pathologic fractures, screening for, 29b
Patient(s)
  autonomy of, 255
  identification of, 592
  personal feelings toward, 430
  satisfaction of, 736
Patient advocates, physicians as, 749
Patient care, 6, 12
  permitting or restricting, 218
Patient confidentiality, 10, 176, 311, 357,
    518–519
  with telephone calls, 492
Patient education, for seizures, 696
Patient welfare, primacy of, 469
Patient-centered medical home, 231–232
PCKD. *See* Polycystic kidney disease
    (PCKD).
PCO_2, in acid-base disorders, 222

PCOS (polycystic ovarian syndrome)
    amenorrhea due to, 547b–548b
    diagnostic criteria and long-term health
        risks of, 551
    weight gain and obesity due to, 525b
PD. *See* Parkinson disease (PD).
PDA (posterior descending artery)
    anatomy of, 81–82, 82f
    angiographic views of, 83–84, 84f, 86f
PE. *See* Pulmonary embolism (PE).
Peak flow meter assessment, for dyspnea,
        147
Pelvic ultrasound, for amenorrhea, 542b
Penetration, in chest radiographs, 189–190
Pentamidine, hypoglycemia due to,
        511b–512b
Peptic stricture, dysphagia due to, 309b
Peptic ulcer disease (PUD), 314b–315b
    evidence-based medicine for, 320
Per diem payments, 154
Perforated viscus, abdominal pain due to,
        283b
Periampullary tumors, 355
Pericarditis, 74b
Perilymphatic fistula, 733b
Peripartum cardiomyopathy, 100
Peripheral bone density measurements, for
        fragility fracture, 556b–558b
Peripheral catheter, bloodstream infection
        related to, 652b–653b
Peripheral neuropathy
    with nausea and vomiting, 296
    weakness due to, 743b–744b
Peripheral smear
    Auer rods in, 369, 370f
    for excessive bleeding or clotting,
        389–390
    of hemolytic anemia
        autoimmune, 373–374
        microangiopathic, 372–373, 373f
    of hereditary spherocytosis, 374, 374f
    importance of, 368–374
    nucleated red blood cells on, 371,
        372f
    platelet clumping on, 371, 372f
    of pseudothrombocytopenia, 371, 372f
    schistocytes on, 372–373, 373f
    spherocytes on, 373–374, 374f
    of thrombocytopenia, 370–371, 371f
    white blood cells in, 368–370
        basophils as, 369
        eosinophils as, 369
        lymphocytes as, 368
        monocytes as, 369
        myeloblasts as, 369
        neutrophils as, 369, 369f
Peripheral vascular imaging, for
        hypertension, 128b
Peritonitis, 282
Pertussis, 54, 621b, 623

PET. *See* Positron emission tomography
        (PET).
PFA-100, for excessive bleeding or clotting,
        390
pH, 220
PH (pulmonary hypertension), 99b–100b
Pharmaceutical companies, disclosing
        relationship with, 102
Pharyngitis, 618, 621b–622b, 623
Phenytoin (Dilantin)
    bone loss due to, 554
    for status epilepticus, 692b–693b
Pheochromocytoma
    hypertension due to, 134b
    hypoglycemia due to, 516
    incidentally discovered, 463b
PHI (protected health information),
        518–519
Philadelphia chromosome, 364b–365b
Phlebotomy, home, 243–244
PHN (postherpetic neuralgia), 597b–598b,
        602
Phosphorus, with polyuria and polydipsia,
        500
Phyllodes tumor, 419
Physical activity, 31b
    for diabetes mellitus type 2, 502b–503b
    for weight gain and obesity, 523
Physical inactivity, 31b
Physical therapist, for acute joint pain,
        577
Physician, impaired, 43–44
Physician-patient joint decision making,
        468
Pigmented skin lesions, 449–459
    due to actinic keratosis, 455b
    due to basal cell carcinoma, 452b
    case on, 449
    clinical entities for, 452b–456b
    community education in, 459
    differential diagnosis of, 449b
    due to keratoacanthoma, 456
    due to malignant melanoma,
        453b–454b
    excision margins for, 457
    due to metastatic carcinoma, 456
    due to nevus(i)
        atypical, 455b
        benign, 456b
        giant hairy, 456
        of Ota and Ito, 456
        Spitz, 456
    patient care for, 449
        clinical thinking in, 449–450
        history in, 450
        imaging considerations in, 452b
        physical examination in, 450–451
        preoperative and postoperative
            discussions in, 458
        tests for consideration in, 451

Pigmented skin lesions *(Continued)*
  speaking intelligently on, 449b
  due to squamous cell carcinoma, 453b
  zebra zone for, 456b
Pills, identification of, 57b
Pituitary adenoma, 545b–546b
PKD1, 249b–250b, 272b
PKD2, 249b–250b, 272b
Plain radiographs
  of chest. *See* Chest radiograph(s).
  for fragility fracture, 556b–558b
  for skin and soft tissue infections, 607b
Plasma aldosterone concentration (PAC), for adrenal mass, 462b
Plasma renin activity (PRA), for adrenal mass, 462b
Platelet aggregation disorders, 394
Platelet clumping, 371, 372f
Platelet disorders, acquired qualitative, 394
Platelet transfusions, for acute myeloid leukemia, 385
Pleural effusion
  dyspnea due to, 151b
  solitary pulmonary nodule due to interlobular, 184b
PNES (psychogenic non-epileptic seizure), 693b
Pneumococcal vaccine, 30b–31b
Pneumonia
  community-acquired, 157b–159b
    determining patients' wishes regarding mechanical ventilation for, 165
    evidence-based practice guidelines for, 165
    prediction rule to identify low-risk patients with, 164
    preempting future anxieties by discussion of natural course of, 164–165
  hospital-acquired, 650b, 654b–655b
  ventilator-associated, 654b–655b
Pneumonitis, aspiration, 164
Pneumothorax
  chest pain due to, 75b
  dyspnea due to, 151b
Podagra, 570
POI (primary ovarian insufficiency), 548b–549b
Polyarteritis, microscopic, 172b–173b
Polycystic kidney disease (PCKD), 272b
  clinical thinking on, 270
  empathy in discussing impact of, 277
  evidence-based medicine for, 276
  hematuria due to, 249b–250b
  history of, 270
  physical examination for, 270
  screening for, 277–278

Polycystic ovarian syndrome (PCOS)
  amenorrhea due to, 547b–548b
  diagnostic criteria and long-term health risks of, 551
  weight gain and obesity due to, 525b
Polycythemia vera (PV)
  elevated blood count due to, 363b
  history of, 362
  low-dose aspirin for, 366
  physical examination for, 362
  tests for consideration in, 363
Polydipsia. *See* Polyuria and polydipsia.
Polymyositis, 746b–747b
Polypectomy, colonoscopic, 330, 332
Polyuria and polydipsia, 497–507
  case on, 497
  clinical entities for, 501b–504b
  due to diabetes insipidus, 503b–504b
  due to diabetes mellitus
    empowering patients to manage their disease in, 506
    evidence-based medicine for, 505
    gestational, 503b
    involving families in patient care plan for, 506
    type 1, 501b
    type 2, 502b–503b
  differential diagnosis of, 497b
  due to hypercalcemia, 504b
  patient care for, 498
    clinical thinking in, 498
    history in, 498–499
    physical examination in, 499
    tests for consideration in, 499
  psychogenic (primary), 505
  speaking intelligently on, 497b–498b
  zebra zone for, 505b
Porphyria, acute intermittent, 289
Positron emission tomography (PET)
  for dementia, 678b
  for malignant melanoma, 452b
  for movement abnormalities, 701b
  of neck mass, 442
Post-activation facilitation, 489b–490b
Posterior descending artery (PDA)
  anatomy of, 81–82, 82f
  angiographic views of, 83–84, 84f, 86f
Posterior reversible encephalopathy syndrome (PRES), 722
Posteroanterior (PA) view, 189
Post-exercise facilitation, 489b–490b
Postherpetic neuralgia (PHN), 597b–598b, 602
Postictal state, 690b–691b
Postoperative discussion, for pigmented skin lesions, 458
Postoperative ileus, 299b–300b
Postrenal azotemia, 199b–200b, 201
Post-streptococcal glomerulonephritis, 172b–173b

Potassium, with polyuria and polydipsia, 500
Potassium chloride (KCl), for hypokalemia, 237b–238b
Potassium disorder(s)
   history for, 234
   hyperkalemia as, 238b–239b
   hypokalemia as, 237b–238b
PPARx (Partnership for Prescription Assistance), 61
PQRST method, of pain assessment, 712
PR (progesterone receptor), in breast cancer, 416b–418b
PR interval, 121
PRA (plasma renin activity), for adrenal mass, 462b
Practice guidelines
   evidence-based, 165
   in medical decision making, 55–56
Practice-based learning and improvement, 6, 13
Preauthorization, for medications, 61
Prednisone
   bone loss due to, 554
   for immune thrombocytopenic purpura, 390b–391b
   for temporal arteritis, 721b–722b
Pregnancy
   abdominal pain during, 292
   gestational diabetes mellitus during, 503b
   with seizures, 696
Pregnancy test, for amenorrhea, 541, 552
Prehypertension, 125
Preoperative discussion, for pigmented skin lesions, 458
Preoperative tumor markers, for testicular mass, 432b, 434
Prerenal azotemia, 199b–200b, 200
PRES (posterior reversible encephalopathy syndrome), 722
Prescription assistance program, 61
Presyncope, 727–728
Preventive medicine, 24–35
   case on, 24, 24b–25b
   evidence-based medicine for, 32b–33b
   interpersonal and communication skills for, 33b
   patient care for, 25
      clinical thinking in, 25
      history in, 25–26
      imaging considerations, 26b
      physical examination in, 26
      tests for consideration in, 26
   practice-based learning and improvement in, 32b–33b
   professionalism in, 33b–34b
   screening and prevention strategies in, 26b–31b
      for breast cancer, 26b–27b

Preventive medicine (Continued)
   for cervical cancer, 28b
   for colorectal cancer, 27b–28b
   for depression, 31b
   for diabetes, 29b
   diet and exercise as, 31b
   DXA scan as, 29b
   for HIV, 29b, 33
   for hypertension and obesity, 30b
   immunization as, 30b–31b
   for ischemic strokes and coronary artery disease, 29b
   for lipids, 29b
   for prostate cancer, 32b
   tests to consider in, 29b
   for thyroid disease, 29b
   for tobacco use and alcohol misuse, 31b
   unnecessary, 34
   speaking intelligently in, 25b
   systems-based practice of, 34b
   zebra zone for, 32b
Prevotella, bacterial vaginosis due to, 640b–641b
Primary ovarian insufficiency (POI), 548b–549b
Primum non nocere, 469
Prinzmetal angina, 77
Procedure, patient refusal of, 255
Process improvement, 255
Prodrome, of seizures, 690b–691b
Professionalism, 6, 13
Progesterone receptor (PR), in breast cancer, 416b–418b
Prognosis
   communication to patient of, 310–311
   delivering news of worsening, 492
Progressive supranuclear palsy (PSP), 703b–704b
Prolactin, in amenorrhea, 541, 552
Prolactinoma, amenorrhea due to, 543b–544b
Prostate cancer, 421–431
   active surveillance for, 423
   brachytherapy for, 423
   case on, 422
   external-beam radiation therapy for, 423
   Gleason score for, 422–423
   hormonal therapy for, 423
   radical prostatectomy for, 423
   recurrent/metastatic
      clinical thinking in, 424
      differential diagnosis of, 424b, 426b–427b
      history of, 424–425, 428–429, 429f
      imaging considerations for, 425b
      palliative care and hospice for, 428, 430–431
      patient care for, 424
      physical examination for, 425

Prostate cancer *(Continued)*
　　self-regulation of personal feelings
　　　　toward patients with, 430
　　tests for consideration for, 425
　　screening for, 32
　　speaking intelligently on, 422b–423b
Prostatectomy, radical, 423
Prostate-specific antigen (PSA)
　　screening for, 32
　　with weight loss, 532
Prostatitis, 262b–263b
Protected health information (PHI),
　　518–519
Proteinuria, with edema, 212
Prothrombin time (PT)
　　for excessive bleeding or clotting, 390
　　for GI bleeding, 314
　　for jaundice, 349
　　for pigmented skin lesions, 451
Protozoal pathogens, lymphadenopathy due
　　to, 442
PSA (prostate-specific antigen)
　　screening for, 32
　　with weight loss, 532
"Pseudoachalasia," 307b
Pseudodementia, 682b–683b
Pseudogout, 574b
　　history of, 570
　　physical examination for, 570
Pseudo-hyperkalemia, 238b–239b
Pseudo-hypertension, 126
Pseudomonas aeruginosa, hospital-acquired
　　pneumonia due to, 654b–655b
Pseudomonas species
　　hospital-acquired UTIs due to,
　　　　650b–652b
　　rash due to, 601–602
　　skin and soft tissue infections with, 613
Pseudothrombocytopenia, 371, 372f
Pseudotumor
　　cerebri, 719b–720b
　　solitary pulmonary nodule due to, 184b
PSI model, for pneumonia, 157b–159b
Psoriasis, 51
Psoriatic arthritis, 585b–587b
PSP (progressive supranuclear palsy),
　　703b–704b
Psychogenic non-epileptic seizure (PNES),
　　693b
Psychogenic polydipsia, 505
Psychogenic purpura, 394
Psychological care, for patient with chronic
　　problems, 268
PT. *See* Prothrombin time (PT).
PTH. *See* Parathyroid hormone (PTH).
PTHrP (parathyroid hormone–related
　　protein), in hypercalcemia of
　　malignancy, 486b–488b
PTT (partial thromboplastin time), for
　　pigmented skin lesions, 451

PUD (peptic ulcer disease), 314b–315b
　　evidence-based medicine for, 320
Pugh scoring system, for liver disease, 355
Pulmonary angiogram, for hemoptysis, 168
Pulmonary causes, of chest pain, 65b
Pulmonary disease(s)
　　chest radiograph for, 188–196
　　cough as, 155–166
　　dyspnea as, 145–154
　　hemoptysis as, 166–177
　　pulmonary nodule as, 177–188
Pulmonary edema, 148b–149b
Pulmonary embolism (PE)
　　chest pain due to, 74b–75b
　　cough due to, 54
　　dyspnea due to, 148b
　　hemoptysis due to, 174b–175b
Pulmonary hypertension (PH), 99b–100b
Pulmonary nodule, solitary. *See* Solitary
　　pulmonary nodule (SPN).
Pulmonary-renal syndrome, 172b–173b
Pulse oximetry, for dyspnea, 146
Punch biopsy
　　of pigmented skin lesions, 451
　　of rash, 604
Purpura
　　immune thrombocytopenia, 390b–391b
　　psychogenic, 394
　　thrombotic thrombocytopenic
　　　　acute kidney injury due to, 204b–205b
　　　　altered mental status due to, 672
　　　　excessive bleeding due to, 393b
　　　　plasma exchange *vs.* plasma infusion
　　　　　　for, 394
PV. *See* Polycythemia vera (PV).
Pyelonephritis
　　dysuria due to, 260b–261b
　　hospital-acquired, 650b–652b

Q
QRS complexes, 118, 118f, 121
Qualitative fecal fat, with diarrhea, 338
Quinine, hypoglycemia due to, 511b–512b

R
R waves, 118
RA (rheumatoid arthritis), 582b–583b
　　cardiovascular morbidity and mortality in
　　　　women with, 591
　　physical examination for, 580
Radiation safety, for patients and families,
　　538
Radiation therapy
　　for breast cancer, 416b–418b
　　for prostate cancer, 423
Radical prostatectomy, 423
Radioactive iodine, radiation safety with,
　　538
Radiofrequency catheter ablation, for atrial
　　fibrillation, 108b–109b

Radionuclide scintigraphy, for GI bleeding, 322–323
Radio-opaque foreign bodies, on chest radiographs, 194–195
Random plasma glucose, for polyuria and polydipsia, 499
Rapid antigen detection test (RADT), for streptococcal pharyngitis, 618
Rapid plasma reagin (RPR) titer, for dementia, 677
Rasburicase, for tumor lysis syndrome, 474b–476b
Rash
  due to atopic *vs.* non-atopic eczema, 51
  case study on, 48–49
  clinical entities for, 50b
  due to dermatitis
    allergic contact, 51
    atopic, 50b, 51
    nummular, 51
    seborrheic, 50b
  differential diagnosis of, 49b
  infections presenting with, 595–604
    accurate documentation of medical information for, 603
    due to bacterial pathogens, 601–602
    case on, 595
    clinical entities for, 597b–601b
    clinical thinking on, 596
    differential diagnosis of, 595b
    due to disseminated gonococcal infection, 600b–601b
    due to fungal pathogens, 602
    history of, 596
    due to Lyme borreliosis, 598b–599b
    due to medication allergy, 603
    patient care for, 596
    physical examination for, 596–597
    punch biopsy for, 604
    due to Rocky Mountain spotted fever, 599b–600b
    speaking intelligently on, 595b–596b
    tests for consideration for, 597
    due to varicella zoster virus, 597b–598b, 602
    due to viral pathogens, 601
    zebra zone for, 601b–602b
  patient care for, 49
    clinical thinking in, 49
    history in, 49
    physical examination in, 49
    tests for consideration in, 49
  due to psoriasis, 51
  speaking intelligently on, 49b
  zebra zone for, 51b
Rate control, for atrial fibrillation, 108b–109b, 114
RBCs (red blood cells), nucleated, 371, 372f

RCA (right coronary artery)
  anatomy of, 81–82, 82f
  angiographic views of, 83–84, 84f–85f
Reactive arthritis, 585b–587b
Rectal exam
  for back pain in cancer patient, 425
  for constipation, 325
  for GI bleeding, 313
Red blood cells (RBCs), nucleated, 371, 372f
Referred pain, in back, 42
Reflex testing, for weakness, 739
Reiter syndrome, 585b–587b
Relatives, caring for, 186, 537
Renal angiomyolipoma, 270, 275b
Renal artery imaging, for hypertension, 128b
Renal artery stenosis, 136b–137b
Renal biopsy
  for hematuria, 247
  for renal mass, 271
Renal cancer, 270, 274b–275b
Renal cell carcinoma, 270, 274b–275b
Renal disease(s)
  acquired cystic, 270, 273b
  acute kidney injury as, 199–210
  dysuria as, 256–268
  and edema, 212
  hematuria as, 244–255
  hypertension due to, 132b
  intrinsic, 199b–200b, 201
  medullary sponge kidney as, 270, 273b–274b
  polycystic. *See* Polycystic kidney disease (PCKD).
  renal mass as, 269–278
Renal failure
  arthritis due to oxalate crystal deposition in, 575
  in cancer patients, 470, 470b
Renal injury, acute. *See* Acute kidney injury (AKI).
Renal mass, 269–278
  due to acquired cystic kidney disease, 270, 273b
  due to angiomyolipoma, 270, 275b
  case on, 269
  clinical entities for, 272b–275b
  differential diagnosis of, 269b
  due to hamartoma, 270
  incidentally discovered, 465b–466b
  due to medullary sponge kidney disease, 270, 273b–274b
  due to metanephric adenomas, 276
  patient care for, 269
    clinical thinking in, 269–270
    history in, 270
    imaging considerations in, 271b
    physical examination in, 270–271
    tests for consideration in, 271

Renal mass *(Continued)*
due to polycystic kidney disease, 272b
clinical thinking on, 270
empathy in discussing impact of, 277
evidence-based medicine for, 276
history of, 270
physical examination for, 270
screening for, 277–278
due to renal cancer, 270, 274b–275b
speaking intelligently on, 269b
due to tuberous sclerosis, 270, 275b
due to von Hippel–Lindau disease, 270, 276
zebra zone for, 276b
Renal sonogram, for hematuria, 247b
Renal tubular acidosis (RTA), 228b
Renal ultrasound
for acute kidney injury, 202b
for edema, 213b
for renal mass, 271b
Renovascular disease, 136b–137b
Repetitive nerve stimulation (RNS), for weakness, 739
Resource allocation, 210
Respiratory acidosis, 220, 221t
Respiratory alkalosis, 220, 221t
Respiratory exam
for arrhythmias, 106
for chest pain, 69
Restrictive cardiomyopathy, 99b
Reticular pattern, on chest radiographs, 191–192
Reversible cerebral vasoconstriction, 722
Reynolds' pentad, in cholangitis, 353b
Rheumatoid arthritis (RA), 582b–583b
cardiovascular morbidity and mortality in women with, 591
physical examination for, 580
Rheumatoid factor (RF), 580
Rheumatoid nodule, 184b
Rheumatologic disease(s)
acute joint pain as, 569–577
chronic joint pain as, 578–592
Rhinitis, allergic, 54b
Rhinosinusitis, viral, 619b
and acute community-acquired bacterial sinusitis, 620b
Rhythm control, for atrial fibrillation, 108b–109b, 114
Rickettsia rickettsii, Rocky Mountain spotted fever due to, 599b–600b
Right coronary artery (RCA)
anatomy of, 81–82, 82f
angiographic views of, 83–84, 84f–85f
Right-sided heart failure, 92
RNS (repetitive nerve stimulation), for weakness, 739
Rocky Mountain spotted fever (RMSF), 599b–600b
Rotation, in chest radiographs, 189–190

RPR (rapid plasma reagin) titer, for dementia, 677
RTA (renal tubular acidosis), 228b
Rubella, 601
Rubeola, 601

S
Safety precautions, for seizures, 696–697
Salicylate(s), hypoglycemia due to, 511b–512b
Salicylate intoxication, acid-base disorders due to, 227b
Salmeterol, for COPD, 152
Sarcoidosis
chronic joint pain due to, 590
jaundice due to, 355
lymphadenopathy due to, 401b–402b
pancytopenia due to, 384
weakness due to, 747
SBO (small bowel obstruction)
nausea and vomiting due to, 293b–294b, 298b–299b
water-soluble contrast agent for, 302
SBP (systolic blood pressure), 125
SCAs (spinocerebellar ataxias), 707
SCC. *See* Spinal cord compression (SCC).
SCC (squamous cell carcinoma), 453b
of head and neck, 443b
SCD (sudden cardiac death), due to hypertrophic cardiomyopathy, 98b–99b
Schatzki ring, 309b
Schistocytes, on peripheral smear, 372–373, 373f
Schwannoma, acoustic, 734
Scintillating scotoma, due to migraine, 716b–717b
SCLC (small cell lung cancer), 170b–171b
Screening, 26b–31b
breast cancer, 26b–27b
cervical cancer, 28b
colorectal cancer, 27b–28b, 334
for depression, 31b
for diabetes, 29b
DXA scan for, 29b
for HIV, 29b, 33
for hypertension and obesity, 30b
for lipids, 29b
prostate cancer, 32
tests to consider for, 29b
for thyroid disease, 29b
for tobacco use and alcohol misuse, 31b
unnecessary, 34
Scrotal exam, for testicular mass, 433
Scrotal mass. *See* Testicular mass.
SCS (subclinical Cushing syndrome), 461b–462b
SE (status epilepticus), 692b–693b, 695
Seborrheic dermatitis, 50b
Seborrheic keratoses, paraneoplastic, 486

Secretagogues, hypoglycemia due to,
510b–511b
Seizures, 687–697
aura prior to, 691b–692b
case on, 687
clinical entities for, 690b–693b
differential diagnosis of, 687b
vs. acute dystonic reaction, 695
vs. hypoglycemia, 694
vs. migraine, 694
vs. panic attacks, 694
vs. sensory TIA, 694
vs. sleep disorders, 694
vs. syncope, 694
driving restrictions for, 697
generalized, 688
primary, 688
secondarily, 688
tonic-clonic, 690b–691b
and menstrual period, 696
and oral contraceptives, 696
partial, 688
complex, 688, 691b–692b
simple, 688, 691b
patient care for, 688
clinical thinking in, 688
history in, 689
imaging considerations in, 690b
physical examination in, 689
tests for consideration in, 689
postictal state after, 690b–691b
and pregnancy, 696
prodrome of, 690b–691b
psychogenic non-epileptic, 693b
safety precautions with, 696–697
speaking intelligently on, 687b–688b
due to status epilepticus, 692b–693b,
695
zebra zone for, 694b–695b
Self-assessment form, for competencies,
15b
Self-care, physician's commitment to, 218
Seminomas, 434, 435b
Sentinel lymph node biopsy, for melanoma,
451
Sepsis, jaundice due to, 355
Septic arthritis
clinical thinking on, 570
diagnosis of, 575b–576b
gonococcal, 571, 572b–573b, 576–577
nongonococcal, 571b–572b
physical examination for, 570
rarer forms of, 575
speaking intelligently on, 569b
Septic joint. *See* Septic arthritis.
Seronegative spondyloarthropathies,
585b–587b
Serotonin syndrome, 657
Serum chemistries. *See* Metabolic panel.
Serum creatine kinase, for weakness, 739

Serum creatinine
for edema, 212
for polyuria and polydipsia, 500
Serum ketones
in acid-base disorders, 222
for polyuria and polydipsia, 500
Serum osmolality
in acid-base disorders, 222–223
with polyuria and polydipsia, 500
Serum prolactin, for amenorrhea, 541, 552
Serum protein electrophoresis (SPEP), for
fragility fracture, 556
Serum testosterone, for amenorrhea, 541
Sexual history
for acute joint pain, 576–577
for dysuria, 257, 267–268
five "Ps" for, 634
for genital ulcers, 627, 634
Sexually transmitted disease(s) (STDs),
625–635
case on, 625–626
chancroid as, 631b–632b
clinical entities for, 628b–632b
differential diagnosis of, 626b
granuloma inguinale (donovanosis) as,
632
herpes simplex virus as, 627,
628b–629b, 633
HIV screening for, 635
infection control for partners of patients
with, 268
lymphogranuloma venereum as, 627,
632
maintaining clarity and understanding
nuances in discussing, 645
patient care for, 626
clinical thinking in, 626–627
confidentiality in, 634
history in, 627
physical examination in, 627
tests for consideration in, 627
screening for, 638
speaking intelligently on, 626b
syphilis as, 627, 630b–631b
urethritis due to, 259b
zebra zone for, 632b
Sexually transmitted infections. *See*
Sexually transmitted diseases
(STDs).
Shingles, 597b–598b
Shingles vaccine, 30b–31b, 602
Shortness of breath. *See* Dyspnea.
Shy-Drager syndrome, 702b–703b
SIADH (syndrome of inappropriate secretion
of antidiuretic hormone),
paraneoplastic, 485, 488b–489b
Sibutramine, for weight gain and obesity,
523
Sick sinus syndrome, 113
Sickle cell disease, 254

Side conversations, during procedures, 79
Sideroblastic anemia, 48
Sigmoid volvulus, 325, 329b
Sigmoidoscopy, 27b–28b
  for constipation, 325
Sign of Leser-Trélat, 486
Sinus rhythm, 119–120
Sinusitis, acute community-acquired bacterial, 620b, 623
Six Sigma, 255
Skin
  metastases to, 456
  pigmented lesions of. See Pigmented skin lesions.
Skin abscess, 609b–610b
Skin and soft tissue infection(s) (SSTIs), 604–615
  abscess as, 609b–610b
  with Aeromonas hydrophila, 613
  with atypical mycobacteria, 613
  case on, 604
  cellulitis as, 608b–609b
  clinical entities for, 608b–613b
  with Clostridium septicum, 613
  with Cryptococcus neoformans, 613
  diabetic foot infections as, 612b–613b, 614–615
  differential diagnosis of, 605b
  erysipelas as, 609b
  extent of erythema with, 606–607
  and hematuria, 246
  with methicillin-resistant Staphylococcus aureus, 614–615
  necrotizing fasciitis as, 611b
  patient care for, 605
    clinical thinking in, 605
    history in, 605–606
    imaging considerations in, 607b
    physical examination in, 606–607
    tests for consideration in, 607
  with Pseudomonas species, 613
  risk factors for, 605–606
  speaking intelligently on, 605b
  due to sporotrichosis, 613
  with Vibrio vulnificus, 613
  zebra zone for, 613b
Skin biopsy
  for pigmented lesions, 451
  for rash, 604
Skin cancer, 449–459
  actinic keratosis and, 455b
  atypical nevus and, 455b
  basal cell carcinoma as, 452b
  case on, 449
  community education on, 459
  differential diagnosis of, 449b, 452b–456b
  giant hairy nevus and, 456
  keratoacanthoma as, 456

Skin cancer (Continued)
  malignant melanoma as, 453b–454b
    ABCDE of, 451
    excision margins for, 457
    imaging considerations for, 452b
    sentinel lymph node biopsy for, 451
    wide local excision for, 451
  patient care for, 449
    clinical thinking in, 449–450
    history in, 450
    imaging considerations in, 452b
    physical examination in, 450–451
    preoperative and postoperative discussion in, 458
    tests for consideration in, 451
  risk factors for, 450
  speaking intelligently on, 449b
  squamous cell carcinoma as, 453b
SLE (systemic lupus erythematosus), 583b–585b
  chronic joint pain due to, 583b–585b
  edema due to, 216
  pancytopenia due to, 384
Sleep apnea
  dyspnea due to, 150b
  hypertension due to, 136b
Sleep disorders, vs. seizures, 694
Sleep study, for weight gain and obesity, 522
SLR (straight-leg raising) test, 40
  for back pain in cancer patient, 425
SMA (superior mesenteric artery) syndrome, 301
Small bowel obstruction (SBO)
  nausea and vomiting due to, 293b–294b, 298b–299b
  water-soluble contrast agent for, 302
Small cell lung cancer (SCLC), 170b–171b
Smoking
  and hematuria, 246
  and osteoporosis, 555
  screening for, 31b
Smoking cessation
  communicating importance of, 153
  evidence-based medicine in, 32
Social media, communication via, 33–34
Sodium
  with acute kidney injury
    fractional excretion of, 202
    urine, 202
  with polyuria and polydipsia, 500
Soft tissue, on chest radiographs, 188, 189f, 194
Soft tissue abscess, 609b–610b
Soft tissue infections. See Skin and soft tissue infection(s) (SSTIs).
Solitary pulmonary nodule (SPN), 177–188
  due to arteriovenous malformation, 184b
  border of, 180
  due to bronchogenic cyst, 184b

Solitary pulmonary nodule (SPN)
  (Continued)
  calcification of, 180
  case on, 177
  clinical entities for, 181b–184b
  coccidioidal, 183b
  defined, 178
  density of, 180
  differential diagnosis of, 177b
  due to dirofilariasis, 182b
  due to fibroma, 184b
  growth of, 180
  due to hamartoma, 182b–183b
  Histoplasma, 184b
  incidentally detected, 466b–467b
    delivering unexpected news about,
      185–186
    standardized follow-up for, 186, 187t
  patient care for, 178
    algorithm for, 178b, 179f
    chest radiographs in, 180, 190, 190f
    clinical thinking in, 178
    history in, 178–180
    physical examination in, 180
    tests for consideration in, 180
  due to primary lung cancer, 181b–182b
    Early Lung Cancer Action Program for,
      185
  due to pseudotumor/interlobular pleural
    effusion, 184b
  rheumatoid, 184b
  risk factors for, 178–180
  size of, 180
  speaking intelligently on, 178b
  zebra zone for, 184b
Somatic complaints, exploring underlying
    reasons for, 43
SPEP (serum protein electrophoresis), for
    fragility fracture, 556
Spherocytes, on peripheral smear, 373–374,
    374f
Spherocytosis, hereditary, 374, 374f
Spinal cord compression (SCC)
  back pain due to, 426b
  history of, 472–473
  as oncologic emergency, 476b–477b
  physical examination for, 473
Spinal cord injury, 742b–743b
Spinal metastases, 426b
Spinal stenosis, 42
Spine, "bamboo," 585b–587b
Spinocerebellar ataxias (SCAs), 707
Spirometry, for dyspnea, 147
Spironolactone, for polycystic ovarian
    syndrome, 547b–548b
Spitz nevus, 456
Splenomegaly. *See* Lymphadenopathy and
    splenomegaly.
SPN. *See* Solitary pulmonary nodule (SPN).
Spondylitis, ankylosing, 585b–587b

Spondyloarthropathies
  inflammatory, 42
  seronegative, 585b–587b
Sporothrix schenckii, skin and soft tissue
    infections with, 613
Sporotrichosis, skin and soft tissue
    infections due to, 613
Spreading cortical depression, due to
    migraine, 716b–717b
Sputum analysis, for cough, 156
Squamous cell carcinoma (SCC), 453b
  of head and neck, 443b
SSc (systemic sclerosis), 588b–590b
SSS (superior sagittal sinus) thrombosis,
    719b
SSTIs. *See* Skin and soft tissue infection(s)
    (SSTIs).
ST segment, on ECG, 122
Staphylococcal toxic shock syndrome,
    601–602
Staphylococcus aureus
  cellulitis due to, 608b–609b
  hospital-acquired pneumonia due to,
    654b–655b
  methicillin-resistant, 609b–610b,
    614–615
  skin and soft-tissue abscess due to,
    609b–610b
Status epilepticus (SE), 692b–693b, 695
STDs. *See* Sexually transmitted disease(s)
    (STDs).
Steatorrhea, 341b–342b
ST-elevation myocardial infarction (STEMI),
    67, 71b–72b
Stem cell transplant, for pancytopenia,
    386
Stereotactic biopsy, of breast mass, 414
Still disease, adult-onset, 590
Stomach, watermelon, 320
Stomach cancer, 319b–320b
Stool cultures, for diarrhea, 337
Stool electrolytes, with diarrhea, 338
Straight-leg raising (SLR) test, 40
  for back pain in cancer patient, 425
Strawberry cervix, 639b–640b
Strength testing, for weakness, 739
Streptococcal pharyngitis, 618, 621b–622b
Streptococcus agalactiae, cellulitis due to,
    608b–609b
Streptococcus pneumoniae
  acute community-acquired bacterial
    sinusitis due to, 620b
  otitis media due to, 622b–623b
Streptococcus pyogenes
  cellulitis due to, 608b–609b
  erysipelas due to, 609b
  necrotizing fasciitis due to, 611b
  pharyngitis due to, 621b–622b
  skin and soft-tissue abscess due to,
    609b–610b

Stress echocardiography, for congestive heart failure, 93
Stress-induced cardiomyopathy, 77
Stricture, benign, jaundice due to, 353b–354b
Stroke, 740b–741b
  atrial fibrillation and risk of, 108b–109b
  protocol for, 674–675
  quality improvement for, 750
  tissue plasminogen activator for, 748
Structured dialogue, 447
Struvite stones, 251b–252b, 265b–266b
ST-segment depression, in NSTEMI, 72b
Subarachnoid hemorrhage
  altered mental status due to, 670b–671b
  headache due to, 38, 714b–715b
Subclinical Cushing syndrome (SCS), 461b–462b
Subclinical hypercortisolism, 461b–462b
Substance abuse, hypertension secondary to, 133b–134b
Substance withdrawal, altered mental status due to, 669b
Sudden cardiac death (SCD), due to hypertrophic cardiomyopathy, 98b–99b
Sulfonamides, hypoglycemia due to, 511b–512b
Sumatriptan, subcutaneous, for migraine, 722
Superficial spreading melanoma, 453b–454b
Superior mesenteric artery (SMA) syndrome, 301
Superior sagittal sinus (SSS) thrombosis, 719b
Superior vena cava syndrome (SVCS), 479
Support groups, for Parkinson disease, 709–710
Supraventricular tachycardia (SVT), 112b–113b
Surveillance
  for prostate cancer, 423
  for testicular cancer, 438–439
SVCS (superior vena cava syndrome), 479
SVT (supraventricular tachycardia), 112b–113b
Sweat chloride test, 162b–163b
Sweet syndrome, 490
Syncope
  pre-, 727–728
  vs. seizures, 694
Syndrome of inappropriate secretion of antidiuretic hormone (SIADH), paraneoplastic, 485, 488b–489b
Syphilis
  dementia due to, 677
  genital ulcers due to, 627, 630b–631b
Systemic infection, altered mental status due to, 669b–670b

Systemic lupus erythematosus (SLE), 583b–585b
  chronic joint pain due to, 583b–585b
  edema due to, 216
  pancytopenia due to, 384
Systemic sclerosis (SSc), 588b–590b
Systems-based practice, 6, 14
Systolic blood pressure (SBP), 125

T
T waves, 118, 118f
T₄ (thyroxine), free
  for amenorrhea, 552
  for weight loss, 532
Tachycardia, 119
  atrioventricular nodal reentrant (junctional reciprocating), 110b–111b
  atrioventricular reentrant (or reciprocating), 111b–112b
  multifocal atrial, 110b
  signs associated with, 104
  supraventricular, 112b–113b
  ventricular, 112b–113b
    ECG of, 120, 121f
Tachycardia-bradycardia syndrome, 113
Tagged RBC scan, for GI bleeding, 314b
Tako-tsubo cardiomyopathy, 77
Tardive parkinsonism, 706b
TB (tuberculosis)
  cough due to, 160b
  hemoptysis due to, 168b–169b
TCC (transitional cell carcinoma), 250b–251b
Tdap (tetanus-diphtheria-pertussis) vaccine, 30b–31b
TdP (torsades de pointes), 113
Team approach, for diabetic foot infections, 614–615
Teamwork, 9–10
Technical terms, in communication with patient, 405
Telephone calls, patient confidentiality with, 492
Temporal arteritis, 38, 721b–722b
Tender points, in fibromyalgia, 587b–588b
Tension headache, 37b
Teriparatide, for osteoporosis, 558b–559b
Test, patient refusal of, 255
Testicular exam, maintaining appropriate patient relations in performing, 438
Testicular mass, 431–439
  case on, 431
  clinical entities for, 435b–436b
  communicating effectively about potential diagnosis for, 437–438
  differential diagnosis of, 431b
  due to epididymo-orchitis, 436
  evidence-based medicine for, 437
  due to hematocele, 436

Testicular mass *(Continued)*
  due to hydrocele, 432b
  due to inguinal hernia, 432b
  due to nonseminomatous germ cell
    tumors, 434, 435b–436b
  patient care for, 432
    clinical thinking in, 432
    health information resources on,
      438–439
    history in, 432–433
    imaging considerations in, 434b
    metastatic workup for, 432b
    physical examination in, 433, 438
    tests for consideration in, 434
    tumor markers for, 432b, 434
  due to seminomas, 434, 435b
  speaking intelligently on, 432b
  due to varicocele, 432b
  zebra zone for, 436b
Testing, preparing patients for possibility
  of, 55
Testosterone, serum, for amenorrhea, 541
Testosterone deficiency, osteoporosis due
  to, 554, 556
Tetanus-diphtheria-pertussis (Tdap)
  vaccine, 30b–31b
Thalassemia, 48
Thiamine, for status epilepticus,
  692b–693b
Thrombocytopenia
  drug-induced, 392b
  peripheral smear of, 370–371, 371f
  pseudo-, 371, 372f
Thrombocytosis, 365
  essential
    elevated blood count due to, 364b
    history of, 362
    physical examination for, 362
    tests for consideration in, 363
Thrombotic thrombocytopenic purpura
  (TTP)
  acute kidney injury due to, 204b–205b
  altered mental status due to, 672
  excessive bleeding due to, 393b
  plasma exchange *vs.* plasma infusion for,
    394
Thyroid cancer, 445b–446b
  anaplastic, 445
  differentiated, 445
  medullary, 445
  neck mass due to, 445b–446b
Thyroid disease
  and edema, 212
  screening for, 29b
Thyroid function testing
  for constipation, 325
  for dyspnea, 147
  for hypertension, 127

Thyroiditis, autoimmune (Hashimoto),
  524b–525b
Thyroid-stimulating hormone (TSH)
  with altered mental status, 667
  in amenorrhea, 541, 552
  in dementia, 677
  in edema, 212
  in electrolyte disorders, 234
  with fragility fracture, 556
  with weakness, 739
  with weight gain and obesity, 522
  with weight loss, 532
Thyrotoxicosis, 534b
Thyroxine (T_4), free
  for amenorrhea, 552
  for weight loss, 532
TIA (transient ischemic attack)
  vs. seizures, 694
  weakness due to, 741b
Timeliness, 9
TIMI risk score, 71b–72b
Tinea pedis, and cellulitis, 606
Tinidazole
  for trichomoniasis, 639b–640b
  for urethritis, 642b–643b
TIPS (transjugular intrahepatic
    portosystemic shunt), for
    esophagogastric varices, 318b
Tissue plasminogen activator, for acute
  ischemic stroke, 748
TLS. *See* Tumor lysis syndrome (TLS).
TMP-SMX (trimethoprim-sulfamethoxazole),
    for hospital-acquired UTIs,
    650b–652b
Tobacco use, screening for, 31b
Tonic phase, of seizures, 690b–691b
Tonic-clonic seizures, generalized,
    690b–691b
Tophi, 570
Torsades de pointes (TdP), 113
Toxic shock syndrome, rash due to, 601–602
Toxicology screen
  for acid-base disorders, 222
  for hypertension, 127
Toxin exposure, and hematuria, 246
Transabdominal ultrasound
  for abdominal pain, 291
  for jaundice, 350b
Transfusion reaction, hemolytic, 387
Transient ischemic attack (TIA)
  vs. seizures, 694
  weakness due to, 741b
Transitional cell carcinoma (TCC),
    250b–251b
Transjugular intrahepatic portosystemic
    shunt (TIPS), for esophagogastric
    varices, 318b
Transthoracic echocardiography (TTE)
  for congestive heart failure, 93
  for weight loss, 532b

Transthoracic needle aspiration (TTNA), of solitary pulmonary nodule, 181
Transvaginal ultrasound, for amenorrhea, 542b
Trauma, to breast, 419
Treatment, patient's right to refuse, 395
Tremor, essential, 704b–705b
  vs. Parkinson disease, 700
Treponema pallidum, 630b–631b
Trichomonas, urethritis due to, 642b–643b
Trichomonas vaginalis, 639b–640b
  vulvovaginitis due to, 261b–262b
Trichomoniasis, 639b–640b
Trimethoprim-sulfamethoxazole (TMP-SMX), for hospital-acquired UTIs, 650b–652b
Troponins, serum
  for chest pain, 67, 69
  for congestive heart failure, 92
Trousseau sign, for pancreatic adenocarcinoma, 354b
Trypanosoma cruzi
  congestive heart failure due to, 100
  dysphagia due to, 307b
TSH. See Thyroid-stimulating hormone (TSH)
TTE (transthoracic echocardiography)
  for congestive heart failure, 93
  for weight loss, 532b
TTNA (transthoracic needle aspiration), of solitary pulmonary nodule, 181
TTP. See Thrombotic thrombocytopenic purpura (TTP).
Tuberculosis (TB)
  cough due to, 160b
  hemoptysis due to, 168b–169b
Tuberous sclerosis, renal mass due to, 270, 275b
Tubulointerstitial nephritis, 249b
Tumor lysis syndrome (TLS), 474b–476b
  history of, 472
  physical examination for, 473
  tests for considerations for, 473
Tumor markers, for testicular mass, 432b, 434
Tyrosine kinase inhibitors, clinical trials of, 367

U
UA (unstable angina), 67, 73b
UAG (urine anion gap), in acid-base disorders, 222
UGI (upper gastrointestinal) series, for nausea and vomiting, 297b
Ulcer(s)
  diabetic foot, 612b–613b, 614–615
  genital, 625–635
  peptic, 314b–315b
    evidence-based medicine for, 320

Ulcerative colitis
  diarrhea due to, 339b–340b
  enteropathic arthritis in, 585b–587b
Ultrasound
  for abdominal pain, 291–292
  for acute kidney injury, 202b
  for amenorrhea, 542b
  of breast mass, 411b
  for dysphagia, 307
  for dysuria, 258b
  for edema, 213b
  for jaundice, 350b
  for nausea and vomiting, 297b
  of renal mass, 271b
  of testicular mass, 434b
Unexpected finding, balancing concern with reassurance for, 255
Unexpected news, delivery of, 185–186
Unified Parkinson's Disease Rating Scale (UPDRS), 700
Unnecessary care, 303–304
Unnecessary procedures, patient or family demands for, 217–218
Unstable angina (UA), 67, 73b
UPEP (urine protein electrophoresis), for fragility fracture, 556
Upper endoscopy
  for dysphagia, 306
  for weight loss, 532b
Upper gastrointestinal (UGI) series, for nausea and vomiting, 297b
Upper respiratory tract infections (URIs), 616–625
  acute bronchitis as, 621b
  acute community-acquired bacterial sinusitis as, 620b
  appropriate use of antibiotics for, 617, 624–625
  case on, 616
  cavernous sinus thrombosis as, 623
  clinical entities for, 619b–623b
  differential diagnosis of, 616b
  diphtheria as, 623
  and hematuria, 246
  nonspecific, 619b
  otitis media as, 622b–623b
  patient care for, 617
    clinical thinking in, 617
    history in, 617–618
    physical examination in, 618
    tests for consideration in, 618
  pertussis as, 623
  pharyngitis as, 618, 621b–622b, 623
  speaking intelligently on, 616b
  viral rhinosinusitis or common cold as, 619b
  zebra zone for, 623b
Ureaplasma urealyticum, bacterial vaginosis due to, 640b–641b
Uremia, acid-base disorders due to, 226b

Ureteral diversion, acid-base disorders due to, 230
Urethral diverticulum, dysuria due to, 265b
Urethral smears and cultures, for dysuria, 258
Urethral stricture, dysuria due to, 264b–265b
Urethritis, 642b–643b
  dysuria due to, 259b
  nongonococcal, 642b–643b
  physical examination for, 637
Uric acid levels, for tumor lysis syndrome, 473
Uric acid stones, 251b–252b, 265b–266b
Urinalysis
  for acid-base disorders, 223
  for acute kidney injury, 202
  for altered mental status, 667
  for chronic joint pain, 580
  for dysuria, 258
  for edema, 212
  for hematuria, 246
  for hypertension, 127
  for nausea and vomiting, 296
  for polyuria and polydipsia, 500
Urinary tract infection (UTI), hospital-acquired, 649–650, 650b–652b
Urinary tract obstruction, 207b
Urine anion gap (UAG), in acid-base disorders, 222
Urine culture
  for dysuria, 258
  for hematuria, 246
Urine cytology
  for dysuria, 258
  for hematuria, 247
Urine electrolytes, in acid-base disorders, 222
Urine eosinophils, for acute kidney injury, 202
Urine ketones, in acid-base disorders, 222
Urine microalbumin-to-creatinine ratio, for polyuria and polydipsia, 500
Urine microscopic examination, for hematuria, 246
Urine osmolality, with polyuria and polydipsia, 500
Urine protein electrophoresis (UPEP), for fragility fracture, 556
Urine sediment
  in acid-base disorders, 223
  with acute kidney injury, 202
Urine sodium, with acute kidney injury, 202
Urine toxicology screen
  for altered mental status, 667
  for arrhythmias, 107
  for weight loss, 532
URIs. See Upper respiratory tract infections (URIs).

UTI (urinary tract infection), hospital-acquired, 649–650, 650b–652b

V
Vaccines, 30b–31b
Vaginal smears and cultures, for dysuria, 258
Vaginitis, 635–646
  atrophic, 644
  due to bacterial vaginosis, 640b–641b
  Candida, 638b–639b, 644
  case on, 635
  clinical entities for, 638b–643b
  desquamative inflammatory, 644
  differential diagnosis of, 636b
  direct testing for, 646
  empiric treatment of, 646
  due to mucopurulent cervicitis, 642b–643b
  patient care for, 636
    clinical thinking in, 636
    history in, 636–637
    physical examination in, 637
    tests for consideration in, 637
  speaking intelligently on, 636b
  due to trichomoniasis, 639b–640b
  zebra zone for, 644b
Vaginosis, bacterial, 640b–641b
Valacyclovir
  for genital herpes, 628b–629b, 633
  for varicella zoster virus, 597b–598b
VAP (ventilator-associated pneumonia), 654b–655b
Variant angina, 77
Varicella, 597b–598b
Varicella zoster, 597b–598b
Varicella zoster vaccine, 30b–31b, 602
Varicella zoster virus (VZV), 597b–598b
Varices, esophagogastric, 318b
Varicocele, 432b
Vascular auscultation
  for arrhythmias, 106
  for chest pain, 69
  for hypertension, 126–127
Vascular dementia, 680b
Vascular parkinsonism, 705b
Vasopressin, in diabetes insipidus, 503b–504b
Venous Doppler, of lower extremities, for dyspnea, 147b
Venous obstruction, and edema, 212
Venous sinus thrombosis, 719b
Ventilator-associated pneumonia (VAP), 654b–655b
Ventricular fibrillation, 121, 121f
Ventricular flutter, 120, 121f
Ventricular hypertrophy, 122
Ventricular tachycardia (VT), 112b–113b
  ECG of, 120, 121f
Vertical reads, 4–5

Vertigo, 726–736
    due to acoustic neuroma, 734
    due to basilar artery migraine, 734
    benign paroxysmal positional,
        730b–731b
        Dix-Hallpike maneuver for, 729f
        Epley maneuver for, 730b–731b, 734
        reassurance for, 735
    case on, 726
    due to cerebellar/brainstem infarct or
        hemorrhage, 732b–733b
    clinical entities for, 730b–733b
    defined, 727
    differential diagnosis of, 726b
    due to Meniere disease, 731b–732b
    and nystagmus, 728t
    patient care for, 727
        clinical thinking in, 727
        history in, 728
        imaging considerations in, 730b
        physical examination in, 728, 729f
        tests for consideration in, 729
    due to perilymphatic fistula, 733b
    speaking intelligently on, 727b
    due to vestibular neuritis, 731b
    zebra zone for, 734b
Vestibular neuritis, 731b
VHL (von Hippel–Lindau) disease, renal
    mass due to, 270, 276
Vibrio vulnificus, hemorrhagic bullous
    cellulitis due to, 613
Video capsule endoscopy, for GI bleeding,
    314
Viral arthritis, 575b
Viral pathogens
    lymphadenopathy due to, 442
    rash due to, 601
Viral pharyngitis, 621b–622b
Viral rhinosinusitis (VRS), 619b
    and acute community-acquired bacterial
        sinusitis, 620b
Visceral leishmaniasis, 384
Vital signs
    for acid-base disorders, 221
    for acute kidney injury, 201
    for altered mental status, 665
    for arrhythmias, 106
    for GI bleeding, 313
    for hypertension, 126
    for nausea and vomiting, 295
Vitamin B_{12} deficiency
    dementia due to, 677
    megaloblastic anemia due to, 380b–381b
Vitamin D, and osteoporosis, 554–555,
    558b–559b
Vitamin D deficiency
    hypocalcemia due to, 240b
    osteomalacia due to, 560b–561b
Vitamin K deficiency, excessive bleeding
    due to, 393b

Volume contraction, and metabolic
    alkalosis, 228b–229b
Volume depletion
    acute kidney injury due to, 203b
    with nausea and vomiting, 296
Volvulus, 325, 329b
Vomiting. See Nausea and vomiting.
von Hippel–Lindau (VHL) disease, renal
    mass due to, 270, 276
von Willebrand syndrome, acquired, 394
V/Q scan, for pulmonary embolism, 74b–75b
VRS (viral rhinosinusitis), 619b
    and acute community-acquired bacterial
        sinusitis, 620b
VT (ventricular tachycardia), 112b–113b
    ECG of, 120, 121f
Vulvovaginal candidiasis (VVC), 638b–639b,
    644
Vulvovaginitis, 261b–262b
VZV (varicella zoster virus), 597b–598b

W
Water deficit, 236b–237b
Watermelon stomach, 320
Water-soluble contrast agent, for adhesive
    small bowel obstruction, 302
WBCs. See White blood cell(s) (WBCs).
Weakness, 737–750
    due to amyotrophic lateral sclerosis, 747
    case on, 737
    clinical entities for, 740b–747b
    delivering bad news on, 748–749
    differential diagnosis of, 737b
    due to Guillain-Barré syndrome,
        744b–745b
    imaging considerations in, 740b
    due to malignancy, 484, 484b,
        489b–490b
    due to multiple sclerosis, 741b–742b
    due to myasthenia gravis, 745b–746b
    due to myopathy, 746b–747b
    due to neurosarcoidosis, 747
    patient care for, 738
        clinical thinking in, 738
        history in, 738
        physical examination in, 738–739
        tests for consideration in, 739
    due to peripheral neuropathy,
        743b–744b
    speaking intelligently on, 737b–738b
    due to spinal cord injury, 742b–743b
    due to stroke, 740b–741b
        quality improvement for, 750
        tissue plasminogen activator for, 748
    due to TIA, 741b
    zebra zone for, 747b
Wegener granulomatosis, 172b–173b
Weight gain and obesity, 519–528
    case on, 519–520
    clinical entities for, 523b–525b

Weight gain and obesity *(Continued)*
  conditions exacerbated by, 522
  due to Cushing syndrome, 523b–524b
  differential diagnosis of, 520b
  evidence-based medicine for, 526
  exogenous, 523b
  due to growth hormone deficiency, 526
  hypertension due to, 136b
  due to hypothyroidism, 524b–525b
  monogenic, 526
  patient care for, 520
    being nonjudgmental in, 527
    clinical thinking in, 520–521
    ensuring access to emergency services
      in, 527–528
    getting to know your patient in, 527
    history in, 521
    physical examination in, 521–522
    tests for consideration in, 522
  due to polycystic ovarian syndrome, 525b
  screening for, 30b
  speaking intelligently on, 520b
  truncal, 521–522
  zebra zone for, 526b
Weight loss, 529–538
  due to adrenal insufficiency, 535
  due to anorexia nervosa, 534b–535b
  due to cancer, 533b
  case on, 529
  clinical entities for, 533b–535b
  due to congestive heart failure, 534b
  differential diagnosis of, 529b
  HIV-associated, 536

Weight loss *(Continued)*
  maintenance of, 526
  patient care for, 530
    clinical thinking in, 530
    history in, 530–531
    imaging considerations in, 532b
    physical examination in, 531
    tests for consideration in, 531
  speaking intelligently on, 530b
  due to thyrotoxicosis, 534b
  zebra zone for, 535b
Weight loss medications, 523
West Nile virus infection, 601
Whipple triad, 510
White blood cell(s) (WBCs), on peripheral
    smear, 368–370, 369f–370f
White blood cell (WBC) count
  for abdominal pain, 282
  for altered mental status, 667
  elevated. *See* Elevated blood counts.
Wide local excision, for melanoma, 451
Wilson disease, movement abnormalities
    due to, 707
Withdrawal, altered mental status due to,
    669b

Z
Zanamivir, for influenza, 619b
Zenker diverticulum, 301
Zoledronic acid (Zometa), for hypercalcemia
    of malignancy, 486b–488b, 491–493
Zoster, 597b–598b
Zoster vaccine, 30b–31b, 602